Medicine at a Glance

EDITED BY

Patrick Davey

Consultant Cardiologist
Northampton General Hospital
Northampton, and
Honorary Senior Lecturer
Department of Cardiovascular Medicine
John Radcliffe Hospital
Oxford

Second Edition

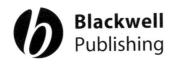

Blackwell
Publishing

© 2006 by Blackwell Publishing Ltd
Blackwell Publishing, Inc., 350 Main Street, Malden, Massachusetts 02148-5020, USA
Blackwell Publishing Ltd, 9600 Garsington Road, Oxford OX4 2DQ, UK
Blackwell Publishing Asia Pty Ltd, 550 Swanston Street, Carlton, Victoria 3053, Australia

First published 2002
Second edition 2006
2   2007

Library of Congress Cataloging-in-Publication Data

Medicine at a glance / edited by Patrick Davey.—2nd ed.
    p. ; cm.—(At a glance)
  Includes index.
  ISBN 978-1-4051-3393-7 (alk. paper)
  1. Clinical medicine—Handbooks, manuals, etc.   2. Diseases—Handbooks, manuals, etc.   I.
Davey, Patrick.   II. Series: At a glance series (Oxford, England)
  [DNLM: 1. Clinical Medicine—Handbooks.   WB 39 M48975 2006]
  RC55.M388 2006
  616—dc22
                                   2005029873

ISBN 978-1-4051-3393-7

A catalogue record for this title is available from the British Library

Set in 9/11½pt Times by Graphicraft Limited, Hong Kong
Printed and bound in India by Replika Press Pvt. Ltd

Commissioning Editor: Vicki Noyes
Editorial Assistant: Caroline Aders
Development Editor: Geraldine Jeffers
Production Controller: Kate Charman

For further information on Blackwell Publishing, visit our website:
http://www.blackwellpublishing.com

Contents

Preface

Medicine is a wonderful and exciting subject. Partly this excitement comes from the pure unadulterated intellectual joy of understanding the functioning of humans in health and disease better, an understanding based on a powerful and growing biological science, one which pushes the frontiers of our knowledge back at an accelerating rate with each passing year. The most amazing advances have been made in the treatment of many illnesses; what is true today for them may be true tomorrow for most diseases. Advances in basic sciences feed through into 'landmark' clinical trials at an ever increasing rate; indeed rarely a week goes by without another key experiment or trial being published. For this reason, now is perhaps the most exciting time ever to be involved in medicine. The medical student rapidly becomes a part of this seething intellectual community. This in itself is reason enough to study medicine.

Medicine, however, is not just about science. It is a profoundly human subject. Indeed, the opportunity to directly study human suffering and then immediately to relieve it is, in large part, what separates medicine from other subjects. Other disciplines try to understand suffering; this almost always occurs from a distance, in the abstract, by the inspection of data, or by the use of philosophical argument. Medicine, being practical, sees and feels human suffering. Most doctors experience human suffering every day of their working lives. This can lead to a far more profound understanding of humans and of the communities in which we all live. Our experience of human suffering has a profound impact on us. Doctors' experience of suffering can itself make them into better people, more humane, more understanding and more tolerant.

The study of medicine is therefore an adventure, but one that requires hard work. Furthermore, what is worth studying is worth excelling in. It should be the aim of every student of medicine to be an outstanding clinician. What makes for excellence in clinical medicine? In part, it is the ability to turn symptoms rapidly into the right diagnosis, to then turn the diagnosis into a treatment plan, then to communicate all this effectively and accurately to a patient and their family. No book can teach you this entirely by itself. Books, however, can help, and the prime aim of this book is to help you reach a diagnosis, and to introduce you to some of the principles of treatment.

How is a diagnosis established? First, the patient's symptoms are fully explored, so as to completely understand what patients are actually experiencing. Second, a full examination is undertaken, to reveal diagnostic clinical signs. Third, the history and physical examination are synthesized, so that important facts are emphasized and unimportant ones rejected. This synthesis allows one to establish a differential diagnosis, ordered according to probability. This differential diagnosis is narrowed down to a diagnosis using appropriate investigations. Accurate diagnosis allows for effective treatment. *This book will help you acquire all these skills.*

There is an aphorism in medicine that in 80% of cases the history establishes the diagnosis, in 10% the examination does, and only in 10% of cases do investigations provide the answer. *History taking* is a real skill, one which you should work hard to acquire; you only have to see an experienced clinician take a history to realize the beauty and skill of a concise and accurate history taking. The acquisition of this skill will be amply rewarded over the years. Do not be deluded into thinking that just because history taking uses a skill we are all familiar with, which is speech, that it is easy. It is not, and it requires time, patience and diligence to acquire. *This book will help you acquire this vitally important skill.* The critical aspect of history taking is to make sense of it as you go along, and not just to ask questions 'by rote'. How do you do this? Well, to understand the nuances of the history, you need to know quite a lot about diseases, particularly those most prevalent in your local community. An understanding of epidemiology helps. Thus 'browsing' through the third part of the book as background reading will help. Use spare moments during the day to do this. However, though acquiring background knowledge will help, I think the very best way to learn medicine is to 'hang' your facts around individual patients, as this really 'fixes' information down in the memory. Thus, whenever you see a patient, look up their symptoms in this book, so as to understand better how symptoms are turned into a diagnosis. You will learn most if for each and every case you see you draw up a differential diagnosis, ordered according to probability. Stick your neck out! This means that you will have a personal investment in the diagnosis; you will feel proud when you are right. This is a good feeling, and will encourage you! When you are wrong, you will learn, and this is more important. Indeed, it is true to say that you will learn more from your mistakes than from your triumphs. When wrong, you should always ask 'why?' Was my reasoning defective? Did I miss a vital part of the history? Did I misinterpret a sign? The most important part of any case is to ask, 'What have I learnt from this case?' It may relate to your knowledge of the biology of the disease, to your clinical skills, to communication, to how the hospital works, etc. You can learn from each and every case. If you take the opportunity to do so you will make an outstanding doctor. Good luck.

Patrick Davey

List of contributors

Chris B. Bunker
Professor of Dermatology & Consultant Dermatologist
Chelsea & Westminster, Royal Marsden Hospitals &
Imperial College School of Medicine
London

Keith Channon
Professor of Cardiovascular Medicine & Honorary Consultant Cardiologist
Department of Cardiovascular Medicine
University of Oxford
John Radcliffe Hospital
Oxford

Patrick Davey
Consultant Cardiologist
Northampton General Hospital
Northampton, and
Honorary Senior Lecturer
Department of Cardiovascular Medicine
John Radcliffe Hospital
Oxford

Suzanne Donnelly
Formerly of Department of Rheumatology
St George's Hospital
London

Peggy Frith
Consultant Ophthalmic Physician
The Radcliffe Infirmary
Oxford

Jonathan Gleadle
Lecturer in Nephrology
The Wellcome Trust
Centre for Human Genetics
Oxford

Mark Juniper
Consultant Physician
Great Western Hospital
Swindon

David Keeling
Consultant Haematologist
Oxford Haemophilia Centre
The Churchill Hospital
Headington
Oxford

David Lalloo
Reader in Tropical Medicine
Liverpool School of Tropical Medicine
Liverpool

Tim J. Littlewood
Consultant Haematologist
Department of Haematology
The John Radcliffe Hospital
Oxford

Angus Patterson
Consultant Clinical Oncologist
Belfast City Hospital
Belfast

Richard Penson
Director of Clinical Research in Medical Gynecologic Oncology
Massachusetts General Hospital
Boston
USA

Jeremy Shearman
Consultant Gastroenterologist
Department of Gastroenterology
Warwick Hospital
Warwick

Gavin Spickett
Consultant in Clinical Immunology, Allergy & General Medicine
Regional Department of Immunology
Royal Victoria Infirmary
Newcastle-Upon-Tyne

David Sprigings
Consultant Cardiologist
Northampton General Hospital
Northampton

Kevin Talbot
MRC Clinician Scientist, Department of Human Anatomy and Genetics,
Honorary Consultant Neurologist
Department of Clinical Neurology
University of Oxford
Radcliffe Infirmary
Oxford

Helen E. Turner
Consultant Endocrinologist
Endocrinology Department
Radcliffe Infirmary
Oxford

Katherine Whybrew
General Practitioner
Bristol

Matt Wise
Consultant in Intensive Care Medicine
University Hospital of Wales
Cardiff

Paul Wordsworth
Professor of Rheumatology
Nuffield Orthopaedic Centre
Windmill Road
Oxford

List of abbreviations

ABPA	allergic bronchopulmonary aspergillosis
ACE	angiotensin-converting enzyme
ACTH	adrenocorticotrophic hormone
ADEM	acute disseminated encephalomyelitis
ADH	antidiuretic hormone
ADPKD	autosomal dominant polycystic kidney disease
AF	atrial fibrillation
AFB	acid-fast bacilli
AFP	α-fetoprotein
AIDS	acquired immune deficiency syndrome
AIHA	autoimmune haemolytic anaemia
AIN	acute interstitial nephritis
ALL	acute lymphoid leukaemia
ALT	alanine transaminase
AMA	American Medical Association
AMI	acute myocardial infarction
AML	acute myeloid leukaemia
ANA	antinuclear antibody
ANCA	antineutrophil cytoplasmic antibody
ANF	antinuclear factor
APC	activated protein C
APKD	adult polycystic kidney disease
APTT	activated partial thromboplastin time
AR	aortic regurgitation
ARDS	adult respiratory distress syndrome
ASD	atrial septal defect
ASO	anti-streptolysin O
AST	aspartate transaminase
ATN	acute tubular necrosis
AV	atrioventricular
AVM	arteriovenous malformation
AVNRT	AV nodal re-entrant tachycardia
AVRT	AV re-entrant tachycardia
BCE	basal cell carcinoma/epithelioma
BiPAP	bi-positive airway pressure
BMI	body mass index
BMZ	basement membrane zone
BOOP	bronchiolitis obliterans organizing pneumonia
BP	blood pressure
BPH	benign prostatic hypertrophy
BPPV	benign paroxysmal positional vertigo
CABG	coronary artery bypass graft surgery
CAD	coronary artery disease
CAH	congenital adrenal hyperplasia
cAMP	cyclic adenosine monophosphate
CAPD	continuous ambulatory peritoneal dialysis
CCU	coronary care unit
CEA	carcinoembryonic antigen
CFS	chronic fatigue syndrome
CHAD	cold haemagglutinin disease
CHART	continuous hyperfractionated accelerated radiotherapy
CIDP	chronic idiopathic demyelinating polyneuropathy
CJD	Creutzfeldt–Jakob disease

CK	creatine kinase
CLD	chronic liver disease
CLL	chronic lymphoblastic leukaemia
CML	chronic myeloid leukaemia
CMML	chronic myelomonocytic leukaemia
CMV	cytomegalovirus
COAD	chronic obstructive airway disease
COPD	chronic obstructive pulmonary disease
COX	cyclo-oxygenase
CPAP	continuous positive airway pressure
CPR	cardiopulmonary resuscitation
CREST	calcinosis, Raynaud's, oesophagitis, sclerodactyly telangiectasia
CRH	corticotrophin-releasing hormone
CRP	C-reactive protein
CSF	cerebrospinal fluid
CSM	Committee of Safety in Medicine
CT	computed tomography
CVA	cerebrovascular accident
CVT	cerebral venous sinus thrombosis
CYP	cytochrome P450
DCIS	ductal carcinoma *in situ*
DCM	dilated cardiomyopathy
DHF/DSS	dengue haemorrhagic fever/dengue shock syndrome
DIC	disseminated intravascular coagulation
DKA	diabetic ketoacidosis
DM	diabetes mellitus
DMSA	$[^{99m}Tc]$mercaptosuccinic acid
DNA	deoxyribonucleic acid
DU	duodenal ulcer
DVT	deep vein thrombosis
EAA	extrinsic allergic alveolitis
EATL	enteropathy-associated T-cell lymphoma
EBV	Epstein–Barr virus
ECT	electroconvulsive therapy
EMA	endomysial antibodies
EMD	electromechanical dissociation
EN	erythema nodosum
ENA	extractable nuclear antigen
ENT	ear, nose, throat
ERCP	endoscopic retrograde cholangiopancreatography
ESR	erythrocyte sedimentation rate
ESRF	end-stage renal failure
5FU	5-fluorouracil
FAP	familial adenomatous polyposis
FBC	full blood count
FDPs	fibrin degradation products
FEV_1	forced expiratory volume in 1 s
FFP	fresh frozen plasma
FRC	functional residual capacity
FSGS	focal segmental glomerulosclerosis
FSH	follicle-stimulating hormone

FTD	frontotemporal dementia	**LCIS**	lobular carcinoma *in situ*
FUO	fever of unknown origin	**LDH**	lactate dehydrogenase
FVC	forced vital capacity	**LEMS**	Lambert–Eaton myasthenic syndrome
		LFT	liver function test
γGT	γ-glutamyl transferase	**LMN**	lower motor neuron
G6PD	glucose-6-phosphate dehydrogenase	**LMWH**	low-molecular-weight heparin
GBM	glomerular basement membrane	**LP**	lumbar puncture
GCS	Glasgow Coma Score	**LV**	left ventricular
G-CSF	granulocyte colony-stimulating factor		
GFR	glomerular filtration rate	**MALT**	mucosa-associated lymphoid tissue
GH	growth hormone	**MCA**	middle cerebral artery
GHRH	growth hormone-releasing hormone	**MCV**	mean cell volume
GI	gastrointestinal	**MELAS**	**m**itochondrial **e**ncephalopathy, **l**actic **a**cidosis, **s**troke-like episodes
GN	glomerulonephritis		
GnRH	gonadotrophin-releasing hormone	**MEN**	multiple endocrine neoplasia
GORD	gastro-oesophageal reflux disease	**methyl-THF**	methyl tetrahydrofolate
GPI	general paralysis of the insane	**MGUS**	monoclonal gammopathy of uncertain significance
GSS	Gerstmann–Sträussler–Scheinker syndrome	**MI**	myocardial infarction
GTN	glyceryl trinitrate	**MND**	motor neuron disease
GU	gastric ulcer	**MODY**	maturity-onset diabetes in the young
		MR	mitral regurgitation
5-HT	5-hydroxytryptamine (serotonin)	**MRCP**	magnetic resonance cholangiopancreatography
HAART	highly active anti-retroviral therapy	**MRSA**	methicillin-resistant *Staphylococcus aureus*
HAV	hepatitis A virus	**MRI**	magnetic resonance imaging
HBV	hepatitis B virus	**MS**	multiple sclerosis
β-hCG	β-human chorionic gonadotrophin	**MSA**	multiple system atrophy
HCV	hepatitis C virus	**MSH**	melanocyte-stimulating hormone
HHM	humoral hypercalcaemia of malignancy	**MSU**	midstream urine
HIV	human immunodeficiency virus	**MVR**	mitral valve prolapse
5HIAA	5-hydroxyindoleacetic acid		
HIT	heparin-induced thrombocytopenia	**NADPH**	reduced nicotinamide adenine dinucleotide phosphate
HLA	human leukocyte antigen	**NG**	nasogastric
HLPP	hereditary neuropathy with liability to pressure palsies	**NGU**	non-gonococcal urethritis
HMG-CoA	hydroxymethylglutaryl-coenzyme A	**NSAID**	non-steroidal anti-inflammatory drug
HMSN	hereditary motor and sensory neuropathy	**nvCJD**	new variant Creutzfeldt–Jakob disease
HNF	hepatocyte nuclear factor		
HNPCC	hereditary non-polyposis colon cancer	**OCP**	oral contraceptive pill
HONK	hyperosmolar non-ketotic coma	**OGD**	oesophago-gastroduodenoscopy
HPOA	hypertrophic pulmonary osteoarthropathy	**OSA**	obstructive sleep apnoea
HRCT	high-resolution computed tomography		
HS	hereditary spherocytosis	**PA**	pernicious anaemia
HSP	Henoch–Schönlein purpura	**PAN**	polyarteritis nodosa
HUS	haemolytic uraemic syndrome	**PBC**	primary biliary cirrhosis
		PCOS	polycystic ovary syndrome
IBD	inflammatory bowel disease	**PCP**	*Pneumocystis carinii* pneumonia
IGF	insulin growth factor	**PE**	pulmonary embolism
INR	international normalized ratio	**PEEP**	positive end-expiratory pressure
IRMAs	intraretinal microvascular abnormalities	**PEFR**	peak expiratory flow rate
ITP	immune thrombocytopenic purpura	**PEG**	percutaneous endoscopic gastrostomy
ITU	intensive therapy unit	**PGE$_1$**	prostaglandin E$_1$
IVC	inferior vena cava	**PKD**	polycystic kidney disease
IVDA	intravenous drug abuse	**PML**	progressive multifocal leukoencephalopathy
IVF	*in vitro* fertilization	**PNH**	paroxysmal nocturnal haemoglobinuria
IVIG	intravenous immunoglobulin	**PPAR-γ**	peroxisome proliferator-activated receptor
IVU	intravenous urogram	**PPD**	purified protein derivative
		PPGRs	post-prandial glucose regulators
JVP	jugular venous pressure	**PR**	per rectum
		PRV	polycythaemia rubra vera
***K*co**	carbon monoxide transfer factor	**PSC**	primary sclerosing cholangitis

PT	prothrombin time	SVC	superior vena cava
PTC	percutaneous transhepatic cholangiography	SVT	supraventricular tachyarrhythmia
PTCA	percutaneous transluminal coronary angioplasty		
PTH	parathyroid hormone	T3	triiodothyronine
PTHrP	PTH-related peptide	T4	thyroxine
PTP	post-transfusion purpura	TB	tuberculosis
PUD	peptic ulcer disease	TIBC	total iron-binding capacity
		TED	thromboembolic disease
RA	refractory anaemia	TIH	tumour-induced hypercalcaemia
RAEB	refractory anaemia with excess blasts	TIPSS	transjugular portosystemic shunt
RAEB-t	refractory anaemia with excess blasts in transformation	TLC	total lung capacity
		TNFα	tumour necrosis factor α
RARS	refractory anaemia with ring sideroblasts	TOE	transoesophageal echocardiography
RAS	renal artery stenosis	tPA	tissue plasminogen activator
RA	rheumatoid arthritis	TPN	total parenteral nutrition
RBC	red blood cell	TRH	thyroid-hormone-releasing hormone
REM	rapid eye movement	TSH	thyroid-stimulating hormone
RIF	right iliac fossa	TT	thrombin time
RNA	ribonucleic acid	TTE	transthoracic echocardiography
RP	retinitis pigmentosa	TTP	thrombotic thrombocytopenic purpura
RPGN	rapidly progressive glomerulonephritis	TURP	transurethral resection of the prostate
RSM	restrictive cardiomyopathy		
RUQ	right upper quadrant	UC	ulcerative colitis
RV	right ventricular; residual volume	U&Es	urea and electrolytes
		UFH	unfractionated heparin
SA	sinoatrial	UMN	upper motor neuron
SACDOC	subacute combined degeneration of the cord	UTI	urinary tract infection
SAH	subarachnoid haemorrhage	UV	ultraviolet
SBP	spontaneous bacterial peritonitis		
SCC	squamous cell carcinoma	$\dot{V}/\dot{Q}$	ventilation–perfusion
SCLC	small cell carcinoma of the lung	VC	vital capacity
SHD	subdural haemorrhage	VEGF	vascular endothelium growth factor
SIADH	syndrome of inappropriate secretion of antidiuretic hormone	VEPs	visual evoked potentials
		VIN	vulval intraepithelial neoplasia
SIMV	synchronized intermittent mandatory ventilation	VIP	vasoactive intestinal peptide
SLA	soluble liver antigen	VSD	ventricular septal defect
SLE	systemic lupus erythematosus	VWF	von Willebrand's factor
SMA	smooth muscle antibody	VZV	varicella-zoster virus
SRH	stigmata of recent haemorrhage		
SSSS	staphylococcal scalded skin syndrome	WCC	white cell count
STD	sexually transmitted disease	WPW	Wolff–Parkinson–White syndrome

Acknowledgements

The Editor, Contributing Authors and Publishers would like to thank all those people who gave their time and expertise to advise us during the writing process of both the first and second editions. The specialist reviewers and medical students who reviewed material for the first edition were invaluable in shaping the final book and we would like to thank them unreservedly for their contribution.

In addition, we would like to acknowledge the following individuals and companies for their kind permission to re-use material. Although the majority of the artwork in *Medicine at a Glance* is new, some tables and figures have been redrawn from other sources and have been used with permission of the publishers. The Editor and Publishers have made every effort to contact all the copyright holders to obtain their permission to reproduce copyright material. However, if any have been inadvertently overlooked, the Publisher will be pleased to make the necessary arrangements at the first opportunity.

Books

R. Baran & R. Dawber (2001) *Diseases of the Nails & their Management* (2nd edn), Blackwell Science.

R. Baran, D. de Berker & R. Dawber (1997) *Manual of Nail Disease & Surgery*, Blackwell Science.

S. Bourke & R. Brewis (1998) *Lecture Notes on Respiratory Medicine* (5th edn), Blackwell Science.

R. Champion *et al.* (1998) *Rook's Textbook of Dermatology* (6th edn), Blackwell Science.

H. Chapel, M. Heaney, S. Misbah, N. Snowden (1999) *Essentials of Clinical Immunology* (4th edn), Blackwell Science.

C. Haslett *et al.* (1999) *Davidson's Principles & Practice of Medicine* (18th edn), Churchill Livingstone.

J. Hunter & J. Savin (1994) *Clinical Dermatology* (2nd edn), Blackwell Science.

V. Hoffbrand, P. Moss & J. Pettit (2001) *Essential Haematology* (4th edn), Blackwell Science.

D. Howlett & B. Ayers (2004) *The Hands on Guide to Imaging*, Blackwell Publishing.

P. Kumar & M. Clark (eds) (1998) *Clinical Medicine* (4th edn), W.B. Saunders.

R. Leach (2004) *Critical Care Medicine at a Glance*, Blackwell Publishing.

A. Mehta & V. Hoffbrand (2000) *Haematology at a Glance*, Blackwell Science.

J. Munro & C. Edwards (2000) *McLeod's Clinical Examination* (10th edn), Churchill Livingstone.

M. Nelson, Department of Medical Illustration and Photography, Chelsea & Westminster Hospital, London.

J. Olver & L. Cassidy (2005) *Ophthalmology at a Glance*, Blackwell Publishing.

K. Patton (2000) *Handbook for Anatomy and Physiology*, Mosby

E. Rubenstein & D.D. Federman (eds) (2002) *Scientific American Medicine*, Webmd.com.

S. Sherlock and J. Dooley (2002) *Diseases of the Liver and Biliary System* (11th edn), Blackwell Science.

M. Snaith (ed.) (1999) *ABC of Rheumatology*, BMJ Publishing Group.

D. Weatherall (ed.) (1995) *Oxford Textbook of Medicine* (3rd edn), Oxford University Press.

J.D. Waye, D. Rex & C. Williams (2003) *Colonoscopy: Principles and Practice*, Blackwell Publishing (figures used are by Dr Michael Macari).

Journals

J. Bruix *et al.* (2001) Clinical management of hepatocellular carcinoma. Conclusions of the Barcelona-2000 EASL conference. European Association for the Study of the Liver. *J Hepatol*, **35**(3), 421–430.

D. Horskette *et al.* (2004) Guidelines on diagnosis, prevention and treatment of infective endocarditis executive summary: The task force on infective endocarditis of the European Society of Cardiology. *Eur Heart J*, **25**, 267–276.

R. Marchioli *et al.* (2001) Assessment of absolute risk of death after myocardial infarction by use of multiple-risk-factor assessment equations: GISSI-prevenzione mortality risk chart. *Eur Heart J*, **22**, 2085–2103.

E.S. Soteriodes *et al.* (2002) Incidence and prognosis of syncope. *New Engl J Med*, **347**, 878–885.

R. Thadhani, M. Pascual, J.V. Bonventre (1996) Acute renal failure. *New Engl J Med*, **334**(22), 1451.

Other

Special thanks to Dr Mansel Heaney for providing cANCA figure for Chapter 132.

Data for graphs for incidence of leukaemia, Chapter 165, are from *Cancer Statistics Registrations: registrations of cancers diagnosed in 2001 England*, Office for National Statistics, Crown copyright 2004.

Data for graphs for Chapter 178 are from *Cancer deaths: site of cancer, sex and age; death rates per million population*, 1971–1995, Office for National Statistics, 1996, Crown copyright.

Figure of pain scales in Chapter 183 are from *Institutionalising Pain Management Project*, University of Wisconsin and Clinics Home Health Agency, Madison WI, USA.

Introduction

1 How to be a medical student

THE HIPPOCRATIC OATH

I SWEAR by Apollo the physician, and Aesculapius, and Health, and All-heal, and all the gods and goddesses, that, according to my ability and judgment, I will heed this oath and this stipulation to reckon him who taught me this Art equally dear to me as my parents, to share my substance with him, and relieve his necessities if required; to look upon his offspring in the same footing as my own brothers, and to teach them this Art, if they shall wish to learn it, without fee or stipulation; and that by precept, lecture, and every other mode of instruction, I will impart a knowledge of the Art to my own sons, and those of my teachers, and to disciples bound by a stipulation and oath according to the law of medicine, but to none other. I will follow that system of regimen which, according to my ability and judgment, I consider for the benefit of my patients, and abstain from whatever is deleterious and mischievous. I will give no deadly medicine to any one if asked, nor suggest any such counsel; and in like manner I will not give to a woman a pessary to produce abortion. With purity and with holiness I will pass my life and practise my Art. I will not cut persons laboring under the stone, but will leave this to be done by men who are practitioners of this work. Into whatever houses I enter, I will go into them for the benefit of the sick, and will abstain from every voluntary act of mischief and corruption; and, further from the seduction of females or males, of freemen and slaves. Whatever, in connection with my professional practice or not, in connection with it, I see or hear, in the life of men, which ought not to be spoken of abroad, I will not divulge, as reckoning that all such should be kept secret. While I continue to keep this oath unviolated, may it be granted to me to enjoy life and the practice of the art, respected by all men, in all times! But should I trespass and violate this oath, may the reverse be my lot.

In 1948 in Geneva the World Medical Association drew up a modern version of the oath.

At the time of being admitted a member of the medical profession:

I solemnly pledge myself to consecrate my life to the service of humanity;

I will give my teachers the respect and gratitude which is their due;

I will practise my profession with conscience and dignity;

*T*he health of my patient will be my first consideration;

I will respect the secrets which are confided in me, even after the patient has died;

I will maintain by all the means in my power, the honour and the noble traditions of the medical profession;

*M*y colleagues will be my brothers;

I will not permit considerations of religion, nationality, race, party politics or social standing to intervene between my duty and my patient;

I will maintain the utmost respect for human life from the time of conception; even under threat I will not use my medical knowledge contrary to the laws of humanity.

I make these promises solemnly, freely and upon my honour.

Good doctors

Medicine can seem a large and daunting subject, not only for reasons of intellectual rigour, but also because so many facts need to be learnt. In learning (and practising) medicine, it is vital to realize that facts alone are not enough! Good physicians have:
- A strong humanity, i.e. an interest in human beings.
- An interest in disease, its causation and treatment.
- An ability to communicate with patients, to obtain a correct and full understanding of their problems and, at the same time, to give accurate information sympathetically about the diagnosis, treatment and prognosis. Good physicians are non-judgemental, empathetic listeners.
- An ability to examine patients and elicit abnormal physical signs.
- An ability to marshal the facts into a coherent story and present them clearly to relevant parties, i.e. 'case' presentation of the history, examination and a structured summary, a probable and differential diagnosis, with plans for further investigations, and treatment.

- An up-to-date knowledge base so that appropriate management (diagnosis + treatment) plans can be made.
- An ability to realize when knowledge/skills are deficient and an ability to learn in response to new knowledge, ideas, etc. from the best source available.
- An ability to acknowledge errors and learn from them. It is important to be open with patients and colleagues as soon as errors/misjudgements are recognized.
- Appropriate technical skills in diagnostic and therapeutic procedures.
- An understanding of economic, social and cultural, political and health-care systems so that the best possible help can be delivered to patients in the most timely fashion. If a deficiency in one or other of these systems damages patients, physicians should seek improvements.
- Excellent managerial and interpersonal skills, with personal, financial and intellectual probity.

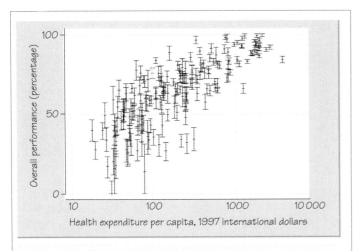

Health care spend related to outcome—different countries can spend the same amounts with very different outcomes, as shown in this graph, where health care expenditure is plotted against health care system performance
(From The World Health Report 2000: health systems: improving performance)

Table 1.1 Health systems have three fundamental objectives, which are:

- Improving the health of the population they serve
- Responding to people's expectations (including personal respect from the system to the patient)
- Providing financial protection against the costs of ill-health

Hippocratic oath and the modern perspective

High ethical and moral standards are an imperative for good practice—the Hippocratic oath and its modern successors aim to codify behaviour. They are guidelines to best behaviour, although medicine is more complex than implied by such phrases. However, regardless of phrasing, the implication that physicians should have the highest ethical, moral and technical standards stands. Society respects physicians, and consequently physicians face social as well as other penalties if performance is poor.

Health-care systems

Health-care systems are imperfect compromises among society's aspirations, wealth, humanity and individual need (figure and Table 1.1). It is vital to understand how any system works, so that it can be used in a patient's best interests. If individual or organizational failure occurs, this should be highlighted to the appropriate responsible individuals, agencies or, rarely, the media.

How to learn

Becoming a doctor means acquiring a set of skills, knowledge and values. How this is best done depends on the individual and the medical school. However, concentrating on one area/skill to the exclusion of others is counterproductive. Facts alone do not make a physician, and nor do learning or technical skills alone. It is the right combination of the above list that 'maketh the physician'. Students need to determine the right balance for themselves, bearing in mind their individual aptitudes, and their medical school's doctrine. A reasonable approach is the 'patient-centred' one, approached in a 'problem-based' fashion,

supplemented by dedicated learning sessions, e.g. seminars, lectures, etc., i.e. students should:

- See patients, so learning communication skills.
- Ascertain symptoms and signs, so learning clerking and examination skills.
- Formulate a diagnosis or differential diagnosis, so learning diagnostic skills. The first part of this book aims to aid in diagnosis, i.e. the turning of symptoms and signs into diseases with names.
- Present findings to attending physicians, so learning presentation skills.
- Formulate investigation and treatment plans, so refining diagnostic and therapeutic skills. The second part of this book aims to help here.
- Observe patients' progress, so determining whether the original diagnosis and therapy were correct. This feedback is an essential component in improving diagnostic and therapeutic skills.

Deficiencies in knowledge and technique are identified at each stage and corrected using information/skills training obtained from books and libraries, electronic resources, physicians, other health-care professionals, patient groups, skills workshops, learning sessions, etc.

Some medical schools have a structured approach to this process, with substantial guidance at each stage; others are less formalized—which appeals more depends largely on you. Which is better is unclear.

How to behave on the wards

It is particularly important when performing ward work to:
- Introduce yourself to the ward staff as well as the patient, so that they know who you are and why you are there.
- Respect patients' privacy, and their right to refuse to see you.
- Ask for consent before seeing a patient.
- If you undress a patient to examine him or her, help him or her to dress again once you have finished.
- Be courteous to nurses and other members of staff (e.g. physiotherapists, ward cleaners, cooks, etc.) at all times.
- Be punctual in attending teaching sessions—you will find that your teachers, who are often busy clinicians, are often late—this is not deliberately done to infuriate you, rather it reflects how hectic their lives are. It is reasonable to wait ~10 min, before 'bleeping' to remind them of the session.
- Write in the notes: different medical schools have different policies on this. Often, however, senior medical students are expected to write in the notes. This is a legal document, so write legibly, never use pejorative phraseology, and sign your name, along with your status as student, legibly at the end. **Never** amend the record at a later time, unless you clearly identify who you are and when the alterations occurred.
- Enjoy yourself!

2 Basic clinical skills

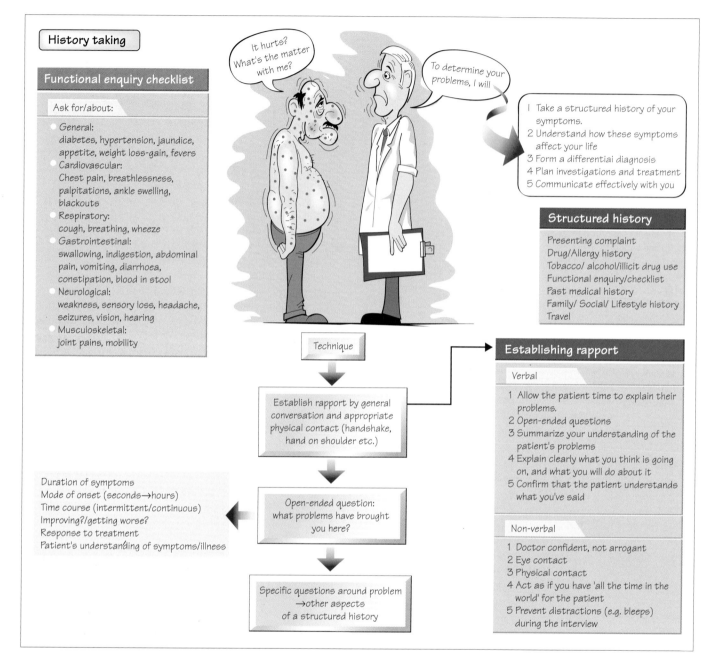

Basic history-taking skills

Competence in the fundamental clinical skills of history-taking and physical examination is crucial to being a good doctor. Diagnostic gold is most often to be found in the history—do not be tempted to cut corners. Your examination of the patient should begin while you are taking the history, and you may need to expand the history in the light of the examination findings.

After the history and examination, you need to be clear about:
• The clinical problems of the patient, i.e. the symptoms and signs placed in coherent groupings (e.g. back pain and progressive weakness of the legs in a man with carcinoma of the prostate).

• The differential diagnosis of these problems (a shortlist of possible diagnoses to account for each clinical problem). As well as the most likely diagnosis (the working diagnosis), you must also consider those other possible diagnoses that are most serious if missed, and most treatable if found.
• The impact of these problems on the patient as a person (e.g. ability to work, look after their family; carry out activities of daily living).
• A plan of action (to include investigation, treatment and what you will say to the patient about the diagnosis and prognosis).

Table 2.1 Checklist for history-taking.

Age, sex, racial origin and occupation

Main symptoms

History of symptoms: mode of onset (abrupt/gradual), time course (constant/intermittent; getting better/getting worse/staying the same), and response to treatment

Current and previous medication including over-the-counter and other non-prescribed remedies: ask women about the oral contraceptive pill and hormone replacement therapy

Allergies to medications and other substances. Also ask about other important adverse effects of medications

Tobacco and alcohol use and use of recreational drugs if the clinical problem suggests that this may be relevant

Functional enquiry (systems review): this is your checklist to make sure that no important symptoms have been overlooked or forgotten by the patient

Past history, under the headings medical, surgical, obstetric-gynaecological, traumatic (bone fractures and other significant injuries) and psychiatric

Family history: establish the age, health or cause of death of parents, siblings and children ('Has anyone in your family had the same problems as you have?'). The family history may be relevant to the diagnosis, and often contributes to an understanding of why certain symptoms may have a particular emotional significance to the patient

Social history including: occupational history ('Which job do you do now? Which job did you do before that? Which job have you done the longest?'). In patients with respiratory symptoms, ask specifically about occupational exposure to dusts, fumes and asbestos

Personal history (general description of lifestyle; if disabled, who are the main carers; use of services such as district nurse; pets and other contact with animals); sexual history (if relevant; begin with an open-ended question such as 'Who are the most important people in your life?'); travel history

Taking the history

Open the interview with a few friendly words of introduction: establishing rapport with the patient is important.
• Begin with an open-ended question ('Perhaps you would start by telling me the problems that led to your coming into hospital') and *listen* to the patient's story, taking notes as the patient talks.
• After a few minutes of listening, you will usually need to clarify points in the history with the intelligent use of questions. This applies particularly to complaints such as dizziness, blackouts, collapse and indigestion—words that are applied to a number of different symptoms.
• Cover all the important areas (see Table 2.1) so that you have a complete picture.

Take stock before performing the physical examination

It is very helpful to try to form a differential diagnosis at the end of the history, which will help focus the examination, and will rule in or out an important diagnosis that you will wish to clarify on examination. You should never perform the physical examination on 'autopilot' but rather adjust it in light of the history and ongoing examination findings. You should always be prepared to interrupt the physical examination to ask further questions if necessary.

Physical examination

You must adapt your method to the circumstances. For most patients, you should examine in detail the system or systems relevant to the clin-

Table 2.2 Checklist for the general examination.

General assessment, including mental state (e.g. lucid, cooperative, anxious, depressed, confused, agitated), nutritional state (body mass index [BMI] = weight in kilograms/[height in metres]^2) < 20, underweight; 20–25, normal weight; 25–30, overweight; > 30, obese); body temperature. Check specifically for:
• Pallor (conjunctival pallor present when haemoglobin is < 10 g/dL)
• Cyanosis (central cyanosis detectable when the oxygen saturation is < 90%, unless anaemia is present, i.e. > 5 g/dL desaturated haemoglobin)
• Jaundice (detectable when bilirubin concentration > 40–50 mmol/L)
• Clubbing (causes include intra-thoracic neoplasms and infection, cyanotic congenital heart disease, inflammatory bowel disease, rarely idiopathic/benign)
• Palpable lumps, including lymph nodes of the head, neck, supraclavicular, epitrochlear, axilla and inguinal regions; thyroid enlargement and nodules; breast lumps
• Abnormalities of the skin, nails and subcutaneous tissues (rash; pigmentation; surgical and other scars; purpura; bruising; lumps; ulceration)
• Metabolic 'flap' of the outstretched hands, from CO_2 retention, decompensated liver disease, uraemia

ical problem, and also perform a rapid, competent general examination. One approach is to perform a general examination by region (e.g. hands–arms–head–neck–chest–abdomen–legs–feet) and then complete a detailed examination of the relevant system or systems. Before you lay hands on the patient, it pays dividends to step back, metaphorically at least, and make a general survey. Does the patient look well or ill and, if ill, in what way? Endocrine disorders are easily missed unless you make a point of thinking of them. Consider hypothyroidism, thyrotoxicosis, acromegaly and Cushing's syndrome. Table 2.2 gives a checklist for general examination.

Examination of systems

• **Cardiovascular system**: pulse rate/rhythm; blood pressure (BP); jugular venous pressure (JVP) (height and waveform); carotid pulse upstroke and volume; inspection/palpation of the precordium; auscultation of the heart; palpation of the abdominal aorta and peripheral pulses; auscultation for carotid, abdominal and femoral bruits; percussion and auscultation of the lung bases; sacral and peripheral oedema. Signs of endocarditis (splinter haemorrhages, fever). An ECG is part of the cardiac physical examination.
• **Respiratory system**: character of the voice; presence and quality of cough; sputum character and quantity; respiratory rate; presence of stridor or wheeze; examination of the upper respiratory tract (nose, tonsils, pharynx, trachea); inspection, palpation, percussion and auscultation of the chest. Spirometry and measurement of peak expiratory flow rate.
• **Alimentary and genitourinary systems**: inspect the lips, tongue, teeth and gums; inspection, palpation, percussion and auscultation of the abdomen (including hernial orifices); examine external genitalia; inspection and digital examination of the anorectum; vaginal examination. Testing of stool for blood and stick testing of urine.
• **Nervous system**: evaluation of the mental state, speech and other higher cerebral functions; examination of the skull and spine; testing of the cranial nerves; ophthalmoscopy; examination of the motor system—limbs, trunk, stance and gait; examination of the sensory system.
• **Musculoskeletal system**: examination of the limb joints and spine for swelling, deformity, tenderness and restriction of movement; examination of the bones for deformity and tenderness and of the muscles for

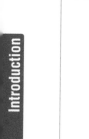

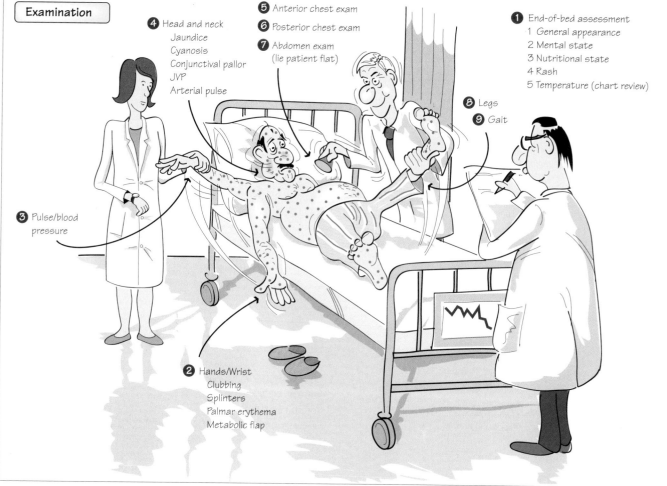

Examination

④ Head and neck
Jaundice
Cyanosis
Conjunctival pallor
JVP
Arterial pulse

⑤ Anterior chest exam
⑥ Posterior chest exam
⑦ Abdomen exam
(lie patient flat)

① End-of-bed assessment
1 General appearance
2 Mental state
3 Nutritional state
4 Rash
5 Temperature (chart review)

⑧ Legs
⑨ Gait

③ Pulse/blood
pressure

② Hands/Wrist
Clubbing
Splinters
Palmar erythema
Metabolic flap

wasting and tenderness; observation of the patient standing, walking and turning.

Rapid neurological/rheumatological examination

If neurological or musculoskeletal disease is not suspected the minimum examination is to:

• Inspect the hands, for wasting of the intrinsic muscles and joint abnormalities, test the power of finger abduction, check light touch sensation over the hands; gently stroke the skin and ask the patient if this feels normal and equal on both sides.

• Ask the patient to hold the arms outstretched with palms down and fingers abducted, and to make piano-playing movements (upper motor lesions cause the movements to be performed more slowly or clumsily), then to turn the palms up and maintain the posture with the eyes closed (upper motor lesions cause the arm to drift downwards and into pronation).

• Put the wrist, elbow, shoulder joints through their range of movement (for muscle tone, and to detect restriction of joint movement), test the power of shoulder abduction (proximal limb weakness is a feature of myopathies). Ask the patient to put the hands behind the head with the elbows back (to assess the glenohumeral, acromioclavicular and sternoclavicular joints). Check the finger-nose test.

• Check cervical spine movements (ask the patient to touch the ear on to the shoulder).

• Check visual acuity, fields, eye movements, pupils and fundi.

• Put the hip, knee and ankle joints through their range of movement (including rotation of the hip joint with the knee flexed—to assess muscle tone and detect restriction of joint movement); test the power of hip flexion.

• Inspect the feet: test the power of ankle dorsiflexion. Check light touch sensation over the feet: gently stroke the skin and ask the patient if this feels normal and equal on both sides. Check the heel-knee-shin test; test the tendon reflexes and plantar responses.

• Observe the patient standing, walking and turning.

Presenting the case

The cardinal virtues here are brevity, clarity and enthusiasm. Your presentation should last ≤ 5 min. If your listener wants more detail, he or she will ask for it. Always include the age and occupation of the patient in your opening remarks. Don't mention the sex and racial origin of the patient if you are presenting the case in his or her presence. Begin with a short summary of the patient's problems; this is especially important in patients with chronic illness who may have multiple medical and social problems. You should then deal, in turn, with information from the history, the findings on examination, your differential diagnosis and the plan of action.

Diagnosis
1 What is diagnosis?

Diagnosis is the central intellectual activity of medicine. It is the process whereby we turn data about the patient into the names of diseases ('diagnoses'). A diagnosis is important because it serves as a guide to action, and it helps us foretell the future ('prognosis'). The data we bring to the diagnostic process is of many types: elements in the history (e.g. headache), an examination finding (e.g. enlargement of the spleen) or a test result (e.g. microcytic anaemia).

2 Why can diagnosis be difficult?
So if diagnosis is simply about mapping data onto diseases, why is it difficult?
• Most manifestations of disease are not specific to one diagnosis, e.g. breathlessness can be caused by heart, lung or neurological disease.
• There are > 3500 manifestations of disease, which may occur singly or in combination, and with different time courses and there are > 500 disease processes.
• Distinguishing between normal and abnormal may be difficult, e.g. is increasing breathlessness due to the ageing process or a disease process?
• The data is often unreliable or partial (e.g. elements in the history may be forgotten by the patient, misinterpreted by the doctor); physical signs may be overlooked or misinterpreted; test results may be wrong (e.g. may belong to another patient).
• Patients may have more than one disease (multiple pathology).
• What is an unlikely diagnosis in many will turn out to be the diagnosis in a few.
• Some symptoms are medically inexplicable.
• Humans make mistakes in the analysis of data.

3 How do we go about making a diagnosis?
The presenting complaint is the key to the diagnosis, and it is usually the case that the problem that took the patient to the doctor reflects a key part of the pathological process going on in that patient. Accordingly the best place to start the diagnostic process is with the presenting complaint, to ensure that the diagnostic analysis accounts for the presenting symptom(s). Only under very unusual circumstances (which nonetheless do occur) should the presenting complaint be ignored. How does one analyse the presenting complaint?
• Analysis by body region: this method works well for many complaints of pain, e.g. headache, chest pain and abdominal pain.
• Analysis by system: this method works well for breathlessness, weakness, etc.
• Analysis by organ: e.g. breast lump.

4 Stages on the way to a diagnosis
One cannot just proclaim the diagnosis; an intellectual exercise needs to be undertaken, which can be approached in a number of different ways:
• Syndromic diagnosis: grouping together of the major data elements. For example, effort-dependent retrosternal chest pain brought on reliably by exercise and relieved promptly by rest is classed as the syndrome of angina.
• Differential diagnosis: a short list of possible diseases that could account for these data elements (to include the most treatable and most important not to miss). For example, angina may be caused by atheromatous coronary disease, aortic stenosis, (very rarely) pulmonary hypertension, syndrome X (inadequate vasodilator reserve), asthma, non-cardiac chest pain, gastro-oesophageal reflux.
• Working diagnosis: the diagnosis on which you will base your immediate management decisions (e.g. what treatment to give), e.g. angina due to aortic stenosis.
• Diagnostic testing: selection of those tests that will help sort out

between the possible diseases, e.g. a cardiac ultrasound, exercise stress test, etc.
• Final diagnosis: the diagnosis when all the information is in, e.g. symptomatic aortic stenosis.

A further example would be headache with fever in a 23-year-old medical student just returned from India, with thrombocytopenia. The differential diagnosis includes malaria, typhoid, bacterial meningitis and viral meningitis. The working diagnosis is malaria. Investigations show malarial parasites on thick blood film, normal CSF, blood culture negative. Thus, the final diagnosis is falciparum malaria.

5 Reasoning about diagnosis
• Probabilistic reasoning; many diagnoses can be made on the basis of a syndromic diagnosis and the underlying probability of disease. For example, anginal type chest pains in an elderly man living in the UK is almost always due to atheromatous coronary disease.
• Does the diagnosis provide a coherent explanation of what has happened to the patient, i.e. the time course of the illness, the important positive and negative findings, e.g. clinical examination and investigations?

6 Interpretation of diagnostic tests
An ideal test is completely specific and sensitive (i.e. all those with the disease have the abnormal test, none without do). If a test result seems inconsistent with most other aspects of the clinical situation, it is usually best to degrade the value of the test result than the value of the clinical circumstances.

7 Co-ordinating diagnoses with the safe care of the patient
In an ideal world one can make the right diagnosis immediately. However, often the situation is less than ideal, either as tests are not available (e.g. middle of the night, wrong sort of hospital, etc.) or take too long to come back (e.g. blood cultures). In these situations, one nonetheless needs to proceed, treating what is probable, and what might be dangerous.
• Data gathering should continue unimpeded throughout.
• Observation is an underused technique. Many illnesses are self-limiting, others move slowly. If the likelihood of either is high, observation (with or without further investigations) may be appropriate.
• Trial of treatment; this is important in dangerous illnesses, or those proceeding rapidly.
• Correction of abnormal physiology is crucial in those with life-threatening disease, for example, volume replacement in gastro-intestinal bleeding.

8 Mistakes in diagnosis
Failure to establish the correct diagnosis is common, and results from:
• Lack of knowledge (e.g. not knowing of diagnoses such as oesophageal rupture, cerebral venous sinus thrombosis).
• Inexperience of the 'fuzziness' of many diagnoses (e.g. pulmonary embolism, acute coronary syndrome).
• Jumping to conclusions.
• Accepting one diagnosis without excluding others (e.g. fever, elevated right hemidiaphragm and right basal lung shadowing after laparoscopic appendicectomy—diagnosis of pneumonia—subphrenic gas ascribed to laparoscopy—CT showed subphrenic abscess).
• Failure to reconsider diagnosis as more data becomes available, e.g. continued fever in a presumed self-limiting illness.

3 The critically ill patient

The key features of the clinical assessment of the critically ill patient

Clinical Assessment
Airway
Breathing
Circulation
Disability (neurological status)
Exposure (full patient examination)
Review of notes/charts of physiological variables and trends

Simple scales have the advantage that they are easier for inexperienced healthcare workers to use and show less interobserver variability than more complicated scales like the Glasgow Coma Score (Chapter 69 Coma)

Simple Assessment of Conscious Level (AVPU, ACDU)

A	Alert	A	Alert
V	Responds to Voice	C	Confused
P	Responds to Pain	D	Drowsy
U	Unresponsive	U	Unresponsive

Criteria for calling an emergency team (for example, an ITU outreach service or, less attractive, the 'crash team') to a sick patient

Possible Criteria for Calling a Medical Emergency Team

Airway
Partial or complete obstruction
Impaired Protection: Reduced conscious level

Breathing
Respiratory arrest
Respiratory rate <8 or >20
Acute hypoxia: PaO_2 <8kPa or SaO_2 <90% or FIO_2 >0.5
Acute hypercapnia: $PaCO_2$ >6.5kPa, pH <7.3

Circulation
Cardiac arrest
Heart rate <40 or >120
Systolic Blood Pressure <90mmHg despite treatment
Acidosis: pH <7.3, lactate >2.0 mmol/L, Base deficit >−4
Urine output <0.5mL/kg/h

Conscious Level
GCS <12 or drop of 2 or more points
Recurrent or prolonged seizures

Other
Failure to respond to treatment
Uncontrolled pain

Example of an early warning scoring system for critically ill patients. Scores >5 can be used for triggering an emergency medical team

Score	3	2	1	0	1	2	3
HR		<40	40–50	51–100	101–110	111–129	>130
BP	<45%	<30%	<15%	Normal for patient	>15%	>30%	>45%
RR		<8		9–14	15–20	21–29	>30
TEMP		<35		35–38.4		<38.4	
CNS				A	V	P	U
URINE	Nil	<0.5mL/kg/h	<1mL/kg/h		>1.5mL/kg/h		

Recognition of the critically ill patient

Though the severity of illness and associated patient mortality varies widely between individuals (and demographics such as age, and co-morbid illness, such as diabetes, previous infirmity, etc. are all crucial) when approaching a potentially sick patient, like in all other patients, the taking a history, performing an examination and ordering appropriate investigations are essential in order to make the correct diagnosis and to institute appropriate therapy.

Sometimes critical illness is obvious from the end of the bed. Often however, critical illness is recognized by alterations in key physiological variables, rather than 'just' by the patient 'looking' sick.

Maintenance of adequate airway, breathing and circulation are prerequisites for survival. Accordingly, simple physiological observations such as heart rate, systolic blood pressure, oxygen saturations, respiratory rate, level of consciousness, urine output and temperature define in-patient mortality. Mortality can be directly correlated with the number of abnormalities rising from 0.7% (30-day mortality) with none, 4.4% with one, 9.2% with two to 21.3% with three or more.

Many patients who suffer a cardiorespiratory arrest or are admitted to intensive care have a documented decline in these physiological variables prior to these events, which often goes unrecognized. It is therefore important to have a system for recognizing critically ill patients, ensuring sufficient monitoring takes place in a designated area, instituting appropriate therapy and calling for additional help or expertise if required. In some cases it might be the realization that the patient is in the process of dying and the patient's symptoms should be palliated.

Examination of the critically ill patient

Dysfunction of the airway, breathing or circulation can lead to immediate death and so the patient assessment should focus on these systems.

Airway Obstruction of the airway is an emergency and unless rectified leads to rapid hypoxia and death within minutes. It is therefore pointless making an examination of the circulation in a hypotensive patient with an obstructed airway; indeed the hypotension may be the consequence of airway obstruction.

- **Complete airway obstruction** leads to paradoxical chest and abdominal movements so that the chest moves in on inspiration and the abdomen out (as opposed to both moving out in normal breathing) and *vice versa* on expiration. Accessory muscle use and a tracheal tug are present. No movement of air is present at the mouth either audibly or by feeling with a hand at the patient's mouth.
- **Partial airway obstruction** leads to noisy breathing with detectable movement of air at the mouth. Stridor indicates obstruction at the larynx or above, while snoring often occurs when the tongue obstructs the pharynx.

In the majority of patients simple measures resolve airway obstruction. Blood, vomit, secretions or foreign bodies may be removed by suction. If consciousness is impaired, loss of muscle tone causes the tongue to fall back and obstruct. A chin lift or jaw thrust opens the airway; occasionally an airway adjunct such as an oropharyngeal (Guedel) or nasopharyngeal airway is required. If these simple methods fail then endotracheal intubation or *rarely* a surgical cricothyroidotomy is required.

Breathing Visual examination is extremely informative with respiratory rate being one of the most important observations. A rate < 8 or > 20 per minute should alert the examiner to severe illness. Expansion of the chest should be compared bilaterally, as well as depth, abdominal breathing, accessory muscle use and tracheal tugging (respiratory pattern). Abnormal expansion usually accompanies underlying disease (collapse, consolidation, effusion, pneumothorax). The inspired oxygen concentration should be noted and oxygen saturations on pulse oximetry recorded (cyanosis is often a late sign); if indicated, a blood gas is performed. The latter provides information on adequacy of ventilation ($PaCO_2$) and oxygenation (PaO_2 and A-a gradient). Respiratory acidosis (pH < 7.3, PCO_2 > 6.5 kPa) or failure of oxygenation (SaO_2 < 90% or PaO_2 < 8 kPa on high flow oxygen) requires urgent intervention. Treatment is discussed in Chapter 88 (Respiratory failure) —all critically ill patients need oxygen saturations maintained above 90%.

Circulation Important parameters of the circulatory examination are blood pressure, pulse, capillary refill, limb temperature, urine output and level of consciousness. A 'normal' blood pressure may represent hypotension in some patients and it is therefore useful to know the patient's usual pressure. Hypotension may also be a late sign when homeostatic mechanisms fail to compensate and is usually preceded by an abnormal pulse (often tachycardia). Normal capillary refill is less than 2 seconds and prolongation suggests inadequate tissue perfusion. An arterial blood gas may be indicated and show metabolic acidosis with a raised lactate if the circulation is inadequate (Base excess > −4 or lactate > 2 mmol/L). Treatment of circulatory abnormalities is discussed in Chapters 9 (Shock) and 217 (Fluid replacement therapy).

Disability Neurological status is assessed by examining the pupils and the level of consciousness (GCS or simple scales such as AVPU or ACDU). Hypoglycaemia should be excluded in all sick patients.

Exposure A general examination should be made with particular attention to drains and wound sites. The temperature should be recorded.

As the patient is examined specific immediate life-saving therapies or investigations may be initiated, such as a chest drain in a patient with a tension pneumothorax, before other parts of the examination are undertaken. Adequate monitoring in an appropriate area also needs to be ensured. If the patient is being seen for the first time a full assessment of the notes needs to be undertaken.

Examination of the charts of the critically ill patient

It is important to examine the patient's charts, which record physiological variables of blood pressure, pulse, temperature, respiratory rate, oxygen saturations, consciousness level and urine output over time. While the absolute values are important **equal value is attached to the trends and response to treatment**. As emphasized earlier the number of physiological abnormalities defines mortality. Earlier recognition of patient deterioration would be expected to prevent unexpected cardiac arrests and admissions to intensive care. It is likely that the introduction of severity triggers or early warning scoring systems and medical emergency teams will become more widespread in hospitals in the future, in order to reduce the morbidity and mortality of critically ill patients in addition to making better end-of-life decisions.

Admission to intensive care

This is a key decision in the management of the sick patient; clearly, patients who benefit from ITU should go there, whereas those who don't shouldn't. However, discriminating these two groups reliably is often not possible, and will require judgement. Obtaining patients' and relatives' views of ITU, in the light of data on outcomes, is crucial to the decision to admit to ITU. Most ITU admissions should be the consequence of discussions between the consultant looking after the patient and the consultant intensivist.

Treatment of the critically sick patient

This is covered in other chapters. Often the crucial question is 'how much treatment', rather than 'what sort of treatment'. This aspect requires great judgement, and excellent communication skills; indeed, in this area perhaps more than any other, the ability to know when to discontinue therapy, when not escalate treatment, and when to implement terminal care at just the right stage are what defines clinical excellence. As relatives often have inappropriately high expectations about the outcome of intensive care therapy, it is important to be realistic (and kind) at all times.

Clinical Presentations at a Glance

4 Chest pain

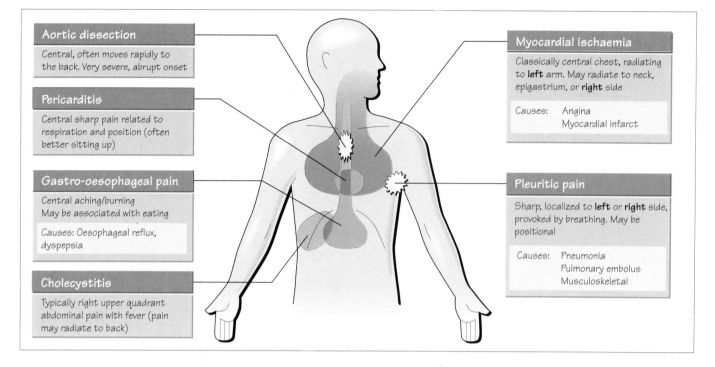

Aortic dissection

Central, often moves rapidly to the back. Very severe, abrupt onset

Pericarditis

Central sharp pain related to respiration and position (often better sitting up)

Gastro-oesophageal pain

Central aching/burning
May be associated with eating

Causes: Oesophageal reflux, dyspepsia

Cholecystitis

Typically right upper quadrant abdominal pain with fever (pain may radiate to back)

Myocardial ischaemia

Classically central chest, radiating to **left** arm. May radiate to neck, epigastrium, or **right** side

Causes: Angina
          Myocardial infarct

Pleuritic pain

Sharp, localized to **left** or **right** side, provoked by breathing. May be positional

Causes: Pneumonia
          Pulmonary embolus
          Musculoskeletal

Determining the origin of chest pain is a common clinical problem which can present a diagnostic challenge. The greatest concern is whether the pain relates to heart disease. This thought dominates the clinical and investigative approach. Most pains are diagnosed by a full history, sometimes aided by the examination. The diagnostic approach involves determining the nature of the pain, how long it has been present, typical provoking and relieving factors, and the presence of risk factors for heart/lung disease.

Typical myocardial ischaemic pain (cardiac pain)

Myocardial ischaemia is a clinical diagnosis, made on the history and supported by finding risk factors for atheromatous coronary disease (see pp. 144–147). There are two forms of ischaemic chest pain: angina and myocardial infarction.

Typical angina is a heavy pain or discomfort felt retrosternally, which may radiate to the neck, and is often associated with heaviness in the left arm. Some patients have atypical symptoms, such as pain in unusual places (e.g. the right chest, shoulder blade), although isolated left-sided chest/submammary pain is rarely angina. A key diagnostic feature is the **relationship of symptoms to effort**. For genuine angina, whatever its location, pain is reliably brought on by effort, and relieved by less than 5 min of rest. Angina is described clinically as stable, crescendo or unstable. In **stable angina**, symptoms are only provoked by effort and readily relieved by rest. In **crescendo angina**, the amount of effort required to provoke symptoms decreases rapidly over several weeks, although symptoms do not occur at rest. In **unstable angina**, symptoms come on unpredictably, either with minimal exertion or at rest. Angina is usually the result of ischaemic heart disease, although it may be caused by aortic stenosis and, very rarely, by severe pulmonary hypertension. In those with coronary artery disease, the occurrence of

crescendo or unstable angina means that the underlying coronary obstruction has increased, usually because of thrombus formation. This is associated with a greatly increased risk of myocardial infarction.

Myocardial infarction (MI) pain typically comes on over a few minutes. Although feeling identical to angina, it is often very severe, and differs from angina in lasting 20 min or more and not being relieved by nitrates. Sweating, nausea and vomiting are very common, and when present greatly increase the chance that symptoms are caused by a myocardial infarct rather than angina. Anginal pain suggesting unstable angina or MI, but without definite diagnosis of MI, is termed an **acute coronary syndrome**.

Aortic dissection

Aortic dissection pain is usually unheralded and of abrupt (instantaneous) onset, unlike MI pain which evolves over minutes, is very severe and is described as having a 'tearing' quality. The location of the pain reflects the site of the origin of the dissection and the spread of the pain reflects the propagation of the dissection plane along the aorta. Thus, classically, dissection of the ascending aorta starts in the anterior chest and rapidly (less than a few minutes) moves into the neck and then the back. Dissections originating in the aortic arch start as neck pain, and those in the descending thoracic aorta as interscapular or shoulder pain.

Pleuritic pain

Pleuritic pain is defined as a 'sharp', 'catching' chest pain, exacerbated by respiration, particularly extreme inspiration. When severe, patients breathe shallowly to avoid pain. There are two causes:
• **Pleural pain**: this is 'pleurisy' localized to one side of the chest, not position dependent. A pleural rub may be heard. Achieving a diagnosis depends on defining the associated symptoms and signs. Pleurisy occurs with pneumonia (fever, cough, tachypnoea and bronchial

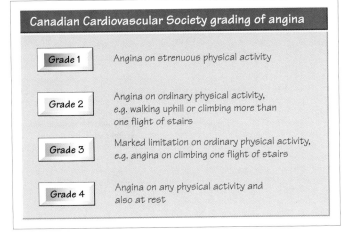

Canadian Cardiovascular Society grading of angina

Grade 1 — Angina on strenuous physical activity

Grade 2 — Angina on ordinary physical activity, e.g. walking uphill or climbing more than one flight of stairs

Grade 3 — Marked limitation on ordinary physical activity, e.g. angina on climbing one flight of stairs

Grade 4 — Angina on any physical activity and also at rest

breathing), pulmonary embolus (breathlessness, tachycardia, cyanosis and no bronchial breathing) and pneumothorax (absent breath sounds).
• **Pericardial pain**: as with pleurisy, pericardial pain is worse on deep inspiration, but unlike pleurisy it is located in the centre of the chest, is positional in nature, and typically is worse lying down and relieved by sitting. A pericardial rub may be heard on auscultation, which may be positional, quite localized or intermittent. Pericarditis occurs with viral infections, post-myocardial infarction and in autoimmune diseases.

Musculoskeletal chest pain

Very common. There may be a history of physical injury or unusual exertion, although this is found surprisingly infrequently. Pain is provoked by arm/chest movement and lasts many hours. Although pains may be exacerbated by effort, rest does not reliably relieve them.

Examination may show localized tenderness. This diagnosis should be considered only once more serious diagnosis has been excluded, because chest wall pain and coronary disease may coexist.

Gastro-oesophageal pain

Several different gastrointestinal pains can cause diagnostic confusion with cardiac pain:
1 Oesophageal reflux causes a retrosternal burning, travelling from the epigastrium upwards. There may be frequent belching, odynophagia or, if a stricture has occurred, dysphagia. Reflux is particularly frequent in obese individuals who smoke, just the population in whom coronary disease is found!
2 Oesophageal spasm, often provoked by oesophageal reflux, can be very difficult to distinguish from cardiac pain, because it causes a retrosternal tightness/heaviness which may be severe. It may, however, be relieved by liquid antacids (e.g. milk) or cold drinks.

The key to the diagnosis of gastrointestinal pain is its clear relationship with food, and the absence of a relationship between the onset of the pain and exertion. Confusingly, some oesophageal reflux (and spasm) can be provoked by exercise, although such pain often resolves only slowly on resting. This can lead to diagnostic confusion with angina—if the risk of coronary artery disease is high, a cardiac origin to the pain should be actively excluded.

Gall bladder disease

Classic biliary colic is felt in the epigastrium and cholecystitis in the right upper quadrant of the abdomen. However, biliary disease may also be felt in the chest and confused with angina. Typically attacks of pain are intermittent, unrelated to exertion, and may be severe. Eating certain particularly fatty foods can precipitate them. It is more common in women than in men, diagnosed on ultrasonography and by the exclusion of anginal syndromes.

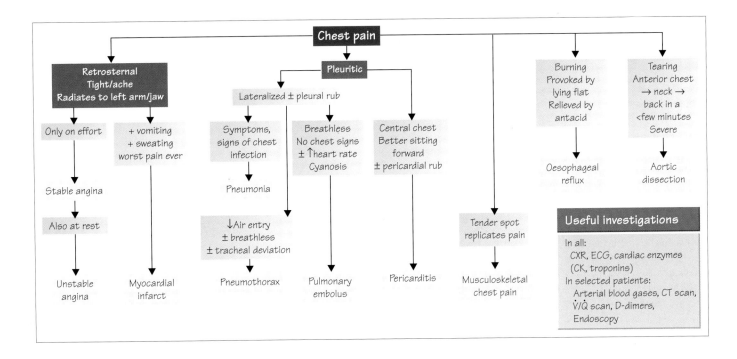

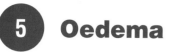

5 Oedema

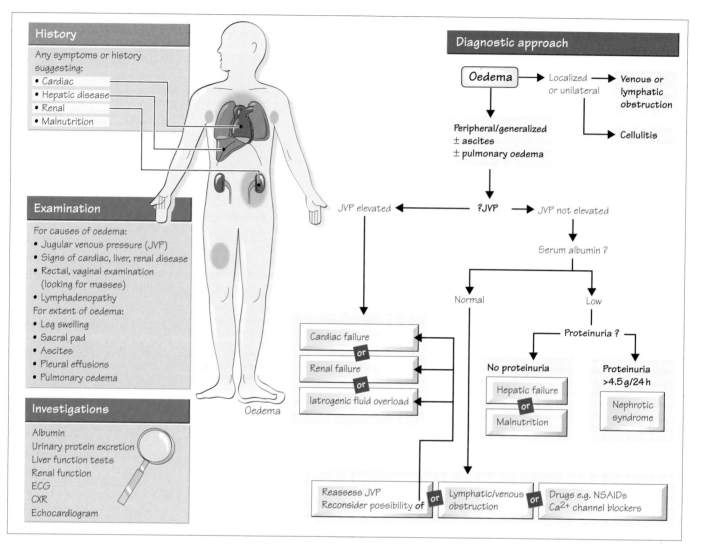

Oedema ('an abnormal build-up of fluid in the tissues') can be a presenting feature of many serious medical conditions, notably congestive heart failure, liver failure, malnutrition and the nephrotic syndrome. Peripheral oedema can also result from venous or lymphatic obstruction or from excessive administration of salt and water. Agents such as non-steroidal anti-inflammatory drugs (NSAIDs) and calcium channel blockers can also produce peripheral oedema.

Presentation

Patients present complaining of swelling of the legs. In severe cases oedema extends to cause abdominal swelling (from ascites), sacral oedema, pleural effusions, pulmonary oedema and even facial swelling. Oedema is often, although not always, posturally dependent, and in bed-bound individuals it may be confined to the sacrum.

Diagnosis

Accurate history taking is vital. Symptoms and signs of cardiac, liver and renal disease should be sought. Two questions are the key to the diagnosis: Is the oedema unilateral or bilateral? Is the venous pressure raised or not? It is also important to determine whether oedema is present in other sites. Oedema diffusely affecting the whole body suggests a low serum albumin, or 'leaky' capillaries, rather than heart failure.

Bilateral leg oedema

In bilateral leg oedema, the diagnosis rests in determining whether the venous pressure is elevated and whether there are signs of liver disease, severe immobility or malnourishment.

- **Heart failure**: leg oedema occurs from right-sided heart failure and is always associated with a high jugular venous pressure (JVP) (Table 5.1). Hepatomegaly is often seen, as are signs of underlying cardiac pathology. If the oedema is mild in the legs, but severe in the abdomen, pericardial constriction should be considered.
- **Liver failure**: leg oedema is caused by a low serum albumin (usually < 20 g/dL). There may be signs of chronic liver disease, such as spider naevi, leuconychia, gynaecomastia, dilated abdominal veins indicating portal hypertension, and bruises (impaired liver synthetic function). The JVP is not elevated. In severe chronic liver disease (e.g. cirrhosis), liver enzyme tests may be only mildly disturbed, although the pro-

Table 5.1 Causes of oedema.

Bilateral oedema
Congestive cardiac failure
Hepatic failure
Renal failure
Nephrotic syndrome
Malnutrition
Immobility
Drugs (NSAIDs, calcium channel blockers)

Unilateral oedema
Lymphatic obstruction
Venous obstruction (usually DVT; rarely, external compression)
Venous valve incompetence from previous DVT
Cellulitis
Ruptured Baker's cyst
Localized immobility, e.g. hemiparesis

thrombin time (PT) is often prolonged (> 20 s). In acute liver failure, the patient is usually very unwell, cerebral disturbance is prominent and liver function tests are usually grossly abnormal.

• **Renal failure**: oedema is caused by either a low serum albumin (nephrotic syndrome, where the urine is frothy and contains 3–4+ of protein on dipstick testing—confirmatory tests include estimation of serum albumin (usually < 30 g/dL), urinary protein (usually > 4 g/24 h) and serum creatinine and urea) or an inability to excrete fluid (nephritic syndrome, associated with hypertension and low urine output).

• **General immobility**: the patient is usually elderly, and obviously immobile from general infirmity or cerebrovascular disease. The JVP is down, and there are no signs of liver or renal disease.

• **Malnutrition**: any chronic illness may be associated with a catabolic state and a degree of malnutrition that can be severe enough to depress serum albumin and cause leg oedema.

• **IVC compression**: rarely, bilateral leg oedema can be caused by compression on the inferior vena cava (IVC). This can be diagnosed by ultrasonographic studies of the abdomen, using colour flow Doppler to determine blood flow and computed tomography (CT), and occurs:

• in extreme obesity
• in severe (tense) ascites from whatever cause
• with extensive venous thrombosis in the IVC, such as occurs in malignancy, or as a complication of the nephrotic syndrome.

Unilateral leg oedema

One-sided leg swelling is likely to have a local underlying cause, such as:

• A **deep venous thrombosis** (DVT) in the leg causes a slow onset

(more than a few hours) of unilateral leg pain, swelling, with skin warmth, and possibly tenderness in the calves and along the veins, particularly the great saphenous vein. As symptoms/signs are unreliable for diagnosis, all patients with suspected DVTs should undergo definitive investigations (vein ultrasonography or venography) and be examined for complicating pulmonary embolisms (PEs) (see Chapter 7).

• **Ruptured Baker's cyst**: a Baker's cyst is a knee joint bursa that juts into the popliteal fossa and usually occurs in rheumatoid arthritis. It may rupture and cause sudden-onset leg pain and calf swelling. Ultrasonography is diagnostic.

• **Cellulitis**: consists of an intense spreading skin erythema, sometimes well demarcated, occasionally tracking up the line of the lymphatics. It is often very painful and is associated with a temperature, and raised erythrocyte sedimentation rate (ESR), C-reactive protein and white count. The organism is usually one of the staphylococci or streptococci species, and is occasionally grown from blood cultures, although rarely from skin swabs.

• **Lymphatic obstruction** results in a 'woody' form of unilateral oedema, sometimes described as 'non-pitting'. It is very rare in the West, and when found is usually the result of carcinomatous invasion and obliteration of the draining lymph nodes, e.g. in metastatic melanoma. In Africa lymph obstruction is very common, often bilateral, and caused by filarial infestation.

• **Pelvic tumours** can unilaterally compress veins, causing unilateral oedema.

• **Localized immobility** can cause unilateral leg oedema, e.g. long-standing hemiparesis.

Investigations

These vary depending on the features established by history and examination but determination of serum albumin, urinary protein loss, liver function tests, creatinine, ECG, chest X-ray and echocardiography are often appropriate.

Treatment

Therapy is directed at correcting the underlying cause. In bilateral oedema diuretics are often used to promote salt and water excretion, although their use should be balanced against the risk of hypovolaemia and worsening renal function, postural hypotension and falls. Several different classes of diuretic agent are used (see Table 5.2). The use of a loop diuretic in combination with a thiazide can produce a pronounced diuretic effect that is useful in resistant oedema. Spironolactone, a competitive aldosterone antagonist, produces a mild natriuresis and potassium retention, and is utilized in conditions with secondary hyperaldosteronism such as liver cirrhosis with ascites. Spironolactone and amiloride are 'potassium-sparing' diuretics, in contrast to the loop and thiazide diuretics which promote potassium depletion.

Table 5.2 Diuretics used in treating oedema.

Class	Example	Diuretic potency	Na$^+$/K$^+$ lowering potential
Thiazide	Bendroflumethiazide	+	++/+
Loop	Frusemide	+++	+/+++
K$^+$ sparing	Amiloride	±	±/0
	Spironolactone	±	±/0

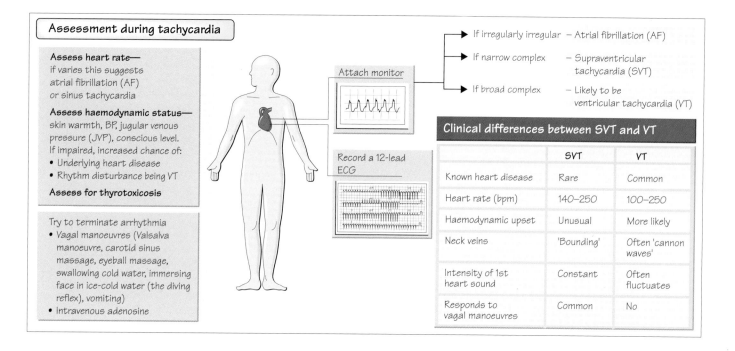

Assessment during tachycardia

Assess heart rate—
if varies this suggests atrial fibrillation (AF) or sinus tachycardia

Assess haemodynamic status—
skin warmth, BP, jugular venous pressure (JVP), conscious level. If impaired, increased chance of:
• Underlying heart disease
• Rhythm disturbance being VT

Assess for thyrotoxicosis

Try to terminate arrhythmia
• Vagal manoeuvres (Valsalva manoeuvre, carotid sinus massage, eyeball massage, swallowing cold water, immersing face in ice-cold water (the diving reflex), vomiting)
• Intravenous adenosine

Attach monitor

Record a 12-lead ECG

If irregularly irregular – Atrial fibrillation (AF)

If narrow complex – Supraventricular tachycardia (SVT)

If broad complex – Likely to be ventricular tachycardia (VT)

Clinical differences between SVT and VT

	SVT	VT
Known heart disease	Rare	Common
Heart rate (bpm)	140–250	100–250
Haemodynamic upset	Unusual	More likely
Neck veins	'Bounding'	Often 'cannon waves'
Intensity of 1st heart sound	Constant	Often fluctuates
Responds to vagal manoeuvres	Common	No

Palpitations are an awareness of the heart beat, either due to an abnormal appreciation of the normal heart beat or from a tachyarrhythmia (bradyarrhythmias never cause palpitations). For diagnosis, it is helpful to establish the mode of onset (instantaneous or over several minutes) and the rate and rhythm (ask the patient to tap out the palpitations using a hand). Distinguishing features include:

1 'Awareness of sinus tachycardia' palpitations: here the heart rhythm is normal, but the heart beats more rapidly and strongly than usual; this occurs with exercise, fear or psychological distress, including anxiety. The diagnosis is established by finding a characteristic history. Palpitations start and stop over many minutes, unlike genuine tachyarrhythmias, which start instantaneously. They are regular and relatively slow (heart rate < 100 beats/min). There is often a background of anxiety (work, relationship stress, etc.), which is worse immediately before an attack. Vagal manoeuvres are unhelpful and syncope never occurs.

Causes of a sinus tachycardia include:
• *Physiological*—exercise; anxiety
• *Common pathologies*—sepsis/fever; pain; heart failure; respiratory distress; haemodynamic compromise; anaemia; thyrotoxicosis
• *Rare*—phaeochromocytoma; sinus node re-entrant tachycardia—diagnosed by 'fixed' heart rate on 24-h taping.

2 Tachyarrhythmia-associated palpitations: here the heart beats more quickly than usual as a result of a tachyarrhythmia or extra beats. The characteristic history of a genuine tachyarrhythmia is of sudden (i.e. instantaneous) onset fast palpitations, which last for a very clearly defined period of time (usually minutes rather than hours), and may (although not reliably) stop as suddenly as they started. Anxiety may occur, but does so during, not before, an attack. Vagal manoeuvres are helpful for supraventricular arrhythmias, and there is often a history of severe heart disease in ventricular arrhythmias. Syncope may occur.

After the event patients may pass abnormally large volumes of urine. A number of different tachyarrhythmias have additional characteristic features:

• **Supraventricular tachycardia** (either AV re-entrant tachycardia [AVRT] or AVNRT [AV nodal re-entrant tachycardia]): these often start during the teenage years. Syncope is very unusual. Post-event polyuria, from atrial natriuretic factor release resulting from atrial stretching during the attack, may occur.

• **Atrial fibrillation**: characteristically the palpitations are felt 'all over the place' or are 'irregularly irregular'. Syncope is very rare (unless the patient has a very fast ventricular response to the atrial fibrillation) but, as this arrhythmia occurs in those with heart disease, breathlessness resulting from associated heart failure is common.

• **Ventricular tachycardia**: patients are often although not always known to have heart disease. Syncope is common, although not universal. Vagal manoeuvres are unhelpful.

• **Extrasystoles**: patients usually do not feel the extra-systole, but feel the post-extra-systolic beat, which is of increased contraction. They thus feel that the heart misses a beat, then 'restarts' with a thump. Patients often say that they are 'worried that their heart may not restart'.

The most helpful investigation in palpitations is an ECG recorded during an attack, and the aim of investigation should be to obtain such an ECG. If attacks are prolonged, this is straightforward. If short-lived, then a 24-h Holter monitor may be useful if attacks are frequent (every 24–48 h). For infrequent attacks, a variety of electronic recorders are available which the patient can apply during the episode. Whatever the cause of the palpitation, patients with a structurally normal heart generally have a good prognosis, whereas impaired ventricular function generally mandates more aggressive investigation and treatment.

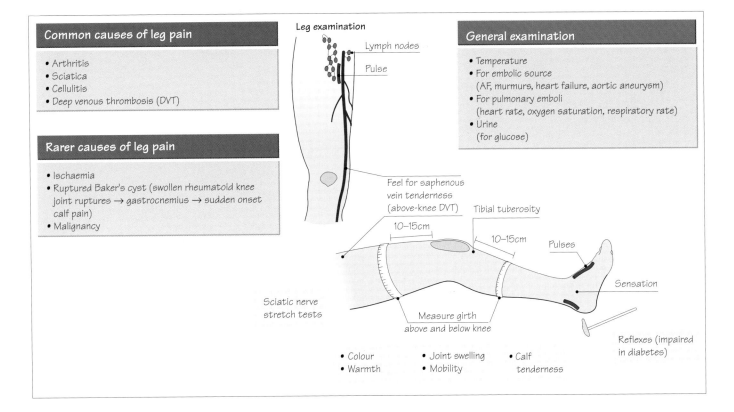

Common causes of leg pain

- Arthritis
- Sciatica
- Cellulitis
- Deep venous thrombosis (DVT)

Rarer causes of leg pain

- Ischaemia
- Ruptured Baker's cyst (swollen rheumatoid knee joint ruptures → gastrocnemius → sudden onset calf pain)
- Malignancy

Leg examination

Lymph nodes

Pulse

Feel for saphenous vein tenderness (above-knee DVT)

Tibial tuberosity

10–15cm

10–15cm

Pulses

Sensation

Reflexes (impaired in diabetes)

Sciatic nerve stretch tests

Measure girth above and below knee

- Colour
- Warmth
- Joint swelling
- Mobility
- Calf tenderness

General examination

- Temperature
- For embolic source (AF, murmurs, heart failure, aortic aneurysm)
- For pulmonary emboli (heart rate, oxygen saturation, respiratory rate)
- Urine (for glucose)

As for all symptoms, a clear description of the site, nature and duration of pain, with provoking and relieving factors, along with a careful examination, is usually sufficient to establish the diagnosis. The following are the common causes of leg pain.

- **Deep venous thrombosis**: patients notice a gradually increasing (over hours) unilateral calf (more rarely thigh) ache and often calf (thigh) swelling. Absent swelling does **not** exclude a deep venous thrombosis (DVT), although the greater the swelling the more likely it is. Normal D-dimer levels **exclude** the diagnosis. Only those with raised D-dimers should go on to have definitive imaging: venography (painful, but the gold standard) or ultrasonography (less reliable for below-knee DVT). The risk of PEs is very low in below-knee and significant in above-knee DVTs. Accordingly, below-knee DVTs do not mandate anticoagulation, although surveillance imaging every few days is **essential** to ensure that the clot has not propagated more proximally. All patients may need anticoagulation to relieve symptoms. DVTs may indicate a procoagulant state (see p. 342), either genetic or acquired. The incidence of recurrent DVTs/PEs is 10% per annum (i.e. 20% after 2 years, 50% after 5 years, etc.). A case for long-term anticoagulation can therefore be made.
- **Cellulitis** (see p. 422)
- **Arterial disease**: chronic arterial insufficiency presents with **intermittent claudication**—pains felt in the calves and/or the buttocks, brought on by exercise and rapidly (i.e. in less than 1 min) relieved by rest. Examination shows reduced or absent arterial pulses, findings confirmed by Doppler measurements. Patients with **critical ischaemia** have pain at rest. Hanging the leg over the edge of the bed relieves symptoms (gravity improves perfusing pressure). **Acute leg ischaemia** presents as a painful leg, and examination shows absent pulses and a bluish discoloration. Causes include *in situ* thrombosis (usually in long-standing claudication), or **arterial embolus**, from the heart (consider recent MI, atrial fibrillation or mitral stenosis) or a diseased aorta (e.g. abdominal aortic aneurysm; much more rarely from aortic dissection). Doppler measurements and peripheral angiography are diagnostic. Treatment is immediate heparin, removal of any embolic clot (which should be sent for histology, because a few are embolized atrial myxomas or lung tumours) using a Fogarty catheter, arterial reconstructive surgery or amputation, along with diagnosis and treatment of any cardiac problem.
- **Leg ulcers** (see p. 128)
- **Arthritis**: symptoms have often been present for months or years. Pain is usually (not always) localized to the affected joint and worse on joint movement or weight bearing, although hip osteoarthritis may cause sufficient nocturnal pain to wake the patient. **Septic arthritis** presents acutely with systemic symptoms (fever, malaise, shivers) and a hot, red, swollen joint with painful, globally restricted movements. Joint aspiration is diagnostic (see p. 392).
- **Nerve root compression**, especially sciatic nerve compression from a prolapsed intervertebral disc ('sciatica'), is common—pain characteristically radiates all the way down the back of the leg (see p. 381).

Clinical Presentations at a Glance

8 Heart murmurs

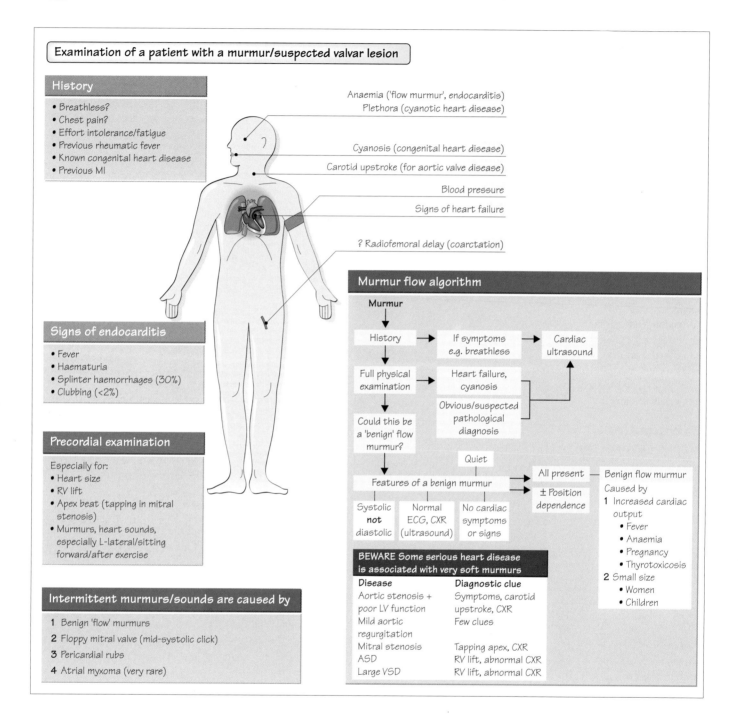

Examination of a patient with a murmur/suspected valvar lesion

History

- Breathless?
- Chest pain?
- Effort intolerance/fatigue
- Previous rheumatic fever
- Known congenital heart disease
- Previous MI

Anaemia ('flow murmur', endocarditis)
Plethora (cyanotic heart disease)

Cyanosis (congenital heart disease)
Carotid upstroke (for aortic valve disease)

Blood pressure
Signs of heart failure

? Radiofemoral delay (coarctation)

Signs of endocarditis

- Fever
- Haematuria
- Splinter haemorrhages (30%)
- Clubbing (<2%)

Precordial examination

Especially for:
- Heart size
- RV lift
- Apex beat (tapping in mitral stenosis)
- Murmurs, heart sounds, especially L-lateral/sitting forward/after exercise

Intermittent murmurs/sounds are caused by

1 Benign 'flow' murmurs
2 Floppy mitral valve (mid-systolic click)
3 Pericardial rubs
4 Atrial myxoma (very rare)

Murmur flow algorithm

Murmur

History → If symptoms e.g. breathless → Cardiac ultrasound

Full physical examination → Heart failure, cyanosis

Obvious/suspected pathological diagnosis

Could this be a 'benign' flow murmur?

Quiet

Features of a benign murmur → All present / ± Position dependence

Systolic **not** diastolic | Normal ECG, CXR (ultrasound) | No cardiac symptoms or signs

Benign flow murmur
Caused by
1 Increased cardiac output
- Fever
- Anaemia
- Pregnancy
- Thyrotoxicosis
2 Small size
- Women
- Children

BEWARE Some serious heart disease is associated with very soft murmurs

Disease	Diagnostic clue
Aortic stenosis + poor LV function	Symptoms, carotid upstroke, CXR
Mild aortic regurgitation	Few clues
Mitral stenosis	Tapping apex, CXR
ASD	RV lift, abnormal CXR
Large VSD	RV lift, abnormal CXR

Murmurs are commonly found on routine physical examination. Although most are benign, not resulting from cardiovascular disease ('flow murmur'—see figure), occasionally they are important clues to the presence of heart disease, such as: valvar disease, left ventricular dysfunction (functional mitral regurgitation [MR]), intracardiac shunts (atrial septal defect [ASD] and ventricular septal defect [VSD]). Very occasionally, other malformations, such as an arteriovenous malformations (AVM) or coarctation of the aorta are responsible for murmurs.

Valvar heart disease is common, important and in most cases asso-

ciated with murmurs. The characteristics of a murmur depend on: the flow velocity, the nature and size of the orifice and the direction of the flow.

As a rule, narrow atrioventricular (AV) valves cause diastolic murmurs, and leaking AV valves cause systolic murmurs; the reverse is true for the pulmonary and aortic valves. Murmurs radiate in the direction of the blood flow across the diseased valve (e.g. aortic stenosis murmurs radiate to the neck, and mitral regurgitation caused by anterior mitral leaflet prolapse radiates to the back). The intensity of a murmur is directly proportional to the pressure gradient and the size of the orifice, unless cardiac function is compromised.

Chronic scarring and calcification make a valve orifice smaller (stenosis) whereas destructive disease processes (e.g. endocarditis, vasculitis) make a valve incompetent (regurgitation). Stenosis of a valve causes pressure overload on the cardiac chamber pumping blood through the valve; regurgitation results in volume overload to compensate for the leak.

Aetiology of valvar lesions

- **Congenital**: increasingly common as those with congenital heart disease survive longer, as a result of better childhood surgery and medicines. The most common adult presentation of a congenital lesion is that of a bicuspid aortic valve, which is asymptomatic for many years, but predisposes to early (from 40 years onwards) calcific aortic stenosis.
- **Rheumatic fever** causes scarring, thickening and calcification of valves over subsequent decades. Affects mitral more than aortic valves. Common in elderly people and in developing countries, but rare in developed countries.
- **Degenerative valve disease**: acquired calcific aortic stenosis in elderly people is the best example of a degenerative lesion. Myxomatous degeneration of mitral valve leads to destruction of leaflets and chordal rupture.
- **Infection**: endocarditis causes destruction of the valve structure and valvar regurgitation, never stenosis.
- **Prosthetic**: artificial valves may degenerate (biological prostheses calcify) or leak as a result of valve dysfunction or dehiscence of the surgical sutures (paraprosthetic leak). Endocarditis is especially high risk with prosthetic valves.

Investigations

- **Chest X-ray**: shows shape of heart, identifies chamber enlargement.
- **ECG**: may reveal atrial fibrillation, left atrial enlargement (mitral valve disease) or left ventricular hypertrophy (aortic valve disease).
- **Echocardiography**: this is the most important investigation in (suspected) valvular heart disease, and is used to assess cardiac chamber size and function, valve morphology and opening. Doppler echocardiography measures blood flow velocity, which is then used to calculate pressure gradients across narrow valves and the severity of regurgitation from leaky valves. Colour Doppler turns echo signals from turbulent blood flow into a two-dimensional colour picture, and is particularly useful for assessing valvar leaks. Standard cardiac transthoracic echocardiography (TTE) with modern equipment produces high-quality images and (usually) sufficient information. Transoesophageal echocardiography (an ultrasound probe is placed in the oesophagus) produces very-high-resolution images of the heart, because there are no intervening structures (unlike the ribs and lungs for transthoracic echocardiography) and is particularly useful when transthoracic images are inadequate, for left atrial or mitral valve pathology, or for prosthetic valves.
- **Cardiac catheterization**: enables accurate direct measurement of pressure in cardiac chambers. High-quality echocardiography has largely replaced cardiac catheterization as a routine investigation. However, coronary angiography is still used to diagnose concomitant coronary artery disease when surgery is being considered.

Treatment

The general principles underlying the treatment of all patients with valvar disease are to do the following:

Table 8.1 Cardiac conditions in which antimicrobial prophylaxis is indicated.

Prosthetic heart valve
Complex cyanotic congenital heart diseases
Surgically constructed systemic or pulmonary conduits
Acquired valvular heart disease
Mitral valve prolapse with valvular regurgitation or severe valve thickening
Non-cyanotic congenital heart disease (except for secundum type ASD)
Hypertrophic cardiomyopathy
Endocarditis prophylaxis is needed for:
- procedures that cause oral bleeding
- procedures that breach or potentially breach respiratory or gastrointestinal mucosa
- procedures that potentially traumatize the urinary tract epithelium
- prolonged vaginal delivery

Reproduced with permission from the European Society of Cardiology from their journal, *European Heart Journal*.

- **Monitor for those symptoms** that indicate a need for surgery. It is important to realize that a valve lesion alone is not an indication for valve replacement because many patients live for decades with medically treated valvular disease.
- **Document left ventricular function**, which if it deteriorates may, even in the absence of symptoms, indicate a need for surgery.
- **Maintain left ventricular function**, e.g. using angiotensin-converting enzyme (ACE) inhibitor therapy in regurgitant lesions.
- **Slow progression** of the stenosis/regurgitant leak, e.g. using antihypertensive therapy in the aortic regurgitation associated with hypertension.
- **Treat any complicating rhythm disturbances**, e.g. atrial fibrillation is a very common rhythm disturbance in all forms of valvar heart disease, and can be treated using digoxin and β-blockers to control the ventricular response.
- **Prevent complications** such as endocarditis, e.g. using prophylactic antibiotics when 'dirty' procedures, such as dental work, are carried out (see Table 8.1).
- **Prevent systemic thromboembolism**, e.g. using warfarin in atrial fibrillation.

Surgical treatment

The indications for surgical therapy are intrusive symptoms (breathlessness, exercise limitation), despite medical therapy, or progressive deterioration in left ventricular function occurring in the absence of symptoms (e.g. as in mitral regurgitation). The different forms of surgery are:

- **Commissurotomy** is used for congenital aortic or pulmonary stenosis, and some cases of rheumatic mitral stenosis.
- **Valve repair** is possible in some cases of mitral valve regurgitation.
- **Valve replacement** with a prosthetic valve. There are two sorts of prosthetic valve: first, synthetic **mechanical** valves (usually a composite of metal and other synthetic material), which require lifelong anticoagulation to prevent thromboembolism. They are very durable and last for more than 20 years. The second form of prosthesis is a valve from an animal (**xenograft**) or human (**homograft**). No long-term anticoagulation is needed because the thromboembolic risk is lower, they have better haemodynamic function, although they are less durable, and they may last only 10 years or less.

9 Shock

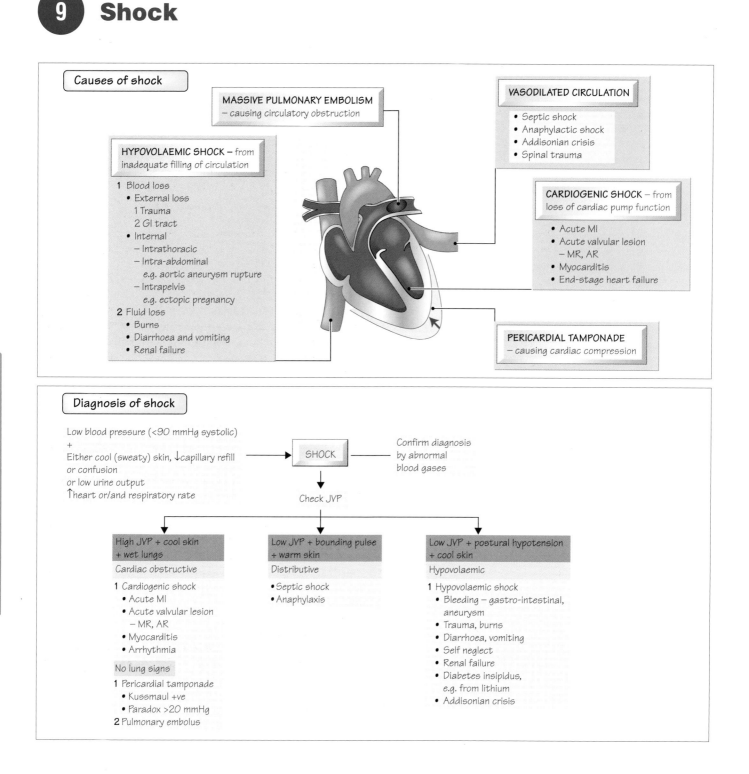

Causes of shock

MASSIVE PULMONARY EMBOLISM
– causing circulatory obstruction

VASODILATED CIRCULATION
- Septic shock
- Anaphylactic shock
- Addisonian crisis
- Spinal trauma

HYPOVOLAEMIC SHOCK – from inadequate filling of circulation

1 Blood loss
  - External loss
    1 Trauma
    2 GI tract
  - Internal
    – Intrathoracic
    – Intra-abdominal
      e.g. aortic aneurysm rupture
    – Intrapelvis
      e.g. ectopic pregnancy
2 Fluid loss
  - Burns
  - Diarrhoea and vomiting
  - Renal failure

CARDIOGENIC SHOCK – from loss of cardiac pump function
- Acute MI
- Acute valvular lesion
  – MR, AR
- Myocarditis
- End-stage heart failure

PERICARDIAL TAMPONADE
– causing cardiac compression

Diagnosis of shock

Low blood pressure (<90 mmHg systolic)
+
Either cool (sweaty) skin, ↓capillary refill
or confusion
or low urine output
↑heart or/and respiratory rate

→ SHOCK → Confirm diagnosis by abnormal blood gases

Check JVP

High JVP + cool skin + wet lungs	Low JVP + bounding pulse + warm skin	Low JVP + postural hypotension + cool skin
Cardiac obstructive	Distributive	Hypovolaemic

High JVP + cool skin + wet lungs

Cardiac obstructive

1 Cardiogenic shock
  - Acute MI
  - Acute valvular lesion
    – MR, AR
  - Myocarditis
  - Arrhythmia

No lung signs

1 Pericardial tamponade
  - Kussmaul +ve
  - Paradox >20 mmHg
2 Pulmonary embolus

Low JVP + bounding pulse + warm skin

Distributive

- Septic shock
- Anaphylaxis

Low JVP + postural hypotension + cool skin

Hypovolaemic

1 Hypovolaemic shock
  - Bleeding – gastro-intestinal, aneurysm
  - Trauma, burns
  - Diarrhoea, vomiting
  - Self neglect
  - Renal failure
  - Diabetes insipidus, e.g. from lithium
  - Addisonian crisis

Shock is characterized by hypoperfusion and subsequent tissue dysoxia leading to a switch from aerobic to anaerobic metabolism and lactic acidosis. All forms of shock have a high mortality and it is therefore important to make an early diagnosis and institute aggressive treatment. The following types of shock have been characterized:
- **Cardiogenic**: ventricular (usually left) pump failure (MI, acute valve dysfunction)

- **Hypovolaemic**: loss of circulating volume with normal cardiac function (trauma, GI bleed, pancreatitis, severe diarrhoea, burns)
- **Distributive**: reduced systemic vascular resistance with normal cardiac function (sepsis, anaphylaxis, Addisonian crisis, spinal trauma)
- **Obstructive shock**: impaired ventricular filling or obstruction of outflow tract (PE, tension pneumothorax, cardiac tamponade)

Clearly more than one form of shock may be present in the same patient. Frequently myocardial depression occurs in the latter stages of other shock states such as sepsis or hypovolaemia, especially if severe acidosis is present.

Successful outcome depends on early diagnosis and treatment. In some patients the cause may be obvious; for example in a patient with acute myocardial infarction or tension pneumothorax; however, in other cases it may be more subtle, as in massive pulmonary embolism or acute mitral regurgitation. **Tissue hypoperfusion is the hallmark of shock but no single sign or investigation is diagnostic on its own.** Clinical signs of shock such as hypotension, reduced central venous pressure, oliguria and confusion tend to be late features when homeostatic mechanisms can no longer compensate. Tachypnoea, tachycardia, reduced capillary refill and lactic acidosis often occur at a much earlier stage, but are very non-specific. There is an extremely poor correlation between direct measurement of cardiac output and clinicians' ability to estimate whether it is low, normal or high. It is therefore crucial to be able to recognize the acute severely ill patient, consider a diagnosis of shock and institute appropriate investigations early.

Useful investigations in diagnosis and management

- **ECG**: myocardial infarction (ST elevation), pericardial tamponade (low voltage), PE ($S_1Q_3T_3$, right axis, RBBB).
- **Chest X-ray**: pulmonary oedema in cardiogenic shock, enlarged cardiac silhouette (massive PE, cardiac tamponade), tension pneumothorax.
- **Echocardiogram**: cardiogenic shock due to pump dysfunction (MI, myocarditis), acute valve lesions (colour flow Doppler), PE (pulmonary hypertension, right ventricular dysfunction, clot in transit), pericardial tamponade (effusion and right ventricular collapse in systole), hypovolaemia (LV chamber size).
- **Arterial blood gases**: raised lactate and base deficit, as a consequence of tissue hypoperfusion and anaerobic metabolism, correlate with both severity of shock and mortality. These may be abnormal before hypotension, oliguria or confusion are present. Serial measurements are useful in assessing adequacy of treatment.
- **Central ($ScvO_2$) or mixed venous ($SmvO_2$) oxygen saturations**: true mixed venous saturations (from a PA catheter) are 10–15% lower than central mixed venous saturations because of the addition of highly deoxygenated blood from the cardiac veins at the level of the right atrium. When oxygen extraction exceeds delivery, such as in cardiogenic shock, venous saturations are low ($ScvO_2 < 70\%$). However, in septic shock saturations may be normal or elevated because cells are unable to extract the delivered oxygen, or low if there is myocardial depression.
- **Blood tests**:
  Haematology: full blood count (haemorrhage, sepsis/DIC), coagulation (haemorrhage and sepsis/DIC), cross-match (haemorrhage), amylase (pancreatitis).
  Electrolytes: low sodium and raised potassium (Addison's), raised urea (GI haemorrhage, severe diarrhoea).
- **Blood cultures**: to isolate organism in septic shock and tailor subsequent antibiotic choice.

General principles of management

Resuscitation should be prompt, as should measures specific to the underlying diagnosis such as the insertion of a chest drain in tension pneumothorax. However, general principles of resuscitation should not be forgotten. There must be adequate vascular access, the airway should be patent, oxygen applied and adequate ventilation ensured.

Monitoring: whether or not mechanical ventilation is required, the patient should be managed in a critical care area with appropriate monitoring and nursing. A minimum requirement is for ECG, pulse oximetry, respiratory rate, central venous pressure, Glasgow Coma Score, urine output and blood pressure to be monitored. The latter should be continuous through an arterial catheter as both fluid and vasoactive drugs may be required. Furthermore an arterial line will enable serial measurements of pH, lactate and base deficit to be performed, which help guide treatment. Additional haemodynamic monitoring is desirable either in the form of a PA catheter, oesophageal Doppler or pulse contour analysis and provides information on cardiac output and vascular resistance.

Supportive treatment: fluid is, with the exception of cardiogenic shock, requisite in most forms of shock. This may be in the form of crystalloid or colloid (blood products in trauma or haemorrhage); however many UK physicians favour colloid. Fluid should be given rapidly after assessment of intravascular status and the response to a challenge assessed (see Chapter 217). Large volume resuscitation with NaCl-rich fluid may itself cause a metabolic (hyperchloraemic) acidosis. Mechanical ventilation may be required either because of a primary respiratory problem or the inability to protect the airway (GCS < 8). The metabolic demand of breathing increases ten-fold in shock and uses one-fifth of cardiac output. Mechanical ventilation therefore reduces metabolic demand, but positive thoracic pressures can have adverse haemodynamic effects.

Renal replacement therapy in the form of haemofiltration may be required if there is anuria, hyperkalaemia, unresolving acidosis or resistant fluid overload (cardiogenic shock).

Following optimization of intravascular volume, vasoactive drugs may be required to ensure an adequate cardiac output and blood pressure. Inotropes such as adrenaline, dobutamine, dopamine or milrinone may be used in low cardiac output states, while vasoconstrictors such as noradrenaline are required in forms of distributive shock with low systemic vascular resistance.

Specific treatments

- **Cardiogenic**: inotropes, thrombolytics and/or angioplasty, Intra-aortic balloon pump, haemofiltration (fluid removal), surgery (MI, acute valve lesion)
- **Hypovolaemic**: fluids, blood products
- **Distributive**:
  Sepsis—fluid, vasoconstrictors (noradrenaline +/− vasopressin), activated protein C, steroids, antibiotics, inotropes if reduced cardiac output ($ScvO_2 < 70\%$)
  Anaphylaxis/Addison's—steroids
- **Obstructive**: cardiac tamponade (pericardial drain), tension pneumothorax (chest drain), PE (thrombolysis, embolectomy).

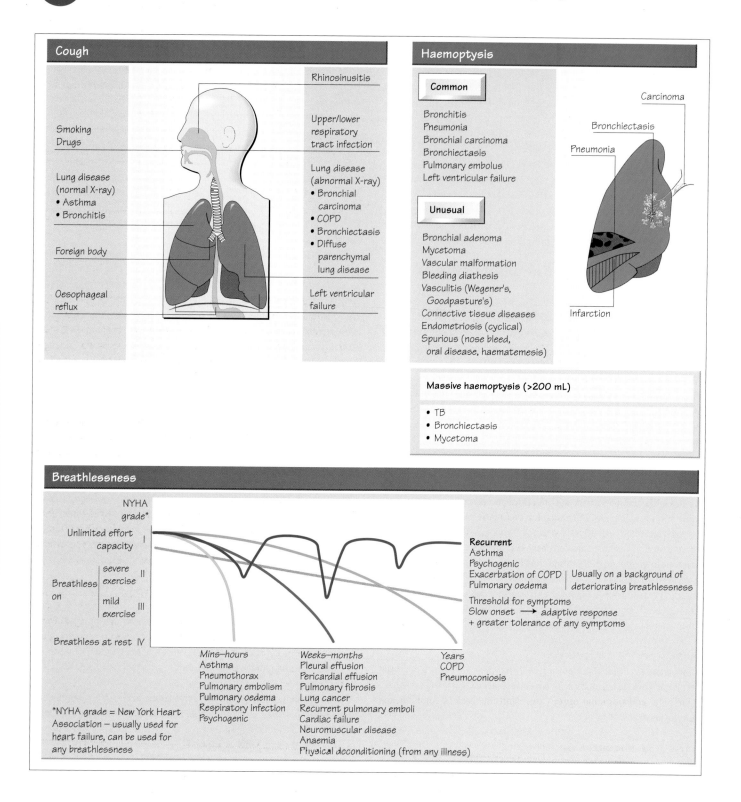

Cough

- Rhinosinusitis
- Smoking / Drugs
- Upper/lower respiratory tract infection
- Lung disease (normal X-ray)
  • Asthma
  • Bronchitis
- Lung disease (abnormal X-ray)
  • Bronchial carcinoma
  • COPD
  • Bronchiectasis
  • Diffuse parenchymal lung disease
- Foreign body
- Oesophageal reflux
- Left ventricular failure

Haemoptysis

Common
- Bronchitis
- Pneumonia
- Bronchial carcinoma
- Bronchiectasis
- Pulmonary embolus
- Left ventricular failure

Unusual
- Bronchial adenoma
- Mycetoma
- Vascular malformation
- Bleeding diathesis
- Vasculitis (Wegener's, Goodpasture's)
- Connective tissue diseases
- Endometriosis (cyclical)
- Spurious (nose bleed, oral disease, haematemesis)

Carcinoma
Bronchiectasis
Pneumonia
Infarction

Massive haemoptysis (>200 mL)
- TB
- Bronchiectasis
- Mycetoma

Breathlessness

NYHA grade*

Unlimited effort capacity — I

Breathless on:
severe exercise — II
mild exercise — III

Breathless at rest — IV

Recurrent
Asthma
Psychogenic
Exacerbation of COPD | Usually on a background of
Pulmonary oedema | deteriorating breathlessness

Threshold for symptoms
Slow onset ⟶ adaptive response
+ greater tolerance of any symptoms

*NYHA grade = New York Heart Association – usually used for heart failure, can be used for any breathlessness

Mins–hours	Weeks–months	Years
Asthma	Pleural effusion	COPD
Pneumothorax	Pericardial effusion	Pneumoconiosis
Pulmonary embolism	Pulmonary fibrosis	
Pulmonary oedema	Lung cancer	
Respiratory infection	Recurrent pulmonary emboli	
Psychogenic	Cardiac failure	
	Neuromuscular disease	
	Anaemia	
	Physical deconditioning (from any illness)	

Breathlessness

Breathlessness is 'an awareness of the act of breathing' and is a common and frightening symptom. The common causes of breathlessness are listed in Table 10.1.

The rate of onset and the pattern of breathlessness (dyspnoea) may be helpful diagnostically (see figure). The characteristic history in some of the different diseases causing breathlessness is outlined below.

Table 10.1 Common causes of breathlessness. Based on Table 4.5 in *Davidson's Principles and Practice of Medicine*, 18th edn, Churchill Livingstone, Edinburgh, 1999.

	Acute breathlessness at rest	Chronic breathlessness on effort
Cardiovascular	Left ventricular failure Acute pulmonary emboli *Mitral stenosis*	Chronic heart failure. 'Angina-equivalent' breathlessness Chronic pulmonary emboli
Respiratory	Acute severe asthma Acute exacerbation of COPD Pneumonia Pneumothorax Adult respiratory distress syndrome Acute anaphylaxis *Inhaled foreign body*	COPD Pleural effusion *Interstitial lung disease* Bronchial cancer *Lymphangitis carcinomatosis*
Other	Psychogenic hyperventilation Fever *Metabolic acidosis* *Neurological disease*	Physical deconditioning Obesity Anaemia *Neurological disease*

Rarer causes are in *italics*.
COPD, chronic obstructive pulmonary disease.

Heart failure

• Dyspnoea is not associated with a wheeze, a characteristic differentiating it from chronic obstructive pulmonary disease (COPD) (unless 'cardiac asthma' is present—bronchospasm provoked by pulmonary oedema). Symptoms from the underlying heart disease also occur.
• In **mild heart failure** breathlessness occurs only on effort.
• In **more advanced heart failure** breathlessness also occurs on lying flat (**orthopnoea**), promptly (< 5–10 min) improved by sitting or standing. When severe, this is called **paroxysmal nocturnal dyspnoea**. There is often ankle oedema—better in the morning, worse at night.

Airway disease

This results in a wheeze when breathless:
• In **COPD**, breathlessness on effort develops progressively over years, often > 5. Patients often also have **chronic bronchitis** (productive morning cough > 3 months/year for 2 years in succession).
• In **asthma**, patients are normal between attacks. Wheezing may be provoked by exercise, pollen (and thus be seasonal), drugs (especially aspirin or β-blockers) or emotion. Symptoms may be worse at night, when a dry cough may occur. Nocturnal symptoms in asthma, unlike those in heart failure, improve slowly (> 30 min) or not at all on sitting/standing.

Respiratory tract infections

Fever and a productive cough are char-acteristic of respiratory tract infections; sore throat occurs in upper respiratory tract infections. In pneumonia, constitutional upset (fever and malaise) is common and pleuritic chest pain may occur.

Pulmonary embolus

Pulmonary embolus presents with sudden onset, i.e. instantaneous breathlessness, in those predisposed (immobile, obese, oral contraceptive pill, postoperative, cancer). Pleuritic chest pain may occur.

Pneumothorax

Pneumothorax presents as a sudden-onset chest pain, often pleuritic in nature, with breathlessness. The diagnosis is made from the physical examination and the chest X-ray.

Lung parenchymal disease

Lung parenchymal disease (interstitial pneumonitis/fibrosis) presents with breathlessness on effort and, when severe, at rest without associated wheeze. Breathlessness, unlike in heart failure, is not strongly dependent on posture. The examination and the chest X-ray are often diagnostic.

Obesity

If severe, obesity can cause breathlessness, both on effort and on lying (orthopnoea, caused by diaphragmatic splinting). Pulmonary embolism, heart failure and obstructive sleep apnoea are all more common in obese individuals.

Physical deconditioning

Physical deconditioning is a potent cause of breathlessness, and often exacerbates breathlessness resulting from other causes. Importantly, most pathological dyspnoea is improved to some extent by physical conditioning. This is helpful therapeutically (rehabilitation).

There are two much rarer causes of breathlessness:
• '**Angina-equivalent' breathlessness**: angina (especially in people with diabetes) is sometimes experienced as breathlessness rather than as chest pain. This is usually caused by severe coronary artery disease.
• **Respiratory failure**: can result from a neuromuscular disease, such as motor neuron disease, or related to obesity (Pickwickian syndrome). Physical examination usually reveals the cause and blood gases show type II respiratory failure (see p. 178).

Breathlessness for 'psychogenic' reasons also occurs (**hyperventilation**). The patient complains that they are 'unable to fill the chest' Associated perioral tingling is a specific symptom. Hyperventilation responds to breathing into a paper bag. **Beware**: many patients breathless from organic disease are frightened and appear anxious. Assume that breathlessness within a hospital is the result of organic disease unless there is incontrovertible evidence to the contrary.

Classification of severity of breathlessness

Although there are many ways of **classifying the severity** of chronic breathlessness (e.g. blood gases, lung volumes, peak oxygen uptake, etc.), the most useful is the **exercise capacity** of the patient at his or her usual pace, e.g. is he or she able to walk 50 m, quarter of a mile or several miles? This is the **key parameter** in understanding the impact of the disease and the severity/extent of the underlying pathology.

Physical examination

The following are diagnostically helpful clues in severe breathlessness. In patients with effort breathlessness alone the signs may be subtle and diagnosis rests on the history and investigations.

- **Skin warmth**. In cardiac dyspnoea (left ventricular [LV] failure, large pulmonary embolus, pericardial effusion) the skin is cool and may be sweaty, whereas in COPD most patients have warm skin with a 'bounding' pulse. A fever may indicate a respiratory tract infection.
- **Heart rate**: severe breathlessness from any cause increases the heart rate. In both left ventricular failure and asthma it can be used as a 'minute-to-minute' guide to the severity of the condition and the effect of treatment.
- **Heart rhythm**.
- **Blood pressure** (BP) itself is rarely diagnostically helpful, but paradox (the difference between inspiratory and expiratory systolic BP: normally < 5 mmHg) is. It is increased in asthma, in severe cases to 15–20 mmHg, and in pericardial effusion (> 20 mmHg).
- **Mucous membranes** for pallor (**anaemia**) and for blueness (**cyanosis**). Patients severely breathless as a result of organic disease are usually centrally cyanosed when breathing air. If not, consider pericardial effusion, anxiety or metabolic acidosis.
- **Jugular venous pressure** (JVP) is a key sign. It is raised in:
  - Heart failure—the most common cause.
  - End-stage COPD (cor pulmonale), when the right heart has failed.
  - Large pulmonary emboli.

  If the JVP is not raised, the breathlessness is less likely to be caused by heart failure, although a normal JVP does not rule out **pure** LV failure.
- **Precordial cardiac examination** may demonstrate a large heart or abnormal LV impulse in most cases of heart failure or a left parasternal lift from right ventricular (RV) hypertrophy (in advanced cardiac failure, cor pulmonale and pulmonary embolus). A third heart sound is universal in LV failure, and its absence when breathless suggests that heart failure is not present. Diagnostic murmurs may be heard.
- **Chest examination**:
  - **Respiratory rate** is increased in most patients who are breathless at rest, although not in respiratory failure resulting from neuromuscular disease (which is very rare). A rise in respiratory rate is often the first sign of any acute illness.
  - **'Hyperinflation'**: a decreased sternal notch-to-trachea distance ('barrel chest') indicates air trapping in the lungs, usually resulting from airway disease (COPD or acute asthma).
  - 'Stony dull' resonance to percussion occurs in pleural effusions.
  - **Wheeze** (see p. 26).
  - **Crepitations**, if 'wet', are often caused by infection (e.g. pneumonia) or fluid (e.g. heart failure), and if 'dry' often indicate pulmonary fibrosis.
  - **Bronchial breathing** indicates consolidation (usually pneumonia).

Investigations

Investigations are directed towards the most likely cause but always include:
- **Chest X-ray**
- **ECG**
- **Spirometry**

- **Haemoglobin**
  The following tests help in specific situations:
- **Blood gases**: usually at rest, sometimes on exercise.
- More detailed lung function tests, including measures of gas exchange (e.g. carbon monoxide transfer factor).
- **Computed tomography** (CT): spiral CT is helpful for diagnosis of pulmonary emboli, and high-resolution thin-cut CT for many interstitial lung diseases.
- **Ventilation/perfusion** ($\dot{V}/\dot{Q}$) scan.
- **Cardiac ultrasonography**.
  These tests are occasionally helpful:
- **Exercise ECG** to determine whether myocardial ischaemia is present, and to document exercise capacity objectively.
- **Cardiac catheterization**: to measure intracardiac pressures and perform coronary angiography.

Treatment

Treatment is for the underlying condition (see relevant chapter). Hyperventilation is treated by reassurance and encouragement of physical fitness.

Cough

'A reflex forced expiration against an initially closed glottis.' The explosive expiration is a protective mechanism for the lung, clearing the lung of harmful substances.

Key points

- Upper respiratory tract infection is by far the most common cause.
- If the chest X-ray is normal, 90% of patients with chronic cough have asthma, gastro-oesophageal reflux disease (GORD) or rhinosinusitis. Empirical treatment for asthma and/or GORD is often helpful because cough may be the only symptom and the two may coexist.
- Persistent cough in a smoker raises the possibility of bronchial carcinoma.

Epidemiology

- Extremely common.
- Prevalence is between 5% and 40%.
- May indicate serious underlying pathology but commonly of little significance, not warranting investigation.

Differential diagnosis

Acute cough (< 3 weeks)

- Viral upper respiratory infection: most common cause is associated sore throat/rhinitis.
- Other acute infections: pneumonia and infective exacerbations of COPD.
- Foreign body: history of choking and sudden onset.

Chronic cough (> 3 weeks)

- Bronchial carcinoma: smoker, weight loss, haemoptysis.
- Asthma: atopy, wheeze, shortness of breath (SOB), nocturnal symptoms, variable peak flow.
- Gastro-oesophageal reflux: heartburn, symptoms on lying flat.
- Rhinosinusitis: headache, nasal blockage, postnasal drip.
- Bronchiectasis: clubbing, copious mucus production, wheeze.
- Diffuse parenchymal lung disease: clubbing, breathlessness.
- Drugs: β-blockers, angiotensin-converting enzyme (ACE) inhibitors.
- Smoking: 50% of those who smoke > 20/day have persistent cough.

Investigations

A new cough lasting > 3 weeks is more likely to be caused by serious disease requiring investigation and treatment. The clinical features often suggest the diagnosis, such as interstitial lung disease, COPD or bronchiectasis.

• **Chest X-ray**: if the cough is chronic or the patient a smoker, this may reveal infection, neoplasm or diffuse lung disease.

• **Spirometry** to diagnose airflow obstruction (peak flow monitoring may be useful in assessing asthma).

• **CT** is used to stage tumours or to diagnose diffuse lung disease.

• **Bronchoscopy** is used to remove a foreign body or for tissue diagnosis of tumours.

• **Oesophageal pH monitoring** is occasionally used to diagnose reflux disease.

In patients with a chronic cough and normal X-ray, sequential empirical treatment with inhaled steroids, antireflux treatment and treatment for rhinosinusitis will provide a 'cure' in a significant percentage of patients.

Haemoptysis

Definition

The coughing of blood from the lungs.

Causes

Minor haemoptysis is common, often related to respiratory tract infection. This resolves quickly and requires no further investigation. Haemoptysis that persists is more likely to indicate underlying serious pathology. Patients should have a chest X-ray; and many will need CT, bronchoscopy and a specialist respiratory opinion.

Clinical approach

Haemoptysis persisting for more than 2 weeks should be investigated (see Table 10.2). A history of smoking (past or present) raises the possibility of lung carcinoma and all patients aged over 40 who smoke should be assumed to have lung cancer until investigation proves otherwise. Serious pathology is more common with increasing age. Associated symptoms or clinical signs may point towards a specific diagnosis.

Table 10.2 Causes of haemoptysis.

Very common	Uncommon
Bronchitis	Bronchial adenoma
Pneumonia	Mycetoma
Common	Rare
Bronchial carcinoma	Vascular malformation
Bronchiectasis	Bleeding diathesis
Pulmonary embolus	Vasculitis (Wegener's granulomatosis,
Spurious (nose bleed, oral	Goodpasture's disease)
disease, haematemesis)	Connective tissue diseases
	Endometriosis (cyclical)

Routine investigation

• **Plain chest X-ray**, blood count (for anaemia from bleeding or chronic disease), clotting profile.

• **Renal biochemistry** because some diseases produce pulmonary haemorrhage and renal failure—so-called 'pulmonary-renal syndromes', e.g. Goodpasture's disease, Wegener's granulomatosis.

• **Liver biochemistry** for evidence of metastatic disease.

• **Special investigations** include high-resolution CT (HRCT) of the chest and bronchoscopy. These together achieve a diagnosis in > 90% of patients.

Management

The key is to find the underlying diagnosis and treat appropriately, or to exclude serious disease. Most haemoptysis is minor or self-limiting, although on occasions bleeding can be severe and uncontrolled.

• Any **coagulopathy** should be corrected. Antifibrinolytic drugs may help.

• In massive haemoptysis, **bronchoscopy** allows identification and local treatment of the bleeding point.

• **Radiological embolization** or **lung resection** may be necessary in life-threatening haemorrhage.

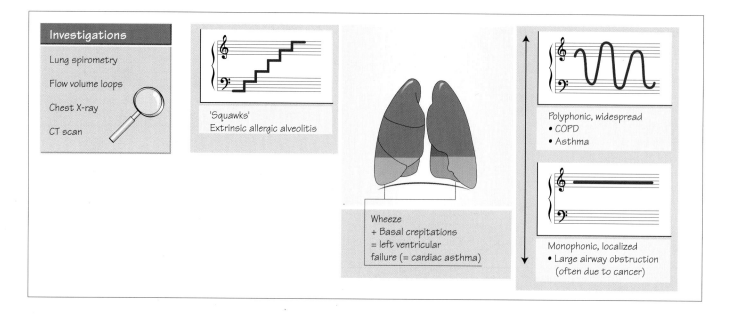

Wheeze is a prolonged sound caused by airway narrowing with apposition of the airway walls. The sound is produced by vibration of airway walls and adjacent tissues. As the airways are generally narrower on expiration, wheeze is more pronounced during the expiratory phase. There are a number of causes of wheeze (Table 11.1).

Wheeze can be divided according to the timing in the respiratory cycle and the actual sound produced (a single note or multiple notes of different pitches):

• **Polyphonic wheeze**: the most common type of wheeze typical of COPD and asthma. Multiple simultaneous different pitched sounds occur during expiration and imply diffuse airway disease.

Table 11.1 Causes of wheeze.

Asthma
COPD
Bronchiectasis
Large airway obstruction
Pulmonary oedema

• **Fixed monophonic wheeze**: a note of single pitch resulting from localized narrowing of a single airway. The sound does not change with coughing and particularly raises the possibility of bronchial carcinoma (see also stridor).

• **Sequential inspiratory wheeze**: otherwise known as 'squawks', caused by vibration after the opening of a previously collapsed airway; they are typical of extrinsic allergic alveolitis.

• **Stridor**: low-pitched monophonic wheeze heard on inspiration and implying local obstruction to the extrathoracic airways (which tend to collapse on inspiration). Often implies carcinoma or foreign body in the major airways.

Investigation

The cause of most wheezes is readily apparent on clinical grounds, and using straightforward tests such as chest X-ray and simple lung function tests. Occasionally diagnostic difficulty occurs—in these situations flow-volume loops may be helpful, as may CT and cardiac ultrasonography.

12 Pleural effusion

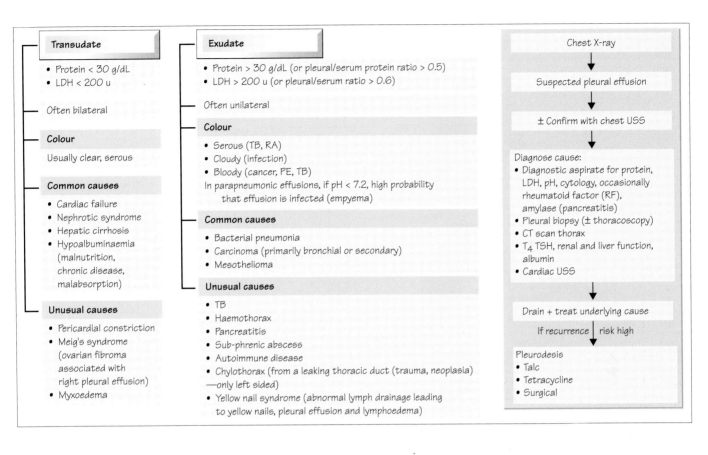

Transudate

- Protein < 30 g/dL
- LDH < 200 u

Often bilateral

Colour

Usually clear, serous

Common causes

- Cardiac failure
- Nephrotic syndrome
- Hepatic cirrhosis
- Hypoalbuminaemia (malnutrition, chronic disease, malabsorption)

Unusual causes

- Pericardial constriction
- Meig's syndrome (ovarian fibroma associated with right pleural effusion)
- Myxoedema

Exudate

- Protein > 30 g/dL (or pleural/serum protein ratio > 0.5)
- LDH > 200 u (or pleural/serum ratio > 0.6)

Often unilateral

Colour

- Serous (TB, RA)
- Cloudy (infection)
- Bloody (cancer, PE, TB)

In parapneumonic effusions, if pH < 7.2, high probability that effusion is infected (empyema)

Common causes

- Bacterial pneumonia
- Carcinoma (primarily bronchial or secondary)
- Mesothelioma

Unusual causes

- TB
- Haemothorax
- Pancreatitis
- Sub-phrenic abscess
- Autoimmune disease
- Chylothorax (from a leaking thoracic duct (trauma, neoplasia) —only left sided)
- Yellow nail syndrome (abnormal lymph drainage leading to yellow nails, pleural effusion and lymphoedema)

Chest X-ray
↓
Suspected pleural effusion
↓
± Confirm with chest USS
↓
Diagnose cause:
- Diagnostic aspirate for protein, LDH, pH, cytology, occasionally rheumatoid factor (RF), amylase (pancreatitis)
- Pleural biopsy (± thoracoscopy)
- CT scan thorax
- T_4 TSH, renal and liver function, albumin
- Cardiac USS
↓
Drain + treat underlying cause
If recurrence ↓ risk high
Pleurodesis
- Talc
- Tetracycline
- Surgical

Definition

A collection of fluid in the pleural space. If the effusion is infected it is called an 'empyema'. If it relates to pneumonia, it is called a 'para-pneumonic effusion'.

Introduction

Pleural effusion is a common problem. The normal parietal pleura produces fluid which is reabsorbed by the visceral pleura. Either excessive fluid production (e.g. as a result of inflammation) or impaired reabsorption leads to an accumulation of fluid. An effusion needs to be at least moderate in size before it produces symptoms of shortness of breath.

Clinical approach

The most common presentation is with breathlessness. Pleural inflammation may cause pain and large effusions may cause cough. The clinical signs are of reduced expansion, stony dullness and reduced breath sounds and vocal resonance. Effusions ≤ 500 mL are difficult to detect clinically. The chest X-ray will show blunting of the costophrenic angle in small collections and more extensive change in the presence of larger effusions. Large effusions are more commonly the result of malignancy.

Investigation

The main distinction to make in determining the cause of an effusion is between high and low protein content (see figure), i.e. exudates versus transudates.

If pleural infection is suspected, the pH of fluid should be measured (pH ≤ 7.2 suggests complicated parapneumonic effusion or empyema, which will only resolve with pleural drainage). Fluid should also be sent for biochemistry (lactate dehydrogenase [LDH]—high in rheumatoid effusions and exudates—and protein estimation), microbiology for culture and cytology.

Management

Treatment of the underlying condition, particularly for transudates:
- Therapeutic large volume aspiration will improve symptoms. Formal drainage with intercostal tubes is often necessary.
- In malignant and other recurrent effusions, agents (tetracycline, talc or bleomycin) can be introduced via an intercostal drain to cause the two layers of pleura to stick together and prevent reaccumulation (pleurodesis).
- Thoracoscopy (under local or general anaesthetic) may be useful in some patients to provide access to the pleura for guided biopsies and subsequent pleurodesis.

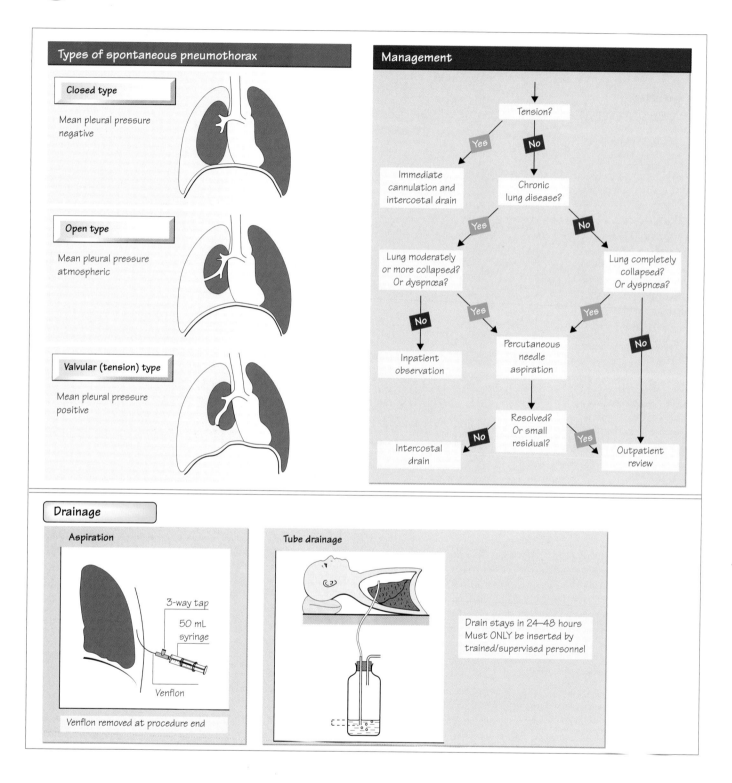

Types of spontaneous pneumothorax

Closed type

Mean pleural pressure negative

Open type

Mean pleural pressure atmospheric

Valvular (tension) type

Mean pleural pressure positive

Management

Tension?

Yes → Immediate cannulation and intercostal drain

No → Chronic lung disease?

Yes → Lung moderately or more collapsed? Or dyspnoea?

No → Lung completely collapsed? Or dyspnoea?

Lung moderately or more collapsed? Or dyspnoea?
No → Inpatient observation
Yes → Percutaneous needle aspiration

Lung completely collapsed? Or dyspnoea?
Yes → Percutaneous needle aspiration
No → Outpatient review

Percutaneous needle aspiration → Resolved? Or small residual?
No → Intercostal drain
Yes → Outpatient review

Drainage

Aspiration

3-way tap
50 mL syringe
Venflon

Venflon removed at procedure end

Tube drainage

Drain stays in 24–48 hours
Must ONLY be inserted by trained/supervised personnel

Definition
The presence of free gas in the pleural space.

Epidemiology
The incidence is 10/100 000 adults per year, males > females, sometimes runs in families. Taller individuals are more prone to primary spontaneous pneumothorax.

Aetiology
• **Primary spontaneous pneumothorax**: implies normal underlying lungs and is caused by rupture of a pleural 'bleb'.
• **Secondary spontaneous pneumothorax** occurs in association with lung disease (COPD, pneumonia, etc.). Rupture of the visceral pleura results in communication between the airway and pleural space.
• **Traumatic** such as stab wounds.

Pathophysiology
The effects of a pneumothorax depend on whether the pleural leak persists or not.
• **'Closed' pneumothorax**: the leak closes as the lung deflates so the amount of air escaping into the pleural space is limited, pleural pressure remains negative and slow resolution will occur even without treatment.
• **'Open' pneumothorax** occurs when persistent communication between the airway and pleural space develops (bronchopleural fistula), seen as a persistent bubbling of the chest drain. The lung cannot re-expand and there is a significant risk of infection developing by transmission of organisms via the airway into the pleural space.
• **A tension pneumothorax** occurs when the leak remains open but acts as a one-way valve between the airway and pleural space. Progressive increase in the volume of gas in the pleural space leads to increase in pressure above atmospheric and compression of the underlying and contralateral lung, the heart and mediastinal shift. Cardiac filling and output decrease and the patient can become extremely unwell and die unless treated urgently.

Clinical features
• **Small pneumothorax** may be asymptomatic.
• **Medium-large pneumothorax**: sudden onset of chest pain with shortness of breath is the most common presentation. There is hyper-inflation with reduced expansion and reduced breath sounds.
• **Subcutaneous emphysema** can occur from an air leak into the skin and subcutaneous tissues, felt as a crackling feeling in the skin. Dramatic facial swelling and airway compromise may occur.
• **Tension pneumothorax** results in pronounced dyspnoea, tracheal deviation, tachycardia and hypotension.

Investigations
• **Chest X-ray** is diagnostic. Mediastinal deviation suggests the presence of tension. The X-ray will also show the presence of any underlying lung diseases.
• **Oxygen saturation** should be measured—usually normal unless there is underlying lung disease.
• **Ultrasonography or CT** are both superior to the plain chest X-ray for detection of small pneumothoraces and are often used after percutaneous lung biopsy.

Management (see figure)
• **Drainage (aspiration or tube)** is not required for small (virtually) asymptomatic primary spontaneous pneumothoraces, but is in all symptomatic patients (initial trial of aspiration is often appropriate). Those with underlying lung disease are at greater risk of complications and should be treated as inpatients. Tension pneumothorax is a medical emergency and requires immediate treatment.
• **Surgical treatment**, with pleural abrasion or pleurectomy to obliterate the pleural space, is used for non-resolving pneumothoraces after tube drainage and for recurrent pneumothoraces.
• **Aeroplane travel**: patients with pneumothorax should not fly for 3 months because the pressure changes lead to expansion of the gas in the pleural space and so to a tension pneumothorax.

Prognosis
With adequate drainage, even in the presence of underlying lung disease, resolution can almost always be achieved. After primary spontaneous pneumothorax, 30% of patients have a further episode within 5 years. After a second episode, the recurrence rate rises above 50% and surgical pleurodesis is therefore usually recommended. Recurrence is extremely unusual following pleurodesis.

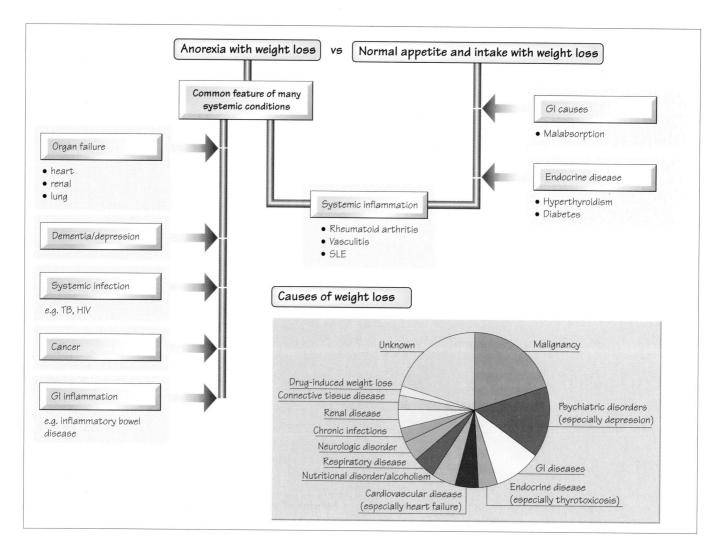

Anorexia with weight loss — vs — Normal appetite and intake with weight loss

Common feature of many systemic conditions

Organ failure
- heart
- renal
- lung

Dementia/depression

Systemic infection
e.g. TB, HIV

Cancer

GI inflammation
e.g. inflammatory bowel disease

Systemic inflammation
- Rheumatoid arthritis
- Vasculitis
- SLE

GI causes
- Malabsorption

Endocrine disease
- Hyperthyroidism
- Diabetes

Causes of weight loss

Pie chart segments: Unknown, Malignancy, Psychiatric disorders (especially depression), GI diseases, Endocrine disease (especially thyrotoxicosis), Cardiovascular disease (especially heart failure), Nutritional disorder/alcoholism, Respiratory disease, Neurologic disorder, Chronic infections, Renal disease, Connective tissue disease, Drug-induced weight loss

Overall approach

Weight loss is a non-specific symptom, which might relate to a gastrointestinal (GI) condition, to systemic pathology or very occasionally to psychiatric pathology.

Epidemiology

Unintentional weight loss is common, and affects 1.3–8% of elderly patients who seek health care. Severe and rapid weight loss ($\geq 7.5\%$ of usual body weight lost in ≤ 6 months) is relatively unusual; it affects 0.45% of the elderly.

Differential diagnosis

See figure and Table 14.1.

Consequences of weight loss

- Weight loss is associated with an increased mortality.
- Some of the increased mortality seen in those who unintentionally lose weight is due to the underlying disease process.
- General consequences: some mortality in those with weight loss is due directly to the consequences of malnutrition on vital structures.

Skeletal muscle mass declines, leading to loss of mobility and increased number of falls. Falls, along with skeletal changes, predispose to hip fractures.

Clinical features

- The overwhelmingly most important aspect is to establish the cause of the weight loss.
- The clinical features of any underlying disease process (see specific chapters) will be present.
- Poor diet is not infrequently the cause of weight loss; a full dietary assessment should be carried out; beware however, as poor diet by itself does not rule out organic disease. It is crucial to determine why the diet is poor: is it due to loss of appetite (which may relate to inflammatory disease including cancer, to depression, to dementia, etc.), or is it due to social factors (poverty, alcoholism, etc.)?
- Often a good question to ask patients with weight loss is whether their appetite is preserved; anorexia and subsequent weight loss often relates to inflammatory disease, whereas weight loss in the presence of a good appetite can relate to malabsorption, thyrotoxicosis, etc.

Table 14.1 Drugs causing weight loss.

Anorexia	Amantadine, amphetamines, antibiotics (e.g. atovaquone), anticonvulsants, benzodiazepines, decongestants, digoxin, gold, levodopa, metformin, neuroleptics, nicotine, opiates, SSRIs, theophylline
Dry mouth	Anticholinergics, antihistamines, clonidine, loop diuretics
Dysgeusia (loss of taste) or dysosmia (loss of smell) or both	Acetazolamide, alcohol, allopurinol, amphetamines, ACE inhibitors, antibiotics (e.g. ciprofloxacin, clarithromycin, doxycycline, ethambutol, griseofulvin, metronidazole, pentamidine, rifabutin, tetracycline), anticholinergics, antihistamines, calcium-channel blockers, carbamazepine, chemotherapy agents, chloral hydrate, cocaine, etidronate, gold, hydralazine, hydrochlorothiazide, iron, levodopa, lithium, methimazole, metformin, nasal vasoconstrictors, nitroglycerin, opiates, penicillamine, pergolide, phenytoin, propranolol, selegiline, sodium cromoglycate, spironolactone, statins, terbinafine, tobacco products, triazolam, tricyclics
Dysphagia	Alendronate, antibiotics (e.g. doxycycline), anticholinergics, bisphosphonates, chemotherapeutic agents, corticosteroids, gold, iron, levodopa, NSAIDs, potassium, quinidine, theophylline
Nausea or vomiting or both	Amantadine, antibiotics, bisphosphonates, digoxin, dopamine agonists, hormone replacement therapy, iron, levodopa, metformin, metronidazole, nitroglycerin, opiates, phenytoin, potassium, SSRIs, statins, theophylline, tricyclics

- Weight loss is a feature of the end-stage of disease processes such as dementia, heart failure and emphysema. Features of these should be sought.
- Drugs not infrequently cause or contribute to weight loss (see Table 14.1). Always take a full drug history.

History
Important questions to be answered concern the following:
- Try and quantify the weight loss; if weights have not been measured, ask about trouser fit/belt tightening. Quantify appetite change.
- Ask about any change in bowel habit (steatorrhoea/constipation).
- Blood from any orifice.
- New pain often provides a clue about the site of pathology.
- Fever, night sweats, headache (non-specific, intra-cranial tumour, temporal arteritis).
- Muscle weakness (non-specific or polymyalgia rheumatica).
- Mood and sleep symptoms of depression (diurnal mood variation, early wakening, anhedonia, etc.).
- Smoking increases the risk of most neoplasms (particularly lung and pancreas) as well as Crohn's disease. Family history of cancer.
- Alcohol abuse is associated with weight loss.
- Travel history and contact with tuberculosis (TB), etc.
- Sexual history and other risks for HIV (intravenous drug use).
- Endocrine symptoms, e.g. thyrotoxicosis.
- If anorexia nervosa is suspected, ask about perception of weight loss and body image.

Examination
Look specifically for:
- Fever.
- Signs of thyroid disease.
- Signs of malnutrition (leukonychia, cheilitis, glossitis, scurvy, pellagra) and objective evidence of weight loss (loose skin, fat and/or muscle loss).
- Lymphadenopathy—generalized as well as Virchow's node (enlarged left supraclavicular node indicating intra-abdominal malignancy).
- Breast examination.
- Abnormalities in respiratory or abdominal examination indicating infection or malignancy.

Investigations
These should be targeted to specific clinical suspicions raised by the history to determine both the cause and the consequence of weight loss:
- **Blood tests**: full blood count (FBC) and raised inflammatory markers (erythrocyte sedimentation rate [ESR]/C-reactive protein [CRP]) often provide non-specific evidence for a worrying cause for weight loss. Urea and electrolytes (U&Es), liver function tests (LFTs) and albumin, Ca^{2+}, vitamin B_{12}, folate, thyroid function, endomysial antibody for coeliac disease, HIV test after counselling.
- **Chest X-ray**: indicated in all patients regardless of respiratory symptoms (for TB, mediastinal lymphadenopathy, metastases, primary or secondary lung carcinoma).
- **Urine examination**: for haematuria (urothelial/renal tumour).
- **Endoscopy**: indicated regardless of upper GI symptoms. Distal duodenal biopsies should be taken if coeliac disease is suspected.
- **Imaging of pancreas and/or ovary**: pancreatic or ovarian carcinoma is a frequent cause of anorexia and weight loss.
- **Faecal microscopy** for faecal fat, indicating malabsorption.
- **Nutritional assessment** is very useful where investigations fail to identify a specific cause and where there are no objective markers of disease (e.g. raised ESR, etc.).

Management
Treat underlying cause. See relevant sections elsewhere. Food supplements may have a role. If no diagnosis reached and weight loss continues:
- Repeat baseline investigations. 'Blind' computed tomography (CT), i.e. without clinical pointers, of the abdomen and pelvis (occasionally of the chest) often leads to a diagnosis, or at least excludes many neoplastic lesions.
- In a few elderly patients with elevated inflammatory indices, an empirical trial of steroids is justifiable although a response is not very discriminatory. Some patients may have TB. If the clinical suspicion is high, empirical anti-TB treatment is justified.

15 Constipation and change in bowel habit

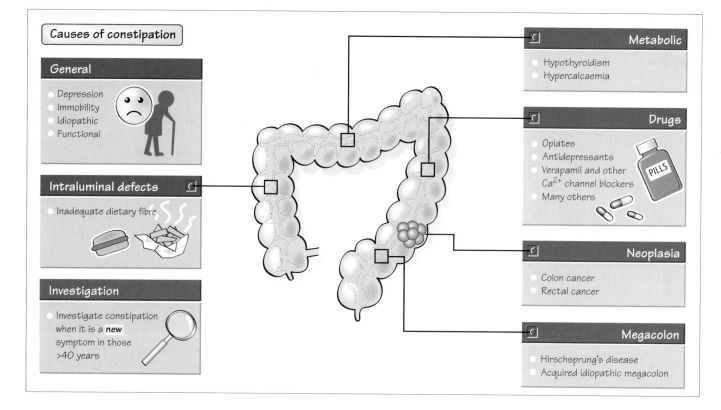

Causes of constipation

General
- Depression
- Immobility
- Idiopathic
- Functional

Intraluminal defects
- Inadequate dietary fibre

Investigation
- Investigate constipation when it is a **new** symptom in those >40 years

Metabolic
- Hypothyroidism
- Hypercalcaemia

Drugs
- Opiates
- Antidepressants
- Verapamil and other Ca²⁺ channel blockers
- Many others

Neoplasia
- Colon cancer
- Rectal cancer

Megacolon
- Hirschsprung's disease
- Acquired idiopathic megacolon

Chronic constipation

Frequency of defecation varies enormously between individuals and in response to dietary and other environmental changes. Patients are often referred when their bowel frequency/habit changes. Although in many circumstances the clinical fear might be the presence of colonic malignancy, benign and functional causes are still more common (Table 15.1).

Overall approach

It is important to ascertain the exact nature of the patients' problem (i.e. consistency, frequency or both). Does the patient harbour concerns of cancer or are they troubled by symptoms?

Clinical features

A clear history is paramount. Important questions include:
- **Over what time period has the patient been constipated?** Often a problem dates back many years and many over-the-counter remedies have been tried (often with varying success).
- **What exactly is the problem?** Has the nature of the problem changed or has the problem become more significantly inconvenient, i.e. needing regular aperients or manual evacuation?
- **Past medical history and particularly obstetric history in women**: pelvic trauma during protracted labour or assisted delivery may present at a later date with defecatory problems.
- **Has there been any rectal bleeding?** This may be due to an innocent cause (e.g. haemorrhoids) but may raise considerable anxiety on a background of constipation.
- **Dietary history** is very important. Patients often take too little regular dietary fibre (i.e. bran) and fluids.

Table 15.1 Differential diagnosis of constipation.

Common
Idiopathic/dietary
Drugs, e.g. *opioid pain-killers, antidepressants, calcium antagonists*
Depression

Uncommon
Colorectal neoplasia
Hypothyroidism
Hypercalcaemia

Rare
Hirschsprung's disease

Examination

This may be unrewarding but a thorough physical examination including rectal examination and sigmoidoscopy is important in providing reassurance.

Investigation

- **Blood tests**: full blood count (FBC), erythrocyte sedimentation rate (ESR), thyroid function, and calcium.
- **Barium enema** is maybe more useful than colonoscopy in symptomatic constipation as it delineates colonic length and diameter in addition to excluding colorectal neoplasia.
- **Transit studies**: in selected cases the passage of radio-opaque markers may distinguish 'slow transit' from problems of the pelvic floor.
- **Anorectal physiology** and **defecating proctography** are useful in selected clinical scenarios only.

Management

Management depends largely on the patient's view of the problem.

Reassurance

If the major concern was colorectal cancer, normal investigations may be sufficient.

Diet and hydration

In those with troublesome symptoms, the first line of treatment is to optimize the patient's intake of fibre and fluids.

Laxatives

• Stimulant laxatives (e.g. senna): in general their use should be limited to short-term constipation (such as that associated with hospitalization). Some patients with chronic constipation may come to depend on stimulants.

• Bulk-forming laxatives (e.g. Fybogel, Isogel): these agents are quite safe but their effect might be limited by the exacerbation of symptomatic bloating.

• Osmotic laxatives (e.g. Movicol, magnesium sulphate) are generally well tolerated and should be considered first-line treatment. Many of these agents are available over the counter (e.g. Milk of Magnesia, Epsom salts). Although lactulose is effectively an osmotic laxative it is of limited benefit and may cause inconvenient colic and wind.

Surgery

In very resistant/recalcitrant cases surgical intervention (e.g. ACE procedure or even subtotal colectomy), may be necessary before patients are able to regain quality of life.

Change in bowel habit in older patients

In the older patient a change in a previously stable bowel habit will often raise specific concerns about the development of colorectal cancer. The following are the particular features of the history suggestive of a significant underlying pathology:

• Anorexia and/or weight loss.

• Nocturnal diarrhoea or pain disturbing sleep.

• Rectal bleeding.

Examination

Although often unrewarding, a full physical examination is mandatory. In particular lymphadenopathy, abdominal masses and organomegaly should be sought, and rectal examination (with faecal occult blood [FOB] testing of stool) and rigid sigmoidoscopy performed.

Management

Evidence of serious underlying disease is sought from an FBC, ESR, iron indices, LFTs, thyroid function; any abnormality here warrants further investigation. **Barium enema** or **colonoscopy** is often used to exclude colorectal cancer in this age group.

Colonic imaging

Barium enema

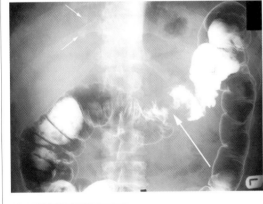

Film from double contrast barium enema in a patient with a large transverse colon carcinoma (see arrow). There is irregular stricturing of the bowel with shouldering apparent. Note lung metastases at lung base (small arrows)

Virtual colonoscopy

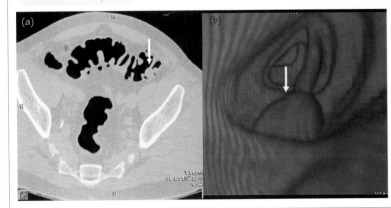

(a)   (b)

Conventional colonoscopy

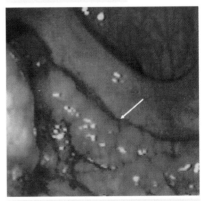

View from conventional colonoscopy confirms irregular morphology of the wall of the rectum. Histological analysis revealed villous adenocarcinoma. Occasionally, very large amounts of fluid are present using a polyethylene glycol preparation and despite supine and prone imaging the entire colonic surface may not be seen. Photo by Dr Michael Macari

Patient who was unwilling to have conventional colonoscopy. Axial image a) shows pedunculated polyp (arrow) in sigmoid. Endoluminal image b) confirms 13mm pedunculated polyp on a stalk (arrow) in the sigmoid colon. When the patient was told of the abnormality he immediately requested endoscopy for removal of the lesion. Photo by Dr Michael Macari

16 Diarrhoea: acute and chronic

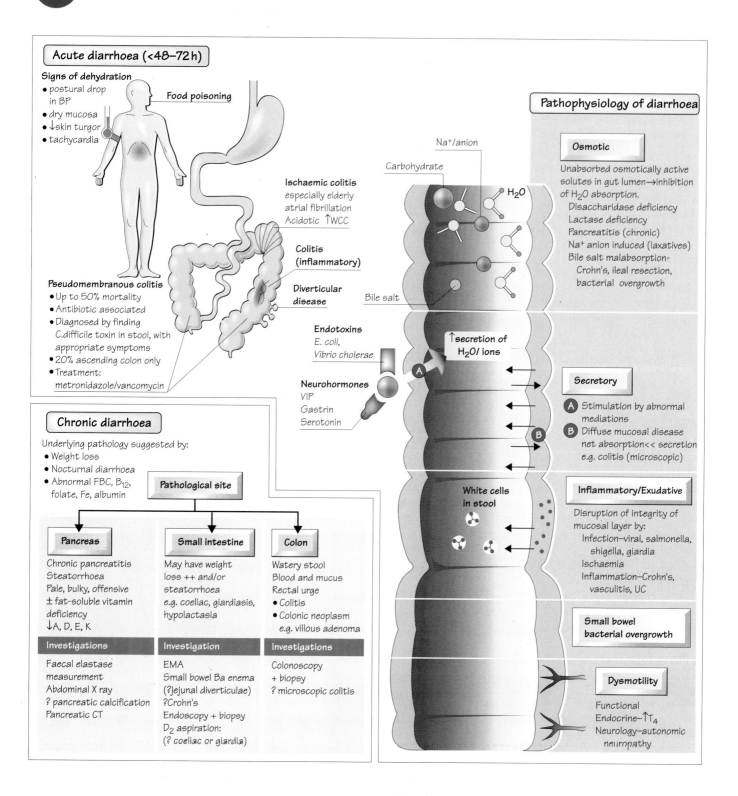

Acute diarrhoea (<48–72h)

Signs of dehydration
- postural drop in BP
- dry mucosa
- ↓skin turgor
- tachycardia

Food poisoning

Ischaemic colitis
especially elderly
atrial fibrillation
Acidotic ↑WCC

Colitis (inflammatory)

Diverticular disease

Pseudomembranous colitis
- Up to 50% mortality
- Antibiotic associated
- Diagnosed by finding C.difficile toxin in stool, with appropriate symptoms
- 20% ascending colon only
- Treatment: metronidazole/vancomycin

Endotoxins
E. coli,
Vibrio cholerae

Neurohormones
VIP
Gastrin
Serotonin

Chronic diarrhoea

Underlying pathology suggested by:
- Weight loss
- Nocturnal diarrhoea
- Abnormal FBC, B_{12}, folate, Fe, albumin

Pathological site

Pancreas

Chronic pancreatitis
Steatorrhoea
Pale, bulky, offensive
± fat-soluble vitamin deficiency
↓A, D, E, K

Investigations

Faecal elastase measurement
Abdominal X ray
? pancreatic calcification
Pancreatic CT

Small intestine

May have weight loss ++ and/or steatorrhoea
e.g. coeliac, giardiasis, hypolactasia

Investigation

EMA
Small bowel Ba enema (?jejunal diverticulae)
?Crohn's
Endoscopy + biopsy
D_2 aspiration:
(? coeliac or giardia)

Colon

Watery stool
Blood and mucus
Rectal urge
- Colitis
- Colonic neoplasm e.g. villous adenoma

Investigations

Colonoscopy
+ biopsy
? microscopic colitis

Pathophysiology of diarrhoea

Na^+/anion

Carbohydrate

H_2O

Bile salt

↑secretion of H_2O/ions

A

B

White cells in stool

Osmotic

Unabsorbed osmotically active solutes in gut lumen→inhibition of H_2O absorption.
Disaccharidase deficiency
Lactase deficiency
Pancreatitis (chronic)
Na^+ anion induced (laxatives)
Bile salt malabsorption-
Crohn's, ileal resection, bacterial overgrowth

Secretory

A Stimulation by abnormal mediations
B Diffuse mucosal disease net absorption<< secretion e.g. colitis (microscopic)

Inflammatory/Exudative

Disruption of integrity of mucosal layer by:
Infection–viral, salmonella, shigella, giardia
Ischaemia
Inflammation–Crohn's, vasculitis, UC

Small bowel bacterial overgrowth

Dysmotility

Functional
Endocrine–↑T_4
Neurology–autonomic neuropathy

Acute diarrhoea
Overall approach

Most acute (< 48–72 h) diarrhoea is infective and relates to food poisoning. Other intestinal pathologies (particularly pseudomembranous colitis) may also present acutely. The differential diagnosis is:

- **Common**: food poisoning; colitis; *Clostridium difficile* toxin-related diarrhoea
- **Uncommon**: ischaemic colitis; diverticular change
- **Rare**: colon cancer, hyperthyroidism, VIPoma.

Clinical features (see figure)

History
- Travel, contacts, take-away/restaurant food (sexual history)
- Recent medications—*Clostridium difficile* toxin-related diarrhoea is common 2 days to 1 month after broad-spectrum antibiotics (particularly cephalosporins) in the infirm elderly patient.

Examination
State of hydration should be determined: even young patients may be considerably volume depleted on admission, with tachycardia and postural hypotension, and may require intravenous saline.

Fever generally suggests an infective cause, but may be present in severe colitis. Markers of chronic disease (clubbing, koilonychia, leukonychia, mouth ulcers, weight loss) may reflect an underlying chronic inflammatory bowel disease. Abdominal examination may reveal non-specific tenderness. Sigmoidoscopy and rectal biopsy may be useful.

Investigations
- **Blood tests**: full blood count (FBC); anaemia or thrombocytosis raise the suspicion of a chronic underlying pathology. A low albumin is a good marker of severity of illness but is non-specific.
- **Stool culture** may identify the responsible organism. *C. difficile* bacteria are found in 5% of normal individuals; diagnosis therefore requires appropriate symptoms in the presence of the toxin rather than the organism alone.
- **Plain abdominal X-ray**: may show features of acute colitis (see p. 222).

Management
- **Rehydration**: the initial management involves resting the gut and giving parenteral rehydration.
- **Treat the underlying cause**: antibiotics or steroids might be indicated if investigations reveal a specific pathogen or evidence of an underlying inflammatory bowel disease. Metronidazole, or vancomycin, is used for pseudomembranous colitis. Relapse occurs in up to 20% and is treated with further courses of metronidazole/vancomycin.

Chronic diarrhoea
Overall approach
Most infectious forms of diarrhoea resolve within 2–3 weeks and any diarrhoea that lasts longer than this warrants further investigation. The differential diagnosis is:
- **Common**: inflammatory bowel disease/colitis; coeliac disease; giardiasis; drugs (e.g. proton pump inhibitors).
- **Uncommon**: hypolactasia; colonic neoplasms, e.g. villous adenomas; thyrotoxicosis.
- **Rare**: endocrine tumours (e.g. Zollinger-Ellison syndrome, which results from a gastrin-secreting tumour).

Clinical features
In difficult cases it may be important to confirm that the patient has true diarrhoea (by stool weights) and not a functional bowel disorder (see p. 243). The specific clinical features suggesting a pathological diarrhoea include: nocturnal diarrhoea; unintentional weight loss; mouth ulcers.

History
The clinical history may give clues about whether the predominant pathology is colonic, small intestinal or pancreatic.

- **Colonic diarrhoea**: watery stool often with blood and mucus. May be associated with urgency of defecation.
- **Small intestinal diarrhoea**: may have features of steatorrhoea (pale, bulky stools that are difficult to flush away) and weight loss.
- **Exocrine pancreatic insufficiency**: steatorrhoea and weight loss are the hallmarks of pancreatic insufficiency. In addition the patient may describe pancreatic pain, which is epigastric (often radiating through to the back) associated with fatty food intolerance.

Examination
- **General appearance**: determine as to whether the patient looks well or not. If possible, corroborate a history of weight loss (loose clothes or skin, belt notches, etc.).
- **Physical signs of malabsorption**: nail changes such as koilonychia, leukonychia. Signs in the tongue and mouth of glossitis, cheilitis and ulcers. Bruising.
- **Abdominal examination**: this should include rectal examination and rigid sigmoidoscopy.

Investigations
Investigations should be chosen depending on the most likely diagnosis on clinical grounds.
- **Blood tests**: usual tests include FBC, ESR, and biochemistry, particularly for serum albumin, vitamin B_{12} and folate. Thyroid function. Tissue transglutaminase or endomysial antibody for coeliac disease.
- **Stool microscopy and culture** ($\times 3$): negative cultures do not exclude giardiasis.
- **Faecal elastase or chymotrypsin** will be low in exocrine pancreatic insufficiency.
- **Abdominal X-ray**: a plain abdominal X-ray may show pancreatic calcification although, if pancreatic insufficiency is suspected clinically, this is better investigated by pancreatic CT and/or endoscopic or magnetic resonance cholangiopancreatography (ERCP or MRCP).
- **Endoscopy, duodenal aspiration and biopsy**: to exclude coeliac disease and giardiasis.
- **Colonoscopy and biopsies**: lower GI endoscopy has the advantage over contrast radiology in that, even if the mucosa looks normal, biopsies might reveal a microscopic colitis (e.g. lymphocytic colitis, collagenous colitis).
- **Hydrogen breath tests**: for hypolactasia (lactose) or small bowel bacterial overgrowth (lactulose).
- **Small bowel imaging**: may show jejunal diverticula *or* intestinal strictures (e.g. Crohn's disease) that might act as a substrate for bacterial overgrowth.
- **24-h stool weights (repeated when fasting)**: although this often appears low on the list of investigations, it remains the most useful way of distinguishing osmotic diarrhoea from a secretory one.
- **Faecal fats**: the collection or estimation of faecal fats as an investigation of malabsorption has now been largely surpassed by the direct measurement of pancreatic enzyme activities (see above).
- **Fasting gut hormones**: if a hormone-secreting tumour is suspected, fasting hormone levels should be measured. If gastrin levels are being measured it is imperative that the patient is not receiving proton pump inhibitors.

Management
Treat specific cause. See relevant sections.

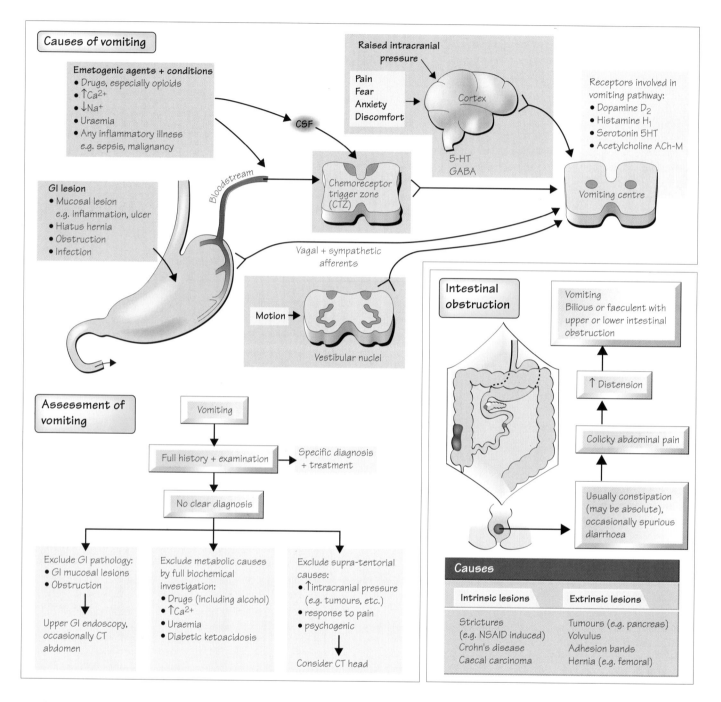

Overall approach

The first step in the assessment of vomiting is to consider whether intestinal obstruction is a possible diagnosis.

Intestinal obstruction is caused by:

- *Intrinsic*
  GI neoplasia, e.g. gastric or colonic carcinoma
  Crohn's disease
  Strictures, e.g. post-surgical; other, including NSAIDs
- *Extrinsic*
  Tumour, e.g. pancreas
  Incarcerated hernia
  Adhesion bands secondary to previous surgery
  Volvulus
- *Pseudo-obstruction*
  Paralytic ileus
  Motility disorders

Clinical features

Key clinical features indicating that vomiting is caused by intestinal obstruction are, first, the presence of colicky abdominal pain and, second, a change in bowel habit (ranging from diarrhoea to absolute constipation).

History
• Ask about the duration of symptoms, anorexia and weight loss (suggests progressive pathology).
• Site of pain (see p. 44).
• Previous intestinal illness or operations.

Examination
General
Observe the general appearance and presence of lymphadenopathy. It is vital to determine the fluid status of the patient from skin turgor, orthostatic hypotension, heart rate and urine output.

Abdominal examination
• Scars from previous surgery raise the possibility of obstruction caused by adhesions.
• Abdominal distension may be present. Absent bowel sounds suggest paralytic ileus (pseudo-obstruction), whereas in most other cases of obstruction bowel sounds are increased. Succussion splash suggests gastric outflow obstruction.
• Tenderness and rebound suggest perforation.
• Palpable inflammatory or neoplastic masses.
• Rectal examination and sigmoidoscopy.

Investigations
• **Blood tests**: FBC/ESR and biochemistry are indicated, partly to determine the effect of vomiting/obstruction on potassium and renal function.
• **Abdominal X-ray**: usually shows features of intestinal obstruction (i.e. dilated fluid-filled loops of bowel) and on occasion may suggest the level of the obstruction (e.g. air absent from the rectum).
• **Endoscopy**: if gastric outflow obstruction is suspected.
• **Water-soluble contrast imaging** may be useful for unresolving problems related to either foregut or hindgut.
• **Barium contrast radiology**: barium follow-through or barium enema is useful in patients whose symptoms resolve (if only partially) with conservative management.

Management
All cases should be managed in conjunction with a GI surgeon.

Initial management
• **Nil by mouth (NBM)**: gut rest is probably the best way to relieve symptoms. A large-bore nasogastric tube (a Ryle's tube) helps to drain obstructed intestinal contents and in cases of protracted large volume vomiting is imperative in preventing aspiration.
• **Intravenous fluids**: patients may be significantly volume depleted/ dehydrated on admission and require substantial fluid resuscitation. Avoid opiate analgesia when possible (as this inhibits intestinal motility).

Subsequent management
• **Laparotomy**: in cases that do not resolve with conservative management a laparotomy may be necessary even before a definitive diagnosis has been achieved.

Vomiting
Overall approach
In the absence of evidence of mechanical obstruction other causes of vomiting should be considered, such as:
• *Metabolic*
  Hypercalcaemia
  Hypoadrenalism (Addison's disease)
  Uraemia
• *Inflammatory disease*
  Visceral inflammation, e.g. hepatitis, pancreatitis, etc.
  Remote infection, e.g. pneumonia
• *Drugs*
  Cytotoxics
  Analgesics (especially opioids)
  Antibiotics
• *Neurogenic*
  Intra-cranial tumours
  Any painful/unpleasant stimulus
  Psychogenic
  Vestibulocochlear disease
• *GI causes*
  Obstruction
  Gastroenteritis

History
Ask specifically about:
• Duration of symptoms, and whether the problem is getting worse.
• Drugs, including those bought over the counter.
• Headache or other features of raised intra-cranial pressure.
• Unusual foods, restaurants, travel.
• Hearing, balance.

Examination
• **General**: overall appearance and the presence of any relevant pathology. State of hydration, particularly postural blood pressure.
• **Abdominal examination**: usually unrewarding but may reveal signs of intestinal obstruction.

Investigation
• **Blood tests**: FBC, ESR; biochemistry, including renal and liver function, sodium, potassium and calcium, amylase.
• **Cortisol**: short Synacthen test, if hypoadrenalism suspected.
• **Chest X-ray**: for infection (including aspiration pneumonia), neoplasm.
• **Endoscopy** is usually indicated in patients with persistent vomiting when no other cause is found.
• **Small bowel imaging** may be indicated in difficult cases to exclude occult subacute obstruction.
• **CT scan of head**: indicated when no other pathology identified.

Management
• Treat the underlying cause.
• **Antiemetics**: empirical treatment with antiemetics may be necessary if physical/mechanical obstruction has been excluded. Domperidone does not cross the blood-brain barrier and is useful for long-term 'as-needed' treatment. Other agents (e.g. metoclopramide, prochlorperazine) are increasingly being replaced by centrally acting serotonin antagonists (e.g. ondansetron).

18 Haematemesis and melaena

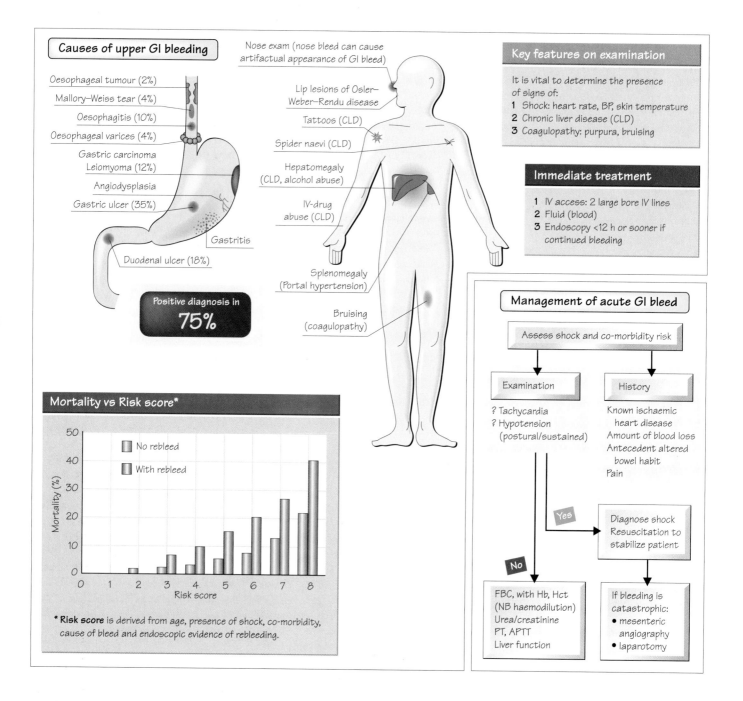

Causes of upper GI bleeding

- Oesophageal tumour (2%)
- Mallory–Weiss tear (4%)
- Oesophagitis (10%)
- Oesophageal varices (4%)
- Gastric carcinoma Leiomyoma (12%)
- Angiodysplasia
- Gastric ulcer (35%)
- Gastritis
- Duodenal ulcer (18%)

Positive diagnosis in 75%

Nose exam (nose bleed can cause artifactual appearance of GI bleed)

- Lip lesions of Osler–Weber–Rendu disease
- Tattoos (CLD)
- Spider naevi (CLD)
- Hepatomegaly (CLD, alcohol abuse)
- IV-drug abuse (CLD)
- Splenomegaly (Portal hypertension)
- Bruising (coagulopathy)

Key features on examination

It is vital to determine the presence of signs of:
1. Shock: heart rate, BP, skin temperature
2. Chronic liver disease (CLD)
3. Coagulopathy: purpura, bruising

Immediate treatment

1. IV access: 2 large bore IV lines
2. Fluid (blood)
3. Endoscopy <12 h or sooner if continued bleeding

Management of acute GI bleed

Assess shock and co-morbidity risk

Examination
- ? Tachycardia
- ? Hypotension (postural/sustained)

History
- Known ischaemic heart disease
- Amount of blood loss
- Antecedent altered bowel habit
- Pain

Yes → Diagnose shock Resuscitation to stabilize patient

No → FBC, with Hb, Hct (NB haemodilution) Urea/creatinine PT, APTT Liver function

If bleeding is catastrophic:
- mesenteric angiography
- laparotomy

Mortality vs Risk score*

Mortality (%) vs Risk score
- No rebleed
- With rebleed

* **Risk score** is derived from age, presence of shock, co-morbidity, cause of bleed and endoscopic evidence of rebleeding.

Overall approach

Haematemesis refers to the vomiting of blood. Blood may be fresh (clots or bright red liquid) or altered by intestinal acid and enzymes, appearing brown and likened to 'coffee grounds'. Vomiting a small amount of altered blood is often a non-specific feature of protracted retching and does not always reflect a significant upper GI haemorrhage.

Melaena refers to a loose, tarry, jet-black stool, with a deeply offensive smell, which sticks to the pan and indicates brisk upper GI haemorrhage with digestion of the blood in the intestine. Solid dark stool that tests positive for occult blood may indicate intestinal bleeding but is not melaena.

Differential diagnosis

- *Common*
  - Peptic ulcer (duodenal, gastric)
  - Mallory–Weiss tear
  - Gastritis, duodenitis, oesophagitis
- *Uncommon*
  - Oesophageal varices/portal hypertensive gastropathy

- *Rare*
  Upper GI malignancy
- *Very rare*
  Angiodysplasia (including the Dieulafoy lesion)
  Aorto-enteric fistula

General clinical features
- **History**: postural dizziness or loss of consciousness in the context of haematemesis or melaena is significant, implying a 'haemodynamically significant bleed'.
- **Drug history** is relevant both to the underlying diagnosis (e.g. aspirin, NSAIDs suggest peptic ulceration) and to treatment (β-blockers, warfarin).

Clinical clues to the diagnosis
A history of dyspepsia makes peptic ulcer more likely. A history of retching and vomitus initially free from blood suggests a Mallory–Weiss tear. Heavy alcohol consumption suggests gastritis (30–40%), peptic ulcer disease (30–40%) or occasionally varices. Weight loss suggests malignancy. Severe bleeding with clots and treatment-refractory shock raises the probability of varices. Previous abdominal aortic surgery raises the possibility of aortoenteric fistula. In young patients with a history of repeated brisk upper GI bleeding (often with haemodynamic collapse) and 'unremarkable' endoscopies, a Dieulafoy lesion should be considered (a submucosal artery, usually on the lesser gastric curve and situated near the cardia, which intermittently causes large GI bleeds).

Examination
General
- General appearance: is the patient cool and clammy, indicating significant peripheral vasoconstriction?
- Pulse and blood pressure, including postural drop. Documentation of the severity of shock is vitally important.
- Signs of chronic liver disease.
- Signs of neoplasia: lymphadenopathy, organomegaly, and recent weight loss.

Abdominal
Infrequently revealing. Epigastric tenderness is most often non-specific. Hepatosplenomegaly and or abdominal ascites raise the possibility of varices.

Predictors of mortality
The following have been demonstrated to be independent predictors of mortality in patients admitted to hospital with haematemesis and melaena:
- Age.
- Co-morbidity: organ failure (renal or hepatic) carries a particularly poor prognosis.
- Shock: tachycardia or hypotension on admission.
- Diagnosis: although varices and upper GI malignancy are rare, they carry a worse prognosis.

- Stigmata of recent haemorrhage: seen at endoscopy. These include blood in the upper GI tract, adherent blood clot or a visible vessel in the base of an ulcer.
- Rebleeding: further evidence of bleeding (more haematemesis or melaena; falling haemoglobin concentration or cardiovascular instability).

Investigations
- **Blood tests**: FBC and crossmatch in case blood transfusion is needed.
- **Urea and creatinine**: a raised urea relative to creatinine (i.e. raised urea/creatinine ratio) is present in significant upper GI haemorrhage and reflects the protein load of fresh blood within the gut, as well as dehydration ('pre-renal' uraemia, p. 268).
- **K^+**: this may be disproportionately high as a result of absorption from blood in the small bowel.
- **Clotting** should be checked in patients on anticoagulants and those with signs of chronic liver disease.
- **ECG, chest X-ray**: early identification of significant cardiopulmonary disease will aid further management.
- **Endoscopy**: may help to establish the diagnosis and allow immediate endoscopic treatment. It also provides prognostic information (i.e. identification of stigmata of recent haemorrhage [SRH]).

Management
All cases should be managed in conjunction with an experienced endoscopist and GI surgeons. If the patient has had abdominal aortic surgery a vascular surgeon should be consulted.

Resuscitation
Early volume replacement (preferably with blood) is vital in patients with shock and coexistent cardiovascular disease.

Central venous pressure (CVP) monitoring
The benefits include safer resuscitation of patients with heart failure and ischaemic heart disease and early recognition of rebleeding (see above).

Endoscopic therapy
In addition to providing a diagnosis endoscopy also allows treatment to bleeding lesions:
- Injection therapy: adrenaline (epinephrine) (1 : 10 000) for peptic ulcers with SRH.
- Heater probe and laser photocoagulation of bleeding vessels, tumours, and ulcers.
- Band ligation of varices has now largely superseded injection sclerotherapy with ethanolamine.

Surgery
Although surgery is less common now than in days before the development of endoscopy, it remains a vital treatment. Surgical intervention should be considered in individuals not responding to resuscitation and those with a clinically significant rebleed, and in those in whom endoscopy has failed or is not feasible. Early consultation with the surgical team always facilitates subsequent management.

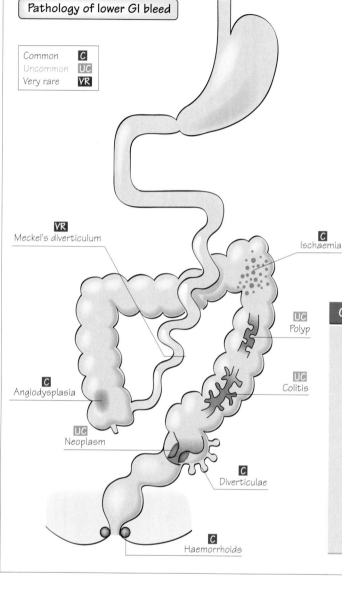

Pathology of lower GI bleed

Common **C**
Uncommon **UC**
Very rare **VR**

VR Meckel's diverticulum
C Ischaemia
UC Polyp
UC Colitis
C Angiodysplasia
UC Neoplasm
C Diverticulae
C Haemorrhoids

Outpatient management of chronic GI bleed

History

?Family history/risks for IBD, neoplasia
Nature of blood loss (see text)
Associated symptoms:
change in bowel habit, pain etc., weight loss

Examine

Abdomen & PR
Liver

Investigation

FBC, ESR, Fe indices
Lower GI scope post barium enema
or
Total colonoscopy, often after acute bleed has settled

Clinical differences between upper and lower GI bleeding

	Upper GI source	Lower GI source
Haematemesis	+++	Never
Melaena	++	Never
Dark red blood PR	+	++
Bright red blood PR	Never	+++
Raised urea/creatinine ratio	++	0 − +
Known ulcerative colitis	0 − +	++
Antecedent altered bowel habit	0 − +	++

Distinguish between acute, heavy, lower gastrointestinal haemorrhage and chronic, persistent, small volume rectal bleeding.

Acute lower GI haemorrhage

Sudden large-volume rectal bleeding most commonly presents in elderly people as a medical emergency with varying degrees of cardiovascular compromise.

Differential diagnosis (Table 19.1)

The common underlying causes are age related and, although they are often in themselves benign, the presence of significant co-morbidity (e.g. ischaemic heart disease) in this group of patients contributes to a significant mortality.

Table 19.1 Differential diagnosis of acute lower GI haemorrhage.

Common
Diverticular change
Colonic angiodysplasia
Ischaemic colitis

Uncommon
Distal colon/rectal carcinoma
Inflammatory bowel disease

Very rare
Meckel's diverticulum

Clinical Presentations at a Glance

Clinical features

The greatest challenge is often to distinguish proximal colonic bleeding from a brisk upper GI bleed. The passage of red blood per rectum is unlikely to be from an upper GI source. Likewise the passage of classic melaena (jet black, tarry, smelly) indicates an upper GI tract lesion. The problem arises when blood appears to be neither one nor the other: in this situation full upper and lower GI tract investigations are appropriate.

History

- **The nature of the bleeding**: was it black 'like tar' (i.e. melaena) or black 'like bramble jelly' (i.e. arising from the proximal colon).
- **Onset**: most commonly the onset of bleeding is sudden, although it is important to elicit whether there had been an antecedent change in bowel habit, which may indicate a colonic neoplasm or colitis.
- **Abdominal pain**: although mild colicky pain is a non-specific finding, severe *and sudden* pain suggests intestinal ischaemia.
- **Significant co-morbidity**: the recognition of significant co-morbidity is important in guiding resuscitation and specific interventions.

Examination

- **State of the circulation (pulse, postural BP)**: any degree of shock must be recognized early and corrected (see below).
- **Abdominal examination**: the absence of a palpable **mass** in the abdomen does not exclude a malignant underlying cause.
- A **bruit** may rarely be heard, indicating mesenteric atheroma and potentially ischaemia.
- **Rectal examination** may identify a low rectal cancer and may be useful in clinically distinguishing lower from upper GI bleeding (melaena = upper). Rigid sigmoidoscopy will often provide very limited views at the time of a large bleed.

Investigations

- **Blood tests**: FBC should be taken, although in acute GI bleeding haemodilution takes several hours, so the haemoglobin level underestimates the severity of the bleed. A clotting profile should be checked if the patient is on anticoagulants or if there are clinical indications of chronic liver disease. Crossmatch if shock is present on admission or if there is significant anaemia. A raised urea/creatinine ratio may indicate an upper rather than a lower GI source.
- **Abdominal X-ray**: a plain abdominal X-ray may show features of ischaemia (localized area of colonic mucosal oedema—sometimes with 'thumb-printing').
- **Lower GI endoscopy**: once resuscitation has been completed and preferably after the acute bleed has subsided. The timing and extent of the endoscopy (i.e. colonoscopy vs. flexible sigmoidoscopy) must be determined on individual clinical grounds. Barium enema may be necessary if the upper limit of bleeding is not identified or total endoscopic examination prevented by technical limitations (e.g. severe diverticular change, ischaemia, stricture).
- **Upper GI endoscopy**: this is often performed at the time of the sigmoidoscopy for formal exclusion of a significant upper GI pathology.
- **Mesenteric angiography**: in persistent heavy colonic bleeding (≤ 2–5 mL/min) angiography can identify areas of angiodysplasia or a bleeding vessel that can be embolized.

Management

- **Resuscitation**: early correction of shock is vital.
- **Treat specific pathology**: in most circumstances colonic bleeding will at least temporarily cease, allowing diagnostic investigations to be performed.

- **Laparotomy**: in catastrophic bleeding, a laparotomy, if possible with on-table colonoscopy, and occasionally a 'blind' colectomy may be necessary.

Chronic rectal bleeding
Overall approach

The recurrent/persistent passage of blood per rectum may present at any age and, in most situations, can be managed as an outpatient.

Differential diagnosis

Although the most common cause of rectal bleeding is benign, appropriate investigations are always indicated in order to make an early diagnosis of colorectal cancer. The differential diagnosis is: 1) Haemorrhoids ('piles'). 2) Colorectal neoplasia (polyps, cancer); more common in the elderly. 3) Distal colitis. 4) Solitary rectal ulcer.

History

The history (particularly the appearance of the blood) often suggests the site of bleeding:
- Bright red 'like tomato ketchup' or dark red 'like bramble jelly' blood suggests, respectively, lower and upper colonic pathology.
- Blood only on the toilet paper and the surface of the stool strongly suggests 'piles' as the source. Blood mixed throughout the stool suggests that the pathology is higher up.
- A change in bowel habit suggests an underlying neoplasm or colitis.
- Bright red bleeding, with mucus discharge and tenesmus (continual feeling of needing to defecate, with a sensation of incomplete defecation) together suggest proctitis.
- A family history of colorectal neoplasia increases the probability (and worry) of this disease.

Examination

Abdominal examination should include identification of any masses or palpable organomegaly and rectal examination for detection of low rectal tumours. All patients should undergo rigid sigmoidoscopy for the detection of rectal polyps/cancer and colitis.

Investigations

- **Blood tests**: FBC, ESR, iron indices—iron deficiency anaemia or raised inflammatory markers should never be ascribed to piles.
- **Lower GI endoscopy**: flexible sigmoidoscopy after an enema should provide good views of the colon as far as the splenic flexure. Total colonoscopy requires full bowel preparation and sedation and is indicated when a proximal colonic neoplasm is suspected clinically, from iron deficiency or the presence of distal colonic polyps.
- **Barium enema** is an alternative to total colonoscopy. A sigmoidoscopic examination (either rigid or flexible) should be performed in addition to exclude a low rectal neoplasm, which might be passed by the enema tube.
- **Virtual colonography** is a form of abdominal spiral CT scan requiring bowel preparation and inflation of the colon with air (or CO_2). Computerized reconstruction of the images generates a 'fly-through' image of the colon comparable to images generated by colonoscopy.

Management

- **Treat specific pathology**: see relevant chapters.
- **Haemorrhoids**: often advice on diet and defecatory habits is sufficient to control symptoms. Injection sclerotherapy, banding and excision may be necessary in some circumstances.

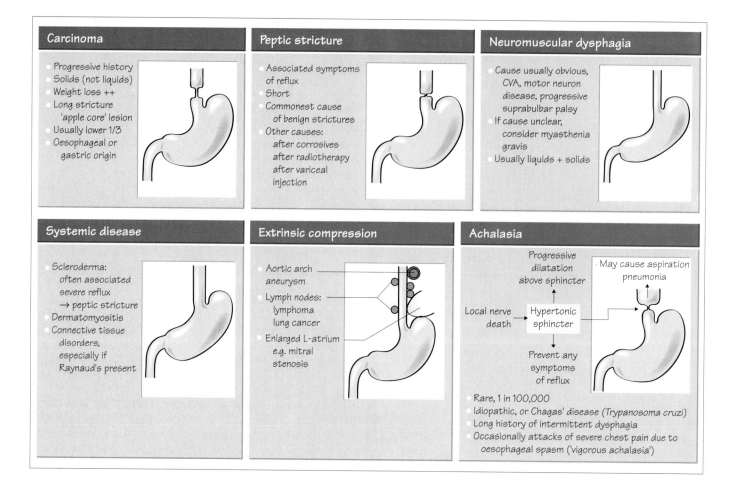

Carcinoma
- Progressive history
- Solids (not liquids)
- Weight loss ++
- Long stricture 'apple core' lesion
- Usually lower 1/3
- Oesophageal or gastric origin

Peptic stricture
- Associated symptoms of reflux
- Short
- Commonest cause of benign strictures
- Other causes: after corrosives after radiotherapy after variceal injection

Neuromuscular dysphagia
- Cause usually obvious, CVA, motor neuron disease, progressive suprabulbar palsy
- If cause unclear, consider myasthenia gravis
- Usually liquids + solids

Systemic disease
- Scleroderma: often associated severe reflux → peptic stricture
- Dermatomyositis
- Connective tissue disorders, especially if Raynaud's present

Extrinsic compression
- Aortic arch aneurysm
- Lymph nodes: lymphoma lung cancer
- Enlarged L-atrium e.g. mitral stenosis

Achalasia
- Progressive dilatation above sphincter
- May cause aspiration pneumonia
- Local nerve death
- Hypertonic sphincter
- Prevent any symptoms of reflux
- Rare, 1 in 100,000
- Idiopathic, or Chagas' disease (Trypanosoma cruzi)
- Long history of intermittent dysphagia
- Occasionally attacks of severe chest pain due to oesophageal spasm ('vigorous achalasia')

Overall approach

Dysphagia relates to difficulty in swallowing which implies oesophageal obstruction. Oadynophagia relates to painful swallowing.

Differential diagnosis (Table 20.1)

Table 20.1 Differential diagnosis of dysphagia.

Common
Oesophagitis and peptic stricture
Oesophageal carcinoma
Gastric cancer at the cardia

Uncommon
Diffuse oesophageal spasm

Rare
Achalasia

Clinical features

Dysphagia is an ominous and frightening symptom and should be investigated at the earliest opportunity.

History

The duration of symptoms and associated heartburn/dyspepsia are useful clinical clues. Progressive symptoms and weight loss are ominous features.

Examination

Examination is often unrewarding. Check for anaemia, weight loss, lymphadenopathy (including Virchow's node behind the head of the left clavicle, indicative of metastatic upper GI cancer).

Investigations

- **General investigations** include FBC and ESR, LFTs and calcium. A chest X-ray may show either a primary or a secondary lung neoplasia.
- **Barium swallow**: this procedure is relatively safe, although there is a small risk of aspiration of contrast into the lungs. This is usually the first test ordered and may demonstrate benign or malignant stricture or dysmotility. All strictures should be biopsied to exclude malignancy, even if the radiological appearances do not suggest this.
- **Endoscopy**: upper GI endoscopy risks oesophageal perforation but allows definitive diagnosis through biopsy and immediate treatment (oesophageal dilatation, placement of stent).

- Other **specific tests** (manometry, pH monitoring, CT) are indicated depending on the results of the above. See sections on reflux and oesophageal carcinoma (see p. 215 and p. 238).

Management

- **Peptic stricture**: strictures associated with reflux oesophagitis occasionally require endoscopic dilatation. Recurrence is probably reduced by treatment with proton pump inhibitors.
- **Oesophageal carcinoma**: see p. 238.
- **Achalasia**: there are a range of treatments for achalasia. Endoscopic injection of botulinum toxin into the lower oesophageal sphincter is relatively safe, but provides only limited relief. Forced pneumatic dilatation carries a risk of oesophageal perforation but provides more lasting relief. Cardiomyotomy (Heller's operation) remains the definitive procedure and can now be performed laparoscopically.
- **Oesophageal dysmotility**: reassurance after exclusion of a malignant underlying cause for the symptoms often helps patients with oesophageal spasm, together with simple advice about diet and nutrition. Calcium antagonists and nitrates also have a role.
- **Neuromuscular dysphagia**: see below.
- **Extrinsic compression** is treated according to the underlying cause.
- **Systemic diseases** producing dysphagia are managed similarly. Scleroderma may produce severe symptoms of reflux, requiring high-dose proton pump inhibition. Benign strictures are dilated endoscopically.

Dysphagia due to cerebrovascular disease

Dysphagia is an important finding in stroke, as it is common (it occurs in some 50–70% of stroke patients); aspiration of food in dysphagic patients is a crucial mechanism contributing to pneumonia, which itself accounts for some 20–40% of stroke-related deaths.

Cerebrovascular disease may interfere with any of the three phases of swallowing:

1 The oral phase, where food is prepared for swallowing (usually by chewing) and then propelled into the oropharynx (the oral propulsive phase)—paralysis of the cranial nerve supplying the tongue, or interference with the cerebellar mechanisms controlling the tongue, may lead to impairment of this phase.

2 The pharyngeal phase, where food is propelled into the oesophagus, by a complex series of reflex events, involving cranial nerves IX–XII.

3 The oesophageal phase, where the bolus of food is propelled down the oesophagus by peristaltic motion.

The signs of dysphagia in stroke patients include: coughing when eating/drinking, recurrent chest infections, weight loss with food avoidance, dehydration. As dysphagia is so frequent in stroke patients, it is crucial to assess swallowing as part of the acute assessment of a stroke. Until this has been done the patient should be 'nil by mouth'.

Swallowing assessment consists of a full neurological examination, with some additional features:

- Assess cranial nerves V, VII–XII.
- Observe jaw movement, mastication, tongue strength and mobility.
- Test the individual functions of the mouth.
- Test for the gag reflex.
- Assess how strong the cough is, as this determines how good the lung is at protecting against infection.
- If the functions of the mouth are intact, ask the patient to swallow; while doing so, place three fingers on the larynx, and assess how it moves during the swallow.
- If all the above are intact, assess how the patient swallows a small amount of water.

If swallowing is impaired, then the patient should not be fed orally; for the very short run, intravenous fluids are appropriate. If swallowing is not satisfactory after a few days, feeding should occur via a nasogastric tube. If swallowing remains impaired after 2–3 weeks, consideration should be given to percutaneous endoscopic gastrostomy (PEG) feeding.

Prognosis: most patients who have acutely impaired swallowing due to a stroke have recovered by 6 months—only a very small proportion need ongoing PEG feeding.

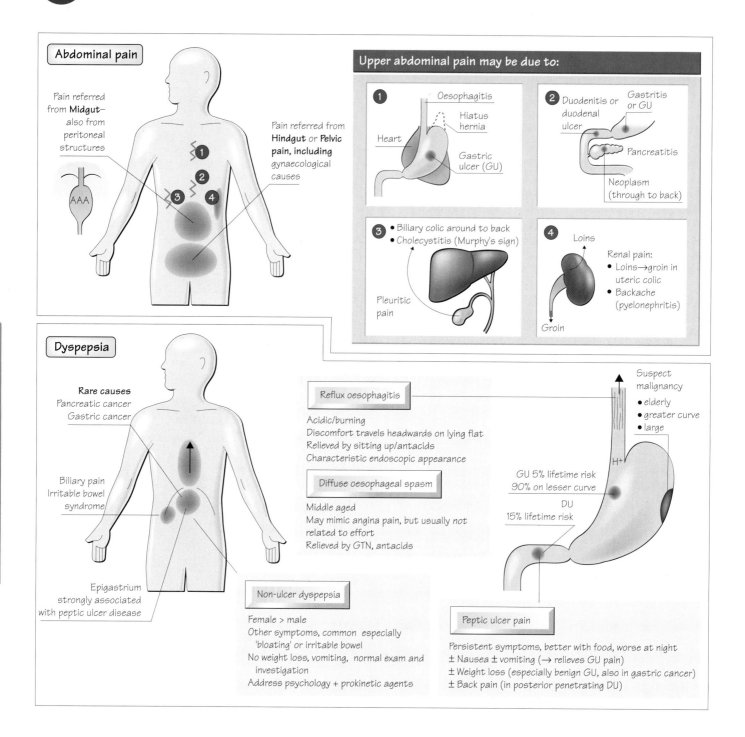

Abdominal pain

A very careful history is mandatory to formulate a differential diagnosis. Pains usually come from within an organ (midline pain, not often localized to the affected viscus) or from irritation of the peritoneal lining (localized to the site of the inflamed viscus). Patients in pain are often frightened. Patience and perseverance initially are rewarded with an earlier and more accurate diagnosis.

History

This is very important. Ask about:
- Onset and duration, the nature and site of the pain.
- Course—getting better, worse or persistent?
- Relationship to eating and defecation.
- Associated symptoms of weight loss, altered bowel habit.
- Precipitants, including alcohol, trauma, drugs.

Certain patterns point to specific sources of pain although there is considerable overlap.

- **Oesophageal pain** has two forms: Dyspepsia relates to acidic sensations and is commonly related to reflux (see p. 215). Oesophageal spasm usually manifests as a tightening felt in the chest, and is sometimes indistinguishable from cardiac pain with radiation into the neck.
- **Biliary pain** (biliary tree and gall bladder) is felt in the right upper quadrant and is colicky in nature. Ask about cholestasis (pale stools, dark urine, jaundice). Pain from the liver itself is unusual, although it may occur in hepatitis, hepatic metastases or right heart failure as a persistent right upper quadrant discomfort from hepatic capsular distension.
- **Pancreatic pain** is usually epigastric, and typically radiates through to the back. Common precipitants include fatty foods and alcohol.
- **Foregut (gastroduodenal) pain** tends to be acidic and situated in the epigastrium.
- **Midgut (small intestinal) pain** is usually colicky and situated periumbilically. It is often associated with bloating, nausea and vomiting.
- **Hindgut (colonic) pain** is also usually colicky in nature but experienced below the level of the umbilicus. Other features may include a change in bowel habit and rectal bleeding. Remember that carcinoma of the caecum is more likely to lead to subacute small bowel obstruction than colonic dysfunction.
- **Peritonitic pain** is more localized because the parietal peritoneum has a rich sensory innervation. The classic example of this is evolving appendicitis. Initially the pain is periumbilical and colicky relating to an inflamed midgut viscus. As inflammation progresses there is local peritonism with persistent pain and tenderness in the right iliac fossa. This may progress to perforation and generalized peritonitis with severe global abdominal pain if left untreated.
- **Loin pain** tends *not* to be related to GI tract pathology but is more likely to arise from the kidneys and ureters.

Other features of the history
It is useful to determine whether the current pain represents an acute problem or a manifestation of a chronic underlying condition (possibly subclinical until then). Previous GI problems or operations suggest an exacerbation of an old problem. Anorexia and weight loss suggests serious pathology.

Examination
General
General appearances. Circulatory state. Markers of chronic disease.

Abdominal
- Areas of tenderness: ask the patient to point to where the pain is maximal. Look for peritonism: guarding and more importantly rebound tenderness.
- Masses, including organomegaly.

Investigations
- **Blood tests**: FBC, ESR, C-reactive protein (CRP), renal function tests; LFTs, calcium; amylase.
- **Abdominal X-ray**: may show intestinal obstruction, vascular calcification (raising the possibility of ischaemia), loss of psoas outline (implying retroperitoneal pathology), and areas of absence gas pattern (bowel loops displaced by a mass). Look for features of a pneumoperitoneum (Wriggler's sign).
- **Erect chest X-ray**: look for the presence of air under the diaphragm.
- **Abdominal ultrasonography**: excellent for the biliary and renal

tracts. Less good for imaging the pancreas and retroperitoneal structures and less sensitive in obese individuals.
- **Abdominal CT** produces better images of the retroperitoneal organs.
- **Barium contrast radiology**: an 'instant' enema (i.e. without bowel preparation) is useful in suspected large bowel obstruction. A gastrografin meal and follow-through is useful in small bowel obstruction.

Management
General measures
- Rest the gut: parenteral rehydration.
- Analgesia: gut-related pain is relatively resistant to simple analgesics. Opioids are effective but are limited by side effects (nausea, constipation, etc.).
- Treat the underlying cause.

No cause identified
If no cause for persistent pain is identified, a diagnostic laparoscopy/laparotomy is occasionally required. Consider several diagnoses:
- Functional GI disorders.
- Munchausen's syndrome: have a very high index of suspicion when patients not resident to the locality present with severe abdominal pain, without convincing clinical or investigative abnormalities. There may be stigmata of multiple previous operations.
- Very rarely myocardial ischaemia presents as upper abdominal pain.
- Rare diseases such as porphyria and familial Mediterranean fever.

Dyspepsia
Dyspepsia refers to symptoms originating from the upper GI tract. These may relate to eating or drinking and include heartburn and pain (usually 'acidic') in the upper abdomen/lower chest, as well as 'bloating', anorexia and vomiting. The most common underlying mechanism is gastro-oesophageal reflux. The figure shows the differential diagnosis of dyspepsia.

History
Symptoms have often been present for some years. Lifestyle factors (smoking, alcohol, weight, 'stress') are relevant for reflux. Cancer incidence increases with **age**, and only becomes significant at age > 45 years. **Dysphagia and weight loss** require urgent investigation.

Examination
Physical examination is usually unrewarding, but may suggest neoplasia (weight loss, lymph nodes, abdominal masses). Abdominal obesity predisposes to reflux.

Investigations
Investigations should exclude serious pathology, principally gastric cancer, as well as establish the diagnosis, when possible. In many the cancer risk is low and empirical treatment without endoscopy is indicated.
- **Blood tests**: a normal FBC and ESR help exclude serious pathology. Positive *Helicobacter pylori* serology might suggest peptic ulcer disease but does not exclude an upper GI malignancy.
- **Endoscopy** is the definitive test for oesophagitis, Barrett's epithelium and peptic ulcer disease. Antral biopsy and urease test for *H. pylori* (CLO test)—see p. 216.
- **Barium swallow/meal** now largely surpassed by endoscopy.

Management
- Treat the underlying cause: see relevant sections (see pp. 215–16).
- Treat the symptoms: see pp. 215–16.

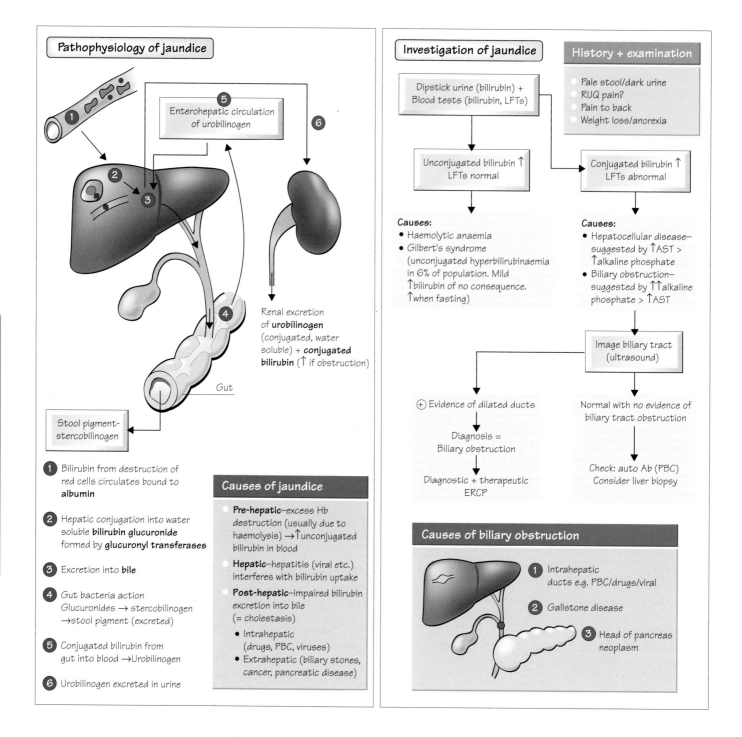

Pathophysiology of jaundice

Enterohepatic circulation of urobilinogen

Renal excretion of **urobilinogen** (conjugated, water soluble) + **conjugated bilirubin** ($\uparrow$ if obstruction)

Gut

Stool pigment-stercobilinogen

1. Bilirubin from destruction of red cells circulates bound to **albumin**

2. Hepatic conjugation into water soluble **bilirubin glucuronide** formed by **glucuronyl transferases**

3. Excretion into **bile**

4. Gut bacteria action Glucuronides → stercobilinogen →stool pigment (excreted)

5. Conjugated bilirubin from gut into blood →Urobilinogen

6. Urobilinogen excreted in urine

Causes of jaundice

- **Pre-hepatic**—excess Hb destruction (usually due to haemolysis) →$\uparrow$unconjugated bilirubin in blood
- **Hepatic**—hepatitis (viral etc.) interferes with bilirubin uptake
- **Post-hepatic**—impaired bilirubin excretion into bile (= cholestasis)
  - Intrahepatic (drugs, PBC, viruses)
  - Extrahepatic (biliary stones, cancer, pancreatic disease)

Investigation of jaundice

Dipstick urine (bilirubin) + Blood tests (bilirubin, LFTs)

History + examination
- Pale stool/dark urine
- RUQ pain?
- Pain to back
- Weight loss/anorexia

Unconjugated bilirubin $\uparrow$ LFTs normal

Conjugated bilirubin $\uparrow$ LFTs abnormal

Causes:
- Haemolytic anaemia
- Gilbert's syndrome (unconjugated hyperbilirubinaemia in 6% of population. Mild $\uparrow$bilirubin of no consequence. $\uparrow$when fasting)

Causes:
- Hepatocellular disease—suggested by $\uparrow$AST > $\uparrow$alkaline phosphate
- Biliary obstruction—suggested by $\uparrow\uparrow$alkaline phosphate > $\uparrow$AST

Image biliary tract (ultrasound)

(+) Evidence of dilated ducts

Normal with no evidence of biliary tract obstruction

Diagnosis = Biliary obstruction

Diagnostic + therapeutic ERCP

Check: auto Ab (PBC) Consider liver biopsy

Causes of biliary obstruction

1. Intrahepatic ducts e.g. PBC/drugs/viral
2. Gallstone disease
3. Head of pancreas neoplasm

Overall approach

Jaundice can result from a range of underlying pathologies varying from an acute short-lived illness (e.g. hepatitis A) to the terminal stages of a chronic disease, which might have been subclinical until that point (e.g. decompensated chronic liver disease).

Aetiology

Jaundice is either 'pre-hepatic', 'hepatic' or 'post-hepatic', although in practice it is often sufficient to restrict one's considerations to whether jaundice is hepatocellular (i.e. hepatic) or obstructive/cholestatic (i.e. post-hepatic) (Table 22.1).

Differential diagnosis

A useful way of considering the differential diagnosis is to clinically distinguish the acute from the chronic conditions and, where possible, to clarify whether the liver injury is hepatocellular or obstructive.

Clinical Presentations at a Glance

Table 22.1 Aetiology of jaundice.

	Acute	Chronic

Hepatocellular	Acute hepatitis
	  Viral hepatitides
	  Drug reactions
	  Budd–Chiari syndrome
		Chronic liver disease
		  Hepatitis B & C
		  Alcoholic disease
		  Autoimmune hepatitis
		  Haemochromatosis

Cholestatic	Biliary obstruction
	  2° biliary disease
	  Pancreatitis
	  Pancreatic carcinoma
		Chronic biliary disease
		  1° biliary cirrhosis
		  1° sclerosing cirrhosis

Table 22.2 Differences between acute and chronic disease underlying jaundice.

	Acute	Chronic
Preceding ill health	0	0–++
Skin signs of chronic liver disease	0	0–++
Encephalopathy	0–+	+–+++
Ascites	0	++
Varices at endoscopy	0	++
Spleen at ultrasound	0	++
Laboratory tests		
MCV	→	↑
Urea	→	↓
Albumin	→ or ↓	↓–↓↓
Prothrombin	→ or ↓	↑–↑↑

Clinical features

The two important clinical features to identify are:
• Is this patient's presentation of an acute illness or a chronic disease (Table 22.2)?
• Is there any clinical evidence of a failing liver?
  These questions can often be answered from a careful history.
• What is the **duration of the illness** and was the patient unwell **before** the jaundice developed? This is often very revealing and may suggest a long period of subclinical ill health before the jaundice.
• Are there clinical **features of cholestasis** (i.e. biliary obstruction)? Pale stools, dark urine and pruritis.
• Has the patient experienced any **pain**? Pain and cholestasis should be considered to be related to gallstones until proved otherwise. The presence of fever and rigors strongly suggests ascending cholangitis as the diagnosis.
• Are there **risk factors** for chronic liver disease? Alcohol—seek corroborative evidence. Travel/contacts—favoured sexual practices. Intravenous drug use—ask specifically. It is useful to know local slang for intravenous drugs such as cocaine (e.g. Coke, Crack, Charlie), heroin (e.g. Brown) and amphetamines (e.g. Speed).
• Are there any **features of liver failure**? Hepatic encephalopathy (reduced attention span, daytime somnolence).

Examination

The depth of the jaundice does not actually matter as much as recognizing features of a failing liver and determining whether there is chronic liver disease.

Recognition of liver failure

Encephalopathy is the clinical hallmark of liver failure. Any degree of confusion/delirium in a jaundiced patient should be considered a manifestation of encephalopathy. The specific clinical sign to seek is the metabolic flap or asterixis. Other bedside measures of encephalopathy include a constructional dyspraxia (e.g. drawing a five-pointed star) or the Trail Test (i.e. a join-the-dots test against the clock).

Features of chronic liver disease

Typically, features of chronic liver disease are considered to be the peripheral stigmata such as palmar erythema, Dupuytren's contracture, spider naevi and gynaecomastia. In practice, the clinical features of portal hypertension, such as ascites and splenomegaly, often represent 'harder' physical signs.

Investigation

• **Blood tests**: FBC—a macrocytosis, thrombocytopenia or low urea may indicate chronic liver disease. A low sodium (not caused by diuretics) is a poor prognostic sign.
• **Liver blood tests**: a low albumin may be non-specific. The transaminases give a clue as to whether the jaundice is predominantly hepatocellular (AST [aspartate transaminase] or ALT [alanine transaminase] > alkaline phosphatase) or cholestatic (alkaline phosphatase or γGT [gamma-glutamyl transferase] > AST), although the picture is often 'mixed'. Normal transaminases suggest the less common conditions of haemolysis or Gilbert's syndrome.
• **Viral hepatitis serology**: hepatitis A IgM is diagnostic of acute hepatitis A. Acute hepatitis B is typified by HBSAg (hepatitis B surface antigen) and detection of hepatitis B DNA. Hepatitis C rarely causes an acute hepatitis but is an increasing cause of chronic liver disease.
• **Autoantibody profile and immunoglobulin**: anti-double-stranded DNA, anti-nuclear, anti-mitochondrial, anti-smooth muscle, anti-liver-kidney microsomal antibodies and serum IgG, IgA and IgM.
• **Liver ultrasonography**: this may help in consolidating a clinical diagnosis. It may show focal liver abnormalities such as metastatic deposits, liver abscesses or vascular abnormalities. It might show evidence of biliary obstruction (i.e. dilated bile ducts) and possibly the underlying cause (i.e. gallstones, pancreatic cancer). It might be normal.
• **MRCP and EUS**: increasingly non-invasive methods such as magnetic resonance cholangiopancreatography (MRCP) and endoscopic ultrasound (EUS) are used to delineate biliary anatomy as a prelude to endoscopic intervention
• **ERCP**: if there is good evidence of biliary obstruction ERCP remains the definitive test in determining whether the obstruction is intra-luminal (i.e. gallstones in the common bile duct [CBD]) or extra-luminal (i.e. malignant stricture from carcinoma of the pancreas). It may also allow relief of the obstruction.
• **Liver biopsy**: liver histology remains the definitive investigation for hepatocellular jaundice and also, in some cases, cholestatic jaundice (e.g. primary biliary cirrhosis, drug-induced intra-hepatic cholestasis). The absolute indications vary.

Management

The management of patients with jaundice depends very much on the underlying cause and whether or not there are clinical features of liver failure. Jaundice itself does not necessarily require hospital admission —many of the underlying conditions and associated complications do.

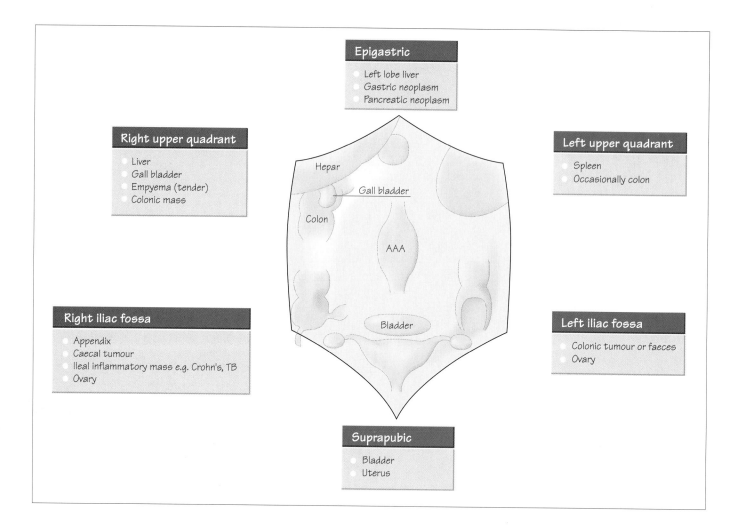

Epigastric
- Left lobe liver
- Gastric neoplasm
- Pancreatic neoplasm

Right upper quadrant
- Liver
- Gall bladder
- Empyema (tender)
- Colonic mass

Left upper quadrant
- Spleen
- Occasionally colon

Right iliac fossa
- Appendix
- Caecal tumour
- Ileal inflammatory mass e.g. Crohn's, TB
- Ovary

Left iliac fossa
- Colonic tumour or faeces
- Ovary

Suprapubic
- Bladder
- Uterus

Labels within figure: Hepar, Gall bladder, Colon, AAA, Bladder

Overall approach

It is uncommon to present solely with a palpable abdominal mass. Usually there are other clinical features such as weight loss or pain, or a change in bowel habit.

Differential diagnosis

The differential diagnosis depends largely on the position of the mass (see figure).

Investigations

• **Blood tests**: FBC, ESR—anaemia, thrombocytosis and raised inflammatory markers suggest an underlying chronic disease process. Biochemistry—abnormal liver blood tests likewise suggest malignancy. The role of tumour markers (e.g. carcinoembryonic antigen [CEA], CA 19–9, α-fetoprotein? [α-FP]) in the diagnosis of malignancy is limited. Their value is greater in monitoring response to treatment and identification of disease relapse.

• **Ultrasonography**: this is very useful for the investigation of liver masses and tumours arising from the kidneys and pelvic organs (ovaries, uterus). It is less useful for characterization of masses arising from the gut or pancreas.

• **CT scan**: CT is very useful for characterization of retroperitoneal masses and is probably more sensitive in identifying intra-abdominal lymphadenopathy. As CT relies on defining tissue planes (i.e. solid tissue against fat), it is probably more sensitive in relatively obese individuals.

• **Biopsy/Aspiration**: if there is doubt about the nature of an intra-abdominal mass, it is usually possible to aspirate cells for cytology or take a percutaneous biopsy under ultrasonic or CT guidance.

• **Laparoscopy, laparotomy**: if the nature of a mass remains obscure, the definitive approach is ultimately a laparotomy and excision. Increasingly, laparoscopy is being used in these circumstances.

Clinical Presentations at a Glance

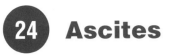

24 Ascites

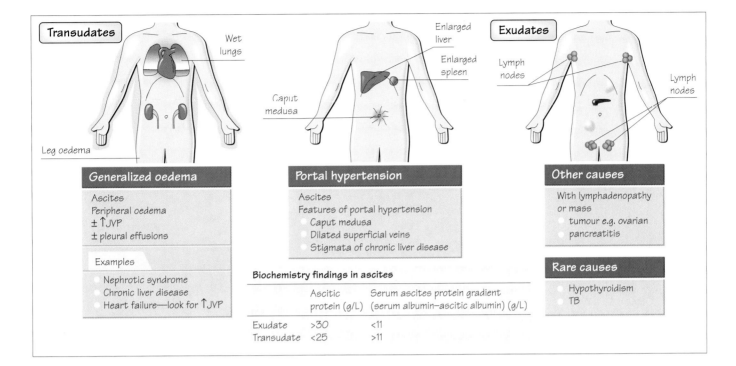

Ascites is the pathological accumulation of fluid within the abdominal peritoneal cavity. Ascites usually reflects the presentation of a chronic disease process that may have been subclinical until that point.

As with other fluid collections ascites is clinically classified as being either an exudate or a transudate (see figure).
• **Exudative ascites** has a high protein content and occurs with inflammatory (e.g. infective) or malignant processes.
• **Transudative ascites** occurs in cirrhosis as a result of portal hypertension and alterations in renal sodium clearance. Pericardial constriction and nephrotic syndrome also cause transudative ascites.

The differential diagnosis most commonly lies between decompensated chronic liver disease and intra-abdominal malignancy. Other conditions that may present with ascites include heart failure, nephrotic syndrome, pancreatitis and tuberculosis.

Clinical features and investigations

There are few features in the history and examination that confidently distinguish between the late presentation of liver disease and malignancy. Notwithstanding this, any historical factor pointing to a liver disease is important. Gross ascites is evident on inspection with pronounced distension of the abdomen, often with eversion of the umbilicus. Lesser degrees of ascites can be demonstrated clinically by eliciting 'shifting dullness'. Helpful investigations include:
• **Examination of the ascitic fluid**: for colour, protein (see above), cell count, bacterial culture and cytology for malignant cells. Ascites is often straw coloured in cirrhosis, bloody in malignancy and cloudy in infection. A leukocyte count of more than > 250 polymorphs/mL is considered diagnostic of bacterial peritonitis regardless of whether or not organisms are subsequently cultured. Cytology (large volume and fresh specimen) may be diagnostic of malignancy. Pancreatitis may present with ascites, so amylase should be measured.
• **Ultrasonography of the abdomen**: to measure liver size (small in cirrhosis), signs of portal hypertension (splenomegaly), and patency of portal and hepatic veins (to exclude hepatic vein thrombosis and the Budd–Chiari syndrome). It is also useful for finding focal abnormalities (suggestive of disseminated malignancy) and for the diagnosis of intra-abdominal tumours (e.g. ovarian).
• **Other blood tests**: biochemistry and liver blood tests looking for markers of liver cirrhosis (low albumin, hyperbilirubinaemia, elevated liver enzymes, low platelets, etc.). Tumour markers if malignancy suspected (especially α-fetoprotein for hepatoma, CA 125 for ovarian carcinoma).

Management

Exudative ascites. Treat underlying cause:
• **Bacterial peritonitis**: antibiotics. In low protein ascites prophylactic antibiotics are of benefit.
• **Malignant ascites**: treat underlying malignancy (commonly ovarian). Therapeutic paracentesis is often needed for symptomatic relief.
Transudative ascites. Treat the underlying cause, and consider:
• Fluid and salt restriction—fluid restriction to ≤ 1–1.5 L/day and a 'no-added salt' diet are usually sufficient.
• Diuretics—usually spironolactone ± furosemide (frusemide).
• Therapeutic paracentesis for refractory ascites (i.e. ascites not responding to diuretic therapy or only with unacceptable drug side effects —hyponatraemia, encephalopathy, etc.).

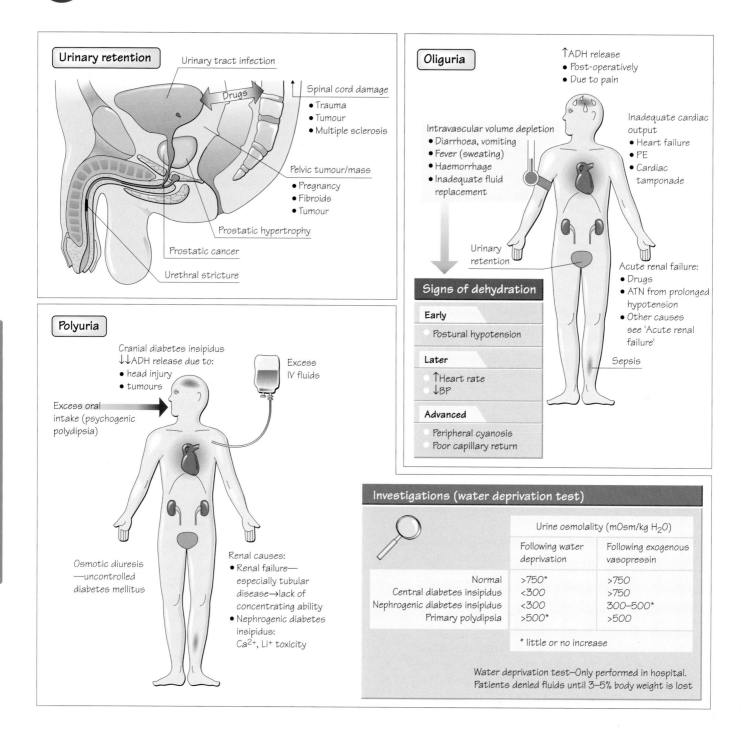

Urinary retention

Urinary tract infection

Drugs

Spinal cord damage
- Trauma
- Tumour
- Multiple sclerosis

Pelvic tumour/mass
- Pregnancy
- Fibroids
- Tumour

Prostatic hypertrophy

Prostatic cancer

Urethral stricture

Oliguria

↑ADH release
- Post-operatively
- Due to pain

Intravascular volume depletion
- Diarrhoea, vomiting
- Fever (sweating)
- Haemorrhage
- Inadequate fluid replacement

Inadequate cardiac output
- Heart failure
- PE
- Cardiac tamponade

Urinary retention

Acute renal failure:
- Drugs
- ATN from prolonged hypotension
- Other causes see 'Acute renal failure'

Sepsis

Signs of dehydration

Early

Postural hypotension

Later

↑Heart rate
↓BP

Advanced

Peripheral cyanosis
Poor capillary return

Polyuria

Cranial diabetes insipidus
↓↓ADH release due to:
- head injury
- tumours

Excess IV fluids

Excess oral intake (psychogenic polydipsia)

Osmotic diuresis —uncontrolled diabetes mellitus

Renal causes:
- Renal failure— especially tubular disease→lack of concentrating ability
- Nephrogenic diabetes insipidus: Ca^{2+}, Li^+ toxicity

Investigations (water deprivation test)

	Urine osmolality (mOsm/kg H_2O)	
	Following water deprivation	Following exogenous vasopressin
Normal	>750*	>750
Central diabetes insipidus	<300	>750
Nephrogenic diabetes insipidus	<300	300–500*
Primary polydipsia	>500*	>500
* little or no increase		

Water deprivation test—Only performed in hospital. Patients denied fluids until 3–5% body weight is lost

Polyuria

Polyuria is defined as excessive urine volume, usually ≥ 3 L/day, and may be accompanied by the symptoms of frequency, nocturia, thirst and polydipsia. The presentation with polyuria requires careful investigation because serious underlying disease may be responsible.

Several conditions may produce polyuria, of which the most common is diabetes mellitus in which increased concentrations of glucose have an osmotic diuretic effect. The causes may be grouped as follows:
1 Excess intake of fluid (primary polydipsia), often associated with psychological disturbance leading to compulsive water drinking. Very rarely, hypothalamic lesions lead to primary polydipsia.
2 An increase in tubular solute load, as with urea in chronic renal failure or glucose from hyperglycaemia caused by diabetes mellitus.
3 Disordered medullary concentration gradient as a consequence of medullary disease (see Chapter 134).
4 A reduction in antidiuretic hormone (ADH) production (diabetes insipidus), after trauma to the head, or tumours or infections of the hypothalamus or pituitary (cranial diabetes insipidus).

Table 25.1 Typical urine findings in conditions that cause acute renal failure.

Condition	Dipstick test	Sediment analysis	Urine osmolality (mOsm/kg)	Fractional excretion of sodium (%)
Prerenal azotaemia	Trace or no proteinuria	A few hyaline casts possible	> 500	< 1
Renal azotaemia				
Tubular injury ischaemia	Mild-to-moderate proteinuria	Pigmented granular casts	< 350	> 1
Nephrotoxins	Mild-to-moderate proteinuria	Pigmented granular casts	< 350	> 1
Acute interstitial nephritis	Mild-to-moderate proteinuria; haemoglobin; leukocytes	White cells and white-cell casts; eosinophils and eosinophil casts; red cells	< 350	> 1
Acute glomerulonephritis	Moderate-to-severe proteinuria; haemoglobin	Red cells and red-cell casts; red cells can be dysmorphic	> 500	< 1
Postrenal azotaemia	Trace or no proteinuria; can have haemoglobin, leukocytes	Crystals, red cells, and white cells possible	< 350	> 1

Source: R. Thadhani, M. Pascual, J.V. Bonventre. Acute renal failure, *N Engl J Med* 1996; 334: 1448–60. © Massachusetts Medical Society.

5 Conditions in which the tubular response to ADH is impaired. These conditions are termed 'nephrogenic diabetes insipidus', and include hypercalcaemia, chronic potassium depletion, lithium toxicity and a rare inherited insensitivity to ADH with X-linked recessive inheritance.
6 After relief of urinary tract obstruction.

Investigations

In a patient with polyuria, the history may provide the diagnosis. If blood glucose is normal, creatinine, calcium and potassium should be determined. If diabetes insipidus is suspected, then a water deprivation test should be undertaken with caution; the patient must not become excessively dehydrated. A water deprivation test involves the restriction of water intake until a 3–5% weight loss has been achieved. Measurements of urinary osmolality and change in urinary osmolality in response to exogenous vasopressin will help establish the diagnosis.

Management

It is important to correct any major water deficit and then to treat the underlying cause. Cranial diabetes insipidus can be treated by the intranasal administration of the vasopressin analogue desmopressin.

Oliguria in the hospital setting

Oliguria is defined as a urine output of less than 0.5 mL/kg weight per h. Many patients in hospital develop a reduced urinary output, postoperative or severely ill individuals. Urine output is a sensitive indicator of fluid status and haemodynamic adequacy. It is particularly important because oliguria may progress to acute renal failure.

In managing the oliguric patient, information can be acquired from the history, examination and investigations. The central issues are whether or not the patient is replete with fluid and excluding urinary retention.

An accurate **history** of fluid intake and output should be obtained. Fluid balance and daily weight charts should be examined; loss of fluid from haemorrhage, diarrhoea, sweating, vomiting, drains and insensible losses all need to be considered. The presence of nausea, pain and thirst should be elicited. Symptoms suggesting urinary retention should be elicited and a urinary catheter passed if there is any doubt.

Examination should include palpation and percussion for a bladder. Signs suggesting fluid depletion or overload should be sought. The signs of fluid depletion include tachycardia, hypotension and, most importantly, postural hypotension, while other signs can include dry mucous membranes, reduced skin turgor, cool peripheries and contracted peripheral veins. Signs of fluid overload can include orthop-noea, peripheral oedema, pulmonary oedema, elevated jugular venous pressure (JVP) and hypertension. A central venous line provides a direct measurement of central venous pressure (CVP) if the fluid status is uncertain.

Investigations and management

Fluid depletion can be accompanied by elevations in haematocrit, serum albuminuria and creatinine (with urea often disproportionately raised), whereas in fluid overload a chest X-ray may reveal pulmonary oedema.

In the oliguric patient, a urinary catheter should be passed or, if present, flushed to exclude blockage. If the situation suggests fluid depletion then intravenous fluid often normal saline should be given. Replacement fluid should be administered until postural hypotension has been abolished and the JVP or CVP is normal. If there is evidence of haemorrhage, then a blood transfusion may be necessary; the source of blood loss should be identified and treated, and clotting times determined. If the patient appears replete with fluid then other causes of shock need to be considered, such as sepsis, myocardial infarction and pulmonary embolism, and other causes of acute renal failure considered. In this situation, an urgent renal tract ultrasound should be requested, mainly to look for signs of renal tract obstruction (e.g. hydronephrosis), but also to look for kidney size (small in long-standing disease).

It is particularly important to avoid agents that may jeopardize renal perfusion (e.g. NSAIDs, or ACE inhibitors), which could be nephrotoxic or accumulate in renal failure.

Urinary retention

Acute urinary retention is a sudden inability to micturate, usually accompanied by pain, the sensation of bladder fullness and a distended bladder. **Chronic urinary retention** is the presence of an enlarged bladder often without difficulty in micturition, and accompanied by frequency, overflow incontinence, bladder distension and sometimes renal failure. Causes can be grouped into those affecting the lumen of the urethra or the urethral wall, compression of the urethra or neurological dysfunction. Urinary tract infection or pain may precipitate retention. Urinary retention is common in elderly men due to benign prostatic hyperplasia or, more rarely, prostate carcinoma; in young adults serious neurological causes may be responsible and require careful investigation. Rectal examination is crucial to assess both the prostate, and anal tone and sensation. In women, urinary obstruction is more likely to be neurological or gynaecological in origin, than urological.

Dysuria, frequency and urgency

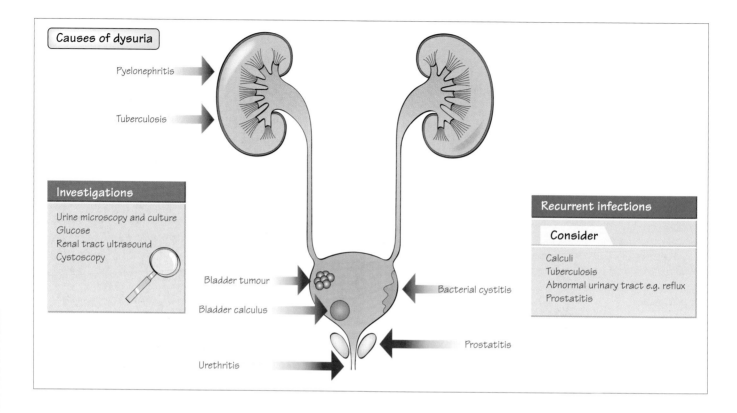

Causes of dysuria

Pyelonephritis

Tuberculosis

Investigations

Urine microscopy and culture
Glucose
Renal tract ultrasound
Cystoscopy

Bladder tumour

Bladder calculus

Urethritis

Bacterial cystitis

Prostatitis

Recurrent infections

Consider

Calculi
Tuberculosis
Abnormal urinary tract e.g. reflux
Prostatitis

Dysuria is painful micturition. Urinary frequency is the increased frequency of the passage of urine. Urgency is an uncontrollable desire to micturate. In adults the most common cause is urinary tract infection, a very common diagnosis in both general practice and hospital patients.

Urinary tract infection (UTI) is commonly looked for in elderly patients (or children) who present with confusion or general deterioration. It is particularly important in all UTIs to ensure that there is pyuria accompanying any bacterial growth from urine, because imperfectly sterile urine collections are common. Bacteriuria is likely to be of clinical significance only when accompanied by pyuria.

Acute pyelonephritis

Urinary tract infection involving the upper urinary tract has systemic features such as fever, which may be very high > 39°C, rigors, malaise, anorexia and flank pain, in addition to the symptoms of dysuria, frequency and urgency. Predispositions include calculi, reflux, obstruction and a neurogenic bladder. Pyelonephritis in an obstructed kidney requires urgent medical attention because of the irreversible loss of renal substance that may occur. The key to diagnosis is the microscopy and culture of urine and blood cultures. There should be pyuria, i.e. > 100 000 white cells/mL, bacteriuria, and often microscopic or even macroscopic haematuria.

Acute cystitis

Urinary tract infection confined to the urinary tract is commonly called acute cystitis. It is more common in women and coliforms are the most common infecting organisms:

- *Escherichia coli* (90% outpatients, 50% of inpatients).
- *Proteus* and *Klebsiella* species (5% outpatients, 20% of inpatients).
- Enterococci (2% outpatients, 7% of inpatients).
- *Pseudomonas* species (0.5% outpatients, 6% of inpatients).

The symptoms may include dysuria, suprapubic discomfort, frequency, urgency, incontinence and microscopic haematuria. Diagnosis, as in pyelonephritis, requires the growth of a pathogenic organism from a midstream specimen of urine, in a quantity sufficient to cause disease, defined as ≥ 100 000 colony-forming units/mL.

Urethritis

This is a condition characterized by dysuria and meatal discharge, and is most commonly caused by sexually transmitted diseases such as gonococci or *Chlamydia* species.

Investigations

The microscopy and culture of urine are critical in the management of patients suspected of having a UTI. Other important investigations, particularly with recurrent infections, may include urine or blood glucose, ultrasonography of the renal tract, plain X-rays of kidney, ureters and bladder, urography or cystoscopy. In recurrent infection, obstruction, prostatitis, renal calculi, diabetes mellitus and bladder dysfunction are potential causes.

Other causes of dysuria, other than acute bacterial infection, are bladder calculi, bladder tumours and tuberculosis (suggested by sterile pyuria in a patient at risk of TB).

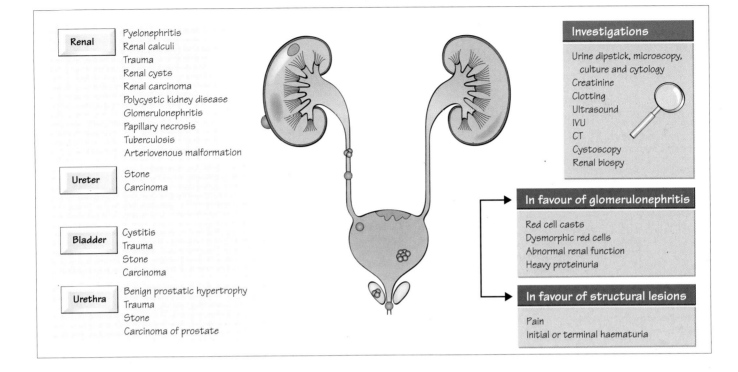

Renal
- Pyelonephritis
- Renal calculi
- Trauma
- Renal cysts
- Renal carcinoma
- Polycystic kidney disease
- Glomerulonephritis
- Papillary necrosis
- Tuberculosis
- Arteriovenous malformation

Ureter
- Stone
- Carcinoma

Bladder
- Cystitis
- Trauma
- Stone
- Carcinoma

Urethra
- Benign prostatic hypertrophy
- Trauma
- Stone
- Carcinoma of prostate

Investigations
- Urine dipstick, microscopy, culture and cytology
- Creatinine
- Clotting
- Ultrasound
- IVU
- CT
- Cystoscopy
- Renal biospy

In favour of glomerulonephritis
- Red cell casts
- Dysmorphic red cells
- Abnormal renal function
- Heavy proteinuria

In favour of structural lesions
- Pain
- Initial or terminal haematuria

Blood can appear in the urine from pathology at any site in the urinary tract. Even small quantities of blood can produce a significantly pink or red coloration in the urine (although this should not be confused with ingested substances that discolour the urine, such as beetroot or rifampicin antibiotic). The small amount of blood found occasionally in urine from patients with glomerulonephritis can make it 'smoky' in appearance. Urinary dipsticks are very sensitive to even very few red cells in the urine. False-positive dipstick tests for blood can be obtained with the presence of free haemoglobin or myoglobin in the urine and by contamination from menstruation. Haematuria can be confirmed by finding more than 3 red blood cells (RBCs) per high power field of spun urine. The continuing presence of microscopic (present on dipstick and seen on microscopy) or macroscopic haematuria (frank blood) requires investigation because it may be the first presentation of a carcinoma of the renal tract or a serious renal disorder.

History and examination

The history should include the timing of haematuria in the urinary stream; blood on commencing urination suggests a urethral cause, whereas terminal haematuria suggests a bladder or prostatic cause. The presence of painful urination suggests a UTI or calculus. Episodes of trauma should be sought, as should systemic features that might indicate a disseminated malignancy or a vasculitis.

The examination must include palpation for abdominal masses, which might represent renal tumours or cysts, a rectal examination for prostatic malignancy and measurement of blood pressure.

Investigations

Once the presence of haematuria has been established, urinary microscopy may indicate whether the source is likely to be glomerular or from elsewhere in the urinary tract. Red blood cells of glomerular origin tend to be dysmorphic and may be accompanied by red cell casts and significant proteinuria. Glomerular disease can affect renal function (see Chapter 131) which should be assessed with plasma creatinine, and is often accompanied by proteinuria. Abnormal urine cytology can suggest the presence of a urinary tract malignancy. If a structural lesion of the renal tract is suspected, imaging can be undertaken with plain radiography looking for radio-opaque calculi (although only a small minority of stones are visible on plain X-ray), ultrasonography looking for renal masses or bladder lesions, intravenous urography (IVU), particularly looking for filling defects within the urinary tract and cross-sectional imaging with computed tomography (CT) or magnetic resonance imaging (MRI). If these investigations fail to demonstrate a cause for the haematuria, a cystoscopy should be performed. If a renal source of the haematuria is suspected (usually because there is proteinuria or biochemical evidence of renal impairment), a renal biopsy may be undertaken which could reveal a glomerulonephritis. The most common renal cause of microscopic or macroscopic haematuria is IgA nephropathy. In this condition the haematuria commonly follows a sore throat. Bleeding disorders are a very rare cause of haematuria but should be looked for if the patient has other sites of abnormal blood loss.

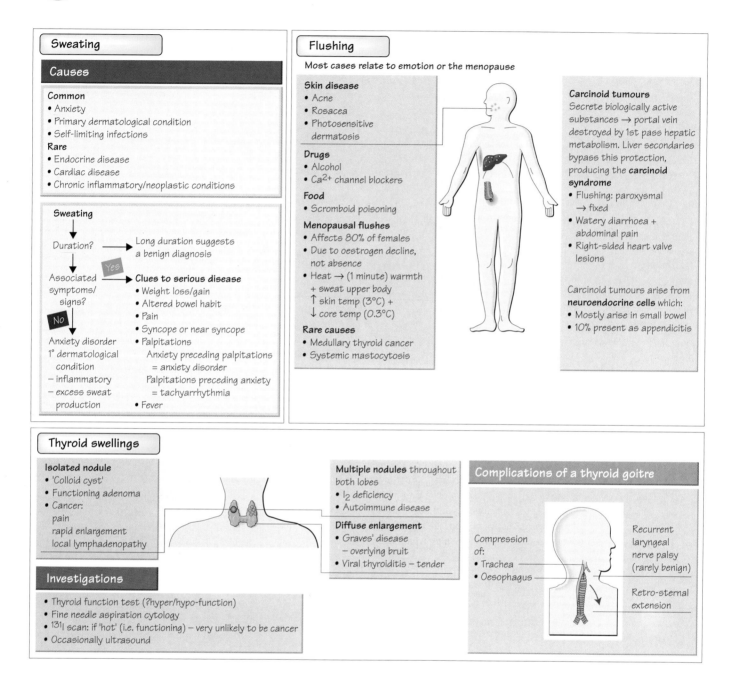

Sweating

Causes

Common
• Anxiety
• Primary dermatological condition
• Self-limiting infections

Rare
• Endocrine disease
• Cardiac disease
• Chronic inflammatory/neoplastic conditions

Sweating
↓
Duration? → Long duration suggests a benign diagnosis
↓
Associated symptoms/ signs? — Yes → Clues to serious disease
• Weight loss/gain
No • Altered bowel habit
Anxiety disorder • Pain
1° dermatological • Syncope or near syncope
condition • Palpitations
– inflammatory   Anxiety preceding palpitations
– excess sweat   = anxiety disorder
production   Palpitations preceding anxiety
                   = tachyarrhythmia
              • Fever

Flushing

Most cases relate to emotion or the menopause

Skin disease
• Acne
• Rosacea
• Photosensitive dermatosis

Drugs
• Alcohol
• Ca^{2+} channel blockers

Food
• Scromboid poisoning

Menopausal flushes
• Affects 80% of females
• Due to oestrogen decline, not absence
• Heat → (1 minute) warmth + sweat upper body ↑ skin temp (3°C) + ↓ core temp (0.3°C)

Rare causes
• Medullary thyroid cancer
• Systemic mastocytosis

Carcinoid tumours
Secrete biologically active substances → portal vein destroyed by 1st pass hepatic metabolism. Liver secondaries bypass this protection, producing the **carcinoid syndrome**
• Flushing: paroxysmal → fixed
• Watery diarrhoea + abdominal pain
• Right-sided heart valve lesions

Carcinoid tumours arise from **neuroendocrine cells** which:
• Mostly arise in small bowel
• 10% present as appendicitis

Thyroid swellings

Isolated nodule
• 'Colloid cyst'
• Functioning adenoma
• Cancer:
   pain
   rapid enlargement
   local lymphadenopathy

Multiple nodules throughout both lobes
• I_2 deficiency
• Autoimmune disease

Diffuse enlargement
• Graves' disease – overlying bruit
• Viral thyroiditis – tender

Complications of a thyroid goitre

Compression of:
• Trachea
• Oesophagus

Recurrent laryngeal nerve palsy (rarely benign)

Retro-sternal extension

Investigations

• Thyroid function test (?hyper/hypo-function)
• Fine needle aspiration cytology
• ^{131}I scan: if 'hot' (i.e. functioning) – very unlikely to be cancer
• Occasionally ultrasound

Sweating

Sweating is a very common problem, but is very rarely serious. The crucial diagnostic features are: how long the problem has been present (the longer it has been there, the more benign the underlying process); presence of any associated symptoms (isolated sweating is rarely serious, and usually indicates a dermatological hypersecretory response rather than any underlying disease process); and is there anxiety during the episode (anxiety normally indicates a panic disorder; very rarely it indicates an underlying phaeochromocytoma).

Differential diagnosis

The most common causes are an anxiety state or a primary dermatological condition. Rarely other disease processes are responsible:
• **Endocrine disease**: thyrotoxicosis, acromegaly, phaeochromocytoma, hypoglycaemia (sweating several hours after last eating, relieved by food), hypogonadism (particularly menopausal).
• **Cardiovascular disease**: paroxysmal tachyarrhythmias cause paroxysmal sweating, although it is very rare for palpitations not to be felt during the event. Very poor left ventricular function causes sweating on effort, as does marked physical deconditioning.

- **Pain**: if severe enough pain induces sweating. Some individuals sweat with mild pain.
- **Inflammatory disease**: including cancer (lymphoma or other malignancies), and chronic infection may cause sweats, particularly at night (see Chapter 36).

Investigations

The aim of any investigation is to exclude serious diagnoses. Laboratory tests: thyroid-stimulating hormone (TSH); inflammatory markers; growth hormone/insulin growth factor 1 (IGF-1) (for acromegaly); urinary catecholamines (for phaeochromocytoma), fasting glucose and insulin (for hypoglycaemia), follicle-stimulating hormone (FSH)/oestradiol + testosterone (for hypogonadism); blood film ± marrow. Other tests: very rarely a 24-h ECG recording (for arrhythmias) may be indicated.

Treatment is for the underlying cause. If no cause is found, cleanliness, antiperspirants and physical conditioning are all that can be recommended.

Flushing

Flushing is very common. The usual causes are emotions in youth. Diseases that may have flushing as a prominent component include:
- **Primary dermatological disease**, especially photodermatosis (see page 129), including autoimmune (systemic lupus erythematosus), metabolic (porphyria), plant related (especially hogweed) and drug induced (especially amiodarone); rosacea.
- **Drugs**: alcohol (especially in those deficient in alcohol dehydrogenase or on disulfiram—Antabuse) and calcium channel blockers commonly cause flushing, as do spicy foods, food allergy and toxin ingestion.
- **Hypogonadism**: most commonly menopause related (see Chapter 150).
- **Carcinoid syndrome**: carcinoid tumours are rare neuroendocrine tumours that are found in the small bowel and the lung. Many are benign. Malignant ones metastasize to the liver, from where they secrete biochemically active substances (principally 5-hydroxytryptamine [5HT; serotonin], but also bradykinin, histamine and other peptides) into the systemic circulation, causing paroxysmal flushing which later becomes fixed, with abdominal pain (cramps) and watery diarrhoea—the carcinoid syndrome. Right-sided valve lesions (tricuspid regurgitation or pulmonary stenosis) occur in 50%. The diagnosis is confirmed by finding hepatic metastasis on liver ultrasound examination and high levels of 5HT metabolites, particularly 5-hydroxyindoleacetic acid (5HIAA) in the urine. Octreotide, a somatostatin analogue that inhibits the release of many gut peptides, is very useful in controlling symptoms. The tumour is remarkably slow growing and patients live for many years.
- **Medullary thyroid carcinoma**: this rare tumour can present as a neck mass, as Cushing's syndrome or as intractable diarrhoea. However, it can also produce a carcinoid-like syndrome. Of the tumours 75% are sporadic in elderly individuals, but 25% relate to genetic cancer syndromes—multiple endocrine neoplasia (MEN).
- **Systemic mastocytosis**: overproliferation of mast cells. May be associated with myeloproliferative disorders or lymphomas. Intermittent release of histamine occurs, causing a syndrome much like scromboid poisoning (see below). Hepatosplenomegaly, portal hypertension and malabsorption also occur.
- **Scromboid poisoning**: histamine is produced by certain bacteria (e.g. *Proteus morgani*) acting to decompose the flesh of scromboid (e.g. tuna, mackerel) or non-scromboid (e.g. sardines, pilchards) fish. Symptoms occur 4 hours after ingestion: flushing, urticarial itching, conjunctival suffusion, abdominal colic; vomiting and diarrhoea may also occur. Treatment is supportive, anti-histamines may help, and symptoms disappear after several hours.

Investigations

Investigation is indicated only if unusual features are present, suggestive of underlying disease. Laboratory tests: FSH + testosterone/oestradiol, urinary 5HIAA for carcinoid syndrome, calcitonin, bone marrow and urinary analysis for histamine excretion in suspected mastocytosis. Treatment is of the underlying cause.

Thyroid swellings

Thyroid nodules occur in 5% (F : M = 5 : 1) and may relate to a thyroid goitre (eu- or hypothyroid), benign adenomas (associated with hyperthyroidism) or malignancy (2% of goitres). Cancer is suggested by known radiation exposure, a family history or voice change (resulting from recurrent laryngeal nerve palsy). Goitres and cancer can cause tracheal (stridor) or oesophageal (dysphagia) compression. Investigation of any thyroid swelling means assessing the following:
- Thyroid status
- Ultrasonography of the thyroid gland. If nodules are found, radionuclide scanning may be indicated—cancer appears as a 'cold' nodule. Fine-needle aspiration cytology is indicated for cold nodules to determine whether cancer is present.

Cancer is treated by excision (good prognosis histology), thyroxine (to suppress TSH, which otherwise promotes tumour growth) and radioactive iodine in hormonally active diseases.

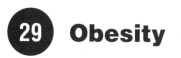

29 Obesity

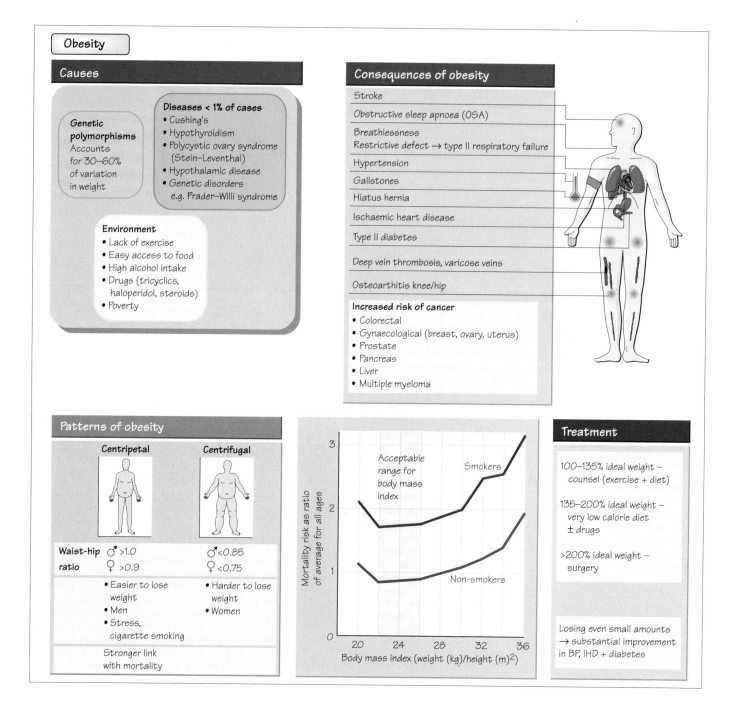

Definition

Obesity is defined as a body mass index (BMI) $> 30 \, kg/m^2$ (BMI = weight (kg)/[height^2 (m^2)]). Normal = 20–25; overweight = 25–30; obese > 30.

Epidemiology

The prevalence of obesity has doubled in the last decade and is now 15% in the UK adult population and up to 50% of certain racial groups.

Aetiopathogenesis of 'simple obesity'

• **Genetic**: genetic effects are complex and polygenic with heritability of 30–60%.

• **Environment**: readily available high-fat, energy-rich diet, associated with a sedentary lifestyle.

• **Neuroendocrine**: neuropeptide Y (hypothalamic hormone stimulating appetite) and leptin (peptide hormone synthesized in adipose tissue which acts in the hypothalamus to suppress food intake and energy

Table 29.1 Multiple endocrine and neurological events involved in the regulation of body weight.

	Afferent signals ↓ appetite or ↑ energy expenditure	Afferent signals ↑ appetite or ↓ energy expenditure
GI tract	Glucagon, cholecystokinin, glucagons-like peptides, bombesin peptides, glucose	Opioids, neurotensin, growth-hormone-releasing hormone, somatostatin
Endocrine system	Epinephrine (β-adrenergic effect), oestrogens	Epinephrine (α-adrenergic effect)
Adipose tissue	Leptin	
Peripheral nervous system	Norepinephrine (β-adrenergic effect)	Norepinephrine (α-adrenergic effect)
Central nervous system	Dopamine, γ-aminobutyric acid, serotonin, cholecystokinin	Galanin, opioids, growth hormone-releasing hormone, somatostatin

These afferent signals act on hypothalamic tracts; involving norepinephrine, serotonin, neuropeptide Y, melanocyte-concentrating hormone, glucagon-like peptide I, corticotropin-releasing hormone

The hypothalamic tracts effect changes, via the sympathetic nervous system, parasympathetic nervous system and thyroid hormone

These systems then affect energy intake and expenditure

expenditure), in association with other neurotransmitters, regulates energy balance, though multiple other pathways are also involved (Table 29.1). Mutations of receptors and transmitters are associated with obesity in mice models and rare cases of severe obesity in humans.

Assessment of the obese patient

The clinical assessment of the obese patient involves:
- **Confirmation of obesity** from the BMI and assessment of the pattern of body fat distribution: centripetal obesity (waist/hip ratio > 0.9 in women, > 1.0 in men) is associated with increased cardiovascular risk.
- **Time course of obesity**: whether the obesity is old or new, any previous treatment for obesity and the family history. Explanation of obesity may also be sought by reference to eating habits and physical activity.
- **Secondary causes**: very rare but should be considered if in recent (less than several) years there has been unexplained weight gain, and/or if there are abnormal physical signs or biochemical tests. Underlying pathology may include Cushing's syndrome (24-h urinary free cortisol), hypothyroidism (TSH), hypothalamic disorder (uncontrolled appetite), Prader–Willi syndrome (deletion of part of the long arm of chromosome 15, resulting in hypogonadism and obesity) or Lawrence–Moon–Biedl syndrome.
- **Overall cardiovascular risk assessment**: from fasting glucose and lipid profile, and other standard risk factors (age, sex, blood pressure, smoking status, alcohol consumption) and presence of vascular disease.

Complications

- **Metabolic complications**: hyperinsulinaemia and insulin resistance ± impaired glucose tolerance/diabetes mellitus; hypertension; ischaemic heart disease (fourfold risk if BMI > 29); cerebrovascular disease; hyperlipidaemia.
- **Hepatic complications:** obesity can lead to fatty infiltration of the liver, which can produce a hepatitis, and eventually lead to cirrhosis.
- **Physical problems**: osteoarthritis, varicose veins, hernias (both hiatal hernia and abdominal hernias), hypoventilation (obstructive sleep apnoea [OSA]—see page 177), operative complications.
- **Increased cancer risk**: breast, ovary, endometrium, prostate, cervix, bowel.

Management

Severely obese individuals need treatment to improve prognosis, improve self-image and minimize symptoms, particularly those arising from physical problems. In men, being 10% overweight increases death rates by 13%, and being 20% overweight by 25%.
- **Behavioural modifications**: these include dietary restriction, exercise and, most importantly, stopping smoking. Alcohol intake should be minimized.
- **Drugs**: amphetamine derivatives (dexfenfluramine, fenfluramine) suppress appetite but have been withdrawn as a result of side effects (cardiac valvulopathy). Orlistat inhibits gastric and pancreatic lipases and reduces fat absorption. Selective serotonin reuptake inhibitors (SSRIs), such as high-dose fluoxetine, can be effective. Sibutramine (serotonin and noradrenaline reuptake inhibitor) increases satiety and reduces food intake. All drugs should be continued only if weight loss of 0.5 kg/week occurs. Most drugs work transiently only.
- **Surgery**: gastroplasty, jaw-wiring and gastric balloon are rarely indicated. Sudden profound weight loss has its own complications, including liver dysfunction and QT interval prolongation, which may predispose to an arrhythmic death.

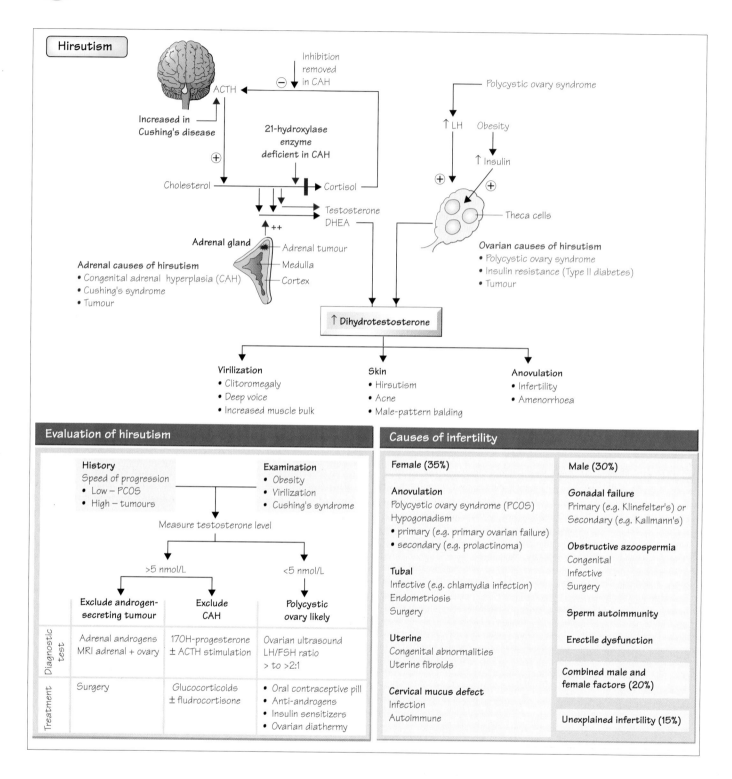

Hirsutism
- Increased in Cushing's disease

ACTH

Inhibition removed in CAH ⊖

21-hydroxylase enzyme deficient in CAH

Polycystic ovary syndrome

↑ LH   Obesity

↑ Insulin

Cholesterol   Cortisol

⊕

Theca cells

Testosterone DHEA

Adrenal gland   ++

Adrenal tumour
Medulla
Cortex

Adrenal causes of hirsutism
- Congenital adrenal hyperplasia (CAH)
- Cushing's syndrome
- Tumour

Ovarian causes of hirsutism
- Polycystic ovary syndrome
- Insulin resistance (Type II diabetes)
- Tumour

↑ **Dihydrotestosterone**

Virilization
- Clitoromegaly
- Deep voice
- Increased muscle bulk

Skin
- Hirsutism
- Acne
- Male-pattern balding

Anovulation
- Infertility
- Amenorrhoea

Evaluation of hirsutism

History
Speed of progression
- Low – PCOS
- High – tumours

Examination
- Obesity
- Virilization
- Cushing's syndrome

Measure testosterone level

>5 nmol/L   <5 nmol/L

	Exclude androgen-secreting tumour	Exclude CAH	Polycystic ovary likely
Diagnostic test	Adrenal androgens MRI adrenal + ovary	17OH-progesterone ± ACTH stimulation	Ovarian ultrasound LH/FSH ratio > to >2:1
Treatment	Surgery	Glucocorticoids ± fludrocortisone	• Oral contraceptive pill • Anti-androgens • Insulin sensitizers • Ovarian diathermy

Causes of infertility

Female (35%)	Male (30%)
Anovulation Polycystic ovary syndrome (PCOS) Hypogonadism • primary (e.g. primary ovarian failure) • secondary (e.g. prolactinoma)	**Gonadal failure** Primary (e.g. Klinefelter's) or Secondary (e.g. Kallmann's)
Tubal Infective (e.g. chlamydia infection) Endometriosis Surgery	**Obstructive azoospermia** Congenital Infective Surgery
Uterine Congenital abnormalities Uterine fibroids	**Sperm autoimmunity** **Erectile dysfunction**
Cervical mucus defect Infection Autoimmune	**Combined male and female factors (20%)**
	Unexplained infertility (15%)

Hirsutism

Hirsutism is common, affects 5% of premenopausal women and usually does not indicate a serious underlying illness. It is defined as excess hair growth in women from increased androgen production or skin sensitivity. Hair growth follows a male pattern, being predominantly facial (moustache or beard), thoracic and abdominal. Male pattern baldness may develop. Serious disease should be suspected in thin women, in rapidly progressive hirsutism, in treatment-resistant hypertension or with severe menstrual disruption. If other features of virilization are present (clitoromegaly, deep voice, male muscle pattern), investiga-

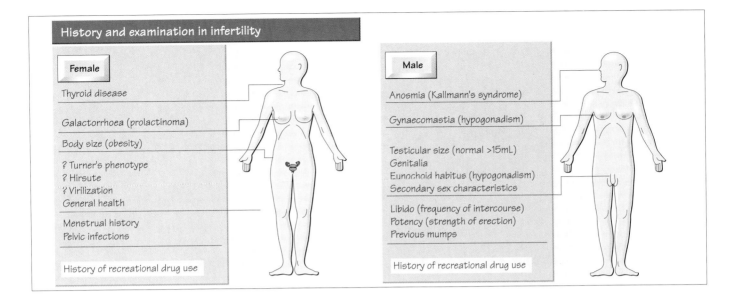

History and examination in infertility

Female
- Thyroid disease
- Galactorrhoea (prolactinoma)
- Body size (obesity)
- ? Turner's phenotype
- ? Hirsute
- ? Virilization
- General health
- Menstrual history
- Pelvic infections
- History of recreational drug use

Male
- Anosmia (Kallmann's syndrome)
- Gynaecomastia (hypogonadism)
- Testicular size (normal >15mL)
- Genitalia
- Eunochoid habitus (hypogonadism)
- Secondary sex characteristics
- Libido (frequency of intercourse)
- Potency (strength of erection)
- Previous mumps
- History of recreational drug use

tions for androgen-secreting tumours are mandatory. The principal causes of hirsutism are listed below, although it is important to realize that hirsutism is often only a minor feature of these conditions:

- **Obesity** is commonly associated with mild hirsutism. Insulin resistance increases virilization. Acanthosis nigricans occurs in morbidly obese individuals.
- **Polycystic ovary syndrome** (PCOS): in its various forms, this affects 10% of women, commonly causing hirsutism. Sufferers often have marked obesity and mild virilization (male pattern hair growth and loss, with acne).
- **Familial or idiopathic hirsutism**, usually in those of Mediterranean descent.
- **Drugs**, particularly androgenic steroids in athletes.
- **Cushing's syndrome** (< 1% of cases): patients rarely present with hirsutism; rather they present with treatment-resistant hypertension and profound hypokalaemia. The physical signs are of thin skin, proximal myopathy and (new and progressive) central obesity.
- **Congenital adrenal hyperplasia** (CAH) is a rare cause of hirsutism (there are 4000 CAH patients in the UK), more common in Jewish people, and usually caused by deficiency of 21-hydroxylase—the enzyme responsible for degrading progesterone (via intermediate metabolites) to corticosterone, cortisol and aldosterone. 17-Hydroxyprogesterone accumulates, is turned into androstenedione and, in turn, to testosterone. Symptoms thus relate in part to corticosteroid deficiency and in part to testosterone excess. Hirsutism occurs and there may be a history of acute adrenal failure when physically stressed. High 17-hydroxyprogesterone levels are found, particularly with ACTH (adrenocorticotrophin hormone) stimulation. Treatment is corticosteroids sufficient to suppress ACTH-mediated 17-hydroxyprogesterone production.
- **Androgen-secreting tumour**: < 1% of cases; can arise from the ovary or the adrenals.

The diagnostic approach is to pick up clues from the history and examination (particularly of marked virilization) and to measure luteinizing hormone (LH)/FSH and androgen levels. Testosterone levels > 5 nmol/L (i.e. significant elevation) imply that a diagnosis of PCOS is unlikely and that of an androgen-secreting tumour or CAH more likely. These need to be formally excluded by hormonal assessment, including stimulation tests and imaging. Treatment of hirsutism, other than that for the underlying cause, involves weight loss, cosmetic approaches (waxing, electrolysis and laser), and insulin-sensitizing drugs (metformin). Anti-androgen therapy may be helpful, usually in conjunction with the combined oral contraceptive pill.

Infertility

Infertility is defined as failure of pregnancy after 1 year of unprotected intercourse. It affects 10–15% of couples.

Investigation of male and female partners is needed for diagnosis. In men the first investigation is semen analysis: normal sperm motility and numbers exclude the man from further investigation. If abnormal sperm are found, FSH and testosterone are measured to investigate the possibility of gonadal failure. If such investigations are normal, then the possibility of obstruction to the spermatic tract should be considered. In the female, midluteal progesterone is measured. Normal levels (> 30 pmol/L) imply normal gonadal function. The problem may then be mechanical and laparoscopy for tubal patency is undertaken. Abnormally low progesterone suggests lack of ovulation, e.g. premature ovarian failure or polycystic ovarian syndrome.

Management

Treatment is for the underlying cause where possible. For anovulation, clomiphene, gonadotrophin-releasing hormone or gonadotrophins are used in low FSH cases (success rate 50–80%), and oocyte donation for raised FSH (50% success rate) cases. Complex stimulatory regimens are needed in male pituitary failure. For tubal or obstructive azoospermia, reconstructive surgery is occasionally possible and, for oligospermia, intracytoplasmic sperm injections (success rate 20% per cycle). Unexplained infertility may respond to *in vitro* fertilization (IVF) (25% success rate/cycle, though rates much lower in women + 40 years).

31 Erectile dysfunction and gynaecomastia

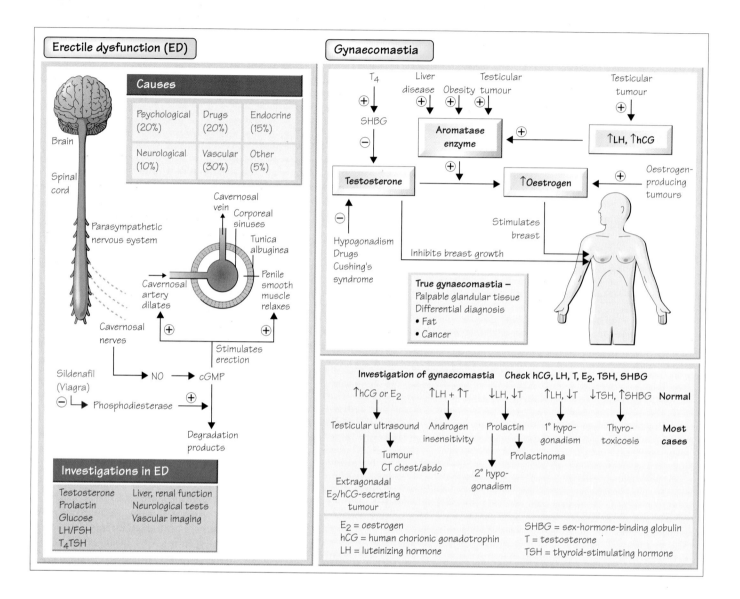

Erectile dysfunction

The normal erection is produced by vasoconstriction of the venous outflow from the penis, resulting in blood distending the corpus cavernosa of the penis. Venous vasoconstriction is the result of activation of sacral autonomic nerves raising levels of venous cyclic adenosine monophosphate (cAMP). Interference with the arterial supply, autonomic nervous system or libido impairs erectile success. Erectile dysfunction (impotence) is defined as an inability to achieve an erection sufficient for sexual intercourse. It affects 10% of males and is caused by the following:

• **Drugs** commonly underlie or exacerbate erectile failure. Particularly important ones are β-blockers, calcium channel blockers and psychotropic agents.

• **Psychological problems**: very common; may cause erectile failure in its own right or complicate a pre-existing medical problem. Impotence is usually variable in severity and morning erections are unaffected.

• **Endocrine disorders**: 30–60% of people with diabetes develop

some degree of erectile failure with diabetes of 6 years' standing, as a result of both neuropathy and vascular disease. Thyroid dysfunction can also impair libido and potency. Androgen deficiency underlies 20% of cases of impotence seen in endocrinology outpatients. Sex drive (libido) is reduced in hypogonadal males.

• **Vascular disease**: peripheral arterial insufficiency involving the terminal aorta is a very common cause for erectile dysfunction. Penis venous insufficiency is, however, a very rare cause of impotence.

• **Neurological disease**: many neurological diseases can be associated with impotence, either directly through damage to the mechanisms involved in erection and ejaculation, or indirectly through psychological mechanisms. Particularly important causes include damage to sacral nerves, as can occur with radical prostrate or pelvic surgery.

• **Other diseases**: structural penile abnormalities such as Peyronie's disease (which results in a curved penis) and microphallus may cause erectile dysfunction. Any chronic debilitating disease can also cause impotence.

Assessment

The key is to diagnose any underlying disease, which may require specific therapy. Absence of early morning erections is a good clue to the presence of underlying organic disease. Symptoms and signs of hypogonadism must be carefully sought (gynaecomastia, decrease in body hair, fatigue, testicular shrinkage, premature osteoporosis). Arterial disease and the factors closely associated with it should be looked for (intermittent claudication, presence of diabetes, hypertension or smoking, presence of foot and leg pulses). General health needs to be assessed, particularly whether liver, renal or neurological disease is present.

Treatment

Any underlying disease should be treated and any causative drug withdrawn.

- **Sildenafil (Viagra)**: inhibits penile phosphodiesterase type 5 and enhances the normal erectile response to sexual stimulation. Contraindicated in recent myocardial infarction/cerebrovascular accident, and if nitrates have been taken ≤ 24 h (profound hypotension can occur).
- **Intracavernous papaverine or prostaglandin E_1 (PGE_1) injection**: these are potent vasoconstrictors and, when injected into the penile venous circulation, they prevent venous efflux, so producing erections. Erections may be persistent and painful (priapism).
- **Vacuum devices**: these work but are cosmetically unattractive.
- **Penile prosthesis**: surgically implanted prosthetic devices can stiffen, or mechanically inflate, the penis; they are useful when other forms of treatment are ineffective, undesirable or contraindicated.

Gynaecomastia

This is enlargement of the male breast as a result of hyperplasia of glandular tissue. It affects 30% of men aged < 30 years and 50% aged > 45 years. It rarely indicates serious underlying disease but if the patient is thin, enlargement is rapid and in particular the glandular tissue is > 5 cm, underlying disease should be suspected.

- **Obesity**: probably the most common cause. Increased peripheral conversion of testosterone to oestrogen by the aromatase enzyme promotes breast growth.
- **Drugs**: a common cause—digoxin, cimetidine, spironolactone, antiandrogens, alcohol, marihuana, etc.
- **Hyperprolactinaemia**: high prolactin levels induce secondary hypogonadism, depressing testosterone levels, allowing for unopposed oestrogen action on the breast.
- **Hypogonadism**: suspect if libido is reduced with erectile dysfunction.
- **Systemic disease**: liver cirrhosis, chronic renal failure.
- **Underlying hormone-secreting tumour**: accounts for 3% of cases of gynaecomastia seen in the endocrine service. The tumour may be testicular (human chorionic gonadotrophin [hCG], oestradiol or aromatase producing), adrenal (oestradiol producing) or a lung/gastrointestinal cancer producing hCG.

Breast cancer, which is rare, may need to be excluded if the breast tissue is hard. Treatment is mainly by reassurance, withdrawal of the offending drug and advice on weight reduction. Drugs may help (antioestrogens, or those that inhibit the aromatase enzyme). Surgical resection is occasionally used.

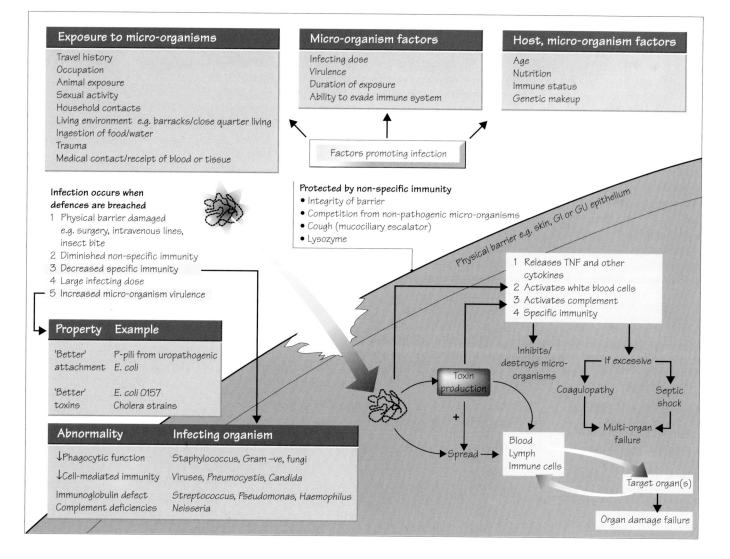

Introduction

Despite antimicrobial agents being available for over 50 years, infections remain a significant health problem. The burden of infectious disease remains enormous as a result of: antibacterial resistance, the emergence of new diseases (e.g. HIV infection) and continuing poverty.

Infections once considered controlled, e.g. tuberculosis, are reemerging as significant problems in both resource-poor and rich countries.

Infection and the development of clinical disease depend on the interaction of a microbial agent and the host. Both must be considered together, e.g. normally non-pathogenic organisms may cause clinical disease in a severely immunocompromised host.

The host

The host influence can be divided into two categories:

1 Factors determining exposure to micro-organisms: assessment of exposure is crucial in evaluating the risk of infection in an individual (or community). One must consider:

- An individual's interaction with his or her environment.

- Particular behaviour that may lead to the acquisition of a potential pathogen.
- Prevalence of infection in a community.

2 Factors influencing infection and development of disease after exposure.

Infection and disease
Non-specific defences

- **Physical barriers**: intact skin and mucosa prevent entry of micro-organisms.
- **Competition** from commensal flora: colonization of body sites by 'normal' bacterial flora prevents colonization with pathogenic micro-organisms.
- **Biological barriers**: e.g. oral lysozyme secretion.
- **Chemical barriers**: e.g. the acidic environment of the stomach.
- **Physical mechanisms expelling bacteria**, e.g. urine flow through the urinary system, the cough reflex and the action of microcilia in the respiratory tract all reduce the risk of bacterial multiplication.

- **Disturbances in non-specific defences** contribute to the risk of infection in hospital, e.g. urinary catheters or intravenous lines breaching skin/mucosal integrity or the effect of antibiotics on bacterial flora.

Specific defences

These comprise the inflammatory response mounted by:
- Neutrophils and phagocytes
- The complement system
- Specific cell-mediated and antibody responses to pathogens

In any infection, always consider whether a patient has had temporary or permanent changes in any of the defence systems (see pp. 312 and 314). Age, immunization, chronic illnesses and drug treatment all affect immunity.

Micro-organisms

Disease may arise from:
- **Endogenous infection**, i.e. micro-organisms that exist on mucosal surfaces or are present in the body as a latent infection. Endogenously acquired infections have become progressively more important in developed countries as populations become more immunocompromised.
- **Exogenous infection** from the environment:
  - Direct exogenous transmission occurs from contact with, or droplet transmission from, an infected host or source (such as soil).
  - Indirect infection may be vector borne, airborne, or result from transmission via infected blood, blood products or organs.

Disease production

Pathogens have evolved strategies to make transmission and establishment in a host more efficient. Different strategies may be utilized by the micro-organism at different points in the establishment of an infection; the following are examples:
- **Mucosal contact**: attachment to epithelial surfaces may be crucial for pathogenesis:
  - Non-specific interactions occur between the hydrophilic bacterial cell surface and the lipophilic endothelial cell surface.
  - Specific interactions also exist: uropathogenic *Escherichia coli* have P-pili—hair-like structures—which adhere to a specific glycolipid receptor on the urothelial cell surface. Influenza virus attaches to cells via the haemagglutinin antigen.
- **Invasion**: pathogens cause damage by invading deeper tissues, either through breaks in the skin or mucosal surface or specific invasion mechanisms:
  - Schistosomal cerceriae are able to penetrate intact skin and subsequently enter the circulation.
  - Enteropathogens utilize a number of different mechanisms to adhere to and then interact with the M cell, leading to transport, invasion and multiplication.
  - *Neisseria meningitidis*, or measles virus, is able to penetrate epithelium.
- **Immune evasion**: some pathogens produce enzymes or have surface components, which bind or inhibit secretory IgA on mucosal surfaces:
  - The polysaccharide capsule of bacteria such as *Streptococcus pneumoniae* or *Haemophilus influenzae* type B helps to resist phagocytosis.
  - *Leishmania*, *Mycobacterium* or *Salmonella* spp. are able to survive and multiply within macrophages.
- **Toxin production** is important in the pathogenesis of some diseases:
  - Cholera toxin activates the adenyl cyclase mechanisms of host intestinal cells, thus producing excretion of large amounts of fluid and electrolytes.
  - The lipopolysaccharide of Gram-negative bacteria (endotoxin) has an important role in the production of the sepsis syndrome.

Potential clinical consequences of infection

Acute
- Cytokine effects: fever, malaise, anorexia, catabolic state, increased white cells and platelets, acute phase response with increased acute phase proteins.
- Circulatory failure (see p. 20).
- Disseminated intravascular coagulation.
- Organ damage and failure, from shock, e.g. renal failure, direct invasion, e.g. pneumonia producing respiratory failure, or by multiple mechanisms, e.g. adult respiratory distress syndrome.

Chronic
- Muscle wasting and weight loss.
- Anaemia of chronic disease: see p. 338.
- Permanent organ destruction: e.g. liver cirrhosis from chronic hepatitis, left ventricular failure after viral myocarditis, permanent paralysis following polio.
- Post-infective phenomena: e.g. lactose intolerance after gastrointestinal infection.

Autoimmune phenomena
- Generalized syndromes: e.g. poststreptococcal phenomena, such as rheumatic fever.
- System specific: the following are examples:
  - Neurological: Guillain–Barré syndrome after a viral infection, cerebellar syndromes after chickenpox.
  - Haematological: haemolytic anaemia after mycoplasma infection.
  - Rheumatological: arthritis after gut or urinary tract infection in genetically predisposed individuals.
  - Dermatological: scarlet fever (rash after streptococcal infection).

Treatment of infection
- Symptomatic support: antipyretics, maintenance of hydration.
- Antimicrobials: either empirical or targeted to identified micro-organisms.
- Removal of sources of infection: e.g. draining abscesses or removing infected lines.
- Circulatory and vital organ support in severe infection.
- Many infections (particularly viral) are self-limiting and do not need specific treatment.

Prevention of infection
- Avoidance of exposure to, or contact with, pathogen.
- Immunization, with either:
  - live attenuated organisms; or
  - killed organisms or components of microbes.

33 Diagnosis of infection

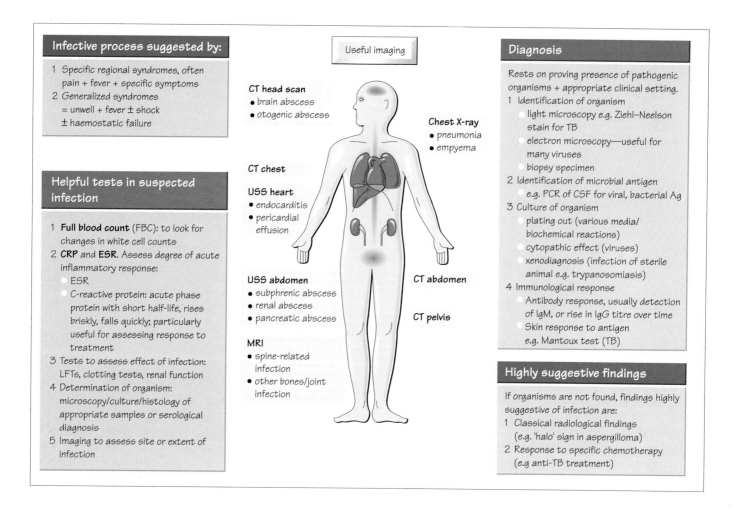

Infective process suggested by:

1 Specific regional syndromes, often pain + fever + specific symptoms
2 Generalized syndromes
= unwell + fever ± shock
± haemostatic failure

Helpful tests in suspected infection

1 **Full blood count** (FBC): to look for changes in white cell counts
2 **CRP** and **ESR**. Assess degree of acute inflammatory response:
   - ESR
   - C-reactive protein: acute phase protein with short half-life, rises briskly, falls quickly; particularly useful for assessing response to treatment
3 Tests to assess effect of infection: LFTs, clotting tests, renal function
4 Determination of organism: microscopy/culture/histology of appropriate samples or serological diagnosis
5 Imaging to assess site or extent of infection

Useful imaging

CT head scan
- brain abscess
- otogenic abscess

CT chest

USS heart
- endocarditis
- pericardial effusion

USS abdomen
- subphrenic abscess
- renal abscess
- pancreatic abscess

MRI
- spine-related infection
- other bones/joint infection

Chest X-ray
- pneumonia
- empyema

CT abdomen

CT pelvis

Diagnosis

Rests on proving presence of pathogenic organisms + appropriate clinical setting.
1 Identification of organism
   - light microscopy e.g. Ziehl–Neelson stain for TB
   - electron microscopy—useful for many viruses
   - biopsy specimen
2 Identification of microbial antigen
   - e.g. PCR of CSF for viral, bacterial Ag
3 Culture of organism
   - plating out (various media/biochemical reactions)
   - cytopathic effect (viruses)
   - xenodiagnosis (infection of sterile animal e.g. trypanosomiasis)
4 Immunological response
   - Antibody response, usually detection of IgM, or rise in IgG titre over time
   - Skin response to antigen e.g. Mantoux test (TB)

Highly suggestive findings

If organisms are not found, findings highly suggestive of infection are:
1 Classical radiological findings (e.g. 'halo' sign in aspergilloma)
2 Response to specific chemotherapy (e.g anti-TB treatment)

Introduction

The initial history and examination usually indicate the most appropriate investigation. In a febrile patient with no obvious source of infection, useful screening investigations include a full blood count (FBC), liver function tests, C-reactive protein (CRP) or erythrocyte sedimentation rate (ESR), blood cultures, urine examination and a chest X-ray.

Full blood count

- **Normochromic/normocytic anaemia** occurs in many chronic infections.
- **Raised neutrophil count** or toxic granulation suggests bacterial sepsis.
- **Raised lymphocyte count**: occurs in many viral infections and some bacterial disorders, e.g. typhoid and brucellosis. Atypical lymphocytes suggest Epstein–Barr (EBV) or cytomegalovirus (CMV) infection.
- **Low neutrophil count**: iatrogenic immunosuppression or infection with typhoid, brucellosis or rickettsial disease. Bad prognostic indicator in severe sepsis.
- **Low lymphocyte count**: consider HIV but common with other acute infections.
- **Low platelet count**: malaria and dengue fever particularly. May reflect disseminated intravascular coagulation in severe sepsis.

- **Eosinophilia** may occur in schistosomiasis and tissue invasion by other parasites.

CRP and ESR

The erythrocyte sedimentation rate (ESR) is the rate at which red cells settle through plasma. It is dependent on age, sex, serum immunoglobulins, especially IgM, acute phase proteins such as fibrinogen, and the shape and nature of the red cell membrane. It increases with age (the normal ESR is ≤ [age/2] + 10). In infection and inflammation it rises only slowly (over 2 weeks). The C-reactive protein (CRP) rises within 4–8 hours after the onset of infection and has a half-life in the circulation of approximately 8 hours. The two tests are not interchangeable. The ESR is sometimes compared to the glycosylated haemoglobin in diabetes (which gives an estimate of the glycaemic control over the previous few weeks), while the ESR gives an average of inflammation over the preceding 2–3 weeks; the CRP, like glucose, gives the picture over the preceding 8 hours.

Liver function tests

Abnormalities in liver function suggest either local infective processes (hepatitis, hepatic abscesses or biliary sepsis) or systemic or disseminated infections.

Microscopy

Direct microscopy of clinical samples allows rapid identification of micro-organisms. Wet preparations are used for urine examination or the detection of parasites in the stool.

Fixed stained preparations

• Gram staining: the size, morphology (cocci or bacilli) and staining characteristics (Gram positive or negative) of bacteria give a clue to their species but definitive identification is rarely possible. Commensal or contaminant organisms in samples make interpretation of microscopy difficult. Microscopy is most useful for samples from normally sterile sites, e.g. cerebrospinal fluid (CSF), joints, etc.

• Specific stains are used to identify some micro-organisms: e.g. Ziehl–Neelsen stain for mycobacteria or Giemsa for parasites such as malaria on a blood slide.

Viruses cannot be identified on standard microscopy but fluorescent linked antibodies visualize viruses in clinical specimens. Electron microscopy is used to identify certain viruses, e.g. rotaviruses in stool or herpes group viruses (varicella-zoster virus) in fluid from chickenpox lesions.

Culture

Culture is the definitive diagnostic method for most bacteria and fungi. Samples are cultured on growth media, whose composition and incubation conditions are varied to isolate particular micro-organisms selectively. Organisms are identified by colonial morphology, growth on specific media and in certain conditions, and by biochemical reactions. Contamination of cultures with normal flora, such as non-pathogenic mouth organisms in sputum samples, may make detection of pathogens more difficult. The use of antibiotic discs on culture plates allows determination of antibiotic sensitivity.

Blood cultures may identify bacteraemia resulting from infection in many different sites of the body. Repeated blood cultures are necessary to detect organisms that do not grow readily or to determine the significance of an initial isolation of a potential contaminating organism. It is rare to need more than three sets of blood cultures. Blood cultures should ideally be taken before starting antibiotics. In 'difficult to diagnose' infection, it is often appropriate to stop all antibiotics and reculture all potentially infected sites, e.g. blood, etc.

Viral culture is useful for isolation of some viruses: cell monolayers are inoculated with appropriate clinical samples. Viral growth may be recognized by specific cytopathic effects or the use of fluorescent antibodies.

Serology

Some organisms, particularly viruses, are difficult to culture. Serology measures the host immunological response to an infection. IgM antibodies or a rise in IgG titre over 10–14 days (acute and convalescent titres) can be considered to be diagnostic of recent infection. Serology is particularly useful in infections such as hepatitis or glandular fever.

Histology

Infection can sometimes be diagnosed only by seeing specific pathological features on examination of tissue. These features include:

• Inclusion bodies in tissue suggesting viral infections such as CMV.

• Granulomas: associated with a number of different infections, including tuberculosis (TB).

• Demonstration of fungi in tissues by the use of specific stains.

Tissue biopsy may sometimes be the only way of making a diagnosis in difficult cases.

Molecular methods

Molecular techniques are becoming increasingly important.

• Nucleic acid hybridization can identify organisms in clinical specimens, e.g. *Chlamydia* or *Neisseria* spp.

• Amplification techniques are useful for detection of small amounts of nucleic acid from organisms that are difficult to culture. The polymerase chain reaction (PCR) is most commonly used in the diagnosis of herpes simplex and meningococcaemia, and to quantify viral load in hepatitis B/C or HIV. The number of applications is expanding rapidly.

• Molecular techniques are now commonly used for the rapid detection of resistance in organisms such as *Mycobacterium tuberculosis*.

Imaging

• **Chest X-ray** can show focal lesions, which are undetectable clinically, and is mandatory in those suspected of having an infection in whom the source is not readily apparent.

• **Abdominal and pelvic ultrasonography** may detect hepatic lesions, identify abdominal nodes and locate intra-abdominal or pelvic abscesses as a source of fever or bacteraemia.

• **Computed tomography** (CT) scans are useful in examining all regions of the body in a search for, or to delineate the extent of, infection. They are a useful early investigation in febrile patients with presumed but unidentified infections, and may identify a source in patients who are bacteraemic with gastrointestinal pathogens. CT also allows for diagnostic sampling and therapeutic drainage in many situations.

• **Magnetic resonance imaging** (MRI) is used in the diagnosis of soft tissue and bony/joint infections.

• **Nuclear imaging**: white cell scans are rarely useful because they do not distinguish acute inflammation from infection, nor detect chronic low-grade infections caused by parasites, viruses, mycobacteria or fungi. They are sometimes helpful in identification of the site of pyogenic inflammation. Newer techniques include the use of radioactively labelled antibiotics.

• **Cardiac ultrasonography** is indicated in suspected bacterial endocarditis, to look for vegetations and assess valve function. If bacteraemia/septicaemia has occurred caused by *Staphylococcus aureus*, early cardiac ultrasonography is mandatory to exclude endocarditis.

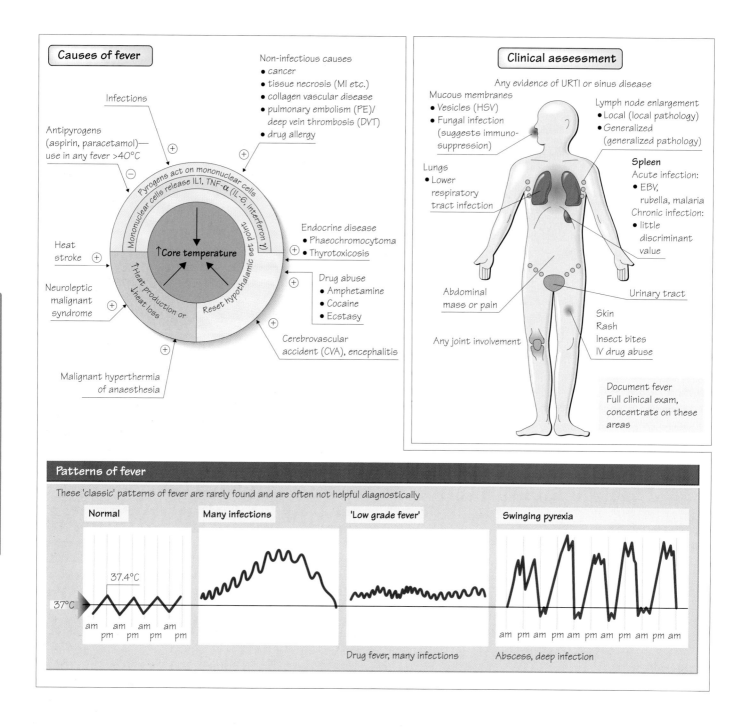

Fever

Fever is a physiological response where the body temperature is increased due to resetting of the normal hypothalamic set point. Normal body temperature varies considerably between individuals (oral range, 36.0–37.7°C) and varies diurnally (peaks—evening; troughs—early morning).

Hyperthermia

Hyperthermia is an elevated body temperature above the hypothalamic set point. It occurs when there is excessive heat production, reduced heat loss or hypothalamic damage. Temperatures > 41°C are rarely the result of infections and usually imply loss of thermoregulation.

Pathogenesis of fever

Fever is produced by the effect of exogenous pyrogens. Infectious agents and their breakdown products or toxins are the most common triggers of fever. Other molecules, such as immune complexes and lymphocyte products, can also elicit a febrile response. These are the basis of fever in malignancy, drug reactions and connective tissue disorders.

Assessment of the patient

History

When evaluating those with possible infection, several important questions should be considered:

• Is the illness likely to represent infection, i.e. are other causes of fever absent or at least unlikely?

• Where is the probable site of infection? Symptoms arising from a particular organ are usually reliable guides to the site of infection. Non-specific symptoms (e.g. fever, muscular aches) may occur in generalized infection (septicaemia or viraemia).

• What are the most likely organisms to be involved? Usually determined by combining the age, immune status, instrumentation and travel history, with the specific symptoms/duration and probable organ affected.

• What organisms has this patient been exposed to? Is there local epidemic disease, e.g. influenza, cholera?

• Are there reasons why this patient might be prone to infection? An immunocompromised host is more prone to infection, including with normally non-pathogenic organisms.

• Is there evidence of tissue or organ damage (kidney, lung, etc.)? This may indicate whether specific supportive therapy (such as mechanical ventilation, blood pressure support) is needed.

A good clinical history is essential and the systems enquiry is particularly useful to establish a focus of infection.

Symptoms

• Duration (acute or chronic) and fever pattern may help diagnose the organism.

• Rigors are uncommon in non-infective causes of fever.

• Weight loss occurs in several chronic infections (TB, endocarditis, intra-abdominal abscesses).

• Symptoms suggest localization.

Exposure to pathogens

Travel history allows an assessment of exposure to potential pathogens. The occupation may be relevant to pathogen exposure, e.g. leptospirosis in sewage workers. Animal contact is relevant in zoonotic infection. Sexual history and intravenous drug usage are also important.

Drug history

Recently prescribed medication, herbal or traditional remedies may cause fever. Previous antimicrobial treatment may modify clinical presentation or make isolation of an organism difficult. Drugs may modify immunity (e.g. corticosteroids). Antipyretics may reduce fever response.

Past medical history

• Other underlying illnesses may increase infection risk.

• Frequent infections suggest an underlying immune problem.

• Immunization history necessary.

• Transfusions for blood-borne viruses.

Family history

If close contacts are also unwell, this may suggest epidemic transmission. History of infection in family may suggest hereditary immune deficits.

Examination and investigation

A careful clinical examination is important, as symptoms may not always be organ specific. Some areas of the examination warrant particular attention (see figure). Routine investigations include:

• FBC, ESR and CRP (see p. 64 and p. 338)

• Blood, urine cultures

• Chest X-ray

• Serological tests

• Ultrasonography/CT-guided diagnosis and aspiration of any suspected abscesses.

If clinical assessment and early investigations do not reveal a cause, take a wide view. Stop all unnecessary drugs, culture all possible sites frequently, consider causes of fever other than infection. Do not give empirical antibiotics, unless the patient is very unwell, when broad-spectrum parenteral antibiotics are indicated.

Very rare causes of hyperthermia

Other than infections (see relevant chapters), important causes of hyperthermia that need to be distinguished from fever include:

• **Neuroleptic malignant syndrome** (NMS): a rare idiosyncratic reaction to antipsychotic agents, promoted by intercurrent illness or dehydration, and characterized by high fever, muscle rigidity, delirium and marked autonomic instability. Muscle enzyme release, e.g. creatine kinase (CK) ('rhabdomyolysis'), which may cause acute renal failure, may occur. Supportive therapy, bromocriptine and dantrolene are all useful. Recurrence is common if major tranquillizers are reintroduced.

• **Malignant hyperthermia of anaesthesia**, incidence of 1 : 15 000 children and 1 : 50 000 adults, occurs in genetically predisposed individuals exposed to suxamethonium or halothane and relates to disordered sarcoplasmic reticulum calcium release. In attacks, cardiac arrhythmias and rapidly rising core temperature with muscle rigidity develop quickly, leading to coma, profound metabolic acidosis and circulatory collapse. The mortality rate is 30%. Dantrolene, which decreases sarcoplasmic reticulum calcium release, is helpful. Susceptible individuals can be identified between attacks, in 'at risk' families, by finding elevated CK enzyme levels. In some, the condition relates to an underlying myopathy.

• **Phaeochromocytoma and thyrotoxicosis**.

• **Drug abuse**: amphetamines, ecstasy, and cocaine.

• **Heat stroke**: can occur in epidemics during hot spells, particularly in people with alcohol problems and people on major tranquillizers, or as a result of exercise when people are fluid deprived or unable to lose heat sufficiently quickly. Patients present with sudden-onset delirium, rapidly progressing to coma. Core temperature is > 41°C: sweating may or may not be present. Extreme tachycardia and hyperventilation are common. Pulmonary oedema with shock and multi-organ failure occurs in advanced cases. The diagnosis is clinical, supported by finding elevated muscle enzymes. Treatment involves removing the patient from the hot environment and giving cool fluids, either sprayed on the skin to encourage heat loss or given intravenously. Shivering, which greatly increases heat production, if prominent should be suppressed with major tranquillizers. Specific organ support may be needed.

• **Cerebrovascular accidents**.

• **Encephalitis**.

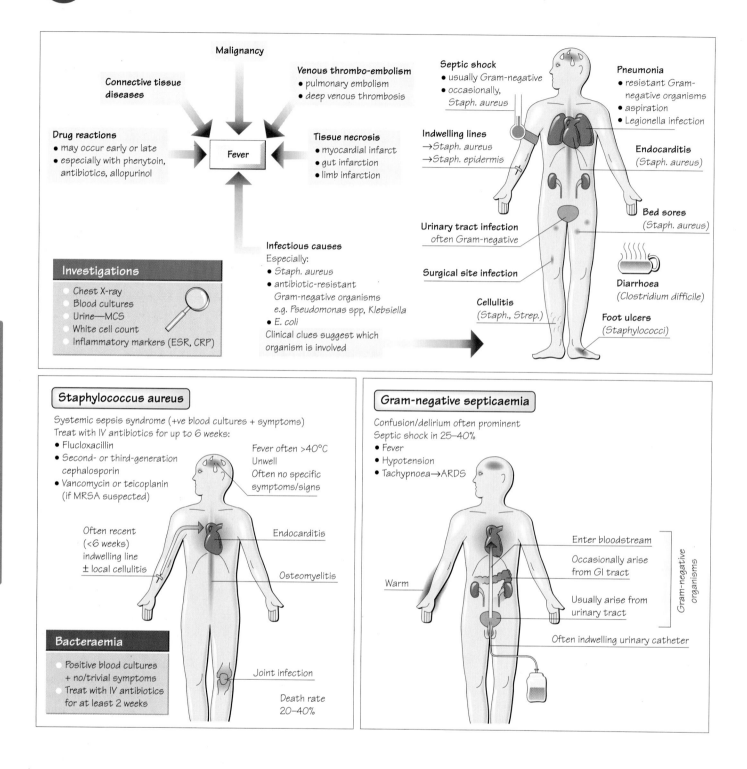

Malignancy

Connective tissue diseases

Venous thrombo-embolism
• pulmonary embolism
• deep venous thrombosis

Drug reactions
• may occur early or late
• especially with phenytoin, antibiotics, allopurinol

Fever

Tissue necrosis
• myocardial infarct
• gut infarction
• limb infarction

Septic shock
• usually Gram-negative
• occasionally, Staph. aureus

Pneumonia
• resistant Gram-negative organisms
• aspiration
• Legionella infection

Indwelling lines
→Staph. aureus
→Staph. epidermis

Endocarditis
(Staph. aureus)

Urinary tract infection
often Gram-negative

Surgical site infection

Bed sores
(Staph. aureus)

Diarrhoea
(Clostridium difficile)

Cellulitis
(Staph., Strep.)

Foot ulcers
(Staphylococci)

Infectious causes
Especially:
• Staph. aureus
• antibiotic-resistant Gram-negative organisms e.g. Pseudomonas spp, Klebsiella
• E. coli
Clinical clues suggest which organism is involved

Investigations
○ Chest X-ray
○ Blood cultures
○ Urine—MCS
○ White cell count
○ Inflammatory markers (ESR, CRP)

Staphylococcus aureus

Systemic sepsis syndrome (+ve blood cultures + symptoms)
Treat with IV antibiotics for up to 6 weeks:
• Flucloxacillin
• Second- or third-generation cephalosporin
• Vancomycin or teicoplanin (if MRSA suspected)

Fever often >40°C
Unwell
Often no specific symptoms/signs

Often recent (<6 weeks) indwelling line ± local cellulitis

Endocarditis

Osteomyelitis

Joint infection

Death rate 20–40%

Bacteraemia
○ Positive blood cultures + no/trivial symptoms
○ Treat with IV antibiotics for at least 2 weeks

Gram-negative septicaemia

Confusion/delirium often prominent
Septic shock in 25–40%
• Fever
• Hypotension
• Tachypnoea→ARDS

Enter bloodstream

Occasionally arise from GI tract

Usually arise from urinary tract

Often indwelling urinary catheter

Warm

Gram-negative organisms

Definition and incidence

Nosocomial means hospital acquired. Hospital-acquired infections affect some 15% of inpatients. Important factors underlying this are:
• Inpatients have underlying conditions that may make their immune system relatively less effective.

• Treatment with antibiotics may select for certain organisms, particularly resistant Gram-negative organisms (e.g. *Pseudomonas* spp.) and *Candida* spp.
• Procedures and care in hospital interfere with the body's natural defences against infection, e.g. intravascular lines, endotracheal tubes.

Significant infection can occur in the absence of fever, particularly in elderly patients, or patients with renal or hepatic disease. Infection should be considered in any patient with changes in clinical state (pulse, blood pressure, mental state).

Nosocomial fever

This may be infectious or non-infectious in origin:

Common infectious causes

- Urinary tract or lower respiratory tract infections, primary and intravascular catheter-associated bacteraemia, sinusitis/middle-ear disease in ventilated patients.
- Surgical wound or intra-abdominal sepsis (may not always present with obvious signs), pressure ulcers/skin infections.
- *Clostridium difficile* diarrhoea is an increasingly common cause of infection; it has a significant mortality and prolongs hospital stay by up to 20 days. Those most commonly affected are:
  - The infirm or very elderly patients (+ 85 years)
  - Those treated with broad-spectrum antibiotics, particularly cephalosporins.
  Diagnosis is by finding *C. difficile* toxin in the stool. Treatment is fluids, oral metronidazole or vancomycin. 10–20% relapse after treatment.

Common non-infectious causes

- Drug fever
- Venous thromboembolism (DVT or PE), resolving haematoma
- Myocardial infarction and infarction of other tissue (particularly intestinal)
- Trauma or surgery

Clinical assessment

- Assessment of immune status.
- History of recent surgical or invasive procedures.
- Examination of lines and catheters.
- Check on new medications and antibiotic therapy.
- Crucial investigations: white cell count, chest X-ray, urinalysis, and urine and blood cultures. Other tests are determined by clinical findings. If diarrhoea is present, *C. difficile* toxin should be assayed.

Specific nosocomial infections

Two groups of pathogens are particularly common causes of nosocomial infections (see Table 35.1):
- *Staphylococcus aureus*, often related to indwelling lines. Patients are usually acutely unwell with high fevers and rigors. The mortality rate is 20–30%. Proven staphylococcal bacteraemia requires prolonged (2–6 weeks) intravenous antibiotic therapy to prevent metastatic infection, especially acute bacterial endocarditis and bone/joint infections, or pulmonary, cerebral and paraspinal abscesses. Persisting blood culture

Table 35.1 Common organisms causing nosocomial fever.

Gram-positive cocci (60–70%)	Gram-negative rods	Fungi (less common)
Coagulase-negative staphylococci	*Escherichia coli*	*Candida* spp.
Viridans streptococci	*Klebsiella pneumoniae*	*Aspergillus* spp.
Staph. aureus	*Pseudomonas aeruginosa*	

positivity despite appropriate antibiotic therapy may indicate endocarditis or tissue abscesses. Methicillin-resistant *Staph. aureus* infection (MRSA) is an increasingly common hospital-acquired pathogen. It is no more virulent than sensitive strains of *Staph. aureus*, but invasive infections require treatment with vancomycin or teicoplanin. Asymptomatic skin colonization can be treated using topical antibiotics.
- Gram-negative organisms, particularly *Escherichia coli*, *Pseudomonas* and *Klebsiella* spp. These usually arise from the urinary or gastrointestinal tract. Around 25–40% of Gram-negative bacteraemias are associated with shock, with a mortality rate of 25%. In addition to fever, chills and hypotension, the earliest sign is often tachypnoea, which may progress to adult respiratory distress syndrome (see p. 211). Mental signs (confusion, delirium) may be prominent. Therapy involves empirical antibiotics, supportive measures and identification and drainage of any collection.

Bacteraemia and line-related infection

Bacteraemia may accompany infections such as urinary tract and pulmonary infections, but may occur with no obvious source. This is often associated with occult infection of intravascular catheters. Complications such as septic thrombophlebitis or endocarditis or metastatic infection may occur. It is important to determine:
- If blood culture isolates are true pathogens or skin flora, repeated blood cultures may help; if cultures persistently grow one organism, it is very likely that this is a true infection.
- Whether an existing intravascular device is infected (inflammation at line site—or using line and peripheral blood cultures).
  Short-term lines should be removed if they are thought to be infected. Precious semi-permanent lines (dialysis or Hickmann lines) can sometimes be treated with trials of antibiotics without removal.

Fever in the neutropenic patient

Common after chemotherapy for haematological or other malignancies: defined as temperature $\geq 38.3°C$ and ≤ 500 neutrophils/mm^3. Infection only proven in 50–60% of patients. Drug- and transfusion-related fevers should be considered. The likelihood and seriousness of infection are increased by the duration and severity of neutropenia.

Special attention should be paid to the common sites of infection: skin; lungs; perioral and pharynx; and perianal area.

Signs of inflammation may be subtle; the absence of neutrophils means that the inflammatory response is blunted. Classic signs of infection (e.g. erythema and induration or an infiltrate on a chest X-ray) may not occur. Bacteraemia may occur in the absence of an obvious source.

Profound or prolonged neutropenia and fever unresponsive to broad-spectrum antibiotics for more than one week increases the likelihood of fungal infection.

Empirical antibiotic regimens are required in all febrile neutropenic patients as a result of the high mortality in this group. Monotherapy (ceftazidime or meropenem) or dual therapy (aminoglycoside + anti-pseudomonal penicillin) is equally effective.

Vancomycin should be considered in the MRSA-colonized patient, if serious line-related sepsis is suspected, or if prophylaxis against Gram-negative organisms has been used (e.g. ciprofloxacin).

If there is no response, consider:
- Changing antibiotics (e.g. adding vancomycin).
- Further investigation for rare causes of fever (herpes simplex virus, cytomegalovirus, *Toxoplasma* spp.).
- Adding antifungal therapy, particularly if no response by 5–7 days.

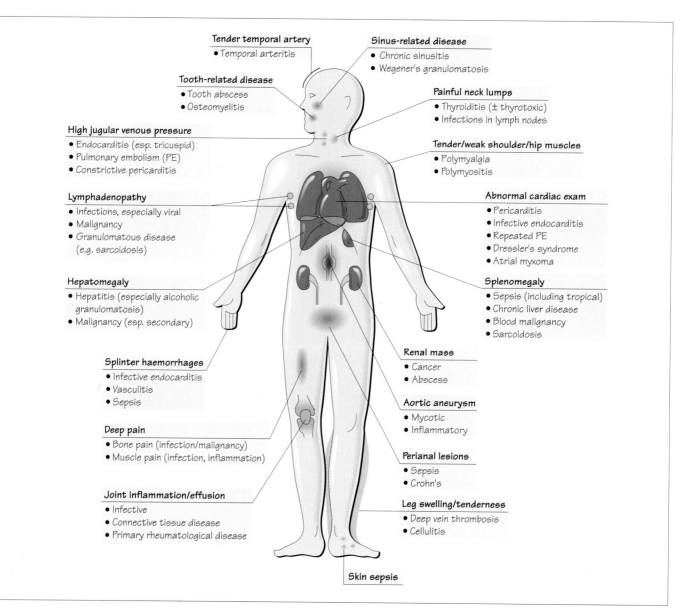

Tender temporal artery
- Temporal arteritis

Tooth-related disease
- Tooth abscess
- Osteomyelitis

High jugular venous pressure
- Endocarditis (esp. tricuspid)
- Pulmonary embolism (PE)
- Constrictive pericarditis

Lymphadenopathy
- Infections, especially viral
- Malignancy
- Granulomatous disease (e.g. sarcoidosis)

Hepatomegaly
- Hepatitis (especially alcoholic granulomatosis)
- Malignancy (esp. secondary)

Splinter haemorrhages
- Infective endocarditis
- Vasculitis
- Sepsis

Deep pain
- Bone pain (infection/malignancy)
- Muscle pain (infection, inflammation)

Joint inflammation/effusion
- Infective
- Connective tissue disease
- Primary rheumatological disease

Sinus-related disease
- Chronic sinusitis
- Wegener's granulomatosis

Painful neck lumps
- Thyroiditis (± thyrotoxic)
- Infections in lymph nodes

Tender/weak shoulder/hip muscles
- Polymyalgia
- Polymyositis

Abnormal cardiac exam
- Pericarditis
- Infective endocarditis
- Repeated PE
- Dressler's syndrome
- Atrial myxoma

Splenomegaly
- Sepsis (including tropical)
- Chronic liver disease
- Blood malignancy
- Sarcoidosis

Renal mass
- Cancer
- Abscess

Aortic aneurysm
- Mycotic
- Inflammatory

Perianal lesions
- Sepsis
- Crohn's

Leg swelling/tenderness
- Deep vein thrombosis
- Cellulitis

Skin sepsis

Most patients presenting with fever have a short-lived acute illness, which is rapidly diagnosed. Persisting fever in the face of initial negative investigations is termed 'fever (pyrexia) of unknown origin (FUO)'. The classic definition of this is 'fever > 38.3°C persisting without diagnosis for 3 weeks including 1 week's investigation in hospital'. Most clinicians have modified this definition in the face of an increasing number of immunocompromised hosts and more rapid diagnostic facilities. Practically, patients with unexplained fever can be divided into categories defined by their immune status:
- Classic fever of unknown origin (FUO; community acquired).
- FUO in the hospital patient (see p. 68).
- FUO in neutropenic and immunosuppressed patient (see p. 69).
- FUO in HIV patient (see p. 74).

Classic fever of unknown origin

May be caused by many different processes (see Table 36.1):
- Infections (25–50%)
- Neoplasms (10–30%)
- Connective tissue/collagen vascular diseases (10–25%)
- Miscellaneous (10–20%)
- Undiagnosed (10–25%)

The relative contribution of different categories depends on the geographical location and the age of the patient: infections are more important in the developing world; neoplasia and connective tissue disorders become more important with increasing age.

Table 36.1 The most common causes of FUO.

Infections
Abscess
Mycobacteria
Endocarditis

Neoplasms
Lymphoma
Solid tumours (gastrointestinal tract, liver, renal cell, sarcoma)
Leukaemia
Other haematological tumours

Connective tissue disease
Temporal arteritis/polymyalgia rheumatica
Polyarteritis nodosa
Systemic lupus erythematosus (SLE)
Still's disease

Infections

Many different infections are implicated in FUO but consider:
1 Systemic infections that are difficult to diagnose, e.g. disseminated mycobacterial disease or culture-negative endocarditis and brucellosis.
2 Localized infections and abscesses where the normal inflammatory or immune response is not able to clear organisms, but the diagnosis is difficult because bacteraemia may not occur. 'Blind' computed tomography (CT) of the abdomen may be helpful to demonstrate sources such as renal, diverticular or pelvic abscesses.

Neoplasms

The majority of neoplasms producing FUO are haematological: fever may precede appearance of lymphadenopathy in lymphoma. In older patients, consider solid tumours, particularly occult gastrointestinal-related neoplasms, such as the pancreas. In women ovarian cancer should be excluded.

Connective tissue diseases

Still's disease is essentially a diagnosis of exclusion. In elderly patients, temporal arteritis/polymyalgia rheumatica is common, but classic temporal artery tenderness and an extremely high erythrocyte sedimentation rate (ESR) do not always occur. If other investigations have not been productive, a 'blind' temporal artery biopsy is sometimes considered.

Miscellaneous

• Drug fever: can occur with many drugs, particularly antibiotics and anticonvulsants. Eosinophilia and a rash may help in the diagnosis.
• Pulmonary emboli (PE): occasionally, repeated PEs cause fever. Breathlessness with a clear chest X-ray should raise the possibility, which can be pursued with spiral CT scan, $\dot{V}/\dot{Q}$ (ventilation/perfusion) scan, etc. The lactate dehydrogenase (LDH) is often raised in this situation.
• Granulomatous disease of the liver, in the absence of an obvious cause, is not uncommon. It may be steroid responsive. Abnormal liver function tests may reflect a hepatological process, but unfortunately may also be a non-specific response to systemic disease, particularly sepsis.
• Factitious fever: psychiatric disorder, often in women and in paramedical professions.

• Habitual hyperthermia: hypothalamic set point may be high—exaggerated diurnal variations in temperature may occur. No pathological significance.

Approach to diagnosis

A comprehensive history and examination are crucial. Establish whether a fever is truly present (a significant proportion of patients have no documented fever at all). The fever pattern may occasionally help. Look for signs accompanying the fever (flushing, sweats, tachycardia, etc.). Determine whether patient is unwell and whether stable or deteriorating. Stop all non-essential drugs.

Investigations

Use localizing symptoms and signs to target investigations.

Routine

Basic screening tests as previously described (p. 67). High ESR and/or C-reactive protein (CRP) suggests a major systemic disease or infection. Normal ESR makes significant infection or collagen vascular disease unlikely. Autoantibody screen (antineutrophil cytoplasmic antibody [ANCA], antinuclear antibody [ANA], rheumatoid factor, complement) may be useful. An abdominal/pelvic CT scan may be helpful, even in the absence of localizing features and should be considered early in the diagnostic process. It may demonstrate abscesses, nodes or malignancy.

Specific

Investigations should ideally focus on abnormalities. Consider:
• Echocardiography.
• Extended blood cultures: brucellosis or fastidious organisms.
• Tissue biopsy: should be aggressively pursued, especially if any organ-specific abnormality is identified. Liver, skin, temporal artery lymph node and bone marrow biopsy can all be helpful.
• Laparotomy is rarely indicated.

Diagnostic trials of therapy

Undiagnosed patients who remain well (no weight loss, stable albumin levels) can be observed. The outcome in this group is extremely good; fever will often spontaneously remit.

A trial of therapy may be indicated in sick or deteriorating patients:
• Antibiotics: blind broad-spectrum antibiotics may be indicated if the patient is unwell or conditions such as culture-negative endocarditis are suspected. A trial of anti-tuberculosis (TB) therapy can be justified if the clinical suspicion is high because TB culture confirmation may take several weeks. Defervescence and an increase in weight are good signs of response to anti-TB therapy. Some anti-TB drugs have broad-spectrum antibacterial activity.
• Corticosteroids: these are occasionally helpful, particularly in elderly patients with a possible temporal arteritis/polymyalgia rheumatica syndrome, or in young patients with Still's disease. Obvious infection and malignancy must be excluded and the fever and ESR/CRP response followed. An initial response does not always prove a non-infectious aetiology; steroid therapy will blunt fevers caused by some infections and may improve systemic symptoms resulting from malignancy. It is crucial, therefore, not to consider steroids until repeated blood cultures have come back as negative, and abdominal CT has ruled out malignancy, and intra-abdominal or pelvic sepsis.

Clinical Presentations at a Glance

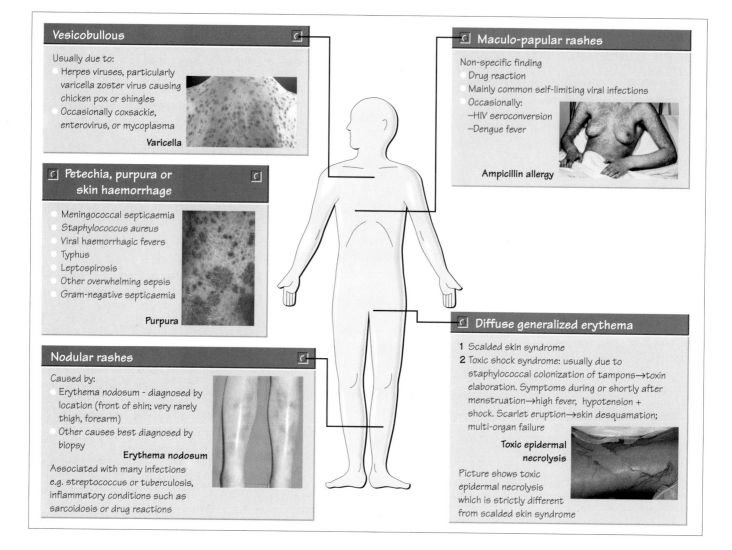

Vesicobullous

Usually due to:
- Herpes viruses, particularly varicella zoster virus causing chicken pox or shingles
- Occasionally coxsackie, enterovirus, or mycoplasma

Varicella

Maculo-papular rashes

Non-specific finding
- Drug reaction
- Mainly common self-limiting viral infections
- Occasionally:
  - HIV seroconversion
  - Dengue fever

Ampicillin allergy

Petechia, purpura or skin haemorrhage

- Meningococcal septicaemia
- Staphylococcus aureus
- Viral haemorrhagic fevers
- Typhus
- Leptospirosis
- Other overwhelming sepsis
- Gram-negative septicaemia

Purpura

Nodular rashes

Caused by:
- Erythema nodosum - diagnosed by location (front of shin; very rarely thigh, forearm)
- Other causes best diagnosed by biopsy

Erythema nodosum

Associated with many infections e.g. streptococcus or tuberculosis, inflammatory conditions such as sarcoidosis or drug reactions

Diffuse generalized erythema

1 Scalded skin syndrome
2 Toxic shock syndrome: usually due to staphylococcal colonization of tampons→toxin elaboration. Symptoms during or shortly after menstruation→high fever, hypotension + shock. Scarlet eruption→skin desquamation; multi-organ failure

Toxic epidermal necrolysis

Picture shows toxic epidermal necrolysis which is strictly different from scalded skin syndrome

---

Patients with fever and a rash are challenging; it is vital to identify those with acute bacterial sepsis who require prompt antimicrobial therapy. Although fever and a rash are most commonly caused by an infection, other processes produce similar clinical syndromes:
- Drug reactions.
- Vasculitis—see page 406.

Some rashes are instantly recognizable; others require a systematic approach for diagnosis. Atypical features of a common disease (e.g. appearance modified by an impaired host immune system) are more likely than rare diseases. Factors that are helpful in diagnosis include:
- Time relationship of fever to rash.
- Drug history.
- Presence of:
  - Mucosal lesions or conjunctivitis
  - Lymphadenopathy or hepatosplenomegaly
  - Arthropathy.

In addition to standard investigations and blood cultures:
- Aspiration of lesions allows Gram smear and culture of organisms in meningococcal, staphylococcal or pseudomonal infections.

- Punch biopsy may reveal organisms, particularly in fungal infections, or demonstrate specific histological features.
- Electron microscopy of vesicle fluid may diagnose herpes virus infections.
- Specific immunofluorescence may be used, e.g. to distinguish herpes simplex from herpes zoster virus infection.

Diffuse erythema

Diffuse erythema is the term given to a widespread reddening of the skin. Scarlet fever, caused by a group A streptococcus, used to be a common cause of a diffuse blanching erythema. Drug eruptions are currently an important cause of fever with diffuse erythema. Important infective causes that should be excluded include:
- **Toxic shock syndrome**, caused by *Staphylococcus* or *Streptococcus* spp., produces generalized erythema, and later desquamation with multiorgan involvement.
- **Scalded skin syndrome** in children, from staphylococcal toxin, produces diffuse erythema, bulla formation and exfoliation.

Vesiculo-bullous

Vesicles are small fluid-filled blisters, whereas bullae are larger fluid-filled blisters. Varicella-zoster infection has two manifestations with vesiculo-bullous rashes:
• **Varicella (chickenpox)** produces vesicles on a halo of erythema, initially clear then cloudy. Successive cropping.
• In **zoster (shingles)**, a dermatomal distribution is found, initially maculopapular, then vesicles, bullae and crusting.

Lesions outside the affected dermatome occur in 5% of the immunocompetent and in the immunocompromised.

Rarer causes of vesiculo-bullous rashes are:
• **Disseminated herpes simplex**: may occur from labial/genital lesions with considerable systemic upset in those with eczema or those who are immunocompromised.
• **Hand–foot–mouth** (Coxsackie virus or enteroviruses): small vesicles in the mouth, and on the hands and feet.
• **Bullous erythema multiforma**: classically mycoplasma and herpes simplex infections; many other agents implicated.
• **Staphylococcal infections:** bullous impetigo.

Petechial–purpuric rashes

Bleeding into the skin has a number of terms—petechiae are small bleeds into the skin, < 1–2 mm in diameter, whereas purpura describes larger areas of bleeding into the skin (> 2 mm in diameter). Skin bleeds larger than about 4 mm are termed ecchymoses. The key purpuric rash to diagnose in acutely sick patients is **meningococcaemia**, which produces a spectrum of rashes from isolated petechiae to multiple purpuric lesions, confluent over the body, associated with complete haemostatic failure and a very high mortality. **Gonococcaemia** typically produces pustular lesions and arthritis, and more rarely mild purpuric rashes; haemostatic failure is unusual and mortality is very low. Other causes of petechial-purpuric rashes include:
• **Staphylococcal endocarditis**: petechiae and purpura may occur, usually immune complex mediated—a 'vasculitic rash'.
• **Disseminated intravascular coagulation** occurs in many severe infections—an important diagnostic clue is spontaneous haemorrhage from old venepuncture sites.
• **Leptospirosis**: skin haemorrhage rarely occurs in very unwell patients.
• **Viral haemorrhagic fevers**, haemorrhages may occur in Lassa, Ebola and Marburg and yellow fever: these patients are very unwell, often jaundiced and very likely to die.
• Petechiae are common in severe dengue infection (**dengue haemorrhagic fever**).

Maculopapular rashes

Macular rashes can be seen, but cannot be felt, i.e. they do not cause any bumps on the skin. The individual spots are usually small—often only a few mm in diameter. Papular rashes can be seen and felt, i.e. there are spots some few mm in diameter, which cause raised lumps on the skin surface. These rashes are extremely common, and can be produced by many pathogens.

Viral infections

These are the most common cause. Although **rubella** (German measles) and **measles** both produce rashes starting on the face, spreading to the trunk, they differ in that, in rubella, the rash is of discrete pink macules, whereas in measles it is maculopapular with lesions (Koplik's spots) in the mouth. Other common childhood viral rashes are the result of **enteroviruses** (diarrhoea and a rash) and **parvovirus** ('slapped cheeks' syndrome). Rarer causes include:
• **Acute HIV infection**: macules, papules or urticaria.
• **Dengue** (uncomplicated): classically, a transitory rash followed by generalized maculopapular rash in second febrile phase.

Rickettsial infections

Maculopapular rashes occur in most rickettsial infections, and an eschar is present in infection by some species.

Mycoplasma and chlamydial infections

These infections may cause maculopapular rashes.

Bacterial infections/spirochaetal

• **Secondary syphilis**: macules that may become papular or pustular. Erosions on oral mucosa, condylomata lata in intertriginous areas.
• **Leptospirosis**: macules, papules or petechiae occur.
• **Meningococcaemia**: initial lesions may be macules before classic petechiae/purpura.

Nodular lesions

Nodular lesions are seen and can be very easily felt—they differ from papules in that they are larger (and often far fewer in number). The most common nodular lesion is **erythema nodosum** (EN), an inflammation of small blood vessels in the deep dermis (a panniculitis), usually on the anterior aspect of the lower leg. EN is often preceded or accompanied by systemic upset (fever and malaise) and sometimes with arthralgia. Lesions never scar and normally heal within 2–3 weeks—much longer and other diagnoses should be sought. Common causes for EN in the UK are:
• Streptococcal infections.
• Sarcoidosis.
• Inflammatory bowel disease.

Worldwide causes commonly include TB and leprosy and, rarely, *Yersinia* sp., hepatitis C, *Histoplasma* and *Coccidioides* spp.

Other nodular rashes are caused by:
• **Disseminated fungal infections**, usually in immunocompromised individuals, most commonly with *Candida*, *Histoplasma* or *Cryptococcus* spp.
• **Mycobacterial disease**: nodular rashes occur occasionally in disseminated TB or atypical mycobacteria.

Other rashes/lesions of importance

• **Typhoid** characteristically results in rose spots (pink papules on the abdomen).
• **Lyme disease** produces a diagnostic lesion (erythema chronicum migrans): the initial macule develops into large flat ring-like lesions.
• *Pseudomonas aeruginosa* can cause ecthyma gangrenosum (erythema surrounded by haemorrhages and necrosis) in neutropenic patients.

Rashes in tropical disease

• **Cutaneous larva migrans**: caused by larvae of the dog or cat hookworm migrating through the skin, resulting in raised scaly erythematous serpiginous lesions in skin that is in contact with ground or sand.
• **Loiasis**: transient, non-erythematous, pruritic, subcutaneous swellings.
• **Onchocerciasis**: nodules and pruritic papules or urticaria.
• **Strongyloides** infection: urticaria and 'larva currens' (evanescent urticarial weals).

38 Fever in HIV-infected patients

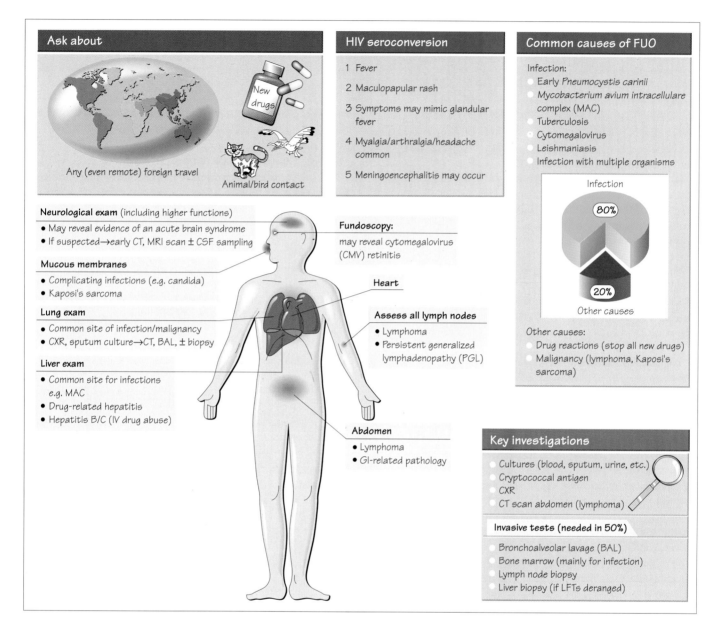

Ask about

Any (even remote) foreign travel

New drugs

Animal/bird contact

Neurological exam (including higher functions)
- May reveal evidence of an acute brain syndrome
- If suspected→early CT, MRI scan ± CSF sampling

Mucous membranes
- Complicating infections (e.g. candida)
- Kaposi's sarcoma

Lung exam
- Common site of infection/malignancy
- CXR, sputum culture→CT, BAL, ± biopsy

Liver exam
- Common site for infections e.g. MAC
- Drug-related hepatitis
- Hepatitis B/C (IV drug abuse)

Fundoscopy:
may reveal cytomegalovirus (CMV) retinitis

Heart

Assess all lymph nodes
- Lymphoma
- Persistent generalized lymphadenopathy (PGL)

Abdomen
- Lymphoma
- GI-related pathology

HIV seroconversion

1 Fever
2 Maculopapular rash
3 Symptoms may mimic glandular fever
4 Myalgia/arthralgia/headache common
5 Meningoencephalitis may occur

Common causes of FUO

Infection:
- Early *Pneumocystis carinii*
- *Mycobacterium avium intracellulare* complex (MAC)
- Tuberculosis
- Cytomegalovirus
- Leishmaniasis
- Infection with multiple organisms

Infection 80%

Other causes 20%

Other causes:
- Drug reactions (stop all new drugs)
- Malignancy (lymphoma, Kaposi's sarcoma)

Key investigations
- Cultures (blood, sputum, urine, etc.)
- Cryptococcal antigen
- CXR
- CT scan abdomen (lymphoma)

Invasive tests (needed in 50%)
- Bronchoalveolar lavage (BAL)
- Bone marrow (mainly for infection)
- Lymph node biopsy
- Liver biopsy (if LFTs deranged)

Fever is common in HIV infections:
- Early HIV infection: fever is a common feature of an acute HIV seroconversion reaction. Appropriate testing should be considered in patients who present with a fever and have risk factors for HIV infection.
- Fever in established HIV infection: fever occurs frequently in patients throughout the course of HIV infection; up to half of patients will present with fever at some point. The source of fever is often obvious on initial investigation and is most commonly the result of either standard or opportunistic infections associated with HIV infection, e.g. bacterial pneumonia, *Pneumocystis carinii* pneumonia (PCP) or infections related to intravenous lines. However, fever may be difficult to diagnose, particularly in late disease.

Fever of unknown origin (FUO) in HIV-infected patients has been defined as fever > 38.3°C lasting more than 4 days in hospital or 4 weeks in outpatients without diagnosis. This usually reflects:
- Systemic infection with few localizing signs or symptoms, e.g. *Mycobacterium avium-intracellulare* complex (MAC) infection.
- Initial stages of an infective process before organ-related signs, e.g. *Pneumocystis carinii*, leishmaniasis or cytomegalovirus (CMV) infection.
- A drug reaction: common because of the increased predisposition to drug reactions in HIV and the polypharmacy often associated with the disease.
- Malignancy, most commonly lymphoma, occasionally Kaposi's sarcoma.

Table 38.1 Most common infections causing FUO in advanced HIV infection.

Mycobacterium avium-intracellulare complex (MAC)
Mycobacterium tuberculosis
Pneumocystis carinii infection (PCP)
Cytomegalovirus (CMV)
Leishmaniasis
HIV infection itself (debated by some)

In contrast to FUO in other hosts, over 80% of patients will have an infection (see Table 38.1) and up to 20% will have more than one cause for their fever.

Approach to the patient
History
The profound immunosuppression of advanced HIV disease means that fever may be caused by unusual organisms or recrudescence of a previously latent infection. A history of potential exposure to such organisms is crucial. Close note should also be taken of:
- Ethnic origin: affects risk of infections such as tuberculosis (TB) or histoplasmosis.
- Travel abroad, even if in the distant past. Mediterranean travel is associated with risks of visceral leishmaniasis; more exotic infection such as with *Penicillium marneffei* may occur in those who have spent time in the Far East.
- Contact with animals or birds.
- Existing prophylactic regimens reduce the chance of, but do not exclude, the diagnosis of conditions such as PCP or MAC.
- Pre-existing serology for *Toxoplasma* sp. and CMV.
- CD4 count: organisms such as CMV or MAC rarely cause disease until CD4 counts are < 100/mm^3.

Examination
This should include particularly:
- Skin and mucosal membranes.
- Lungs.
- Examination of the dilated fundi for evidence of CMV retinitis.
- Examination of lymph nodes.

Few clinical or biochemical findings are specific for a particular disease process, e.g. abnormal liver function may be found in drug reactions, lymphoma or MAC, and lymph node enlargement may occur in MAC or lymphoma. However, abnormalities warrant further investigation.

Diagnosis
Discontinuing drugs, particularly ones started recently, and watching the fever response may be helpful. Routine cultures should be performed but several specific investigations may be helpful:

Non-invasive methods
- Chest X-ray.
- Urine, stool and regular blood cultures.
- Mycobacterial and fungal blood cultures—particularly looking for MAC; 60–80% sensitivity using modern techniques.
- Serum cryptococcal antigen.
- Examination of induced sputum; diagnosis of PCP in asymptomatic patients, *Mycobacterium tuberculosis* and atypical mycobacteria and other respiratory pathogens.
- CT of the abdomen: may show retroperitoneal lymph nodes or masses.

Invasive methods (required in up to 50%)
- Bronchoscopy with bronchoalveolar lavage (BAL), in which small aliquots of saline are flushed in and out of the lung, collecting inflammatory cells and organisms from the lung. Organisms can be identified by culture or specific stains.
- Bone marrow examination: useful for MAC culture and diagnosis of intracellular organisms, e.g. *Histoplasma* spp., cryptococci or leishmaniasis.
- Lymph node biopsy of enlarged nodes: diagnosis of lymphoma or TB.
- Liver biopsy: if there is evidence of liver enzyme abnormality that persists after stopping drug therapy.
- Lumbar puncture should be considered if there is altered mentation or neurological function.

Management
Diagnosis is eventually made in about 80% of cases and appropriate therapy should be instituted. Failure of response should lead to searches for other causes because of the high prevalence of multiple conditions. Empirical therapy is sometimes necessary, particularly in very advanced HIV with < 50 CD4 cells/mm^3 when MAC is common but cannot always be demonstrated.

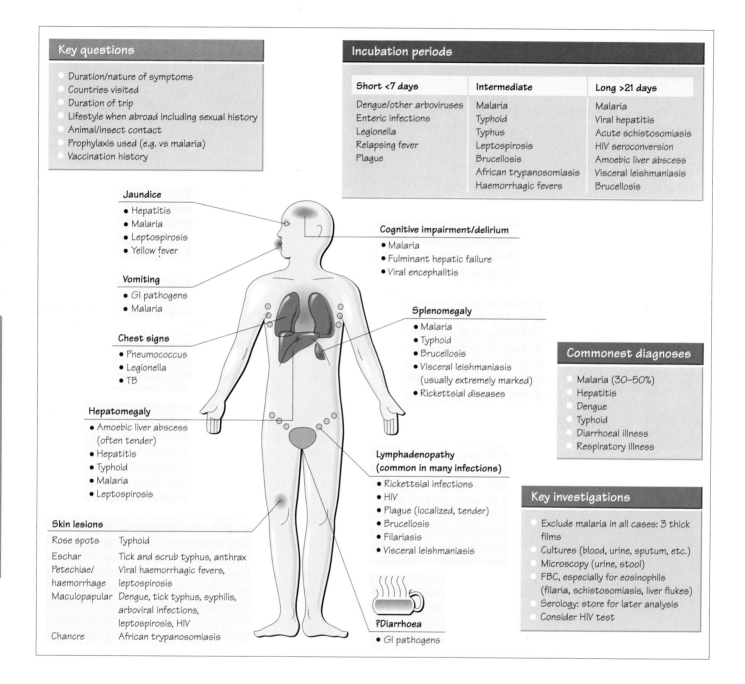

Key questions

- Duration/nature of symptoms
- Countries visited
- Duration of trip
- Lifestyle when abroad including sexual history
- Animal/insect contact
- Prophylaxis used (e.g. vs malaria)
- Vaccination history

Incubation periods

Short <7 days	Intermediate	Long >21 days
Dengue/other arboviruses	Malaria	Malaria
Enteric infections	Typhoid	Viral hepatitis
Legionella	Typhus	Acute schistosomiasis
Relapsing fever	Leptospirosis	HIV seroconversion
Plague	Brucellosis	Amoebic liver abscess
	African trypanosomiasis	Visceral leishmaniasis
	Haemorrhagic fevers	Brucellosis

Jaundice
- Hepatitis
- Malaria
- Leptospirosis
- Yellow fever

Vomiting
- GI pathogens
- Malaria

Chest signs
- Pneumococcus
- Legionella
- TB

Hepatomegaly
- Amoebic liver abscess (often tender)
- Hepatitis
- Typhoid
- Malaria
- Leptospirosis

Skin lesions

Rose spots	Typhoid
Eschar	Tick and scrub typhus, anthrax
Petechiae/ haemorrhage	Viral haemorrhagic fevers, leptospirosis
Maculopapular	Dengue, tick typhus, syphilis, arboviral infections, leptospirosis, HIV
Chancre	African trypanosomiasis

Cognitive impairment/delirium
- Malaria
- Fulminant hepatic failure
- Viral encephalitis

Splenomegaly
- Malaria
- Typhoid
- Brucellosis
- Visceral leishmaniasis (usually extremely marked)
- Rickettsial diseases

Lymphadenopathy (common in many infections)
- Rickettsial infections
- HIV
- Plague (localized, tender)
- Brucellosis
- Filariasis
- Visceral leishmaniasis

?Diarrhoea
- GI pathogens

Commonest diagnoses

- Malaria (30–50%)
- Hepatitis
- Dengue
- Typhoid
- Diarrhoeal illness
- Respiratory illness

Key investigations

- Exclude malaria in all cases: 3 thick films
- Cultures (blood, urine, sputum, etc.)
- Microscopy (urine, stool)
- FBC, especially for eosinophils (filaria, schistosomiasis, liver flukes)
- Serology: store for later analysis
- Consider HIV test

Incidence

As foreign travel has becomes more common, the number of patients presenting with fever following travel has increased considerably. Around 2–3% of travellers report fever during or after a visit to the tropics; 1% of patients have fever after visits to such areas as the Greek islands. Approximately two-thirds of those seek medical advice for fever that persists or first occurs after their return home.

Many of these fevers are not caused by exotic pathogens but reflect ordinary viral, urinary tract or respiratory infections, e.g. infectious mononucleosis (glandular fever—see p. 298) is a common final diagnosis in young travellers. However, significant tropical pathogens, particularly malaria, need to be excluded.

The most common imported infections

- Malaria (see p. 306)
- Hepatitis (see p. 229)
- Dengue (see p. 311)
- Typhoid (see p. 310)
- Diarrhoeal illness (see p. 34)

Up to a quarter of fevers settle spontaneously and are undiagnosed.

Clinical Presentations at a Glance

Making a diagnosis

Assessing the immune status of the traveller is important. Although most travellers are healthy, increasing numbers of elderly or immunocompromised people are travelling abroad. These individuals may be at particular risk of certain infections. In addition to the presenting symptoms, the history should focus on potential exposure to pathogens.

Important questions

• Symptoms or illnesses while away.
• Geographical areas visited and length of time away (possible organisms and incubation periods). Remember that some people travel extensively and history of exposure during previous (as well as most recent) trips is important.
• Kind of trip: business hotel, tourist, living with local people (incidence of tropical disease is much higher in those who have been travelling rough).
• Level of protection against bites by mosquito, ticks, flies. Full immunization history. Malaria prophylaxis and adherence.
• Food and water history (enteric infections, hepatitis).
• Freshwater exposure (schistosomiasis, leptospirosis).
• Sexual activity.
• Illness in fellow travellers (possible single source exposure) or contact with potentially infected individuals (particularly for health workers with potential exposure to haemorrhagic fevers).
• Animal contact (rabies, brucellosis, histoplasmosis—bats in caves).

Important features of examination

• Physical signs are often rather non-specific.
• Establishing fever and sometimes pattern (biphasic in dengue, tertian in untreated malaria).
• Presence of rash, mosquito bites or ticks.
• Jaundice.
• Hepatosplenomegaly and lymphadenopathy.

Important investigations (guided by symptoms)

• Routine screening tests including blood cultures, chest X-ray, urine dipstick and culture.
• Malaria slide (at least three thick films if malaria possible).
• Consider HIV test if sexually active while away.
• Stool examination for ova, cysts and parasites, and culture.
• Look for eosinophilia (schistosomiasis, filariasis, liver flukes).
• Store serum for later serology.

Management

Depends on the underlying condition. Two major initial aims should be:
1 To exclude malaria.
2 To consider whether disease may be transmissible to others, in particular the rare but highly infectious viral haemorrhagic fevers.

Treatment of specific conditions is covered later. Some conditions can be treated on clinical grounds alone; serological confirmation may take several weeks, e.g. the traveller from South Africa with an eschar, maculopapular rash and fever should be treated for African tick typhus.

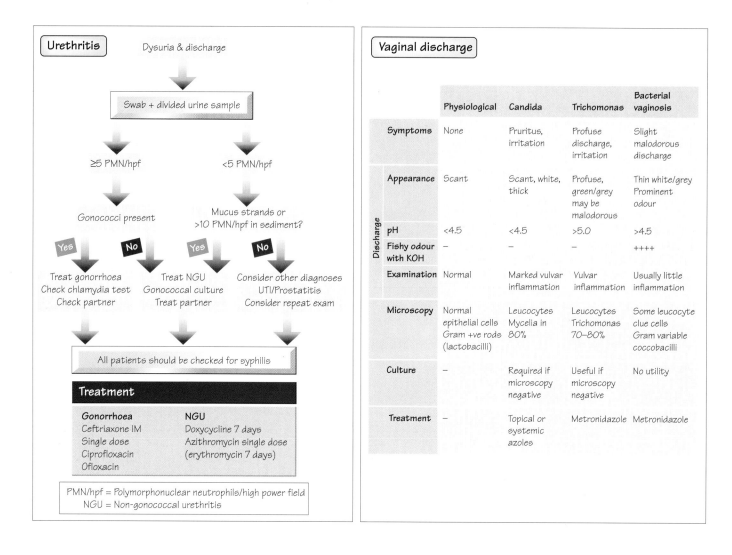

Vaginal discharge

Vaginal discharge is one the most common symptoms that women present with to their general practitioner, and it accounts for over a quarter of referrals to sexually transmitted disease (STD) clinics. All women have a physiological discharge, which varies considerably between individuals. An abnormal vaginal discharge is most commonly caused by infections, but may also be the result of:

• Chemical and physical irritation (e.g. soaps, spermicides, minipads, etc.).
• Allergy and contact dermatitis.
  Other, much rarer, causes include:
• Cervical polyps and other neoplasms.
• Retained tampons.

Infectious causes

Three conditions account for the vast majority of infectious cases:
• Bacterial vaginosis (40–50%).
• *Candida* spp. (20–30%).
• *Trichomonas vaginalis* (15–20%).

Bacterial infection secondary to a foreign body or atrophic vaginitis may also occur and group A streptococci can cause vaginitis with severe systemic symptoms. The other main sexually transmitted pathogens in women, *Neisseria gonorrhoeae* and *Chlamydia* spp., do not usually cause a profuse vaginal discharge, but may occasionally cause an endocervical or urethral discharge which is noted by the patient.

Pathogenesis

Bacterial vaginosis is caused by an imbalance of the organisms of the normal vaginal flora. Lactobacilli are replaced by an overgrowth of mixed flora, including *Gardnerella* species and anaerobes, leading to clinical symptoms. It is associated with complications in pregnant women or those with other gynaecological disease.

Candida species are frequently found in the genital tract of asymptomatic women; the triggers for progression to clinical disease are not understood. Risk factors for candida carriage and disease include pregnancy, diabetes, steroid therapy and antibiotic therapy.

Trichomonas vaginalis, a flagellated protozoan, is usually acquired from sexual contact and causes epithelial cell damage leading to vaginal and vulval inflammation.

Clinical features (see table in figure)

The history and findings on speculum examination sometimes allow a clinical diagnosis, but samples should be taken for microscopy and culture.

Diagnostic tests

A wet mount preparation of vaginal secretions is the most useful investigation. This may demonstrate both organisms and polymorphonuclear cells. Culture is useful for *Candida* and *Trichomonas* infection. Bacterial vaginosis is diagnosed on the basis of three of the following four criteria:

1 Adherent white, non-floccular discharge.
2 Vaginal pH > 4.5.
3 Fishy odours on addition of 10% potassium hydroxide to secretions.
4 Presence of clue cells (vaginal squamous epithelium covered with *Gardnerella vaginalis*).

Management

Oral metronidazole is the drug of choice for both bacterial vaginosis and trichomoniasis: 1-week courses have cure rates of over 90% for both diseases. Partners of patients with trichomoniasis should also be treated. *Candida* spp. can be treated with topical antifungals (e.g. clotrimazole or miconazole) or oral therapy with azoles; good cure rates may be achieved by short courses.

Urethritis

Definition and aetiology

Urethritis is a clinical syndrome consisting of a urethral discharge and dysuria. It is the most common STD syndrome in men. Most cases are caused by infection, but chemical irritants, foreign bodies and some inflammatory conditions may cause similar symptoms. There are two main infectious syndromes in men:

1 Gonococcal urethritis
2 Non-gonococcal urethritis (NGU), caused predominantly by *Chlamydia trachomatis* but also by *Ureaplasma urealyticum* and *Mycoplasma genitalium*.

Urethritis may occur in women, caused by the same organisms, but the concomitant cervicitis dominates the clinical picture. In the UK, NGU is far more common than gonorrhoea, rates for which have steadily declined over the last 30 years. Co-infection with *Neisseria gonorrhoeae* and agents of NGU occurs in approximately 10–30% of men.

Clinical features

Incubation period

• Short (2–7 days) in gonorrhoea.
• Up to several weeks in *Chlamydia* sp.

Urethral discharge

• Often copious purulent yellow or green in gonorrhoea.
• Smaller volume, mucopurulent in *Chlamydia* sp.

Dysuria

Most marked in gonorrhoea:
• Frequency or urgency (symptoms of cystitis rather than urethritis) are **not** a feature.
• Lymphadenopathy does not occur in either disease.

May need to differentiate from upper urinary tract infection, other causes of prostatic disease and herpes simplex infection (external vesicles and enlargement of the local lymph nodes is common).

Complications

• Epididymitis (rarely prostatitis)
• Conjunctivitis
• Reiter's syndrome in NGU (urethritis, uveitis, arthritis)
• Rarely disseminated gonococcal infection (skin lesions, joint swelling)

Examination and diagnosis

Patients should not pass urine for at least 2 hours before examination. Quantity and colour of discharge should be noted. 'Stripping' the urethra by running the thumb along the urethra up to the meatus can often produce discharge. Examine lymph nodes; large or tender nodes make the diagnosis unlikely. Examine epididymis for tenderness or enlargement.

Investigations

A small swab should be passed into the urethra and rolled onto a slide. Gram staining of slide should be performed to look for polymorphs and Gram-negative intracellular diplococci (*Neisseria gonorrhoeae*). Swabs should be plated out on to a gonococcal culture medium *at the bedside*. Swabs should also be taken for chlamydia detection by immunoassays or fluorescent antibody techniques.

Divided urine samples are also useful. The first and second 10-mL aliquots voided after examination should be saved. Mucus threads in the first aliquot suggest urethritis. The sediment after centrifugation of both samples can be examined for cells.

Management (see figure)

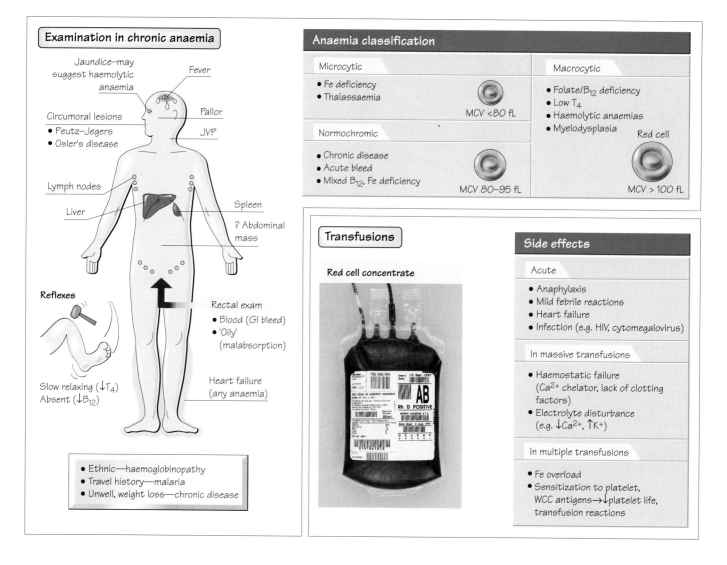

Examination in chronic anaemia

Jaundice—may suggest haemolytic anaemia

Fever

Pallor

JVP

Circumoral lesions
- Peutz–Jegers
- Osler's disease

Lymph nodes

Liver

Spleen

? Abdominal mass

Reflexes

Slow relaxing ($\downarrow T_4$)
Absent ($\downarrow B_{12}$)

Rectal exam
- Blood (GI bleed)
- 'Oily' (malabsorption)

Heart failure (any anaemia)

- Ethnic—haemoglobinopathy
- Travel history—malaria
- Unwell, weight loss—chronic disease

Anaemia classification

Microcytic
- Fe deficiency
- Thalassaemia

MCV <80 fL

Normochromic
- Chronic disease
- Acute bleed
- Mixed B_{12}, Fe deficiency

MCV 80–95 fL

Macrocytic
- Folate/B_{12} deficiency
- Low T_4
- Haemolytic anaemias
- Myelodysplasia

Red cell

MCV > 100 fL

Transfusions

Red cell concentrate

Side effects

Acute
- Anaphylaxis
- Mild febrile reactions
- Heart failure
- Infection (e.g. HIV, cytomegalovirus)

In massive transfusions
- Haemostatic failure (Ca^{2+} chelator, lack of clotting factors)
- Electrolyte disturbance (e.g. $\downarrow Ca^{2+}$, $\uparrow K^+$)

In multiple transfusions
- Fe overload
- Sensitization to platelet, WCC antigens→$\downarrow$platelet life, transfusion reactions

Anaemia is present when the haemoglobin is more than two standard deviations below the mean haemoglobin for that individual. The mean haemoglobin varies with sex and age.

Symptoms

Symptoms depend on the underlying pathology as well as the severity and speed of onset of the anaemia. Mild anaemia often causes no symptoms. Insidious onset anaemia, even if profound, likewise may cause few symptoms. In more severe or rapid onset anaemia, the following may occur:
- Fatigue.
- Peripheral oedema, e.g. swollen feet.
- Breathlessness: particularly if heart or lung disease is present. Anaemia is one cause of decompensation in chronic heart failure.
- Angina, if there is underlying coronary disease, which may have been undetected before the anaemia.

Signs

The physical examination in anaemia is usually unremarkable.

- Pallor (palms of the hands, conjunctiva) may occur, although this is an unreliable sign because many pale people are not anaemic, and many anaemic people are not pale.
- A systolic 'flow' murmur is common.
- There may be evidence of the underlying pathology.
- In long-standing iron deficiency anaemia, koilonychia (spoon-shaped nails) may occur.

Management

Anaemia is a physiological abnormality: not a diagnosis. A final, pathological diagnosis must always be made. The first step in doing this usually involves classifying the anaemia according to red cell size.

Microcytic/hypochromic anaemia: the red cells are smaller than normal (microcytic) and contain less haemoglobin than normal (hypochromic). Common causes are iron deficiency anaemia and thalassaemia trait.

Normochromic and normocytic anaemia: sometimes referred to as 'the anaemia of chronic disease'. The red cells are of normal or just slightly reduced size and have a normal haemoglobin concentration.

Common causes include:
- Chronic infections, e.g. tuberculosis (TB) and osteomyelitis.
- Inflammatory diseases such as rheumatoid arthritis and connective tissue disorders.
- Malignant disease.
- Renal failure.

The anaemia of chronic disease is in part caused by the inhibitory effect of interleukin 1 on erythropoiesis, and by erythropoietin deficiency (the latter especially in renal failure). Iron deficiency often complicates chronic diseases and may explain a lower than expected haemoglobin.

Macrocytic anaemia: the red cells are larger than normal. Common causes include:
- Vitamin B_{12} or folate deficiency.
- Cytotoxic drug treatment, e.g. azathioprine or cyclophosphamide.
- Myelodysplasia (see p. 337).
- Haemolytic anaemias.
- Hypothyroidism: can cause either a normocytic or a macrocytic anaemia.
- Liver disease and alcohol abuse result in a macrocytosis, but not anaemia, unless there is coincidental bleeding or haematinic deficiency.

Investigation

The clinical features and the morphological characteristics of the red cells drive investigations on the blood film (see diagram of red cell morphology on p. 338). The following tests are frequently helpful:

Haematinic status (iron stores, vitamin B_{12} and folate—see p. 318) should be determined; iron status should be evaluated in micro- or normocytic anaemias, and vitamin B_{12}/folate status in macrocytic anaemias. **Beware**: haematinic deficiency is common even when another cause for anaemia is clear (e.g. folate deficiency in haemolytic anaemia, iron deficiency in colon cancer, etc.). Once haematinic deficiency is found, the specific cause (malnutrition, malabsorption, excess use or loss, etc.) should always be determined.

A **blood film** is often diagnostic in primary haematological disease as well as in many systemic diseases. It is therefore mandatory in all anaemias that have not been diagnosed by more simple investigations. Person-to-person discussion with the haematologist often speeds up the diagnostic process.

Blood count for the white or platelet count often helps. A **raised neutrophil count** is common and causes include:
- Bacterial infection
- Underlying chronic inflammatory disease)
- Myeloproliferative process (leukaemia, etc.) when mature (chronic leukaemias) or immature (acute leukaemias) white cells are found.

A **low white count** is commonly seen in patients with acute infections as well as in primary bone marrow diseases such as myelodysplasia.

A **high platelet count** may be reactive to:
- Infection—particularly abscesses
- Chronic inflammatory disorders such as rheumatoid arthritis
- Malignancy
- Bleeding
- Post splenectomy
- Or may be a feature of a primary bone marrow disorder such as a myeloproliferative disease.

A **low platelet count** is found in patients with excess consumption of platelets (e.g. idiopathic thrombocytopenic purpura [ITP] or disseminated intravascular coagulation [DIC]) or in diseases where bone marrow production of platelets is impaired (e.g. acute leukaemia, myelodysplasia).

Other investigations important in some patients with anaemia are:
- Bone marrow examination; this is often helpful and should be discussed with a haematologist.
- Renal and liver biochemistry diagnose underlying organ specific disease.
- Markers of inflammation (erythrocyte sedimentation rate [ESR] or C-reactive protein [CRP]) are often raised in anaemia of chronic disease, e.g. disseminated malignancy, sepsis or vasculitis.
- Thyroid status: hypothyroidism can cause a macrocytic or normocytic anaemia.
- Blood cultures are useful if sepsis is suspected.

Treatment

Treatment is of the underlying disease. In patients with the anaemia of chronic disease, blood transfusion or treatment with recombinant erythropoietin may be of help.

Blood transfusion

Donor and recipients need to be blood group 'matched' for successful transfusion.
- The ABO system: the A and B genes encode enzymes transforming a cell membrane glycoprotein (substance H) into either A or B antigens. Individuals possess either two A or two B genes (AA or BB), one of each (AB), either A or B (AO, BO) or neither (O), and IgM antibodies to the antigen that they do not possess (i.e. anti-B if AA or O, and anti-A if BB or O). To avoid transfusion reactions, patients must receive blood either similar to their own group or from a group 'O' donor (a 'universal donor').
- The rhesus (Rh) system comprises three allelic sets of genes (cC, D (Rhesus positive) and no D (Rhesus negative), and eE).
- Other systems.

Complications of blood transfusion

- Transfusion reactions; immediate or delayed anaphylaxis (see p. 132). Minor reactions (common in those with multiple transfusions) cause (post-) transfusion fever and shorten transfused red cell life.
- Large transfusions may provoke heart or haemostatic failure (blood preservatives chelate calcium, so inhibiting the clotting cascade).
- Viral transmission, especially HIV and hepatitis B or C. Many countries routinely screen all blood for these pathogens.
- Iron overload in those receiving multiple transfusions (e.g. hereditary anaemias).
- Immune suppression. Though there is controversy, there is some evidence that blood transfusion in those with cancer increases the chance of the cancer progressing. This phenomenon is referred to as transfusion-related immunomodulation (TRIM).
- Graft versus host disease: this is a rare disease in which the lymphocytes from the donor blood survive in the blood transfusion recipient, and recognize the recipient as being 'foreign'. This results in an illness called 'graft versus host disease' characterized by skin rash, diarrhoea and biochemical evidence of liver damage, usually early after transfusion. The illness has a high mortality.
- Transfusion-related acute lung injury (TRALI), which usually occurs 1–6 hours after transfusion. The patient becomes breathless and breathes rapidly, and cyanosis may be evident. Examination may shows inspiratory crackles and decreased air entry. Blood gases confirm hypoxaemia. A chest X-ray reveals widespread 'fluffy' infiltrates, consistent with an acute lung injury. There is no specific treatment; mechanical ventilation may be required.

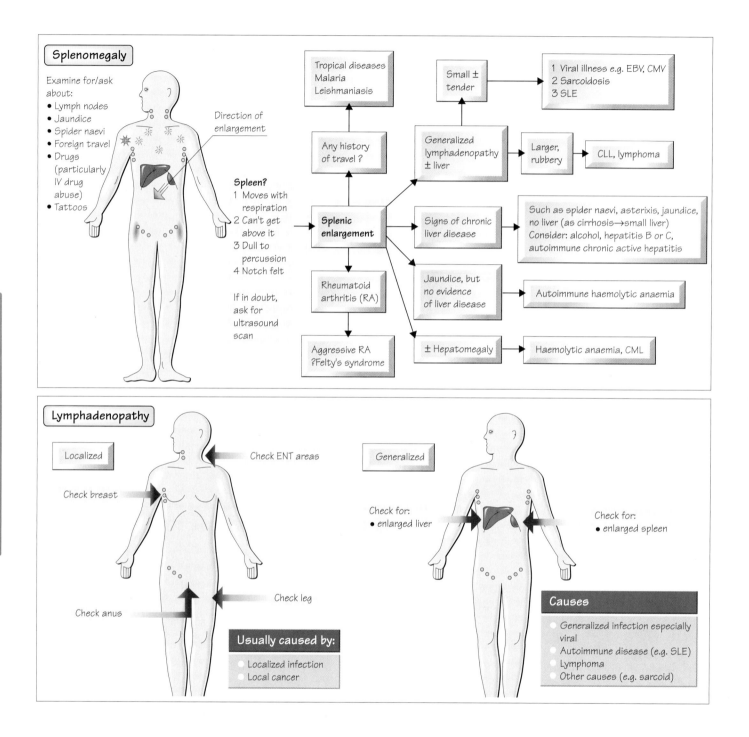

Lymphadenopathy

Local lymphadenopathy often relates to local infection or malignancy, whereas generalized lymphadenopathy has a wider differential diagnosis, including:

• **Infections** including viral, spirochaetal, rickettsial and protozoal ones.

• **Inflammatory disorders**, such as autoimmune conditions, particularly systemic lupus erythematosus (SLE).

• **Malignancy**, e.g. lymphoma.

• **Miscellaneous** diseases such as sarcoidosis.

Many patients with lymphadenopathy referred to hospital are worried that they have cancer.

History and examination

The history and examination should focus on possible sites or sources of infection resulting in lymphadenopathy, the presence of inflammatory or connective tissue diseases such as rheumatoid arthritis, SLE or the potentially more sinister symptoms of weight loss, long-lasting malaise or sweats, which might indicate a malignant disease. Lymph node size and texture give some clues:

- Bulky, hard nodes are suggestive of cancer.
- Soft, mobile, tender nodes point towards infection.

These features can be misleading and it is unwise to make a judgement solely on these findings. It is vital to examine the area drained by the lymph node thoroughly, if necessary, using radiological techniques, e.g. mammography for axillary lymph nodes.

Investigation

A full blood count (FBC), erythrocyte sedimentation rate (ESR), liver function tests and C-reactive protein (CRP) estimation are useful screening tests. Other investigations (e.g. computed tomography [CT]) should be tailored to the clinical situation. A biopsy should be undertaken if there is any suspicion of malignancy causing lymph node enlargement, either a fine needle aspirate (quick and easy, but high error rate) or open or Tru-cut biopsy (invasive but diagnostically reliable).

Splenomegaly

The differential diagnosis for a mass in the left upper quadrant includes renal or colonic masses and, less commonly, a mass of abdominal lymph nodes. Ultrasonography or CT scan can confirm that the mass is a spleen. The spleen needs to enlarge threefold before it can be palpated. Thus, a palpable spleen is always pathological and should prompt thorough investigations to establish the cause. The differential diagnosis of splenomegaly includes:

- Infections: e.g. infectious mononucleosis and malaria.
- Lymphoproliferative diseases: especially chronic lymphoid leukaemia (CLL) and lymphoma.
- Myeloproliferative diseases: particularly chronic myeloid leukaemia (CML) and myelofibrosis.
- Haemolytic anaemias, especially autoimmune haemolytic anaemia (AIHA), hereditary spherocytosis.
- Portal hypertension complicating cirrhosis, or much more rarely without cirrhosis (e.g. portal vein thrombosis, schistosomiasis).
- Autoimmune disease: e.g. SLE.
- Other rarer causes such as sarcoidosis, iron deficiency.

The history and physical signs in addition to the splenomegaly often give a strong pointer towards the correct diagnosis.

- Viral infection, often Epstein-Barr (EBV) or cytomegalovirus (CMV): several days of flu-like symptoms, sore throat and minor generalized lymphadenopathy, often with mild hepatomegaly.
- Toxoplasmosis.
- Liver cirrhosis: features of chronic liver disease may be noted (see p. 233) and, unlike the above disorders, the liver is often small and therefore impalpable.
- Lymphoma: general malaise, weight loss, sometimes night sweats, bulky lymphadenopathy and hepatomegaly.

Investigation

An FBC and film are extremely helpful in ruling many diagnoses in or out:

- **A myeloproliferative disorder**: the haemoglobin is high in polycythaemia rubra vera, the white cell (both mature and immature granulocytes) count is high in CML and the platelet count high in essential thrombocythaemia.
- **Myelofibrosis**: where the bone marrow is replaced by fibrous tissue. Haematopoiesis occurs in extramedullary sites, including the spleen, resulting in massive splenomegaly. The peripheral blood shows leukoerythroblastic features (see p. 338) along with misshapen red cells.
- **A haemolytic anaemia**: the blood count shows anaemia and polychromasia (reflecting increased reticulocytes). Other abnormalities (such as spherocytes) may be present depending on the underlying cause of haemolysis.
- **Viral infection**: reactive lymphocytes in the blood suggest a viral infection.
- **Liver disease**: target cells and a macrocytosis are often seen in liver disease.
- **Lymphoma**: the blood count and film of those with any form of lymphoma may be normal or non-specifically abnormal; it cannot therefore be relied on to rule this diagnosis in or out. However, mild anaemia and rouleaux formation, indicative of a raised ESR, may be present.
- **CLL**: the white cell count will be high with $\geq 5 \times 10^9$/L circulating lymphocytes.

Additional investigations, including lymph node or liver biopsy, are sometimes necessary for diagnosis. Fine needle aspirate or biopsy of the spleen is dangerous and is not recommended. A diagnostic splenectomy is rarely necessary, but should be considered in persistent undiagnosed splenomegaly despite full and thorough investigation. However, CT scanning of the abdomen/thorax in serious conditions associated with splenomegaly often reveals either the diagnosis or lymphadenopathy suitable for percutaneous biopsy.

Complications of splenomegaly

Splenomegaly itself is usually asymptomatic, although sometimes a 'dragging' sensation is felt in the left upper quadrant. Occasionally splenomegaly is complicated by:

- **Infarction**, resulting in a 'pleuritic' pain over the spleen, i.e. the lower lateral aspect of the left chest. The differential diagnosis is from other causes of pleurisy (see p. 12). Repeated infarction (e.g. in sickle-cell disease) or splenectomy causes hyposplenism, which predisposes to overwhelming bacterial (especially pneumococcal) infection (although this is an uncommon complication). Such patients should receive pneumococcal/meningococcal/HIB immunization and life-long prophylactic penicillin (erythromycin in penicillin-sensitive patients).
- **Rupture**: pathological spleens rupture more easily than normal, causing abdominal pain and marked hypotension. Thus, the differential diagnosis of anyone with splenomegaly who becomes hypotensive includes splenic rupture, treated by immediate surgery. A sepsis syndrome should also be considered in hypotensive patients with a large spleen.
- **Hypersplenism**: spleens pool blood in proportion to their size. A normal spleen pools 2% of the blood volume; a very large spleen may pool $\geq 20\%$ of the blood volume, which may result in anaemia, thrombocytopenia (especially in portal hypertension) or even pancytopenia (see p. 326). Diagnosis is by excluding other causes.

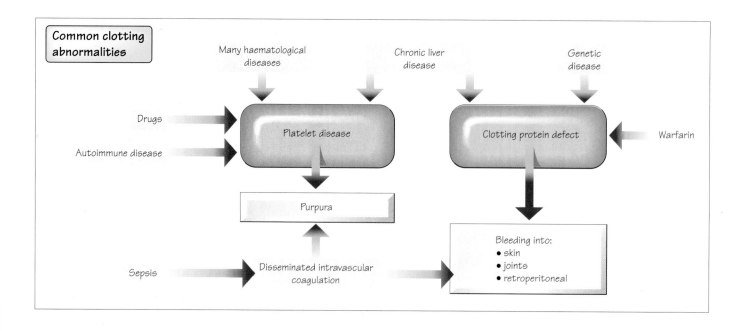

Common clotting abnormalities

The key to assessing a bleeding/bruising problem lies in the history and in particular whether the bleeding has been life-long or is new:

• **Life-long bleeding** suggests an inherited disease, confirmed by ascertaining the bleeding response to remote haemostatic challenges (e.g. operations, dental extractions or postpartum bleeding, although von Willebrand's disease improves with pregnancy). The family history and mode of inheritance should be determined (e.g. X-linked for haemophilia A and B).

• **New bleeding** suggests an acquired problem. This often relates to medical problems, either covert (e.g. hypothyroidism) or overt (e.g. septicaemia or disseminated intravascular coagulation).

A full drug history must always be taken—aspirin and NSAIDs are the most common cause of platelet dysfunction. Other drugs may cause marrow aplasia (see p. 326).

Examination

The main purpose of the physical examination is to exclude any underlying medical disease (e.g. sepsis, leukaemia, etc.) and determine the consequences of bleeding (e.g. haemoarthroses, gastrointestinal blood loss), which in themselves need specific treatment. Any bleeding pattern present should be determined because this relates to the underlying defect.

In platelet defects (quantitative or qualitative), purpura/petechiae are common; other manifestations also seen in von Willebrand's disease are epistaxes and, in women, menorrhagia.

In contrast, in coagulation factor deficiency (e.g. haemophilia) bleeding is usually into muscles or joints.

Investigations

First-line investigations (the 'basic clotting screen') include:
• **Full blood count**: particularly the platelet count; the haemoglobin and white count provide important clues to the presence of marrow aplasia or leukaemia.

• **Coagulation screen**: a prothrombin time (PT: prolonged when any of factors I, II, V, X or VII is deficient/inhibited), activated partial thromboplastin time (APTT, prolonged if any of factors I, II, V, VIII, IX, X, XI or XII is deficient/inhibited) and if indicated a thrombin time (TT, prolonged when fibrinogen is deficient, fibrinogen polymerization is inhibited by fibrin degradation products [FDPs] or if heparin is present). If a prolonged clotting time is found, adding normal plasma (which contains all clotting factors) allows differentiation between bleeding caused by clotting factor deficiency (coagulation corrects) and that caused by inhibition (coagulation does not correct). A common inhibitor is the lupus anticoagulant (see p. 347), which paradoxically is associated with a procoagulant state rather than with bleeding.

• **Factor VIII, von Willebrand's factor (VWF) activity** and **VWF antigen** when inherited disorders are suspected.

• **Bleeding time** after a skin cut 1 mm deep and 1 cm long. Prolonged bleeding occurs with deficient or defective platelets, and is further investigated by *in vitro* platelet aggregation tests.

If bleeding is undeniably abnormal and first-line tests are unremarkable, **second-line investigations** are undertaken. Von Willebrand's disease must be specifically looked for, because basic screening tests can be normal. The bleeding time is a difficult test even in expert hands and is being replaced by *in vitro* alternatives, such as the PFA 100 test. Platelet aggregation can be little affected in storage pool disease, so it is routine to look at the platelet nucleotide content. Factor XIII deficiency and α_2-antiplasmin deficiency are rare autosomal recessive bleeding disorders—neither affects screening tests, so they are considered when there is a good history and first-line tests are negative, especially if there is parental consanguinity.

Treatment

This is of the underlying cause. Specific treatments are outlined in Chapters 172 and 173.

44 Leukopenia

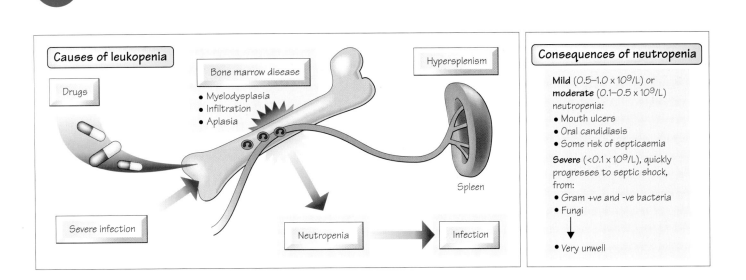

Causes of leukopenia

Drugs

Bone marrow disease
- Myelodysplasia
- Infiltration
- Aplasia

Severe infection

Neutropenia → Infection

Hypersplenism

Spleen

Consequences of neutropenia

Mild ($0.5-1.0 \times 10^9$/L) or **moderate** ($0.1-0.5 \times 10^9$/L) neutropenia:
- Mouth ulcers
- Oral candidiasis
- Some risk of septicaemia

Severe ($<0.1 \times 10^9$/L), quickly progresses to septic shock, from:
- Gram +ve and -ve bacteria
- Fungi

- Very unwell

A decrease in the number of circulating white cells (leukopenia) is not uncommon, and may indicate serious disease that needs immediate diagnosis and treatment.

Neutropenia

Neutropenia means decreased circulating neutrophils (total count $\leq 2.0 \times 10^9$ neutrophils/L). In extreme cases there may be no circulating neutrophils—called agranulocytosis. There are many causes of neutropenia:

- **Drug-induced** neutropenia is the most common cause, and may result in a selective decrease in neutrophils (e.g. carbimazole), or a more general bone marrow depression, a pancytopenia. Examples of the latter include cytotoxic chemotherapy, rheumatological drugs including sulphasalazine, gold and some non-steroidal anti-inflammatory drugs (NSAIDs). Many other drugs have been implicated. Alcoholism may underlie neutropenia.
- **Myelodysplastic syndrome** is common in elderly people (see p. 337).
- **Severe infection** can cause neutropenia, as in pneumococcal pneumonia with complicating septicaemia, where the low white cell count is associated with a worse outlook. The diagnosis is usually obvious. Typhoid and viral infections likewise can depress neutrophil counts.
- **Bone marrow infiltration**, particularly from haematological malignancy, such as leukaemia. Usually affects all cell lines (pancytopenia)—see p. 326.
- **Bone marrow failure** results in pancytopenia, e.g. aplastic anaemia.
- **Hypersplenism** (see p. 83), including Felty's syndrome (rheumatoid arthritis with high-titre rheumatoid factor).
- Very rare causes include cyclical neutropenia.
- **Autoimmune** neutropenia.

Most patients with mild-moderate neutropenia (counts $1.0-2.0 \times 10^9$/L) have no symptoms. However, the lower the count, the greater the risk of infection (neutropenic sepsis): this risk becomes significant when counts are below 0.5×10^9/L and very significant below 0.1×10^9/L.

- Mouth ulceration and oral candidiasis are common in sustained neutropenias.
- Infection can very rapidly (i.e. within hours) become overwhelming, producing severe septic shock (see p. 20).
- Organisms may be 'typical' pathogenic bacteria (e.g. *Staphylococcus aureus*, pathogenic streptococci, Gram-negative bacilli), although low-grade pathogens and fungi are also commonly implicated.
- Treatment involves establishing which organism is responsible (blood cultures), providing circulatory support (fluids, sometimes vaso-constrictors) and, most importantly, giving high-dose broad-spectrum antibiotics without delay.
- Treatment with granulocyte–colony-stimulating factor (G-CSF) may sometimes help to shorten a period of neutropenia, depending on the cause (e.g. especially chemotherapy-induced neutropenia).

Lymphopenia

A decrease in the number of circulating lymphocytes is much rarer than neutropenia. Causes other than haematological malignancy and its treatment are uncommon, and include:

- Autoimmune disease, such as systemic lupus erythematosus (SLE).
- Viral infections, including acute (e.g. Epstein-Barr virus and cytomegalovirus) or chronic infections (e.g. HIV).
- Inherited disease (see p. 314).

Presentation is with other features of the underlying disease or with infection/malignancy. T-cell deficiency predisposes to infection with intracellular pathogens (especially viruses), pyogenic bacteria (e.g. staphylococcal infection), fungi, *Pneumocystis carinii* and protozoa (e.g. *Cryptosporidium* sp.), in addition to increasing the rates of lymphoma and solid organ cancers. B-cell deficiencies predispose to pyogenic bacterial infection.

45 Oncological emergencies

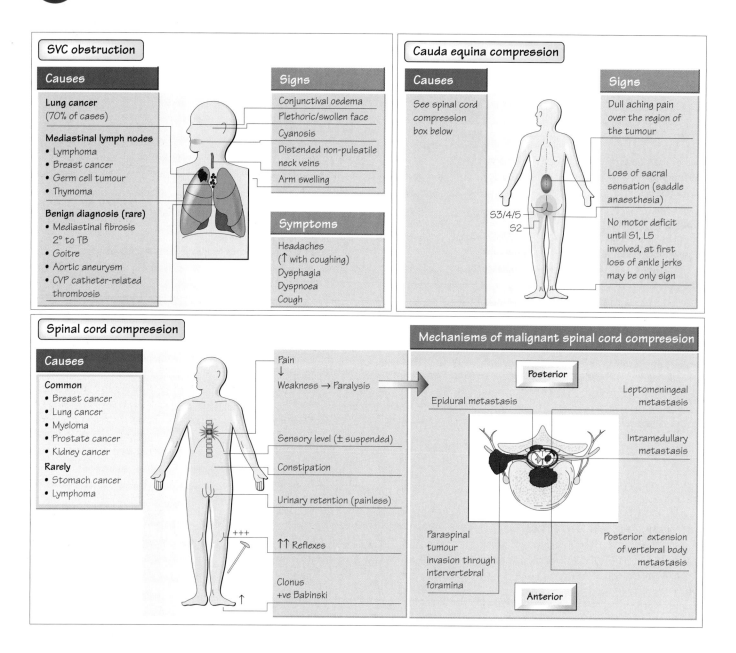

SVC obstruction

Causes

Lung cancer
(70% of cases)

Mediastinal lymph nodes
- Lymphoma
- Breast cancer
- Germ cell tumour
- Thymoma

Benign diagnosis (rare)
- Mediastinal fibrosis
  2° to TB
- Goitre
- Aortic aneurysm
- CVP catheter-related
  thrombosis

Signs

Conjunctival oedema
Plethoric/swollen face
Cyanosis
Distended non-pulsatile
neck veins
Arm swelling

Symptoms

Headaches
(↑ with coughing)
Dysphagia
Dyspnoea
Cough

Cauda equina compression

Causes

See spinal cord
compression
box below

Signs

Dull aching pain
over the region of
the tumour

Loss of sacral
sensation (saddle
anaesthesia)

No motor deficit
until S1, L5
involved, at first
loss of ankle jerks
may be only sign

S3/4/5
S2

Spinal cord compression

Causes

Common
- Breast cancer
- Lung cancer
- Myeloma
- Prostate cancer
- Kidney cancer
Rarely
- Stomach cancer
- Lymphoma

Pain
↓
Weakness → Paralysis

Sensory level (± suspended)

Constipation

Urinary retention (painless)

+++

↑↑ Reflexes

Clonus
+ve Babinski

↑

Mechanisms of malignant spinal cord compression

Posterior

Epidural metastasis

Leptomeningeal
metastasis

Intramedullary
metastasis

Paraspinal
tumour
invasion through
intervertebral
foramina

Posterior extension
of vertebral body
metastasis

Anterior

Superior vena caval obstruction

A clinical syndrome arising from obstruction of blood flow through the superior vena cava (SVC). This thin-walled vessel may be compressed, invaded or thrombosed.

Aetiology

- **Malignant** (usually): from malignant lymph nodes compressing or invading the SVC. Lung cancer is the cause in 70%. The remainder are the result of lymphoma, and more rarely breast cancer and other tumours.
- **Benign** (rarely): mediastinal goitre; aortic aneurysm; iatrogenic, e.g. thrombosis from indwelling central venous catheters; mediastinal fibrosis (histoplasmosis/tuberculosis).

Clinical presentation

Symptoms arise from the increase in venous pressure in the jugular and subclavian veins, and from the local effects of a mediastinal or bronchial tumour; they comprise dyspnoea, facial/arm swelling, headaches (worse on coughing) or head fullness, cough or dysphagia. Signs include non-pulsatile distension of neck and chest wall veins, oedema of face, neck and arms, plethoric facies, dilated veins over upper chest wall, cyanosis and conjunctival oedema (chemosis).

Investigation

SVC obstruction is a medical emergency. Previously patients received immediate radiotherapy, but modern oncological therapy now makes histological diagnosis vital. However, if patients are acutely ill radiotherapy is still given before histological diagnosis.

- Chest X-ray: superior mediastinal widening, pleural effusions, right hilar mass
- Sputum cytology
- Lymph node biopsy (if accessible node palpable)
- Bone marrow examination
- Bronchoscopy
- Mediastinoscopy/thoracotomy
- Computed tomography (CT)-guided, percutaneous, transthoracic, fine needle aspiration.

Management

Bed rest with head elevated, oxygen, and high-dose steroids (dexamethasone). Additional therapy depends on aetiology:

- **Malignant** disease: wire stent insertion followed by radiotherapy for non-small cell lung cancer; chemotherapy for small cell lung cancer, lymphoma and germ cell tumours.
- **Non-malignant** causes are treated by percutaneous angioplasty and wire stent insertion. These are useful in those previously irradiated or in those with lung cancer before radiotherapy.
- **Thrombotic** SVC obstruction: remove the local precipitant of thrombosis (SVC catheter) and consider thrombolysis. Surgery (bypassing the blocked SVC) is rarely indicated and is reserved for non-malignant cases refractory to other therapies.

Prognosis

Patients with SVC obstruction from non-small cell lung cancer often live < 6 months. Presentation with SVC obstruction does not affect prognosis in patients with lymphoma or small-cell lung cancer. Those with non-malignant causes of the syndrome live much longer—reported average being 9 years.

Malignant spinal cord compression

Malignant spinal cord compression is the second most common neurological complication of malignancy after cerebral metastases, and often arises in the pre-terminal phase of the illness.

Pathophysiology and aetiology

The spinal cord and its nerve roots are most commonly compressed anteriorly by posterior extension of haematogenously spread metastases in the vertebral body, extending into the epidural space or through vertebral body collapse. The cord may also be compromised by extension of a paraspinal tumour through the intervertebral foramina, which can occur without evidence of bony involvement. Damage is principally mediated by disruption of small vessel circulation which is precipitated by the changes in pressure within the spinal canal. There may be multiple epidural metastases causing cord compression at different levels. See figure for aetiology.

Clinical presentation

Most patients are known to have malignancy. Spinal cord compression is the first manifestation of cancer in 10%. The thoracic spine is the most common site of compression, followed by the lumbosacral and cervical regions.

Symptoms and signs

- Pain: most common symptom; it may predate neurological signs. Constant, dull, aching pain, which may radiate laterally, and is worse on movement (flexion) or increases in thoracic pressure (sneezing, straining). The involved vertebrae may be tender to percussion.

- Weakness: particularly to the proximal muscles of the lower limbs in an upper motor neuron pattern, although the exact distribution of power loss depends on the site of compression. Deep tendon reflexes are increased and the plantar response is extensor.
- Sensory loss/paraesthesiae: ascending to or just below level of relevant dermatome at level of compression (suspended level).
- Ataxia: loss of proprioception (posterior columns).
- Urinary retention and constipation: late symptoms of autonomic dysfunction.

Investigations

Malignant spinal cord compression is a medical emergency and mandates urgent investigation, i.e. within 24 h of symptom onset.

- **Plain radiographs** may show vertebral body collapse or pedicle destruction.
- Whole spine **magnetic resonance imaging** (MRI) is the investigation of choice. It defines the exact location and disease extent. The whole spine must be examined as multiple sites of compression can occur.
- CT-guided **percutaneous biopsy** if primary unknown.

Treatment

- **High-dose corticosteroids** may improve symptoms and outcome.
- **Radiotherapy** to debulk the tumour is the treatment of choice and reduces pain. There may be some improvement in power, but paraplegia is reversed in only 10–15%. The radiation field includes two vertebrae either side of the site of compression (the site of frequent recurrence).
- **Surgery** has significant morbidity and mortality, but has a role in those without a diagnosis, those with spinal instability, progression of neurological deficit during radiotherapy, compression in a previously irradiated area (spinal cord has already received maximal tolerable radiation dose) or radioresistant disease, and may be associated with better functional outcome and survival.
- **Chemotherapy**: cytotoxic chemotherapy is the treatment of choice in children with chemosensitive tumours, and as an adjunct to radiotherapy in adults with chemosensitive disease. Endocrine therapy may help in prostate and breast cancer.
- **Physiotherapy** is crucial in maximizing any return of neurological function.

Prognosis

The three main predictors of outcome are:
- Pre-treatment neurological status: 80% of those ambulant at diagnosis remain so with urgent treatment. Paraplegia is reversed in < 15% of cases.
- Speed of onset of neurological deficit: disease progressing gradually is more likely to be reversible.
- Tumour type: radiation- and chemotherapy-sensitive disease responds faster and better to treatment. Radioresistant tumours have a poor outcome.

Most patients presenting with malignant spinal cord compression will not achieve ambulation. They are often pre-terminally ill and face the loss of independence that confinement to a wheelchair brings. Maximizing physical and psychological support in this deeply distressing situation is as important as any therapeutic treatment.

Hypercalcaemia (see p. 288)

Fever with neutropenia (see p. 85)

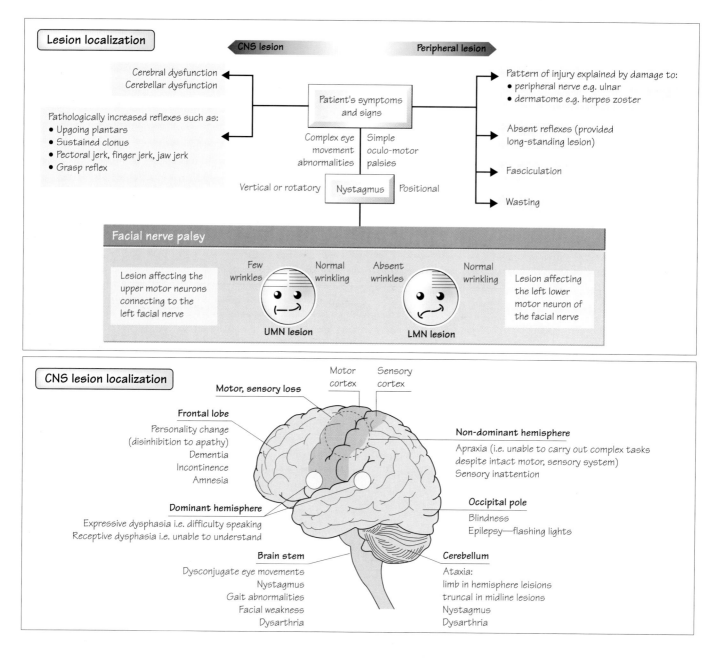

Lesion localization

CNS lesion → Peripheral lesion ←

Patient's symptoms and signs

Cerebral dysfunction
Cerebellar dysfunction

Pathologically increased reflexes such as:
• Upgoing plantars
• Sustained clonus
• Pectoral jerk, finger jerk, jaw jerk
• Grasp reflex

Complex eye movement abnormalities | Simple oculo-motor palsies

Vertical or rotatory | Nystagmus | Positional

Pattern of injury explained by damage to:
• peripheral nerve e.g. ulnar
• dermatome e.g. herpes zoster

Absent reflexes (provided long-standing lesion)

Fasciculation

Wasting

Facial nerve palsy

Lesion affecting the upper motor neurons connecting to the left facial nerve

Few wrinkles | Normal wrinkling

Absent wrinkles | Normal wrinkling

Lesion affecting the left lower motor neuron of the facial nerve

UMN lesion

LMN lesion

CNS lesion localization

Motor cortex | Sensory cortex

Motor, sensory loss

Frontal lobe
Personality change (disinhibition to apathy)
Dementia
Incontinence
Amnesia

Non-dominant hemisphere
Apraxia (i.e. unable to carry out complex tasks despite intact motor, sensory system)
Sensory inattention

Dominant hemisphere
Expressive dysphasia i.e. difficulty speaking
Receptive dysphasia i.e. unable to understand

Occipital pole
Blindness
Epilepsy—flashing lights

Brain stem
Dysconjugate eye movements
Nystagmus
Gait abnormalities
Facial weakness
Dysarthria

Cerebellum
Ataxia:
limb in hemisphere leisions
truncal in midline lesions
Nystagmus
Dysarthria

There are so many different neurological diseases that it is not always possible to make a firm diagnosis from a particular set of signs and symptoms, e.g. there are numerous causes of ataxia—the combination of peripheral neuropathy and ataxia only narrows this down but still leaves a range of possible underlying diagnoses. Neurologists therefore make an anatomical diagnosis followed by an aetiological or pathological diagnosis.

In addition to many acquired diseases, there are also many inherited conditions involving the nervous system. Partly, this is because there are so many genes expressed in the nervous system (40% of the body's 30 000 genes are neurally expressed). Mutation in many of these may be devastating but not lethal, allowing the survival of individuals with genetic disease. Furthermore, the brain undergoes more postnatal maturation than other organs, which requires the expression of new genes. The third important feature of the nervous system is that most cells of the central nervous system (CNS) are non-dividing and therefore abnormal protein products of mutant genes accumulate and cause progressive neurodegeneration.

There are six steps to neurological diagnosis:

1 Knowledge of neuroepidemiology (see Chapter 48). The prior probability of a diagnosis depends on the age of the patient and other factors.

2 In a neurological diagnosis, 80% depends on a good history. The examination contributes 10% and investigations another 10%. Many neurological patients have normal scans, especially those with neurodegenerative diseases.

Clinical Presentations at a Glance

3 Perform a standard, simple examination on every patient. Extend this examination in particular situations.

4 Synthesize the history and examination to decide whether the problem is in the central or peripheral nervous system (including the muscles) or of psychiatric origin or from another system.

5 Only then can you draw up a differential diagnosis, taking into account the location of the problem (brain, spinal cord, nerve or muscle), the onset and progression of symptoms, and the age of the patient.

6 Perform special investigations to confirm your diagnostic hypothesis.

Lesion localization

In clinical practice the key distinction in lesion localization is between the central and the peripheral nervous system (PNS). In diagnostic terms this is far more important than whether the lesion is in a specific brain region.

The cerebral hemispheres

The extent of neurological dysfunction is affected by individual variation, the tempo and nature of the pathological process and cortical plasticity. Hemispheric lesions cause less motor and sensory dysfunction than lesions of equivalent volume in lower structures, and show a less consistent relationship between dysfunction and lesion localization than in the brain stem, spinal cord or PNS:

• **Contralateral hemianaesthesia** arises from damage to the cortical sensory area (see figure) or from damage to thalamocortical connections. It is usually incomplete because somatosensory function is partially represented in both hemispheres.

• **Hemiplegia** may be caused by:
  • lesions of the primary motor cortex (when conscious level is also often decreased)
  • the descending motor tracts in the corona radiata or the posterior limb of the internal capsule, in which conscious level is usually normal
  • the brain stem (rarely), when there are usually associated cranial nerve signs.

• **Bilateral weakness** is unlikely to be the result of a single lesion of the cerebral cortex, except in the context of coma, because the motor pathways for each side of the body are in separate cerebral hemispheres. An extraordinarily rare exception of a single cortical lesion causing bilateral weakness is a midline parasagittal meningioma.

• **Language dominance** is in the left hemisphere in 98% of people (including 60% of left-handed individuals). This is important in deciding whether a lesion is in the left hemisphere.

• **Expressive (Broca's) dysphasia** is caused by lesions of the dominant frontal lobe—patients show a marked decrease in verbal fluency but normal comprehension.

• **Receptive (Wernicke's) dysphasia** is the result of dominant temporal lobe lesions; it is characterized by fluent speech with frequent paraphrasic errors (use of the wrong word) and poor comprehension.

• **Disorders of spatial awareness**, including neglect, are more common in right posterior hemisphere (parietal) disease.

• **Immediate memory** is dependent on the functional integrity of both hippocampi, which lie adjacent to the temporal lobes. These structures are affected in herpes encephalitis and anoxia (e.g. after cardiac arrest or CO poisoning).

• **Executive function** (planning, impulse control, etc.) is probably a diffuse brain function, but selective disorders of executive control have some localizing value for lesions of the frontal lobes.

The cerebellum

The cerebellum functions as a modulator of motor learning and execution to facilitate the smooth integration of movement. Anatomically it is divided into the midline vermis and two hemispheres. The vascular supply of the cerebellum is from the vertebrobasilar system via the posteroinferior cerebellar artery, the anterior inferior cerebellar artery and the superior cerebellar artery:

• Lesions of the vermis cause **truncal ataxia**; lesions of the hemispheres cause **limb ataxia**.

• **Ocular features** of cerebellar disease are usually prominent and include nystagmus, broken smooth pursuit, slow (hypometric) saccadic movement and ocular dysmetria (saccadic overshoot).

• **Cerebellar tremor** is a kinetic tremor with exacerbation at the end of movement, underlining the function of the cerebellum in damping movement.

• Other signs of cerebellar disturbance are **gait ataxia and dysarthria**. The latter is characteristically a disorder of loss of prosody with monotonous, slurred speech.

The brain stem

The brain stem consists of the midbrain, pons and medulla oblongata. There is a concentration of anatomically important structures in a small area, so most lesions of the brain stem are complex.

• Typical features of brain-stem disease are nystagmus and disorders of conjugate gaze, vertigo, facial weakness, dysarthria, gait disturbance and ataxia. All these can occur as a result of disease in other sites, but the constellation together suggests a brain-stem origin.

• Most eponymous vascular brain-stem syndromes are rarely seen in pure form—precise localization has been greatly aided by magnetic resonance (MR) imaging and MR angiography.

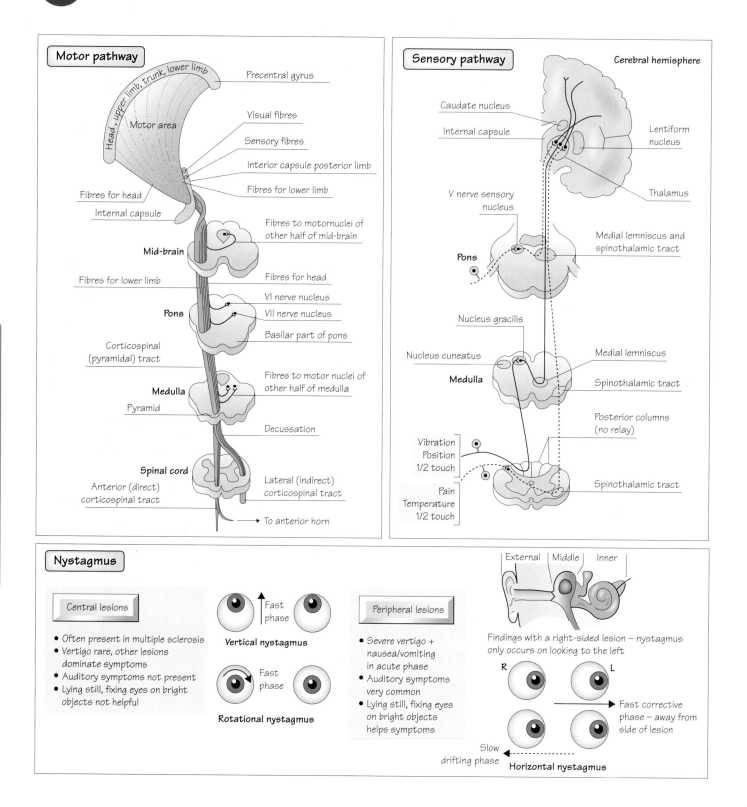

Eye movements

Virtually every region of the brain has some influence on the control of conjugate gaze. Voluntary gaze centres in the frontal lobes and parietal cortex initiate volitional eye movement. These send descending pathways to the brain-stem nuclei, which receive influences from the cerebellum and basal ganglia, and the ascending influences from the spinal cord. There are important internuclear connections. Thus disorders of conjugate gaze may be:

- supranuclear
- internuclear—see p. 99
- nuclear.

Eye movements are also affected by disease of the extraocular muscles and the structures of the orbit, and damage to the peripheral segments of cranial nerves III, IV and VI. Examination of eye movements is thus far more than simply the examination of cranial nerves III, IV and VI. It should be directed at describing the abnormality without assumptions about whether the lesion is in the nerve, the brain stem or higher up. Common patterns of abnormality in conjugate gaze are described in the section on visual disturbance. Nystagmus should be described as occurring in the:
- primary position (the midline) or on
- horizontal or vertical gaze.

In practice it is often difficult to localize nystagmus and it is best to consider it in the context of the rest of the history and examination, before deciding if it is arising from peripheral structures (the labyrinth), the brain stem or the cerebellum. The slow phase of nystagmus is the 'pathological' component and the fast phase is corrective.
- **Peripheral (vestibular) nystagmus** is typically associated with severe symptoms of dysequilibrium, nausea and vomiting, and is often unilateral. The fast phase is away from the lesion because the vestibular apparatus functions to stimulate eye movement towards the contra-lateral side.
- **Central nystagmus**: ipsilateral structures in the brain stem maintain horizontal gaze. Thus, the pathological drift of the eye (the slow phase of nystagmus) is away from the lesion, with a corrective (fast) phase towards the affected side of the brain stem in central nystagmus. Furthermore, central lesions are often bilateral.
- **Cerebellar nystagmus** is similar in that it is probably mediated by cerebellar-brain stem connections.

The spinal cord

The spinal cord is a small structure < 1.5 cm in diameter. There is no anatomical boundary between each side, and many pathological processes are therefore bilateral.

The vascular supply to the spinal cord is of clinical relevance. A single spinal artery supplies the anterior portion of the cord, leaving it vulnerable to ischaemic damage (see p. 380), whereas the posterior part of the cord has a rich anastomotic supply (from posterior spinal arteries).

Weakness caused by spinal cord disease is therefore usually bilateral and associated with a motor and sensory level. At the level of the lesion, there are lower motor neuron signs as evidenced by diminished tendon reflexes and weakness; below the lesion, there are upper motor neuron signs, and above the lesion the limbs are normal.

Descending tracts from the motor cortex travel as the lateral corticospinal tract before synapsing on lower motor neurons in the ventral horns. These cells receive descending influences from the basal ganglia, red nucleus and vestibular apparatus. Lower motor neurons thus serve as a final common pathway for motor function.

The ascending sensory pathways can be divided into:
- spinothalamic tracts, which carry pain and temperature in the contralateral lateral spinothalamic tract and light touch in the ventral spinothalamic tract to synapse in the thalamus;
- gracile and cuneate fasciculi, which carry joint position, sense, kinaesthetic sense, two-point discrimination and light touch on the ipsilateral posterior columns to synapse in the medullary nuclei and on to the thalamus;
- spinocerebellar tracts.

The vertebral level is not the same as the spinal cord level—the cord ends at L1, so it is safe to perform a lumbar puncture in adults in L2–3, L3–4 and L4–5 spaces.

The cord terminates in the conus medullaris and the cauda equina. Conus lesions are characterized by sphincter dysfunction, sensory loss in the perineum and loss of ankle jerks. Cauda equina lesions can involve the same functions, but sphincter disturbance is a late feature and symptoms and signs are usually asymmetrical.

The nerve roots

The identification of lesions at specific spinal root levels requires knowledge of dermatomes and myotomes:
- Root disease is characterized by radicular pain, and sensory and motor dysfunction.
- Particular diseases (e.g. herpes zoster and Guillain–Barré syndrome) have a predilection for nerve roots.
- The most common levels for intervertebral disc prolapse are between the sixth and seventh vertebrae in the cervical region (C7 root compression) and between the fourth and fifth vertebrae in the lumbar region (L5 root compression).
- The effects of root compression at various levels are as follows:
  - C5: weakness of shoulder abduction (deltoid) and forearm flexion (biceps), sensory loss on the lateral aspect of the arm and loss of the biceps jerk;
  - C6: weakness of forearm flexion, finger and wrist extension, loss of the biceps jerk, sensory loss on the lateral surface of the forearm and first and second digits;
  - C7: loss of the triceps reflex, weakness of elbow extension and wrist extension and flexion, sensory loss in the third and fourth digits;
  - C8: weakness and wasting of intrinsic hand muscles, sensory loss in the fifth digit and the medial forearm; there may be an ipsilateral Horner's syndrome;
  - T1: wasting of the small muscles of the hand and ipsilateral Horner's syndrome;
  - L4: weakness of knee extension, loss of the knee jerk and wasting of quadriceps;
  - L5: weakness of knee flexion, ankle dorsiflexion and plantar flexion;
  - S1: loss of the ankle jerk, weakness of dorsiflexion of the great toe.

Lesion localization in peripheral nerve and muscle

See pages 382 and 384.

48 Introduction to neurological diagnosis 3: neuroepidemiology

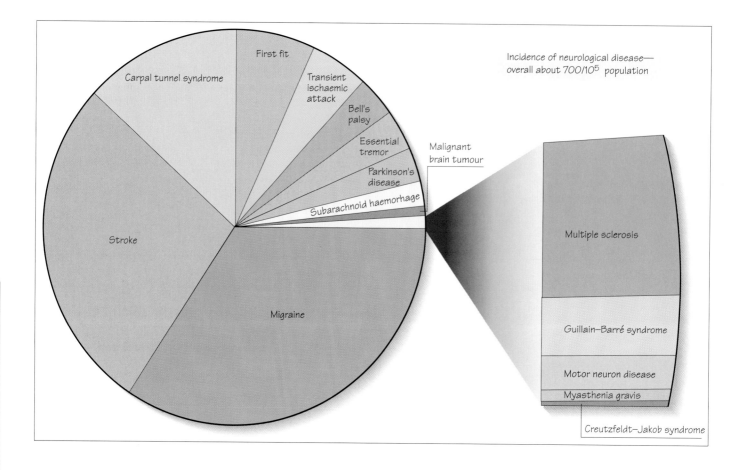

One of the difficulties in learning neurology is that there are apparently a bewildering number of possible conditions and diagnosis for each clinical syndrome, e.g. there are hundreds of different causes of peripheral neuropathy. Therefore, a sensible diagnostician bases the likelihood of a certain diagnosis on the prior probability, or incidence, of that condition. As many conditions are rare, it is reasonable to express this as cases per 100 000 population per year. It will be strikingly apparent from Table 48.1 that the incidence of conditions in general practice is very different from that in a neurology clinic. Although a consultant neurologist (there are 1 per 200 000 people in the UK) will see a patient with a first fit in virtually every clinic, a GP may only see one such patient a year. It is also important to remember that it may be the prevalence of a disorder that gives a true indication of its impact on society as a whole. For example, multiple sclerosis and Parkinson's disease are disorders that do not significantly shorten lifespan in most patients, but last for decades, and therefore they have a high prevalence and impose a high burden on health and social care systems. It will also be immediately apparent that neurology teaching tends to overemphasize rare conditions that many students may never see again.

Table 48.1 Incidence of neurological conditions in the general population.

Condition	Annual incidence per 100 000 population	Time between each new case for a GP
Migraine	250	10 weeks
Stroke	200	12 weeks
Carpal tunnel syndrome	100	6 months
First fit	50	1 years
Transient ischaemic attack	35	17 months
Bell's palsy	25	2 years
Essential tremor	25	2 years
Parkinson's disease	20	2.5 years
Subarachnoid haemorrhage	15	3.3 years
Malignant brain tumour	5	10 years
Multiple sclerosis	5	10 years
Guillain–Barré syndrome	2	25 years
Motor neuron disease	1	33 years
Myasthenia gravis	0.4	125 years
Creutzfeldt–Jakob disease	0.1	500 years

From *Stroke: A Practical Guide.* C.P. Warlow *et al.*, 2nd edn, Oxford: Blackwell Science, 2001.

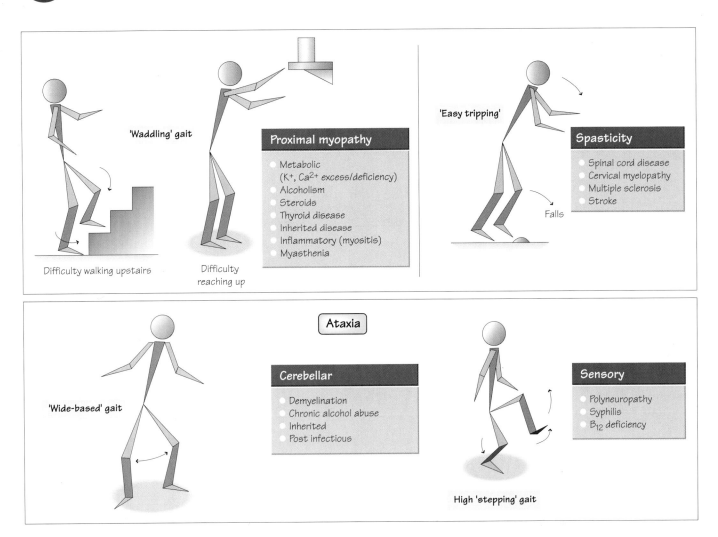

Difficulty walking

Both neurological and non-neurological diseases, e.g. joint disease, can cause difficulty in walking. Analysing gait problems in elderly people carries particular difficulties in interpretation and is complicated by:

- Multiple co-morbidities
- Age-related changes in musculoskeletal function
- Joint disease
- Underlying cerebrovascular disease
- Postural hypotension—see p. 110
- Fear of falling.

A full neurological and rheumatological history and examination are necessary to place all of these contributory factors in context. The most important part of the assessment is to see the patient walking. Invaluable information is obtained by watching the patient get up from the waiting room chair and walk into the consulting room.

Patterns of gait disturbance

Bear in mind that classic gait patterns are present in their pure form only in advanced disease. More frequently a non-specific or mixed gait abnormality is observed.

- Peripheral neuropathies:
  - motor nerve damage—foot drop occurs with a 'high stepping' gait
  - sensory nerve damage, ataxia and sometimes a 'stamping' gait develop.
- Muscle disease usually causes proximal muscle weakness and a 'waddling' gait.
- Spinal cord or upper motor neuron (UMN) damage: The earliest symptom is 'easy tripping up' or difficulty walking on rough ground. Subsequently the leg(s) drag. Examination shows a narrow-based gait, brisk reflexes, often with clonus. The gait is described as being 'stiff', and 'spastic scissoring' together of the legs sometimes occurs.
- Cerebellar disease causes a wide-based, staggering gait (termed 'ataxic'). Midline cerebellar lesions may cause gait ataxia with relatively few signs in the limbs. For causes of ataxia, see overleaf.
- Hemispheric damage causes a contralateral hemiplegic gait, with the contralateral arm held in flexion. In walking, the leg is swung outwards and forwards, in a circular motion—a movement termed 'circumduction'.
- Parkinson's disease causes a stooped posture, with shuffling footsteps and an asymmetrical reduction in arm swing. The gait may be

Clinical Presentations at a Glance

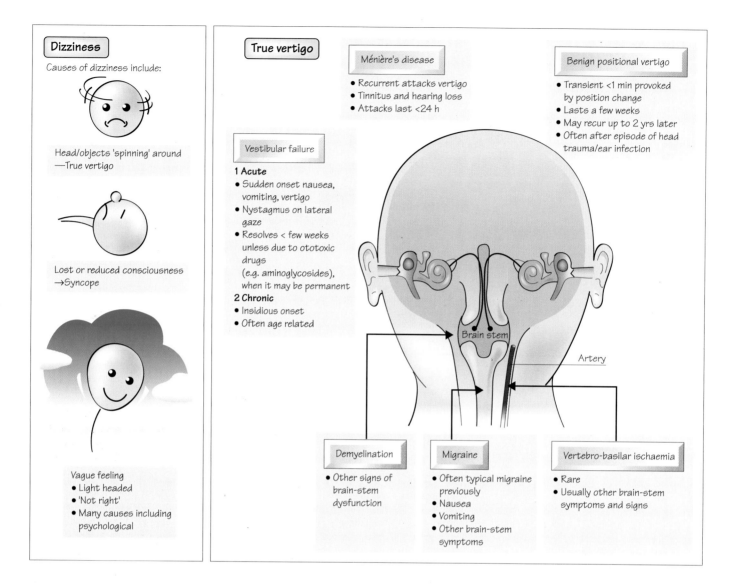

Dizziness

Causes of dizziness include:

Head/objects 'spinning' around
—True vertigo

Lost or reduced consciousness
→Syncope

Vague feeling
- Light headed
- 'Not right'
- Many causes including psychological

True vertigo

Méniėre's disease
- Recurrent attacks vertigo
- Tinnitus and hearing loss
- Attacks last <24 h

Benign positional vertigo
- Transient <1 min provoked by position change
- Lasts a few weeks
- May recur up to 2 yrs later
- Often after episode of head trauma/ear infection

Vestibular failure

1 Acute
- Sudden onset nausea, vomiting, vertigo
- Nystagmus on lateral gaze
- Resolves < few weeks unless due to ototoxic drugs (e.g. aminoglycosides), when it may be permanent

2 Chronic
- Insidious onset
- Often age related

Brain stem

Artery

Demyelination
- Other signs of brain-stem dysfunction

Migraine
- Often typical migraine previously
- Nausea
- Vomiting
- Other brain-stem symptoms

Vertebro-basilar ischaemia
- Rare
- Usually other brain-stem symptoms and signs

'festinant', which means that there is a tendency to hurrying, and turning may be slow and result in postural instability.
• Diffuse vascular disease causes a variety of gait disturbance, including a form of lower body parkinsonism with a wide-based gait, and small steps termed 'marche à petit pas'.
• Gait apraxia is an inability to carry out complex tasks, such as walking, as a result of damage to the part of the brain that integrates complex behaviour. The gait is disordered and the patient is apparently unable to initiate steps, but individual actions, e.g. cycling on a bed, remain intact. It occurs in a number of different cortical diseases, including diffuse vascular disease and also normal pressure hydrocephalus.
• Dizziness—see below.
• **Loss of balance**: may relate to inner-ear disease (often either continuous or episodic), cerebellar disease, dorsal column loss or peripheral sensory neuropathy.

Differential diagnosis of ataxia

Ataxia is defined as incoordination of complex movement, e.g. an inability to walk in a straight line. Anatomically, ataxia is caused by:
• **Lesions of the cerebellum** ('cerebellar ataxia')—wide-based gait, falling to the side of the lesion. A 'kinetic' or intention tremor (brought out by the 'finger-nose' test) is usually present.

• **Disorders of proprioception** ('sensory ataxia') caused by polyneuropathies (see p. 384) or lesions of the dorsal columns (classically, as in tabes dorsalis, causing a 'high stepping' or broad-based gait).
The causes of ataxia are legion and include:
• **Drugs**: anticonvulsants, alcohol, benzodiazepines.
• **Multiple sclerosis**.
• **Cerebellar lesions**: tumours or vascular insults.
• **Inherited disease**: Friedreich's ataxia, spinocerebellar ataxias.
• **Metabolic**: vitamin B_{12} deficiency, heavy metal poisoning.
• **Parainfectious** (more common in children): chickenpox, glandular fever, mycoplasma infection, psittacosis and legionellosis.
• **Paraneoplastic** cerebellar degeneration.

Dizziness

This extremely common problem causes considerable misery to patients, although it rarely has a serious underlying cause. First, establish what is meant by 'dizziness' because this word is used to express a large range of subjective feelings from presyncope or faintness, through vertigo to an odd light-headedness. It is crucial to define the symptom accurately. Although it is always better to let the patient use his or her own words and unwise to put words into patients' mouths, some people

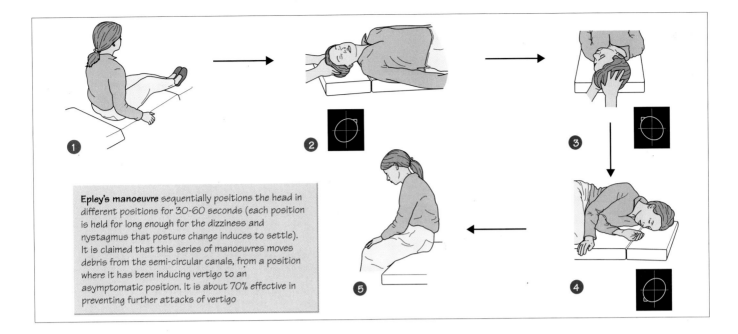

Epley's manoeuvre sequentially positions the head in different positions for 30-60 seconds (each position is held for long enough for the dizziness and nystagmus that posture change induces to settle). It is claimed that this series of manoeuvres moves debris from the semi-circular canals, from a position where it has been inducing vertigo to an asymptomatic position. It is about 70% effective in preventing further attacks of vertigo

have such difficulty describing this symptom that it may be appropriate cautiously to offer some possibilities:

• Do you feel as if you are going to faint? The symptom is likely to represent presyncope (see p. 108).

• Do objects in your vision such as furniture or pictures on the wall actually move around or do you feel as if you are moving? Suggests true vertigo, caused by peripheral pathology affecting the inner ear or cranial nerve VIII, or central pathology affecting the brain stem.

• Do you just have a vague feeling all the time of light-headedness? May represent a variety of problems ranging from hyperventilation through to tension headache. This is sometimes called psychophysical dizziness. It is uncommon to find a clear diagnosis.

• What other symptoms are present? Tinnitus with deafness suggests inner-ear pathology. Nausea and vomiting suggest vestibular or brain-stem disease. Diplopia suggests brain-stem disease. Ataxia—see above.

• What provokes symptoms? If head movement provokes symptoms, then vestibular disease is likely. Provocation on standing suggests postural hypotension.

Once the nature of the symptom has been established, a physical examination should be directed at excluding cardiac arrhythmia or postural hypotension. Then a specific neurological examination should look for evidence of cerebellar and brain-stem disease.

Peripheral causes of vertigo

• **Benign paroxysmal positional vertigo** (BPPV) causes recurrent attacks of transient (lasting seconds) dizziness and vertigo associated with changes in head posture, e.g. lying on the pillow at night. Attacks tend to persist for weeks or months before spontaneously resolving, but may recur. Conventional physical examination is normal. Hallpike's manoeuvre is a specific provocation test performed by bringing the patient from a sitting position down onto their back while turning the head briskly in one direction. If positive, there is nystagmus with rotation towards the side of the lesion and the patient's symptoms are replicated. It is caused by debris in the semicircular canals and can be treated by Epley's manoeuvre (see above).

• **Acute vestibular failure** is a common clinical problem where patients complain of the sudden onset of nausea, vomiting and severe vertigo. On examination there is nystagmus on lateral gaze and ataxia. This condition, which has a good prognosis and tends to resolve over days to weeks, has a variety of synonyms such as 'acute labyrinthitis', and 'vestibular neuronitis' which suggest a possible viral, postviral or inflammatory origin, but betrays our ignorance of the true pathogenesis. It sometimes occurs after an upper respiratory tract infection.

• **Ménière's disease**: recurrent attacks of vertigo, tinnitus and decreased hearing occur in middle life and ultimately may progress to deafness. The attacks build up over minutes, last for hours and then gradually resolve. The key to the diagnosis is to document fluctuating levels of hearing loss.

• **Chronic vestibular failure**: this has a number of causes and presents with a more insidious form of dizziness, which can be rather non-specific in character. Common causes include aminoglycoside toxicity. Age-related vestibular degeneration is increasingly being recognized.

• **Drugs**, such as high-dose aminoglycosides, furosemide (frusemide) can cause vestibular failure.

Central causes of vertigo

• **Vertebrobasilar ischaemia** is a rarer cause of isolated dizziness than usually thought. Attacks of dizziness of abrupt onset and lasting for several minutes are typical. Most patients with vertebrobasilar ischaemia have other symptoms of brain-stem involvement. Brain-stem stroke also usually produces other physical signs.

• **Migraine** can cause transient vertigo. Other symptoms of brain-stem involvement are usual. A migrainous headache may or may not follow.

• **Brain-stem disease**, including multiple sclerosis.

Mixed causes of vertigo

• **Acoustic neuroma** is a benign Schwann cell tumour arising on the vestibular portion of cranial nerve VIII, either isolated or caused by neurofibromatosis type 2 (see p. 378), causing deafness and often vertigo. Brain-stem compression may cause ataxia, and if severe, aqueduct compression and hydrocephalus. Sensation to the cornea is lost. MRI confirms the diagnosis. Surgery may be curative.

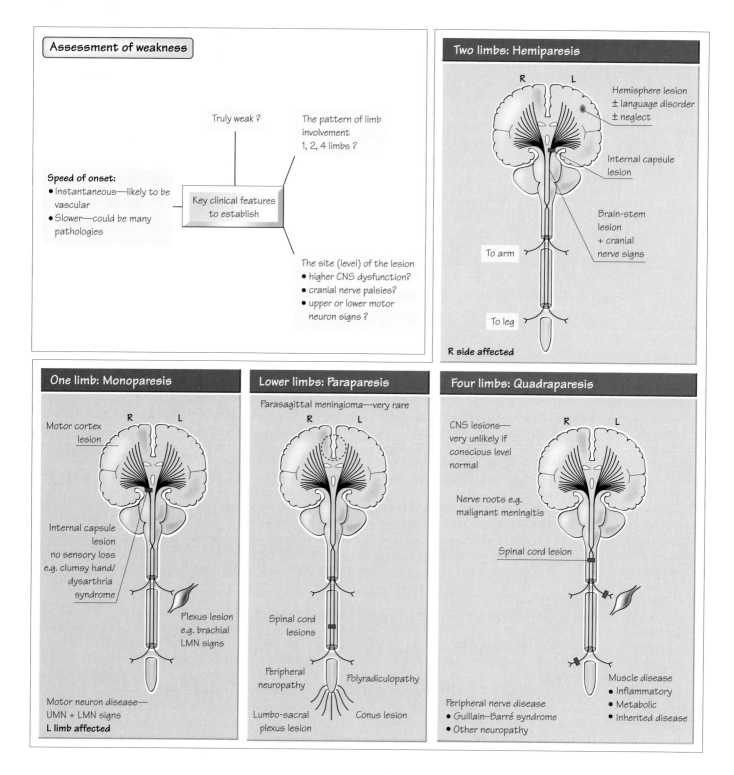

Assessment of weakness

Truly weak ?

The pattern of limb involvement 1, 2, 4 limbs ?

Speed of onset:
- Instantaneous—likely to be vascular
- Slower—could be many pathologies

Key clinical features to establish

The site (level) of the lesion
- higher CNS dysfunction?
- cranial nerve palsies?
- upper or lower motor neuron signs ?

Two limbs: Hemiparesis

R   L

Hemisphere lesion ± language disorder ± neglect

Internal capsule lesion

Brain-stem lesion + cranial nerve signs

To arm

To leg

R side affected

One limb: Monoparesis

R   L

Motor cortex lesion

Internal capsule lesion no sensory loss e.g. clumsy hand/ dysarthria syndrome

Plexus lesion e.g. brachial LMN signs

Motor neuron disease— UMN + LMN signs
L limb affected

Lower limbs: Paraparesis

Parasagittal meningioma—very rare

R   L

Spinal cord lesions

Peripheral neuropathy

Polyradiculopathy

Lumbo-sacral plexus lesion

Conus lesion

Four limbs: Quadraparesis

CNS lesions— very unlikely if conscious level normal

Nerve roots e.g. malignant meningitis

Spinal cord lesion

R   L

Muscle disease
- Inflammatory
- Metabolic
- Inherited disease

Peripheral nerve disease
- Guillain–Barré syndrome
- Other neuropathy

Weakness may be used loosely by patients to include fatigue or tiredness—it is vital to establish that any weakness is genuine, i.e. has led to loss of function (although loss of function may also relate to sensory loss, dyspraxia or incoordination, e.g. as a result of cerebellar disease). It is useful to ask the patient to list the specific activities that cannot be performed (walking, climbing stairs, rising from sitting to standing, reaching above the head, writing, unscrewing lids, etc.). Motor weakness may result from lesions affecting:
- the brain
- spinal cord
- nerve, neuromuscular junction or muscle.

In approaching the diagnosis of weakness it is crucial to establish

Table 50.1

	Upper motor neuron (usually pyramidal tract)	Extrapyramidal or basal ganglia disorders	Lower motor neuron	Muscular	Neuromuscular junction
Pattern of weakness	Limb weakness often incomplete, affecting large movements Most marked in the extensors of upper limb and flexors of lower limb	No true loss of muscle power, but failure of integration of agonist and antagonist muscles Generalized throughout a whole limb	Usually marked, affecting specific muscle groups, except in diffuse polyneuropathies Maximal distally	Usually generalized, unless one muscle is injured Maximal proximally and usually symmetrical: neck and swallowing and eye muscles may be involved	Variable but fatiguable, ptosis and extraocular muscles
Tone	Spasticity: velocity-dependent resistance to movement Clasp knife reflex Clonus	Rigidity	Decreased	Normal or decreased	Normal
Reflexes	Brisk	Normal	Reduced or absent	Normal	Normal or depressed (Eaton-Lambert syndrome)
Muscle appearance	Disuse atrophy after prolonged weakness, but no true wasting	Normal	Segmental wasting; fasciculation if lesion at the level of anterior horn cell	Normal or atrophic	Usually normal

whether the problem is of central or peripheral origin (neuroanatomy—see p. 88). Differences between weakness of central (upper motor neuron [UMN]) origin or peripheral (lower motor neuron [LMN]) origin are outlined in Table 50.1. Finally, bear in mind that coexisting medical conditions such as joint disease can lead to difficulties in interpreting neurological weakness.

Weakness of all four limbs

Depending on the evolution and associated physical signs, generalized weakness is most likely to be due to lesions in one of the following structures:

Cerebral hemispheres

It is very unlikely that a patient with a *normal level of consciousness* and generalized weakness has a hemispheric lesion of the brain.

Brain stem

A pontine haemorrhage or other lesion can lead to complete quadriplegia, including the face (locked-in syndrome). Consciousness is usually markedly depressed in the early stages.

Spinal cord

The degree to which weakness is generalized and affects the upper and lower limbs depends on the level of involvement of the spinal cord. Complete weakness affecting all four limbs occurs only if the spinal lesion is above C5. The pathological diagnosis is often suspected from the speed of onset of symptoms:
- Acute: cord compression, anterior spinal artery thrombosis, and acute transverse myelitis.
- Subacute: intrinsic spinal cord tumours, vascular malformations of the dura, vitamin B_{12} deficiency, and malignant meningeal infiltration.
- Chronic: benign tumours, syringomyelia, and inherited conditions—

hereditary spastic paraparesis (although this usually affects only the legs), spinocerebellar ataxias (e.g. Friedreich's ataxia) and tropical spastic paraparesis caused by human T-lymphocyte virus 1 (HTLV-1) infection.

Nerve roots

Inflammation, such as that caused by viral infection (cytomegalovirus [CMV], varicella-zoster virus [VSV]) of the nerve roots can cause weakness in all four limbs, as can malignant infiltration of the CSF (malignant meningitis).

Polyneuropathy

Diffuse nerve damage can cause weakness of all four limbs, such as occurs in Guillain–Barré syndrome (see peripheral nerve section), chronic inflammatory demyelinating polyneuropathy (CIDP) or inherited neuropathies such as hereditary motor and sensory neuropathy (HMSN). Other causes include critical illness polyneuropathy, diphtheria, sarcoidosis, Lyme disease, borreliosis and amyloid.

Muscle disease

Inflammatory, metabolic or inherited can all produce a diffuse weakness (see p. 382).

Weakness of one limb

This is a difficult problem clinically and can arise from lesions almost anywhere in the nervous system.

Cortical lesions

Cortical lesions affecting the motor pathways to the limbs can start as a problem isolated to one limb. UMN signs are found. Lacunar strokes affecting the basis pontis can give rise to clumsiness and weakness of one hand.

Motor neuron disease

Motor neuron disease not infrequently begins in one limb with foot drop or wasting of the intrinsic hand muscles, although subtle signs can often be seen in other limbs.

Spinal cord lesions

Spinal cord lesions at the appropriate level can give rise to weakness of one leg associated with loss of pain and temperature in the contralateral leg.

Plexopathy

A plexopathy (brachial or lumbosacral) can affect an arm or a leg. Inflammatory diseases such as brachial neuritis or diabetic amyotrophy are examples.

Involvement of multiple large motor nerves (mononeuritis multiplex)

Mononeuritis multiplex can present in one limb or asymmetrically involve several limbs. Mononeuritis multiplex is usually a consequence of an underlying systemic disease process (see table).

Isolated mononeuropathy

An isolated mononeuropathy, e.g. femoral, can give rise to isolated weakness of one limb.

Weakness of one side of the body

A hemiparesis can arise in a wide variety of locations, as outlined below.

Contralateral cerebral hemisphere

Damage to the contralateral cerebral hemisphere can cause weakness down one side of the body, when it may be associated with other physical signs (e.g. language dysfunction in the dominant hemisphere, neglect in the non-dominant hemisphere).

The brain stem

This can cause a number of eponymous syndromes:
• In the midbrain there will be weakness with a contralateral third nerve palsy (Weber's syndrome).
• In the pons, the weakness will be associated with conjugate gaze deviation towards the weak limbs and there may be a contralateral LMN facial weakness.
• In the medulla there may be ipsilateral loss of pain and temperature and a contralateral Horner's syndrome (lateral medullary syndrome of Wallenberg).

The spinal cord (see p. 380)

Weakness of both lower limbs (paraparesis)

• Spinal cord lesion.
• Peripheral neuropathy
• Bilateral involvement of the lumbosacral plexus
• Rarely, bilateral parasagittal lesions in the brain, classically a meningioma (although this is very rare); other bilateral pathologies may also be responsible.

Weakness of both upper limbs

• Spinal cord lesion
• Unusual forms of motor neuron disease
• Bilateral brachial neuritis.

51 Disturbance of vision: a neurological perspective

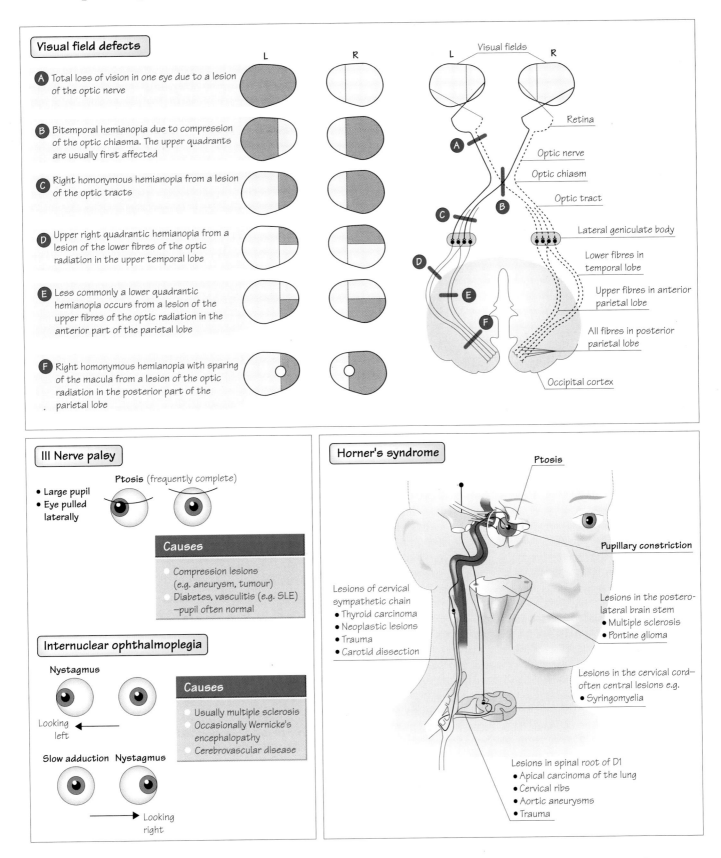

Visual field defects

A Total loss of vision in one eye due to a lesion of the optic nerve

B Bitemporal hemianopia due to compression of the optic chiasma. The upper quadrants are usually first affected

C Right homonymous hemianopia from a lesion of the optic tracts

D Upper right quadrantic hemianopia from a lesion of the lower fibres of the optic radiation in the upper temporal lobe

E Less commonly a lower quadrantic hemianopia occurs from a lesion of the upper fibres of the optic radiation in the anterior part of the parietal lobe

F Right homonymous hemianopia with sparing of the macula from a lesion of the optic radiation in the posterior part of the parietal lobe

Visual fields

Retina
Optic nerve
Optic chiasm
Optic tract
Lateral geniculate body
Lower fibres in temporal lobe
Upper fibres in anterior parietal lobe
All fibres in posterior parietal lobe
Occipital cortex

III Nerve palsy

Ptosis (frequently complete)

- Large pupil
- Eye pulled laterally

Causes

- Compression lesions (e.g. aneurysm, tumour)
- Diabetes, vasculitis (e.g. SLE) –pupil often normal

Internuclear ophthalmoplegia

Nystagmus

Looking left

Slow adduction Nystagmus

Looking right

Causes

- Usually multiple sclerosis
- Occasionally Wernicke's encephalopathy
- Cerebrovascular disease

Horner's syndrome

Ptosis

Pupillary constriction

Lesions of cervical sympathetic chain
- Thyroid carcinoma
- Neoplastic lesions
- Trauma
- Carotid dissection

Lesions in the postero-lateral brain stem
- Multiple sclerosis
- Pontine glioma

Lesions in the cervical cord– often central lesions e.g.
- Syringomyelia

Lesions in spinal root of D1
- Apical carcinoma of the lung
- Cervical ribs
- Aortic aneurysms
- Trauma

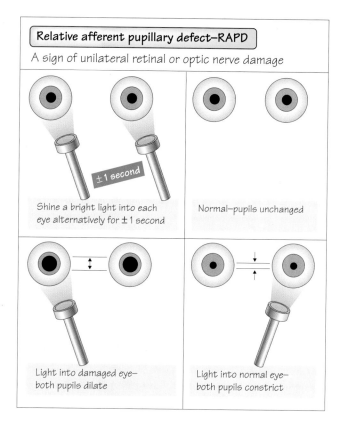

Visual loss

Monocular visual loss

This is a lesion anterior to the optic chiasma:
- The eye—cornea, lens and vitreous, e.g. cataract or vitreous haemorrhage.
- The retina, especially the fovea, e.g. diabetic retinopathy or macular degeneration.
- The optic nerve, e.g. optic neuritis or ischaemic neuropathy.
    Bilateral involvement of these structures causes bilateral visual loss.

Binocular visual loss

This is a lesion at or behind the chiasma:
- The optic chiasma: classically bitemporal.
- The optic radiation: homonymous—either quadrantanopia (superior: temporal lobe, affecting Meyer's loop; inferior: parietal) or hemianopia.
- The visual cortex: homonymous, often hemianopia.

Typical clinical presentations of 'neurological' causes of visual loss

Brief monocular or binocular visual loss

- Amaurosis fugax, brief unilateral blindness lasting minutes (see p. 364).
- Brief transient visual obscurations, caused by idiopathic intracranial hypertension with papilloedema, may occur in one or both eyes. More common in obese young women with headache. The cause is often undefined; some cases are the result of sagittal sinus thrombosis. Acute papilloedema alone has an enlarged blind spot but no visual loss.

Sudden painless loss of vision in one eye

Sudden painless loss of vision in one eye is the result of:
- Anterior ischaemic optic neuropathy: profound irreversible visual loss with a pale swollen optic disc; caused by atheroma emboli or temporal arteritis (p. 412)

- Established retinal arterial or venous occlusion—visible with the ophthalmoscope.

Rapid progressive monocular visual loss

Rapid and progressive monocular loss of vision as a result of optic neuritis typically comes on over a few days. Symptoms range from clouding of vision with a vague central scotoma to marked monocular blindness. Pain is variable, but characteristically occurs on looking to one side. Signs comprise loss of colour vision, a relative afferent pupil defect, papilloedema early on and optic atrophy weeks/months later. Eyesight improves over a few weeks, although diminished colour vision may be permanent. If the brain shows evidence of demyelinating lesions on magnetic resonance imaging (MRI), there is at least an 80% chance of subsequent multiple sclerosis.

Progressive night blindness

Progressive night blindness occurs in retinitis pigmentosa (RP), causes peripheral concentric field loss and spicular pigmentation on fundoscopy. Genetically there are many types, with X-linked or autosomal (dominant or recessive) inheritance. RP is associated with certain neurological syndromes, e.g. Refsum's or Usher's syndromes.

Bitemporal quadrantic or hemianopia

Bitemporal quadrantic or hemianopia is found in a pituitary lesion that compresses the optic chiasma, usually a macroadenoma. This is often slowly progressive and relatively asymptomatic, unless endocrine features are prominent or pituitary infarction occurs (see pp. 283 and 292).

Homonymous hemianopia

Homonymous hemianopia may indicate a structural lesion of the hemisphere affecting the optic radiation or visual cortex (rarely the optic tract). Common causes include infarct, haemorrhage and tumour.

Visual neglect

Visual neglect suggests a parietal lobe lesion, in the presence of intact visual fields.

Visual hallucinations

Visual hallucinations, including macropsia or micropsia, result from disease of the visual cortex.

Migraine (see p. 106)

Double vision

Double vision may be the result of lesions of oculomotor cranial nerves, the brain (usually the brain stem), the neuromuscular junction, muscle or other disease of the orbit (e.g. Graves' ophthalmopathy, head trauma). It is useful to establish the pattern, e.g. worse in one direction, on near or far vision or at different times of the day.

Sixth nerve palsy

In sixth nerve palsy, horizontal doubling, worse in the distance and on looking laterally, occurs. Looking straight ahead, there is a convergent squint as the affected eye is held adducted (unopposed medial rectus action). Causes include raised intracranial pressure, compression of the sixth nerve and microvascular disease. In children, sixth nerve palsy can follow a viral infection.

Fourth nerve palsy

Fourth nerve palsy is rare and causes diplopia on looking down, in and near, i.e. reading, eating and walking down stairs. On examination, there is failure to depress the eye when held in adduction (on abduction the eye is depressed by inferior rectus).

Third nerve palsy

In third nerve palsy diplopia is complex and occurs in most directions. Ptosis (often complete) and pupil dilatation occur (compare Horner's syndrome which has partial ptosis and pupil constriction). The eye is abducted as a result of unopposed lateral rectus action. Caused by compressive lesions, e.g. posterior communicating artery aneurysms, tumours and microvascular disease (hypertension, diabetes—pupil usually spared).

Internuclear ophthalmoplegia

Internuclear ophthalmoplegia is caused by medial longitudinal fasciculus damage, which connects the third and sixth nerve nuclei to allow fluent rapid lateral gaze. There is failure of prompt ipsilateral adduction on saccadic movement, and contralateral abducting nystagmus may be seen. Usually a sign of multiple sclerosis (MS) (especially if bilateral) but can also occur in other inflammatory lesions and vascular events in the brain stem. Frequently asymptomatic.

Brain stem lesions

Diplopia with other cranial nerve signs suggests brain stem disease (or cavernous sinus/orbital apex, depending on which nerves are involved). Isolated nuclear cranial nerve palsies may be found, but failure of conjugate gaze is more common. The eyes may be held in skew deviation; there may be gaze instability, nystagmus or failure of upgaze/downgaze. Causes include MS, stroke or tumour, or Wernicke's encephalopathy.

Cerebellar disease

Cerebellar disease may affect conjugate gaze but instability of vision is the usual symptom, rather than diplopia. Nystagmus is common.

Myasthenia gravis

Myasthenia gravis almost always has eye involvement. Diplopia is a common presentation, usually with ptosis. Any muscles can be affected, but the medial rectus is particularly susceptible. The pattern of doubling and the precise signs found are variable and may include fatigue.

Mitochondrial myopathies

Mitochondrial myopathies can present with chronic progressive external ophthalmoplegia (CPEO) and ptosis. Rarely associated with diplopia, as malalignment is so gradual. Mitochondrial diseases are rare, though important. They can present in multiple different ways (Table 51.1). Damage to the external eye muscles, retina and/or optic nerve is commonly found in the many different forms of mitochondrial disease, and causes defects in vision appropriate for the location of the damage.

Thyroid disease

Thyroid eye disease—see p. 286.

Pupils
Large

- Both pupils enlarge in response to dim lighting, fear, intoxication (e.g. cannabis, deadly nightshade) or death.
- One pupil enlarged may be the result of parasympathetic palsy (e.g. third nerve compression), Adie's pupil or iris paralysis (e.g. dilating drops or trauma).

Small

- Both pupils constrict with bright light, near focus, intoxication (e.g. opiates or cholinesterase inhibitors), or pontine haemorrhage.
- One constricted pupil may be the result of a sympathetic palsy (Horner's syndrome), pilocarpine use or iritis.

Table 51.1 Mitochondrial diseases (prevalence is 10–15 per 100 000, i.e. about 6000–9000 in the UK).

Syndrome	Clinical features
MELAS syndrome *Mitochondrial encephalomyopathy lactic acidosis and stroke like episodes*	Seizures Episodes of unconsciousness with lactic acidosis Stroke-like episodes
PEO *Progressive external ophthalmoplegia*	Ptosis External ophthalmoplegia Limb myopathy Kearns-Sayre syndrome variant; develops age ≤ 20 years, + pigmentary retinopathy, ataxia and heart block
MERRF *Myoclonic epilepsy with ragged red fibres*	Myoclonic epilepsy Cerebellar ataxia Myopathy
NARP *Neuropathy, ataxia and retinitis pigmentosa*	Proximal–muscle weakness Sensory neuropathy Retinal pigmentary degeneration Developmental delay; dementia Ataxia Seizures
LHON *Lebers hereditary optic neuropathy*	Painless subacute visual loss Scotomas Abnormal colour vision
Others, including aminoglycoside induced deafness (AID), maternally inherited Leigh's syndrome (MILS), Pearson's syndrome (PS)	Variable, usually suggested by the title; cardiomyopathy and deafness common in AID, sideroblastic anaemia and pancreatic failure in PS

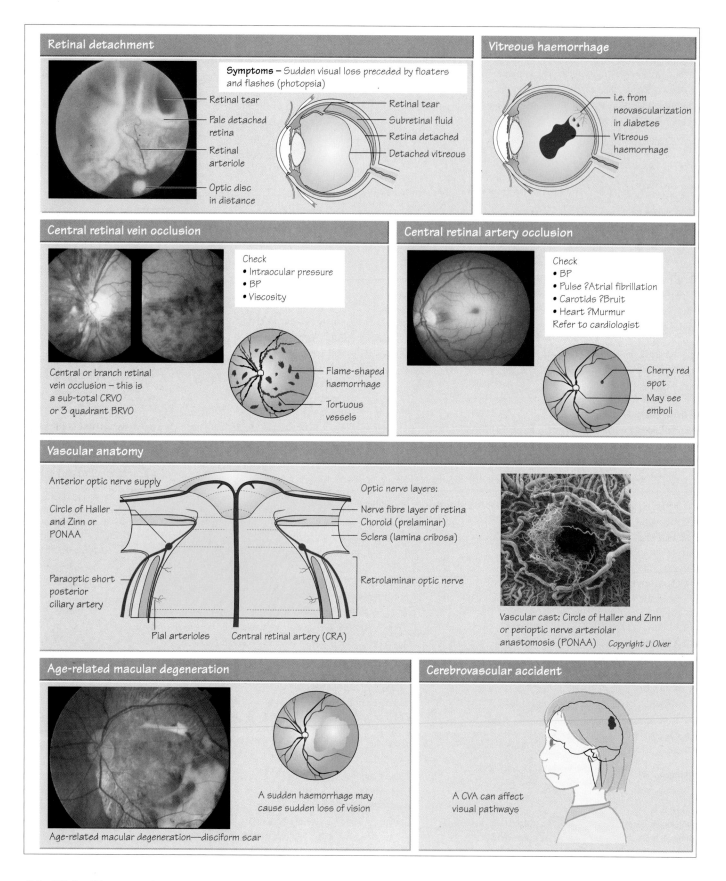

Retinal detachment

Symptoms – Sudden visual loss preceded by floaters and flashes (photopsia)

- Retinal tear
- Pale detached retina
- Retinal arteriole
- Optic disc in distance

- Retinal tear
- Subretinal fluid
- Retina detached
- Detached vitreous

Vitreous haemorrhage

- i.e. from neovascularization in diabetes
- Vitreous haemorrhage

Central retinal vein occlusion

Check
- Intraocular pressure
- BP
- Viscosity

Central or branch retinal vein occlusion – this is a sub-total CRVO or 3 quadrant BRVO

- Flame-shaped haemorrhage
- Tortuous vessels

Central retinal artery occlusion

Check
- BP
- Pulse ?Atrial fibrillation
- Carotids ?Bruit
- Heart ?Murmur
Refer to cardiologist

- Cherry red spot
- May see emboli

Vascular anatomy

Anterior optic nerve supply

Circle of Haller and Zinn or PONAA

Paraoptic short posterior ciliary artery

Optic nerve layers:
- Nerve fibre layer of retina
- Choroid (prelaminar)
- Sclera (lamina cribosa)

Retrolaminar optic nerve

Pial arterioles   Central retinal artery (CRA)

Vascular cast: Circle of Haller and Zinn or perioptic nerve arteriolar anastomosis (PONAA)   *Copyright J Olver*

Age-related macular degeneration

A sudden haemorrhage may cause sudden loss of vision

Age-related macular degeneration—disciform scar

Cerebrovascular accident

A CVA can affect visual pathways

Clinical Presentations at a Glance

The main causes of painless loss of vision are:
- Retinal detachment
- Vitreous haemorrhages
- Certain forms of vascular occlusion.

Retinal detachment
- Sudden (sometimes gradual) painless loss of vision.
- Usually preceded by symptoms of flashing lights (photopsia) and/or floaters and/or visual field defects.
- When the macula is not involved the visual loss involves the peripheral field and visual acuity may be normal.
- Once the macula is involved the central vision is lost.

Management
Laser to retinal hole or retinal surgery ± vitrectomy.

Vitreous haemorrhage
Haemorrhage into the vitreous cavity can result in sudden painless loss of vision. The extent of visual loss will depend on the degree of haemorrhage.
- A large haemorrhage will cause total visual loss.
- A small haemorrhage will present as floaters and normal or only slightly reduced visual acuity.

Aetiology
- Proliferative retinopathy—spontaneous rupture of abnormal fragile new vessels that grow on the retinal surface cause bleeding into the vitreous cavity. The most common cause is proliferative diabetic retinopathy.
- Retinal detachment—a small retinal blood vessel may rupture when the retinal break occurs, bleeding into the vitreous cavity.
- Trauma.
- Posterior vitreous detachment can result in vitreous haemorrhage if, as the vitreous separates from the retina, it pulls and ruptures a small blood vessel.
- Age-related macular degeneration (AMD)—haemorrhage may occur into the vitreous from the abnormally weak vessels forming a subretinal neovascular membrane.

Management
Referral to an ophthalmologist to determine cause and manage any complications (e.g. glaucoma due to red blood cells occluding the trabecular meshwork) that may occur.

Vascular occlusion
Central retinal vein occlusion
Central retinal vein occlusion (CRVO) or a branch retinal vein occlusion (BRVO) often presents with sudden painless loss of vision.

Aetiology
- Systemic hypertension
- Raised intraocular pressure
- Hyperviscosity syndromes
- Vessel wall disease (e.g. diabetes, inflammation such as sarcoidosis).

Management
- As CRVO and BRVO are strongly associated with arteriosclerosis, patients with vein occlusion must have their blood pressure checked, should be examined for evidence of arterial disease (determine from the history whether any symptoms of MI, stroke or claudication; feel all the pulses, listen for arterial bruits), have their intraocular pressure checked and be checked for diabetes and systemic inflammation.
- Young patients presenting with CRVO or BRVO, or older patients in whom there is no obvious cause, should be investigated for hyperviscosity syndromes.

Central retinal artery occlusion
Central retinal artery occlusion (CRAO) or a branch retinal artery occlusion also presents as acute painless loss of vision.

Aetiology
- Very high intraocular pressure, as seen in acute angle-closure glaucoma.
- Arterial embolus from diseased carotid, valvular heart disease, atrial fibrillation; examine the patient carefully considering that some part of the 'arterial organ' is damaged.
- Arterial occlusion from atheroma or inflammation (e.g. giant cell arteritis); consider ordering an ESR.

Non-arteritic anterior (AION) or posterior ischaemic optic neuropathy (PION)
- Results from occlusion or hypoperfusion of the small blood vessels supplying the optic nerve head (AION) or posterior optic nerve (PION).
- In AION the optic disc is swollen; this swelling may be segmental or involve the entire nerve head. There are usually associated splinter haemorrhages at the disc.
- In PION the optic disc looks normal.
- There may be arteriosclerosis and arteriovenous nipping, depending on the cause.
- Risk factors: arteriosclerosis, hypertension, hypotensive episode, smoking, 'disc at risk' (e.g. small optic nerve head with no central cup).

Cerebrovascular accident (CVA)
A haemorrhagic or embolic CVA affecting the visual pathways will present as acute painless visual loss. Depending on the site of the lesion, the patient will have a corresponding field defect on fields to confrontation. (See Chapter 51). It is very rare for the visual loss to be the only, or indeed the dominant, symptom.

Acephalgic migraine
This rare form of migraine presents with transient visual disturbances involving one or both eyes in the absence of headaches.

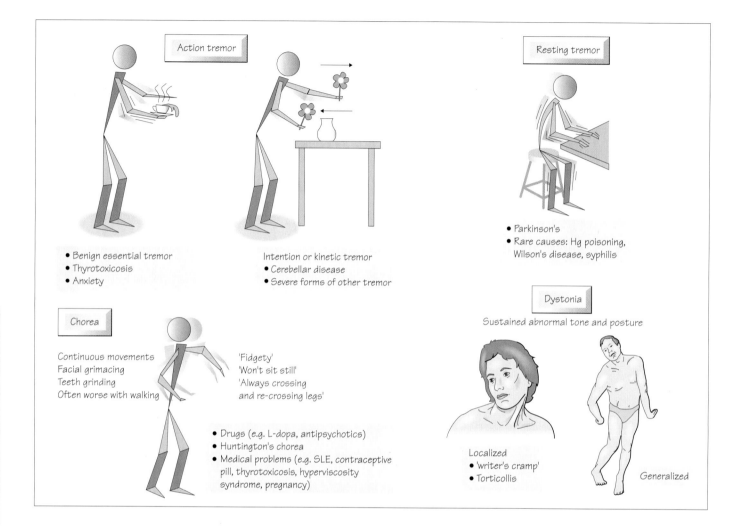

Understanding and interpreting movement disorders depends on having a precise grasp of the terminology used to describe the phenomenology of abnormal movement and posture.

Tremor is the *involuntary, rhythmical oscillation* of a muscle group. It should be distinguished from other involuntary movements such as dyskinesia, chorea, myoclonus, tics and mannerisms (defined below). Measuring the frequency of the tremor is not often of value in distinguishing the cause. There are, in clinical practice, only three common types of tremor (Table 53.1):

1 Resting tremor: if asymmetrical this is almost pathognomonic of idiopathic Parkinson's disease.

2 Postural tremor that is usually the result of essential tremor.

3 Action or kinetic tremor that is a feature of cerebellar dysfunction.

Common causes of tremor
Essential tremor

Essential tremor is usually symmetrical and barely present at rest, becomes pronounced on movement and posture (the rattling of the teacup is suggestive of the diagnosis), and can be relieved by small amounts of alcohol, although this effect wanes with time. It is often associated with a family history and is very rarely disabling.

Cerebellar disease

The characteristic feature of cerebellar tremor is that it is brought out at the end of movement. The head may be involved. Isolated tremor is most unusual and usually there are other signs of cerebellar dysfunction.

Parkinsonism (see Chapter 195)

Parkinson's tremor is of asymmetrical onset, most prominent at rest, and reduced by voluntary action. Head tremor is not characteristic of idiopathic Parkinson's disease, but the jaw is frequently involved.

Drugs and toxins

• Alcohol withdrawal; though tremor is extremely common, and indeed almost universal in alcohol withdrawal, the clinical condition is usually dominated by other features, especially neuro-psychiatric ones, including difficult behaviour, acute confusional state, hallucinations, seizures; patients are not infrequently jaundiced, with other stigmata of liver disease, such as spider naevi, ascites, etc.

• Sodium valproate

• Lithium

• Caffeine

• Heavy metal poisoning.

Table 53.1 Types of tremor and their features.

	Maximal	Distribution	Response to movement	Involvement of head
Essential tremor	Action and postural	Symmetrical	Worse	If severe
Parkinsonian	Rest, abolished by action	Asymmetrical	Abolished	Never (but does involve jaw)
Cerebellar	Kinetic	Symmetrical, frequently head	Accentuated at end of movement	Frequent

Metabolic

- Thyrotoxicosis
- Phaeochromocytoma
- Hepatic encephalopathy
- Wilson's disease; rare (1 in 33 000–100 000), autosomal recessive caused by mutations/deletions of the ATP7B protein encoded by chromosome subbands 13q14.3–q21.1. Fifty per cent present with movement disorders (nearly all patients with neurological symptoms have Kayser-Fleischer rings), the remainder with liver disease, anaemia, or by proband screening.

Other abnormal movements

Myoclonus

This comprises brief, explosive 'electric shock'-like activation of a group of muscles, often involving a whole limb. It is reasonable to think of this as an 'epileptic' phenomenon which can arise from anywhere in the central nervous system, including the brain stem and spinal cord. There are a very large number of causes, ranging from vascular disease, drugs and metabolic derangements to neurodegenerative disease such as spongiform encephalopathies.

Dystonias

These are sustained abnormal tone and posture of a group of muscles, which can be:

- Focal, e.g. writer's cramp, torticollis, now known as 'idiopathic cervical dystonia', and hemifacial spasm.
- Generalized, e.g. generalized torsion dystonia, a condition of abnormal writhing movements, which may be genetic (dominantly inherited) or symptomatic of other conditions (drugs, structural lesions of the brain, neurodegenerative disease).

Chorea

These are continuous random flowing or dancing movements of the extremities, which in it mildest form may be turned into semi-purposeful movements such that the patient just appears fidgety. The definition of the ad hoc Committee on Classification of the World Federation of Neurology is helpful, and states that chorea is 'a state of excessive, spontaneous movements, irregularly timed, non-repetitive, randomly distributed and abrupt in character. These movements may vary in severity from restlessness with mild intermittent exaggeration of gesture and expression, fidgeting movements of the hands, unstable dance-like gait to a continuous flow of disabling, violent movements.'

There are multiple causes including:

- Drug-induced syndromes: chorea not infrequently complicates long-term Parkinson's disease, where long-term treatment with dopamine agonists may be contributory. It also complicates long-term treatment with dopamine antagonists, such as the neuroleptic drugs used for major psychosis.
- Huntington's disease: abnormal movements are the presenting symptom in 50–75% of HD patients. Indeed, choreiform movements can, occasionally, be so profound as to result in severe weight loss due to the high-energy expenditure resulting from nearly continuous motor activity! Chorea is particularly prevalent in those who present at an older age; patients with HD who present in childhood or early adult life tend to have more symptoms from rigidity and seizures than from chorea. Chorea may precede other symptoms, including overt cognitive decline, and/or neuropsychiatric symptoms.
- Sydenham's chorea: this is a complication of rheumatic fever, which most typically occurs some 1–6 months after an acute attack of rheumatic fever. However, it has been described as occurring up to 30 years after the acute attack! This means that the history is often the vital aspect of the diagnosis, rather than the finding of raised anti-streptococcal antibodies. Chorea often occurs in isolation.
- Systemic lupus erythematosus (SLE)
- The oral contraceptive pill
- Hyperviscosity syndromes
- Pregnancy
- Thyrotoxicosis: while tremor is almost universal in hyperthyroidism chorea, though well described, is extraordinarily rare. It usually resolves on successfully treating the overactive thyroid.
- The antiphospholipid syndrome (APS): most patients (= 90%) with APS who develop chorea are female, about 25% develop symptoms either on the pill or when pregnant, it is unilateral in 45%, and 35% have abnormalities on brain MRI scanning.
- There are many other causes including Wilson's disease.

Dyskinesias

These are disorder of movement integration, which may have choreiform or dystonic components. The term is usually used for drug-induced movements caused by neuroleptics, Parkinson's disease or its treatment.

Tics

Tics are stereotyped explosive movements, under partial voluntary control, which are recognizably part of the normal movement repertoire (e.g. blinking or winking).

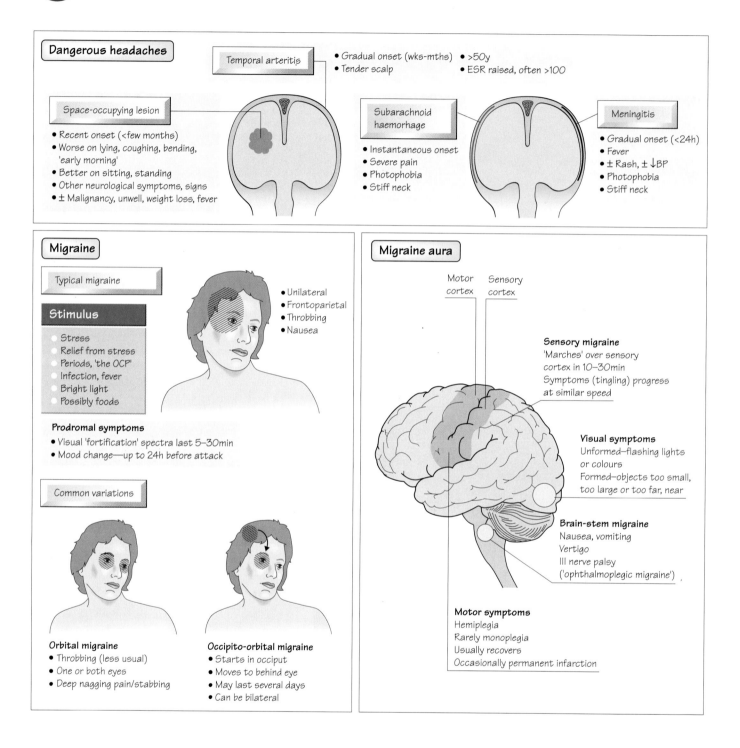

Dangerous headaches

Temporal arteritis
- Gradual onset (wks-mths)
- Tender scalp
- >50y
- ESR raised, often >100

Space-occupying lesion
- Recent onset (<few months)
- Worse on lying, coughing, bending, 'early morning'
- Better on sitting, standing
- Other neurological symptoms, signs
- ± Malignancy, unwell, weight loss, fever

Subarachnoid haemorhage
- Instantaneous onset
- Severe pain
- Photophobia
- Stiff neck

Meningitis
- Gradual onset (<24h)
- Fever
- ± Rash, ± ↓BP
- Photophobia
- Stiff neck

Migraine

Typical migraine

Stimulus
- Stress
- Relief from stress
- Periods, 'the OCP'
- Infection, fever
- Bright light
- Possibly foods

- Unilateral
- Frontoparietal
- Throbbing
- Nausea

Prodromal symptoms
- Visual 'fortification' spectra last 5–30min
- Mood change—up to 24h before attack

Common variations

Orbital migraine
- Throbbing (less usual)
- One or both eyes
- Deep nagging pain/stabbing

Occipito-orbital migraine
- Starts in occiput
- Moves to behind eye
- May last several days
- Can be bilateral

Migraine aura

Motor cortex   Sensory cortex

Sensory migraine
'Marches' over sensory cortex in 10–30min
Symptoms (tingling) progress at similar speed

Visual symptoms
Unformed—flashing lights or colours
Formed—objects too small, too large or too far, near

Brain-stem migraine
Nausea, vomiting
Vertigo
III nerve palsy
('ophthalmoplegic migraine')

Motor symptoms
Hemiplegia
Rarely monoplegia
Usually recovers
Occasionally permanent infarction

Headache is a subjective sensation, so the patient and not the doctor defines its presence or absence. The brain is insensate: pain in the head and face arises from the trigeminovascular system which supplies the meninges. As an isolated symptom (i.e. no other symptoms or neurological signs), it is almost never indicative of structural brain disease (and is referred to as 'primary headache'). The following isolated headaches are exceptions and may indicate underlying disease:

- Explosive onset headache, which may be the result of subarachnoid or intracerebral haemorrhage.
- Headache gradually increasing in severity over several hours with fever, photophobia and neck stiffness (not all components need be present) suggests acute meningitis, a medical emergency. Immediate intravenous antibiotics are given if definitive diagnosis (usually established by lumbar puncture) is unavoidably delayed. Chronic meningitis may cause isolated headache progressive over days to weeks.

- Exertional headache, or headache occurring exclusively on coughing sneezing or stooping, can occasionally be caused by vascular malformations of the brain or lesions of the foramen magnum, e.g. the Arnold–Chiari malformation.
- Postural headache, may indicate abnormalities of cerebrospinal fluid (CSF) pressure (high or low).
- Headache waking the patient from sleep: although most often the result of benign conditions, e.g. migraine, this should prompt a search for a structural lesion by careful physical examination (e.g. for hemiplegia) and consideration of neuroimaging.
- New and continuous headache in those aged over 50 years raises the possibility of temporal arteritis. The scalp may be tender. A raised erythrocyte sedimentation rate (ESR) supports the diagnosis (see p. 413).

Classification of primary headache
Migraine
The core features of migraine are headache, typically but not exclusively unilateral, nausea and vomiting and variable constitutional upset (fatigue, carbohydrate craving, diuresis), which usually lasts < 48 h. There are two main types:

1 Migraine with aura: there is a prodrome of neurological symptoms, evolving gradually over a few minutes, unlike stroke or transient ischaemia where symptoms arise instantaneously. These prodromal symptoms comprise:
- visual phenomena: positive: scintillations, fortification spectra, etc. or negative: scotomata, hemianopia
- altered sensations of the face or limbs
- occasional rare variants such as 'basilar' migraine with double vision and vertigo, ophthalmoplegic and hemiplegic migraine.

2 Migraine without aura: there are no accompanying neurological symptoms or signs but nausea and the other constitutional features are still present.

Acute attacks may respond to simple analgesia if given quickly (paracetamol or high-dose aspirin in soluble form; codeine-based preparations are contraindicated because of nausea and rebound headache). Triptans (e.g. sumatriptan) are usually reserved for severe recurrent attacks and ergotamine is now used rarely. Prophylaxis is indicated for debilitating attacks occurring several times a month and propranolol, sodium valproate and pizotifen have all been shown to work in selected patients.

Tension-type headache
This is an unsatisfactory term, because patients believe that they are being criticized as tense. The relationship to psychosocial stress is uncertain and variable but the symptoms are still disabling. The key features are:
- A dull generalized headache, usually poorly localized (occasionally localized over the eyes), sometimes referred to as a 'fuzzy head'.
- Poor response to over-the-counter analgesia.
- Worsening throughout the day.
- Duration of days to weeks.

Some neurologists consider this to be a variant of migraine and it is not uncommon to find both types of headache in the same patients or to find a cluster of migraines merging into tension headache. They do not usually respond to antimigraine therapy but some respond to low-dose amitriptyline.

Chronic daily headache
This describes patients who have a non-specific, non-disabling headache on most days (4% of the UK population). Unresponsive to simple analgesia and difficult to treat.

Cluster headache
This is more common in men (9 : 1) and characterized by episodes of severe unilateral headache of extreme to excruciating intensity, often arising from sleep. Eye watering may occur. Duration is 10–60 min Patients prefer to move around. Occurs in clusters, typically daily for 6–8 weeks before disappearing completely. Acute treatment is with triptan antimigraine therapy; some respond to high-flow oxygen. Prophylaxis is with lithium. Once started, clusters can sometimes be aborted with a reducing course of prednisolone.

Indomethacin-responsive headaches
These are a group of unusual headache syndromes, which are defined by the specific response to indomethacin. Paroxysmal hemicrania is a unilateral lancinating headache of great severity, which continues throughout the day. Patients describe paroxysms of sharp jabbing, lasting for seconds and often localized behind the eye. If it becomes chronic it is known as 'hemicrania continua'.

Facial pain
- Trigeminal neuralgia causes a unilateral lancinating facial pain in the distribution of the trigeminal nerve (usually maxillary or mandibular), typically arising in middle age. Bilateral symptoms can be the result of multiple sclerosis. Patients usually report that the pain is precipitated by tactile stimulation of the face (shaving, brushing teeth, hot or cold drinks, and the wind). The pain can be difficult to control. Most patients respond to carbamazepine but the effect is not always sustained. A minority of patients have vascular compression of the trigeminal nerve shown by MRI, and may respond to surgical decompression of the posterior fossa.
- Post-herpetic neuralgia: this troublesome condition affects 30% of people after an episode of shingles. Risk factors are age and late treatment with aciclovir. The most common location is in the ophthalmic trigeminal division, but it can occur anywhere. Although it is difficult to treat, carbamazepine or amitriptyline are worth trying. In many, symptoms abate after several years.
- 'Atypical facial pain', by definition, does not have any of the distinguishing features of the aforementioned conditions. Most common in young women. Not associated with physical signs. Amitriptyline is the treatment of choice.

Other causes of headache
- Analgesic overuse headache
- Benign paroxysmal headache (triggered by cold, exertion or coughing)
- Temporomandibular joint dysfunction
- Sinusitis
- Dental caries.

55 Episodic alterations in awareness and consciousness

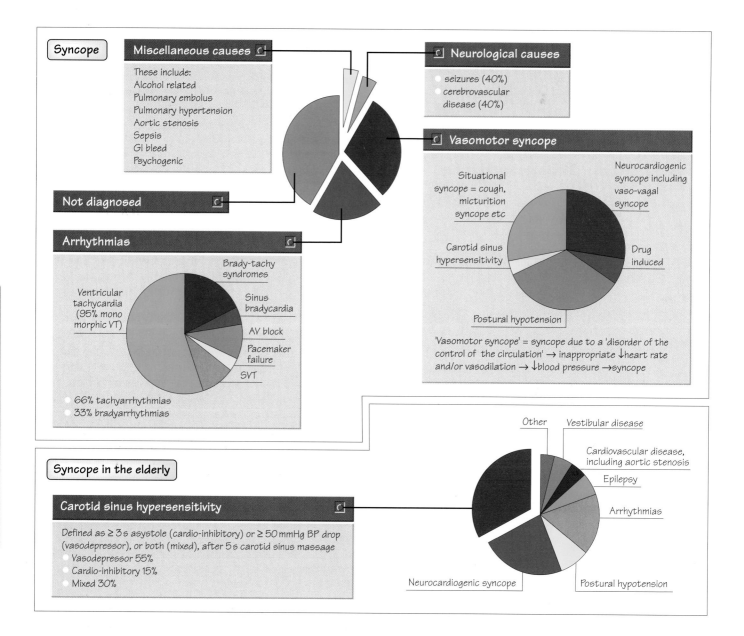

Syncope

Miscellaneous causes [c]

These include:
Alcohol related
Pulmonary embolus
Pulmonary hypertension
Aortic stenosis
Sepsis
GI bleed
Psychogenic

Not diagnosed [c]

Arrhythmias [c]

Brady-tachy syndromes

Ventricular tachycardia (95% mono morphic VT)

Sinus bradycardia

AV block

Pacemaker failure

SVT

- 66% tachyarrhythmias
- 33% bradyarrhythmias

Neurological causes [c]

- seizures (40%)
- cerebrovascular disease (40%)

Vasomotor syncope [c]

Situational syncope = cough, micturition syncope etc

Neurocardiogenic syncope including vaso-vagal syncope

Carotid sinus hypersensitivity

Drug induced

Postural hypotension

'Vasomotor syncope' = syncope due to a 'disorder of the control of the circulation' → inappropriate ↓heart rate and/or vasodilation → ↓blood pressure →syncope

Syncope in the elderly

Carotid sinus hypersensitivity [c]

Defined as ≥ 3 s asystole (cardio-inhibitory) or ≥ 50 mmHg BP drop (vasodepressor), or both (mixed), after 5 s carotid sinus massage
- Vasodepressor 55%
- Cardio-inhibitory 15%
- Mixed 30%

Other

Vestibular disease

Cardiovascular disease, including aortic stenosis

Epilepsy

Arrhythmias

Neurocardiogenic syncope

Postural hypotension

Blackouts and near blackouts are frightening experiences. The most helpful diagnostic approach is to obtain a full history from an accurate witness, because the examination and special investigations often add little. The features of diagnostic value to focus on are:
- What happens immediately before the attack? A prodrome (warning) suggests a vasovagal cause, whereas no warning is a feature of primary generalized epilepsy or Stokes–Adams attacks. Patients with temporal lobe epilepsy (which is rare) can have an unusual prodrome, with any form of hallucination, strange epigastric sensations, and *deja/jamais vu* ('thoughts of having/never having/been here before').
- What does the patient look like during the attack? Abnormal movements suggest epilepsy. Pallor, or an appearance 'as if dead' suggests a

cardiovascular cause. These distinctions are not absolute—for example some 40% of patients with vasomotor forms of syncope have some minor twitching during the attack, and a few (especially those kept in the upright position) have more generalized hypoxic seizures (termed 'secondary hypoxic seizures').
- What is the memory of the attack itself? The remembrance of events during the attack suggests that consciousness was not fully lost. This is often so in minor cardiovascular events, in partial epilepsy (see later) and in hyperventilation.

Did injury occur? Major injury suggests an absence of warning, as well as total loss of consciousness. Attacks with injury are strongly associated with significant underlying pathology.

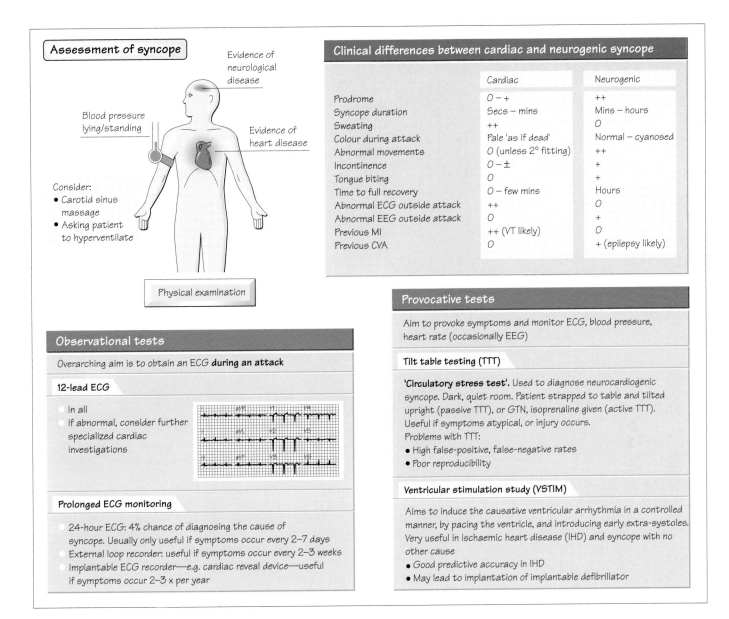

Assessment of syncope

Evidence of neurological disease

Blood pressure lying/standing

Evidence of heart disease

Consider:
- Carotid sinus massage
- Asking patient to hyperventilate

Physical examination

Clinical differences between cardiac and neurogenic syncope

	Cardiac	Neurogenic
Prodrome	0 – +	++
Syncope duration	Secs – mins	Mins – hours
Sweating	++	0
Colour during attack	Pale 'as if dead'	Normal – cyanosed
Abnormal movements	0 (unless 2° fitting)	++
Incontinence	0 – ±	+
Tongue biting	0	+
Time to full recovery	0 – few mins	Hours
Abnormal ECG outside attack	++	0
Abnormal EEG outside attack	0	+
Previous MI	++ (VT likely)	0
Previous CVA	0	+ (epilepsy likely)

Observational tests

Overarching aim is to obtain an ECG **during an attack**

12-lead ECG

- In all
- If abnormal, consider further specialized cardiac investigations

Prolonged ECG monitoring

- 24-hour ECG: 4% chance of diagnosing the cause of syncope. Usually only useful if symptoms occur every 2–7 days
- External loop recorder: useful if symptoms occur every 2–3 weeks
- Implantable ECG recorder—e.g. cardiac reveal device—useful if symptoms occur 2–3 x per year

Provocative tests

Aim to provoke symptoms and monitor ECG, blood pressure, heart rate (occasionally EEG)

Tilt table testing (TTT)

'Circulatory stress test'. Used to diagnose neurocardiogenic syncope. Dark, quiet room. Patient strapped to table and tilted upright (passive TTT), or GTN, isoprenaline given (active TTT). Useful if symptoms atypical, or injury occurs.
Problems with TTT:
- High false-positive, false-negative rates
- Poor reproducibility

Ventricular stimulation study (VSTIM)

Aims to induce the causative ventricular arrhythmia in a controlled manner, by pacing the ventricle, and introducing early extra-systoles. Very useful in ischaemic heart disease (IHD) and syncope with no other cause
- Good predictive accuracy in IHD
- May lead to implantation of implantable defibrillator

- What happens immediately afterwards? Post-event confusion suggests epilepsy, whereas post-event flushing and/or sweating suggests a cardiovascular cause.
- What do witnesses say? This is often the key to diagnosis.
- Are attacks recurrent? If so are they all similar (stereotyped attacks suggest a single underlying aetiology), do they all occur in the standing position (which suggests postural hypotension or neurocardiogenic syncope), on effort (see below), or in the same psychological situation (which suggests vasovagal attacks).
- The patient's age alters the probability of disease: ≤ 30 years: vasovagal syncope and epilepsy are more likely; ≥ 60 years: cardiac causes and micturition syncope are more likely. However, any cause can occur at any age.

Cardiovascular causes of loss of consciousness

Consciousness is disrupted if there is a decrease in the blood supply to the brain, either from a decreased cardiac output or hypotension from inappropriate vasodilatation. Such cardiovascular diseases are characterized by faintness (presyncope, which means that patients feel that they are about to 'blackout') or actual loss of consciousness (syncope) of brief duration (always less than a few minutes), with pallor during the attack, to the extent that the patient may 'appear dead'. Sweating afterwards is a good clue to a cardiovascular aetiology. Full consciousness returns rapidly. The variants of cardiovascular syncope are as follows.

Vasovagal syncope A common cause of altered consciousness at any age with the following features:
- A coherent account of the events leading up to the attack is given by the patient. Attacks may be precipitated by emotional stimuli and often recur in the same context.
- Loss of consciousness is preceded by: 1) a feeling of lightheadedness or dysequilibrium, which is occasionally prolonged; 2) ringing in the ears or a progressive alteration in sound quality; 3) a feeling of warmth or flushing.
- The warning prodrome may be absent in elderly people in whom the picture may be of sudden drop attacks. Younger people often recall slowly falling to the ground before 'blacking out'.

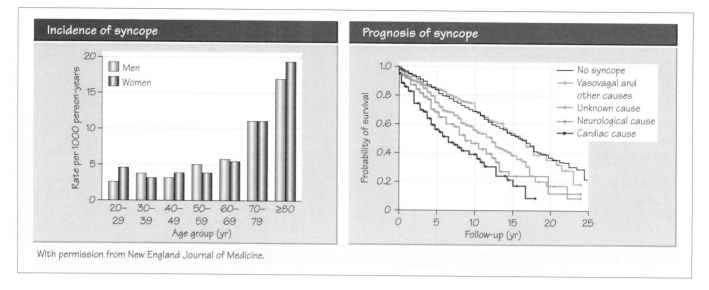

With permission from New England Journal of Medicine.

• The patient is fully orientated as he or she comes round, although may feel weak, nauseated and light-headed. Recovery is complete within minutes. Prolonged confusion raises the suspicion that the attack is epileptic.
• Brief, non-sustained jerking of the limbs is common and those who faint with a full bladder may be incontinent. The diagnosis is complicated in those rare patients who faint and have a secondary anoxic convulsive seizure, from maintenance of the upright position.

Postural hypotension Here the autonomic nervous system fails to prevent blood pressure falling on standing. Characterized by symptoms of vasovagal syncope on standing, never when sitting or lying:
• Patients are usually elderly. The condition may be provoked or exacerbated by drugs (diuretics, antihypertensives, antipsychotics) and dehydration (e.g. fluid deprivation, diuretics, gastrointestinal bleed). Autonomic failure is also a common cause, e.g. diabetic neuropathy.
• The diagnosis is established by demonstrating a progressive fall on standing in blood pressure over 5–10 min.

It differs from hypotensive cardioneurogenic syncope in that the blood pressure fall starts immediately, not after a delay, and there is never any absolute bradycardia. Treatment is for the underlying disease (diabetes, dehydration). If this is not possible fludrocortisone may help.

Micturition syncope Patients usually have prostatic hypertrophy. Prolonged straining to initiate micturition decreases venous return to the heart. Cardiac output falls and syncope results. Syncope prevents straining and thus improves cardiac venous return and output, restoring consciousness. A variant of micturition syncope is cough syncope, which occurs in individuals with chronic lung disease and prolonged paroxysms of coughing. The diagnosis is made from the history alone.

Stokes–Adams Attacks describe a specific pattern of syncope, unheralded (so that patients often injure themselves falling), with complete loss of consciousness, lasting < 2–3 min. The absence of warning means that patients often fall heavily and sustain significant facial or limb injuries, in contrast to patients who simply faint and are not usually injured. Witnesses state that patients become pale, cyanotic and then reactively hyperaemic on recovery. Afterwards there is a rapid (less than a few minutes) restoration of all mental and physical faculties. Attacks are usually the result of the temporary asystole that accompanies the onset of 3° heart block. If not then they may be caused by VT.

Syncopal (pre-syncopal) tachyarrhythmias To cause syncope, tachyarrhythmias must either be very fast or associated with at least moderately severe, structural heart disease. Ventricular tachycardia is the most common underlying rhythm disturbance, although AF is occasionally the culprit. Patients complain of fast palpitations before fainting. Total loss of consciousness is unlikely to last for more than a few minutes, although a depressed conscious level can last much longer. The 12-lead ECG, 24-h ECG taping ('Holter monitoring') or specialized cardiac investigation (e.g. ventricular stimulation study) may be diagnostic. If not, and an arrhythmia seems likely, implantation of a solid-state device to continually record the heart rhythm may be appropriate.

GTN syncope Is the result of excess glyceryl trinitrate (GTN) consumption while the patient is standing. Vasodilatation occurs, resulting in syncope. Patients may have failed to understand the role of GTN, and are taking this inappropriately. More usually GTN syncope is associated with severe cardiac disease: Either unacceptable angina, such that a coronary intervention is required (see p. 152), or impaired left ventricular (LV) function, or aortic stenosis.

Effort syncope Syncope on effort occurs either because the heart cannot increase the cardiac output as a result of a fixed obstruction (such as in severe aortic stenosis commonly, in hypertrophic obstructive cardiomyopathy less commonly and in severe pulmonary hypertension rarely) or because exercise provokes an arrhythmia. Cardiac ultrasonography and exercise testing are usually diagnostic.

Cardioneurogenic syncope Is a confusing term applied to an autonomic reflex, activated only in the standing position, whereby either the heart rate or blood pressure (BP) or both drop sufficiently to cause syncope. Characteristically patients are standing still, feel faint for 30 s to several minutes, and then faint and fall down. Sitting down early on may terminate the attack. The diagnosis is confirmed by replicating symptoms and heart rate/BP changes on tilt-table testing.

Carotid hypersensitivity syndrome Patients have hypersensitive carotid baroreceptors, which are activated inappropriately by neck turning (often when looking upwards). Inappropriate bradycardia, sometimes with reflex vasodilatation, occurs and the patient faints. The diagnosis is confirmed by eliciting symptoms and severe bradycardia on carotid sinus massage.

Terminology Most doctors define syncope as 'loss of consciousness with loss of postural reflexes'. The definition does not imply any particular mechanism. Thus syncope can occur from a cardiac cause, or equally from a neurological one.

Neurological causes of loss of consciousness

Most neurological disease underlying loss of consciousness is **epilepsy**, although very occasionally brain-stem ischaemia is the cause.

Epilepsy resulting in loss of consciousness is classified as generalized epilepsy and is caused by abnormal electrical discharges disrupting the function of the major subcortical structures that maintain consciousness.

• If the abnormal electrical discharges originate in these subcortical structures, unconsciousness occurs immediately and the epilepsy is termed 'primary generalized'. Patients have no warning and instantaneous collapse occurs. **Beware**: the absence of a warning is also a feature of some localized seizures that progress unusually rapidly to secondary generalized seizures.

• If these subcortical structures are involved by electrical discharges spreading from a more distant focus it is termed 'secondary generalized'. In this situation patients often experience some symptoms referable to the first structure involved, i.e. there is usually an aura or attenuated seizures.

• Seizures without loss of consciousness are termed 'partial seizures' and may be simple (normal awareness) or complex (loss of awareness) (for further discussion, see p. 372).

Features that are strongly in favour of epilepsy as a cause of loss of consciousness are:

• A good witness account, although these are disappointingly rare.

• Post-ictal confusion (ictal = the epileptic attack itself) lasting some time, e.g. often for many hours. Post-ictal headache.

• Muscular aching and tongue biting.

• Incontinence, which can also occur in other situations, is suggestive but non-specific.

• Known cerebrovascular disease, i.e. a previous stroke, or a degenerative brain condition increases the probability that a collapse relates to a seizure disorder.

Examination immediately after a seizure may show sleepiness for the first few hours, and bilateral extensor plantar responses for the first day, as well as signs referable to any underlying pathology (see p. 88). Generalized seizures cause peripheral skeletal muscle fibre tearing, so muscle enzymes, e.g. creatine kinase, are often elevated, as are serum prolactin levels for the first day or so. Electroencephalographic (EEG) recordings show abnormal interictal activity in 50% of patients with epilepsy.

Transient Brain-stem ischaemia can result in falls, with loss of consciousness. Conscious level is usually only transiently disturbed (< 1 min). The diagnosis is one of exclusion in a patient with cerebrovascular disease. There are no abnormal movements, the patient does not change colour and no rhythm disturbances are found. This syndrome is very rare, and is overdiagnosed.

Prognosis in syncope

Prognosis in syncope varies greatly—in some patients, syncope is due to highly dangerous pathology (for example, complete heart block), with a very poor natural history (untreated acquired complete heart block leads to death within a few weeks or months). At the other extreme, vasomotor syncope is associated with a normal life expectancy (figure). It is crucial to determine how likely it is that dangerous pathology underlies the syncope. The clues to this can often be obtained fairly easily:

• If the heart is structurally abnormal, and especially if there is damage to the left ventricle following a myocardial infarct, or there is a known cardiomyopathy (or complex congenital heart disease) then a high-grade ventricular arrhythmia could underlie the syncope (e.g. VT). Patients with syncopal VT are likely to experience further attacks, and the concern is that if the first episode of ventricular tachycardia reduced cardiac output enough to cause syncope, the second may reduce myocardial blood flow enough to provoke ventricular fibrillation. Thus syncope from a ventricular arrhythmia is a warning that the patient is at high risk of dying. The clue that VT is the cause of the syncope is the presence of damage to the heart, diagnosed from the history (e.g. previous MI, known heart muscle disease, high alcohol intake, or the presence of multiple risk factors for IHD—e.g. smoking + age + diabetes, etc.), examination, ECG (most patients with structural heart disease have some ECG abnormality). A cardiac ultrasound can be useful.

• Rarely certain genetic diseases underlie dangerous ventricular arrhythmias; the commonest of these is the still rare Brugada syndrome (prevalence 1 in 1000). Other dangerous genetic diseases include hereditary long QT syndrome. Most genetic illnesses cause characteristic abnormalities on the resting ECG—however, often the real clue to their presence is the finding of sudden death in young family members.

Other causes of altered consciousness

• Hyperventilation occurs in young adults and there is usually a history of perioral and peripheral paraesthesiae, anxiety and specific provocations.

• Hypoglycaemia is associated with sweating, anxiety and confusion before loss of consciousness. Drugs for diabetes are the only common cause. Rarely it may be caused by insulin-secreting pancreatic tumours.

• Narcolepsy is not strictly speaking a disorder that leads to loss of consciousness but, because of its curious manifestations, it is often misdiagnosed as epilepsy or patients are labelled as 'functional'. It is fundamentally a disorder of the central nervous system (CNS) regulation of arousal and the cardinal diagnostic feature is a low rapid eye movement (REM) sleep latency. The four aspects to the full-blown narcolepsy syndrome are: 1) excessive daytime somnolence with an irresistible desire to sleep which cannot be overcome; 2) cataplexy: a sudden loss of body tone; this may range from full falling to the ground to as mild a feeling as jaw dropping; it is usually precipitated by emotional stimuli such as jokes or arguments; 3) sleep paralysis; 4) hypnagogic hallucinations.

• Migraine is often associated with mild non-specific feelings of dissociation but can very rarely lead to frank coma.

• Transient global amnesia is a syndrome of obscure aetiology in which there is complete loss of new memory formation for a period of hours. Patients may appear relatively normal to external observers but are disorientated and ask repetitive and inconsequential questions. It may be a migrainous phenomenon but rarely recurs.

• Psychogenic disorder is always a dangerous diagnosis to make, but psychological illness occasionally underlies blackouts. However, most patients with psychological/psychiatric illness who black out have genuine organic diseases. Occasionally patients mimic seizures (i.e. have 'pseudoseizures')—this most commonly occurs in psychologically disturbed patients who also have genuine seizures.

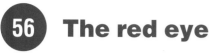

Diagnosis	How common 1 = very common 6 = very rare	Symptoms especially	Signs		Treatment
Conjunctivitis infective dry eye allergic	1 1 2	Sticky Gritty Itchy Stringy discharge		Redness entire surface, eye and two lid linings	Topical chloramphenicol Topical lubricants Topical mast stabilizer
Episcleritis	2	Irritation		Sectorial redness, eye only	None?
Iritis (anterior uveitis)	3	Pain, moderate Photophobia		Redness, eye only around cornea ± small pupil	Topical corticosteroid and dilate
Corneal (keratitis)	4	Pain, sharp Photophobia Watering		Local redness and corneal stain	Topical antiviral
Scleritis	5	Pain, may be severe, may increase on eye movement		Intense redness, eye only	Systemic with corticosteroid and cytotoxic?
Acute glaucoma	6	Pain, aching Vomit		Intense redness, eye only ± large fixed pupil	Topical after diagnosis Acetazolamide also?

Redness of the eye surface is caused by inflammation of its coverings, either the superficial conjunctiva or the episclera that lies beneath, or both.

Is this conjunctivitis?

Do not assume that redness is the result of conjunctivitis, even though this is by far the most frequent cause. If this is a single episode of red eye, the aetiology is usually infective and is most likely to be bacterial, although it could be viral or occasionally chlamydial. It is important to recognize which, because the non-bacterial types need different treatment.

Infective

The eye is not only red but also sticky, to a variable extent—most with bacterial and least with viral infections. There may be mild discomfort and irritation but, if the patient describes actual pain, consider alternative causes such as iritis or a corneal ulcer. Similarly with vision; in conjunctivitis the vision may be slightly blurred by sticky discharge, which

is cleared by blinking or bathing, but the patient usually expects this and should not seem worried about loss of vision.

The straightforward single episode may be treated topically with chloramphenicol drops, hourly for the first day then three times daily for five more. A meta-analysis of large numbers of cases of aplastic anaemia has shown no significant association with ocular chloramphenicol use, so the risk has been unfairly publicized.

If the problem fails to settle rapidly or recurs, consider swab for microbiology, including *Chlamydia* sp. if the patient is sexually active. If this seems possible, refer to a genitourinary medicine (GUM) department because the necessary swabs can be taken properly and treatment with oral erythromycin prescribed.

Viral conjunctivitis does not respond to chloramphenicol. It is less sticky, more uncomfortable and takes longer to settle. The patient needs sympathy and explanation, which may be reinforced if adenovirus can be isolated by swab which goes into transport medium, and takes several days to yield a result.

Dry eye

If symptoms are more chronic and the eyes are described as feeling dry or gritty and worse in heated or smoky atmospheres, the patient may have dryness. In younger patients especially, this might be a sicca syndrome and related to autoimmunity or even sarcoidosis. Extra signs are revealed by Schirmer's strip test or staining the cornea and conjunctiva with fluorescein at the slitlamp.

Allergic

Certain extra symptoms especially suggestive of allergy, either acute or chronic and possibly seasonal, are an itching and stringy discharge. When the patient tries to remove the offending discharge, this emerges from the eye as 'a long string, like melted cheese'!

Could it be episcleritis?

This is relatively common and harmless. The patient notices recurrent redness of part of the eye surface, which settles spontaneously but tends to recur. The eye is uncomfortable but not sticky. Underlying systemic disorders are uncommon and the treatment is usually nothing. Referral to the eye department may settle the dilemma if not the condition.

Can I recognize iritis?

This internal inflammation of the anterior chamber is much less common than either conjunctivitis or episcleritis but is very important to recognize because it needs prompt and correct treatment, and might signify an important underlying disorder. Send suspects to the eye department as definitive diagnosis needs a slitlamp, and treatment is tailored to the intensity of inflammation.

Characteristically the eye is painful and specifically often photophobic, so that looking at light hurts. The patient who has experienced attacks before will recognize them early, but the inexperienced doctor often delays considering the possibility until several days have passed and the eye is more inflamed. Another clue is a small pupil, which may appear stuck or festooned on dilating. The eye is not sticky and is usually most red around the edge of the cornea. There are a number of causes (Table 56.1).

Table 56.1 Causes of iritis.

Idiopathic	50% of cases
Systemic disease	Sarcoidosis
	Ankylosing spondylitis
	Inflammatory bowel disease
	Behçet's syndrome
	Reiter's disease
Infection	Syphilis
	Tuberculosis
	Herpes zoster
	Herpes simplex
	Lyme disease
Auto-immune	Juvenile inflammatory arthritis

Could the cornea be affected?

Keratitis is another uncommon possibility. Characteristic features are photophobia and pain which may be sharp and, if acute, the eye feels as if scratched; watering may also be present. Redness may be localized to the area adjacent to the affected part of the cornea and an ulcer that will stain with fluorescein is sometimes visible to the naked eye. A dendritic, or branching, pattern, seen best with the slitlamp, suggests herpes viral keratitis, typically herpes simplex virus. Two aspects of management are of great importance:

1 Urgent diagnosis is needed, so that effective treatment (anti-viral therapy) can be started early on, to decrease the chance of corneal scarring and impaired vision.
2 Topical steroids promote viral growth, and can lead to a dramatic deterioration in vision in infective keratitis—they should not be given unless keratitis is known not to be present.

Keratitis may also occur in association with graft versus host disease in which corneal malaise is often compounded by dryness. A very rare cause is Cogan's syndrome, associated with deafness and aortitis, with raised systemic inflammatory markers; syphilis would be a differential diagnosis.

Is it possible the red eye could be scleritis?

This ischaemic condition of the eye coat is rare but very important. First, it can result in perforation of the eye if not treated correctly and, second, there is sometimes an associated systemic vasculitis which may threaten other organs, especially the kidney. The usual culprit is rheumatoid arthritis, occasionally Wegener's granulomatosis, microscopic polyarteritis or systemic lupus erythematosus, in that order.

Some rheumatoid patients develop necrotizing disease with no pain but most patients describe an unpleasant ocular ache, which may be severe and characteristically interrupts sleep. The pain is often worse on eye movement. If the posterior part of the eye is involved, the optic nerve may be affected and vision lost as a result.

Treatment for all aspects, including the eye, must be systemic with corticosteroids and possibly a cytotoxic drug such as cyclophosphamide.

Does the remote possibility of acute angle-closure glaucoma need to be considered?

Very rarely the eye pressure may rise acutely and the anterior part becomes ischaemic. Pain is intense and characteristically the patient will vomit, as with acutely raised intracranial pressure. Vision becomes misty and the congested eye feels like a cricket ball rather than its usual squash-ball tension, with a fixed dilated pupil. This is an ocular emergency and needs to be given a slitlamp examination rapidly; delay of over an hour dictates immediate intravenous acetazolamide.

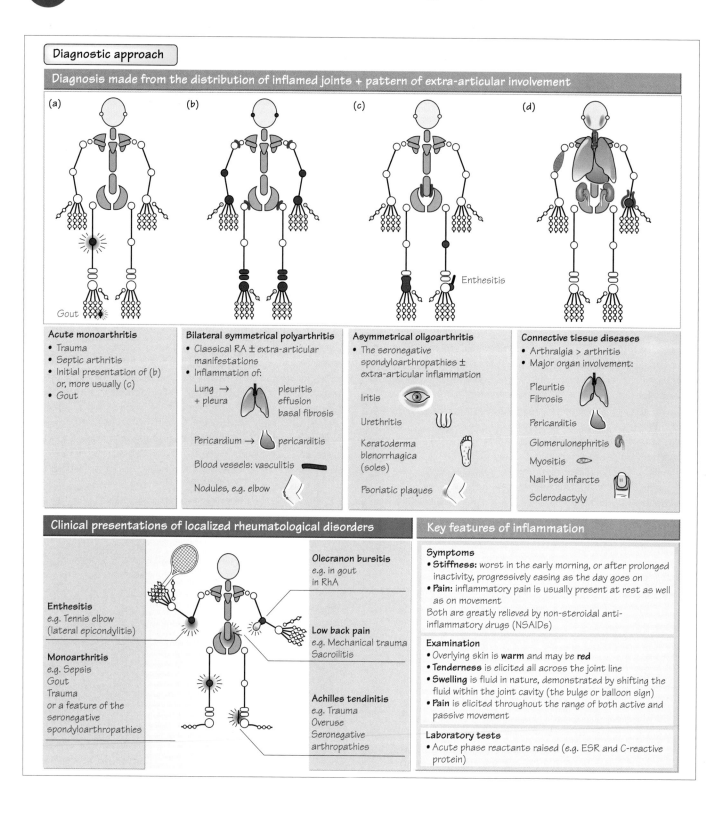

Diagnostic approach

Diagnosis made from the distribution of inflamed joints + pattern of extra-articular involvement

(a)   (b)   (c)   (d)

Enthesitis

Gout

Acute monoarthritis
- Trauma
- Septic arthritis
- Initial presentation of (b) or, more usually (c)
- Gout

Bilateral symmetrical polyarthritis
- Classical RA ± extra-articular manifestations
- Inflammation of:

Lung → pleuritis
+ pleura   effusion
           basal fibrosis

Pericardium → pericarditis

Blood vessels: vasculitis

Nodules, e.g. elbow

Asymmetrical oligoarthritis
- The seronegative spondyloarthropathies ± extra-articular inflammation

Iritis

Urethritis

Keratoderma blenorrhagica (soles)

Psoriatic plaques

Connective tissue diseases
- Arthralgia > arthritis
- Major organ involvement:

Pleuritis
Fibrosis

Pericarditis

Glomerulonephritis

Myositis

Nail-bed infarcts

Sclerodactyly

Clinical presentations of localized rheumatological disorders

Enthesitis
e.g. Tennis elbow (lateral epicondylitis)

Monoarthritis
e.g. Sepsis
Gout
Trauma
or a feature of the seronegative spondyloarthropathies

Olecranon bursitis
e.g. in gout in RhA

Low back pain
e.g. Mechanical trauma
Sacroilitis

Achilles tendinitis
e.g. Trauma
Overuse
Seronegative arthropathies

Key features of inflammation

Symptoms
- **Stiffness:** worst in the early morning, or after prolonged inactivity, progressively easing as the day goes on
- **Pain:** inflammatory pain is usually present at rest as well as on movement
Both are greatly relieved by non-steroidal anti-inflammatory drugs (NSAIDs)

Examination
- Overlying skin is **warm** and may be **red**
- **Tenderness** is elicited all across the joint line
- **Swelling** is fluid in nature, demonstrated by shifting the fluid within the joint cavity (the bulge or balloon sign)
- **Pain** is elicited throughout the range of both active and passive movement

Laboratory tests
- Acute phase reactants raised (e.g. ESR and C-reactive protein)

Diagnosis in rheumatology largely depends on clinical pattern recognition, because the pattern of joint, periarticular structure and connective tissue involvement is usually highly characteristic for a particular condition. Three patterns are recognized:

- **Localized disorders** where there is a single swollen joint/painful area (e.g. gout, low back pain, tennis elbow) are of inflammatory, infectious or mechanical origin and usually present as regional pain syndromes (p. 118).

Clinical Presentations at a Glance

- **Widespread disorders** that cause symptoms predominantly in one component of the musculoskeletal system, e.g. rheumatoid arthritis (RA) if it predominantly affects the joints.
- **Widespread disorders with extra-articular manifestations**: involving many components of the musculoskeletal system and connective tissues, e.g. systemic lupus erythematosus (SLE) which affects joints, skin and serosal surfaces as well as major organs, e.g. the kidney and brain.

Definitions of terms used in rheumatology
- **Monoarticular**: single joint involvement.
- **Oligoarticular**: 2–4 joints involved. Usually large joints of the lower limb, but can affect any joint.
- **Polyarticular**: multiple joints involved, but may start with limited joint involvement. Typically affects the small joints of the hands and feet.
- **Extra-articular**: involvement of structures at sites removed from the joints, e.g. rheumatoid nodules in the skin or lung, rheumatoid scleritis or episcleritis (the eye).

Key points in clinical assessment
The impact and consequences (functional impairment, disability, handicap) of the condition to the patient are integral to the clinical assessment.
- Loss of function and pain are key symptoms in rheumatological diseases; the severity of disability and distribution and intensity of pain should always be fully assessed.
- Depression is common in rheumatic disease (both as primary and secondary phenomenon) and should be specifically sought (p. 432).
- Inflammation is suggested by pain, swelling, early morning stiffness and tenderness. Assessment of activity of inflammation, i.e. those symptoms reversible with agents, which suppress inflammation, is made on the basis of clinical and laboratory findings.
- Distribution of inflamed joints is usually characteristic of particular diseases.
- Extra-articular symptoms may suggest a disease with systemic features and multiorgan involvement.

History
The chronology and impact of symptoms on the patient should be determined. The presenting symptoms usually relate to a joint or area around a joint.
- Pain
- Stiffness
- Deformity
- Loss of function.

These may arise from joints or periarticular structures. Inflammatory characteristics (degree of pain, and duration of early morning stiffness) should be carefully elicited. Extra-articular symptoms may be diagnostically helpful in pointing to those diseases strongly associated with arthritis:
- **Psoriasis**: skin rash (may be limited to the scalp, umbilicus, nails or natal cleft).
- **Systemic lupus erythematosus (SLE)**: skin rashes occur in 70% (p. 409), polyserositis (pericardial or pleural pain; p. 12). Raynaud's syndrome or mouth ulcers.
- **Reactive arthritis or seronegative spondylarthropathies** (p. 402): diarrhoea, urethritis, conjunctivitis.

- **Wegener's granulomatosis**: sinusitis, mononeuritis multiplex, skin ulcers.

In suspected multisystem diseases specific organ involvement (lung, kidney, nervous system) should be sought on clinical grounds and by special investigations. Constitutional symptoms including fever, malaise, weight loss or fatigue may indicate a widespread inflammatory process.

Examination
Examination of the locomotor system is based on the **look, feel, move** paradigm.

Look for attitude (how the joint/affected part is held), swelling, deformity or asymmetry, muscle wasting around the joint, redness of the overlying skin. Determine the pattern of joint disease, e.g. small vs. large, symmetric vs. asymmetric. Characteristic patterns of joint involvement in the major arthritides occur (see figure).

Feel for heat. Determine if swelling is:
- Bony (nodal osteoarthritis)
- Fluid (effusion, synovitis)
- Tissue (rheumatoid nodules).

The site of maximum tenderness elicited by mild/moderate direct pressure (sufficient to blanche the examining finger nail) allows determination of which structures are involved:
- Over joint line: arthritis
- Over periarticular structure, e.g. enthesitis.

Move. Note the pattern and any restriction in joint movement:
- Restriction throughout the range of active and passive motion suggests inflammatory synovitis of the affected joint.
- End-of-range pain and restriction (often with crepitus) suggests OA. Crepitus is a 'creaking' sound on passive movement that usually indicates advanced joint destruction.
- Pain only in specific planes or on specific movements suggests a local periarticular or mechanical problem. Active resisted movements that stress the involved structure can aggravate all tendinitis, enthesitis and bursitis.
- Long-standing disease may produce deformities such as 'fixed flexion' or angular deformities (varus/valgus).

Extra-articular signs
Extra-articular signs may be of diagnostic significance or indicate the extent of multiorgan involvement, particularly in the vasculitides and the connective tissue diseases:
- Systemic: high fever may suggest infection, Still's disease or rheumatic fever but sometimes gout or SLE.
- Skin and appendages: particularly in psoriasis, vasculitis including SLE, RA, scleroderma and dermatomyositis.
- Mucosa: in Crohn's disease and Behçet's syndrome. Mucosal dryness in Sjögren's syndrome.
- Major organ involvement: such as renal, heart or lungs, peripheral nerves or CNS in the vasculitides.

On the basis of the history and examination a presumptive diagnosis can be made (figure), usually confirmed by investigations, including joint X-rays and specific serological tests (see individual chapters).

Management and outcome
Treatment aims to relieve symptoms, maintain (restore) function, and suppress the underlying disease process. The best technique to achieve these aims depends on the disease, its severity and extent. A multidisciplinary approach is required, particularly in the chronic inflammatory disorders. Available techniques include:

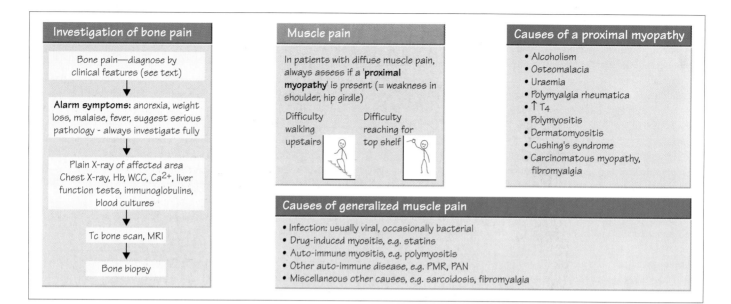

Investigation of bone pain

Bone pain—diagnose by clinical features (see text)

↓

Alarm symptoms: anorexia, weight loss, malaise, fever, suggest serious pathology - always investigate fully

↓

Plain X-ray of affected area Chest X-ray, Hb, WCC, Ca²⁺, liver function tests, immunoglobulins, blood cultures

↓

Tc bone scan, MRI

↓

Bone biopsy

Muscle pain

In patients with diffuse muscle pain, always assess if a '**proximal myopathy**' is present (= weakness in shoulder, hip girdle)

Difficulty walking upstairs

Difficulty reaching for top shelf

Causes of a proximal myopathy

- Alcoholism
- Osteomalacia
- Uraemia
- Polymyalgia rheumatica
- ↑ T4
- Polymyositis
- Dermatomyositis
- Cushing's syndrome
- Carcinomatous myopathy, fibromyalgia

Causes of generalized muscle pain

- Infection: usually viral, occasionally bacterial
- Drug-induced myositis, e.g. statins
- Auto-immune myositis, e.g. polymyositis
- Other auto-immune disease, e.g. PMR, PAN
- Miscellaneous other causes, e.g. sarcoidosis, fibromyalgia

Immunology and radiology in rheumatic diseases

Patterns of nuclear staining for antinuclear antibodies can be clinically helpful, though rarely are diagnostic

Pattern appearance	Disease association
Homogeneous (diffuse)	Common pattern
Rim of nucleus (peripheral; annular)	SLE
Nucleolar	Scleroderma SLE
Speckled	SLE Sjögren's syndrome Mixed connective tissue disease
Centromere (dividing cells only)	Limited systemic sclerosis (CREST syndrome)

SLE, systemic lupus erythematosus

Rheumatoid factors are autoantibodies against antigenic determinants of the Fc fragment of IgG
- They may be IgM, IgG or IgA class
- Only measurement of IgM RF is clinically useful
- IgM RF is usually measured by agglutination tests, and expressed as the serum dilution where agglutination still occurs (e.g. 1 in 40, 80, 160, 320 etc.)
- They occur in rheumatic diseases (e.g. in 70% of rheumatoid arthritis, 40% of SLE, 30% systemic sclerosis) – in RA they are of most use in prognosis rather than diagnosis (high titre = adverse prognosis)
- They also are found in:
  - Viral infections e.g. EBV infections)
  - Chronic inflammatory diseases (e.g. tuberculosis)
  - Neoplasms
  - 5% of healthy individuals

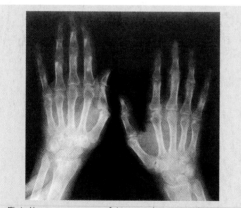

Plain X-rays are very useful in any chronic condition involving joints, and often show characteristic changes. This X-ray of hands with rheumatoid arthritis demonstrates erosive changes in the proximal interphalangeal joints (IPJ) of the thumbs, the metacarpophalangeal joint (MCPJ) of the left thumb, several of the carpal bones and the wrist and distal ulnar joint of the left hand. In addition there is characteristic juxta-articular osteopenia.

Antibodies to different components of extractable nuclear antigens (ENA) can be diagnostically helpful

Antigen	Molecular target	Clinical relevance*
'Smith' (Sm)	Common core proteins of U1, U2, U4, U5, U6—s RNPs	Alone or with RNP antibody—a subset of SLE (20%)
Ribonucleoprotein (RNP)	U1—s RNP	High titre—mixed connective tissue disease (100%)
Ro (SS-A)	60-kDa small RNP-binding Ro RNAs	ANA-negative SLE Neonatal lupus and congenital heart block Subacute cutaneous lupus
La (SS-B)	Transcription terminator of Ro RNAs	Primary Sjögren's syndrome
Scl-70	Topoisomerase I	Systemic sclerosis (20%)
Jo-1	Histidyl-transfer RNA synthetase	Myositis, arthritis—often with pulmonary fibrosis

*Figures in brackets show percentage of patients in disease category who have demonstrable antibody. U, uridine rich; s RNP, nuclear ribonucleoproteins.

- General measures, including education and advice, physiotherapy and occupational therapy for joint protection measures, e.g. splinting and local application of heat. The provision of aids and appliances when function is impaired can help dramatically.
- Intra- or periarticular steroid injections.
- Drugs: including, anti-inflammatory medications and disease modifying drugs for inflammatory conditions (e.g. methotrexate, sulphasalazine for RA, cyclophosphamide for SLE renal disease).
- Biological therapies: anticytokine therapies and anti-adhesion molecule therapies. Anti-TNF therapy is now widely used in RA and typically induces remission in a quarter of patients within 3 months. Two-thirds of patients improve by at least 20% and one-quarter by 70% within 6 months.
- Surgery (joint fusion, replacement, synovial resection) is useful to reduce pain, and to stabilize joints.

Bone pain

Bone pain arises when there is destruction of the integrity of normal bone. Pain arising from bone has the following characteristics:
- Pain is deep seated and intense
- Characteristically unremitting and disturbs sleep
- Is present independent of movement or posture
- Is often poorly responsive to simple analgesia or non-steroidal anti-inflammatory drugs (NSAIDs).

Differential diagnosis of bone pain

- Fracture
  - Traumatic
  - 'Stress' (e.g. related to excess physical activity, such as marathon running, etc.)
  - Atraumatic (osteoporotic)
- Osteonecrosis (avascular necrosis)
- Neoplasia
  - Primary tumour: benign or malignant (e.g. osteoid osteoma, or osteosarcoma)
  - Secondary tumour: commonly from breast, lung, thyroid, and renal or prostate primary. Myeloma can present as bone pain, commonly from crush fractures to vertebral bodies.
- Metabolic
  - Paget's disease of bone
  - Osteomalacia

- Infection
  - Osteomyelitis.

Investigation of bone pain is shown in the figure.

Muscle pain

Pain arising from muscles is extremely common. Symptoms may be localized (e.g. due to trauma/overuse) or more diffuse (in the context of a systemic process). Muscle pain:
- Is usually felt as a dull ache, i.e. the muscle hurts = myalgia.
- Is often associated with weakness of the affected muscle group. If there is intrinsic weakness of the muscle due to intrinsic muscular disease the process is a myopathic one.
- May be associated with tenderness of the muscles.
- Often affects equivalent groups in the upper and lower limb girdles if due to a systemic process.

Differential diagnosis of muscle pain

Different patterns suggest different illnesses:
- Predominant weakness (usually painless) of muscle groups suggests a myopathy (see p. 382).
- Predominant muscular ache, and tenderness with stiffness in the proximal muscle groups suggests polymyalgia rheumatica (PMR).
- Predominant pain and tenderness with secondary weakness suggests:
  Either trauma or overuse if symptoms are local; or
  Inflammation (myositis) if there are widespread symptoms, e.g. polymyositis or dermatomyositis.

Management of muscle pain

The aim is to clearly demarcate the symptoms of pain, tenderness, stiffness and weakness as well as the extent and distribution of muscle involvement. The physical examination may elicit evidence of muscle tenderness and weakness. Investigations in inflammatory myositis show:
- Elevation of inflammatory markers CRP and ESR (may be > 100 in PMR).
- The muscle enzyme creatine kinase may be markedly raised (aldolase and AST are less specific).
- Electromyography (EMG) may be helpful.
- Diagnostic muscle biopsy with special staining.
  Treatment is determined by the cause. Trauma/overuse responds to rest and simple analgesics (e.g. paracetamol) or NSAIDs. Most inflammatory diseases require corticosteroids.

58 Low back pain and other regional pain syndromes

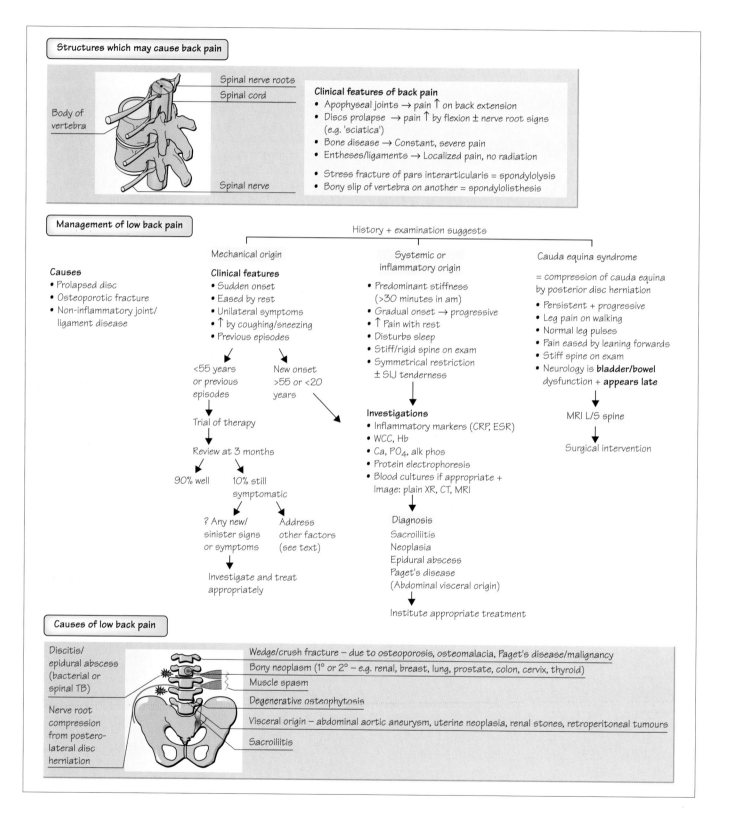

Structures which may cause back pain

- Spinal nerve roots
- Spinal cord
- Body of vertebra
- Spinal nerve

Clinical features of back pain
- Apophyseal joints → pain ↑ on back extension
- Discs prolapse → pain ↑ by flexion ± nerve root signs (e.g. 'sciatica')
- Bone disease → Constant, severe pain
- Entheses/ligaments → Localized pain, no radiation

- Stress fracture of pars interarticularis = spondylolysis
- Bony slip of vertebra on another = spondylolisthesis

Management of low back pain

History + examination suggests

Causes
- Prolapsed disc
- Osteoporotic fracture
- Non-inflammatory joint/ligament disease

Mechanical origin

Clinical features
- Sudden onset
- Eased by rest
- Unilateral symptoms
- ↑ by coughing/sneezing
- Previous episodes

<55 years or previous episodes

New onset >55 or <20 years

Trial of therapy

Review at 3 months

90% well   10% still symptomatic

? Any new/ sinister signs or symptoms

Address other factors (see text)

Investigate and treat appropriately

Systemic or inflammatory origin
- Predominant stiffness (>30 minutes in am)
- Gradual onset → progressive
- ↑ Pain with rest
- Disturbs sleep
- Stiff/rigid spine on exam
- Symmetrical restriction ± SIJ tenderness

Investigations
- Inflammatory markers (CRP, ESR)
- WCC, Hb
- Ca, PO_4, alk phos
- Protein electrophoresis
- Blood cultures if appropriate + Image: plain XR, CT, MRI

Diagnosis
Sacroiliitis
Neoplasia
Epidural abscess
Paget's disease
(Abdominal visceral origin)

Institute appropriate treatment

Cauda equina syndrome

= compression of cauda equina by posterior disc herniation

- Persistent + progressive
- Leg pain on walking
- Normal leg pulses
- Pain eased by leaning forwards
- Stiff spine on exam
- Neurology is **bladder/bowel** dysfunction + **appears late**

MRI L/S spine

Surgical intervention

Causes of low back pain

Discitis/ epidural abscess (bacterial or spinal TB)

Nerve root compression from postero-lateral disc herniation

Wedge/crush fracture – due to osteoporosis, osteomalacia, Paget's disease/malignancy
Bony neoplasm (1° or 2° – e.g. renal, breast, lung, prostate, colon, cervix, thyroid)
Muscle spasm
Degenerative osteophytosis
Visceral origin – abdominal aortic aneurysm, uterine neoplasia, renal stones, retroperitoneal tumours
Sacroiliitis

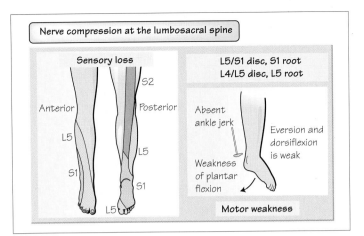

Nerve compression at the lumbosacral spine

Sensory loss

Anterior — L5, S1

Posterior — S2, L5, S1, L5

L5/S1 disc, S1 root
L4/L5 disc, L5 root

Absent ankle jerk

Weakness of plantar flexion

Eversion and dorsiflexion is weak

Motor weakness

Low back pain is common and disabling. The lifetime incidence is 65–80%, representing about 10% of rheumatological problems in general practice. The economic cost in 1990 was $US24 bn in the USA.

Aetiology and nomenclature

The different causes of low back pain are:
• **Mechanical** low back pain arising from an anatomic structure such as muscle, ligament or intervertebral disc due to trauma, deformity or degenerative change.
• **Systemic illness** such as inflammatory spondylitis, infection, malignancy or Paget's disease.
• **Sciatica** is pain that radiates from the buttock down the back of the leg and into the foot, often accompanied by paraesthesia in the same distribution. It is usually due to compression of a lumbosacral nerve root by a protruding intervertebral disc.

Symptoms

• Mechanical back pain causes localized symptoms, which may be referred to other sites around the pelvic girdle and upper legs. It does not extend below the knee unless there is additional nerve root compression causing sciatica. In this case symptoms and signs in the anatomical distribution of the sciatic nerve occur (see figure).
• Central canal narrowing (large central disc prolapse and/or osteophyte formation) may cause compression of the cauda equina, giving rise to distinct symptoms of bilateral leg claudication. Bladder/bowel dysfunction constitutes a medical emergency.
• Lateral recess stenosis may occur as a result of posterolateral protrusion of the disc, osteophyte around a degenerate zygo-apophyseal joint or a combination of the two. Sciatica is prominent on standing or walking for any length of time: nocturnal pain in the leg (with or without paraesthesia) typically wakes the patient in the early hours and may be eased by walking around. Neurological signs may be minor or absent.
• Features suggestive of systemic/inflammatory illness (malaise, fevers, weight loss) or cauda equina compression (paraparesis, bladder involvement) should prompt complete systemic examination and investigations (see algorithm in figure).

Natural history of low back pain

Most episodes of low back pain are self-limiting and not incapacitating.
• 90% are due to 'mechanical' back pain.
• 50% are better 1 week after onset.

• < 10% have pain persistent > 6 months. These enter a 'chronic pain cycle', are the least likely to return to full employment/activity and account for 80% of the costs incurred in care.
• 10% are due to underlying systemic or inflammatory illness.

Clinical approach

The aims of the clinical evaluation are:
• Discrimination between mechanical and systemic causes.
• Identification of features which suggest the need for advanced imaging studies ± early surgical referral.

Examination

Routine back examination is shown in the figure. Pointers towards serious underlying disease include:
• Patients with systemic or inflammatory features.
• Those > 55 or < 25 years old with new-onset low back pain.
• Those unresponsive to a 6–8-week trial of therapy for mechanical low back pain.

Management (see figure)

Initial treatment: Simple analgesia ± NSAIDs. Bed rest in the acute phase (≤ 48 h) with early mobilization, followed by a graded exercise programme.

Unresponsive patients with no new physical findings:
• Identification of occupational, physical and psychosocial contributions. Patient-tailored rehabilitation programme.
• Identification of specific anatomic lesions causing pain (e.g. facet joints, disc lesions, nerve roots, bones).

Where such lesions can be identified, the following may be useful:
• **Facet joint injection** with local anaesthetic and corticosteroids. This may be therapeutic, or helpful in localizing a painful segment prior to spinal fusion.
• **Local anaesthetic injections** around nerve roots to confirm compression at specific levels prior to surgical decompression, particularly when there are lesions at multiple levels.
• **Chemonucleolysis** by intradisc injection of chymopapain to relieve compression symptoms from a bulging disc.
• **Surgery** is performed to relieve nerve compression by disc herniation using the technique of partial laminectomy/discectomy. It may be combined with spinal fusion at the corresponding level.

Regional pain syndromes

Regional rheumatic pain syndromes are very common. They may be difficult to diagnose with confidence. In particular pain arising in a localized area, such as the shoulder or hip, presents a clinical challenge. Pain may arise in any of the articular or periarticular structures, or may be referred from a more distant organ or structure.

Differential diagnosis

The differential diagnosis of regional pain is dependent on a good knowledge of the regional anatomy and a precise history and examination. The differential diagnoses for pain around the hip, shoulder and wrist are shown in the figure.

General approach
History
• Details of all factors relevant to pain—nature and severity, radiation, factors which relieve or exacerbate, movements which provoke pain.
• Causative factors such as trauma or overuse related to work or leisure.

- Features suggestive of a more widespread inflammatory or systemic condition.

A complete neuromuscular examination is performed: **Look** for swelling, redness, muscle wasting, posture in which affected part is held. **Feel** carefully localize where tenderness is maximal. **Move** carefully and so determine the range of passive, then active motion around the appropriate joints. Note which movements provoke pain.

Ask the patient to perform these movements against resistance. Lesions such as tendinitis, enthesitis and bursitis are often more painful on movement against resistance.

Principles of management

- Exclude serious systemic disease and infection by appropriate tests, e.g. synovial fluid microscopy for crystals from gouty bursitis or microorganisms from septic bursitis.
- Educate the patient regarding avoidance or correction of mechanical triggers. Reassure.
- Advise on an appropriate level of activity/exercises.
- Splinting (particularly for synovitis and tenosynovitis).
- Analgesia, including intralesional steroid/local anaesthetic.

Prognosis and outcome

Many of these conditions are self limiting and respond well to simple measures as above. Most will be asymptomatic within 12–18 months of onset. Those who receive prompt advice and therapy usually do better. A small percentage of cases fail to settle, and it may be necessary to alter work or sporting techniques.

Back examination

Examine patient while standing

- **Gait**; look for any abnormality whilst walking and turning, and note whether walking aids are required. Normal gait involves stance (60%) and swing (40%) phases

- **Back**; look for any abnormality including scoliosis, which is described by the side of the vertebral concavity; cervical lordosis, thoracic kyphosis, and lumbar lordosis are normal [i.e. looking at the patient from the side, with the patient facing to the right, a lordosis is a curve shaped like a closing bracket ')', whereas a kyphosis is shaped like an opening bracket '(']

- Check for any localized tenderness in the spine (press, and then 'bang' on each of the vertebral processes in turn) – local tenderness may indicate infection

- Look at the progression of the thoracic kyphosis; a useful measure is the distance from the wall to the tragus (ear lobe) when the patient stands with his/her back to the wall

- Forward bending; measure the increase in length between L5/S1 vertebrae and points 10 cm above and 5 cm below (Schober's test) – it should be ≥ 4 cm [incidentally, the finger to floor distance on bending forward is not a good measure of spinal stiffness as it may vary with hip mobility]

- Lateral flexion; ask the patient to reach down laterally to the knee joint. This can normally be achieved, but may be restricted in ankylosing spondylitis

- Hyperextension; which is arching the back backwards. Usually 10° from the vertical can be achieved

Examine patients while sitting

- Cervical spine; examine for flexion (i.e. bending the neck forward), extension (i.e. bending the neck backwards), lateral flexion (i.e. tilting the head to one side), and rotation (i.e. moving the head to the left and right). The angle attained is measured from the face forward position – normal ranges are; flexion and extension, 70°, lateral flexion, 40°, rotation, 80°

Pelvis examination

Examine while standing

- Look for asymmetry of the pelvis, which may suggest unequal leg length

- Trendelenburg's test. Ask the patient to stand on one leg – a dropped pelvis on the side of the raised leg (= +ve Trendelenburg test) suggests muscle weakness or hip pathology

Examine while supine

- Sacro-iliac tenderness; press the anterior superior iliac spines gently apart. This will cause sacro-iliac pain if they are inflamed. With the patient prone, press on the sacrum – this will cause pain if there is sacro-iliac joint inflammation

- True and apparent leg lengths. Measure from the anterior superior iliac spine and umbilicus, respectively, to the medial malleolus; an apparent difference may indicate lateral tilting of the pelvis

- Hip flexion; bring the leg in towards the chest with the knees flexed – the normal limit is 110°

- Hip extension; with the patient prone, extend the hip – the normal range is 0-30°. This will exacerbate the symptoms if there is nerve root irritation, as the femoral nerve will be stretched

- Internal and external rotation, abduction and adduction of the hip. Rotate each hip internally (normal range 25°), and externally (normal range 45°) with the hip flexed, then measure the range of abduction (normal range 50°) and adduction (normal 30°)

- Traction manoeuvres. Assess the sciatic nerve by straight leg raising (and record the angle of elevation). Dorsiflex the foot whilst raised (Lasègue's test). This will exacerbate symptoms of lumbosacral root compression

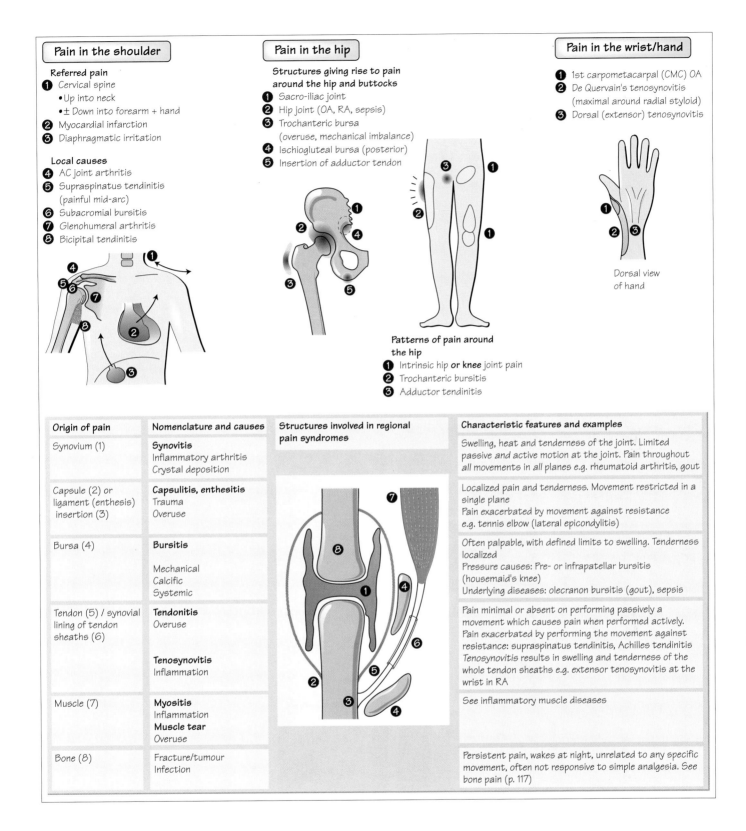

Pain in the shoulder

Referred pain
1. Cervical spine
   • Up into neck
   • ± Down into forearm + hand
2. Myocardial infarction
3. Diaphragmatic irritation

Local causes
4. AC joint arthritis
5. Supraspinatus tendinitis (painful mid-arc)
6. Subacromial bursitis
7. Glenohumeral arthritis
8. Bicipital tendinitis

Pain in the hip

Structures giving rise to pain around the hip and buttocks
1. Sacro-iliac joint
2. Hip joint (OA, RA, sepsis)
3. Trochanteric bursa (overuse, mechanical imbalance)
4. Ischiogluteal bursa (posterior)
5. Insertion of adductor tendon

Patterns of pain around the hip
1. Intrinsic hip **or knee** joint pain
2. Trochanteric bursitis
3. Adductor tendinitis

Pain in the wrist/hand

1. 1st carpometacarpal (CMC) OA
2. De Quervain's tenosynovitis (maximal around radial styloid)
3. Dorsal (extensor) tenosynovitis

Dorsal view of hand

Origin of pain	Nomenclature and causes	Structures involved in regional pain syndromes	Characteristic features and examples
Synovium (1)	**Synovitis** Inflammatory arthritis Crystal deposition		Swelling, heat and tenderness of the joint. Limited passive *and* active motion at the joint. Pain throughout all movements in all planes e.g. rheumatoid arthritis, gout
Capsule (2) or ligament (enthesis) insertion (3)	**Capsulitis, enthesitis** Trauma Overuse		Localized pain and tenderness. Movement restricted in a single plane Pain exacerbated by movement against resistance e.g. tennis elbow (lateral epicondylitis)
Bursa (4)	**Bursitis** Mechanical Calcific Systemic		Often palpable, with defined limits to swelling. Tenderness localized Pressure causes: Pre- or infrapatellar bursitis (housemaid's knee) Underlying diseases: olecranon bursitis (gout), sepsis
Tendon (5) / synovial lining of tendon sheaths (6)	**Tendonitis** Overuse **Tenosynovitis** Inflammation		Pain minimal or absent on performing passively a movement which causes pain when performed actively. Pain exacerbated by performing the movement against resistance: supraspinatus tendinitis, Achilles tendinitis Tenosynovitis results in swelling and tenderness of the whole tendon sheaths e.g. extensor tenosynovitis at the wrist in RA
Muscle (7)	**Myositis** Inflammation **Muscle tear** Overuse		See inflammatory muscle diseases
Bone (8)	Fracture/tumour Infection		Persistent pain, wakes at night, unrelated to any specific movement, often not responsive to simple analgesia. See bone pain (p. 117)

59 Introduction to dermatology

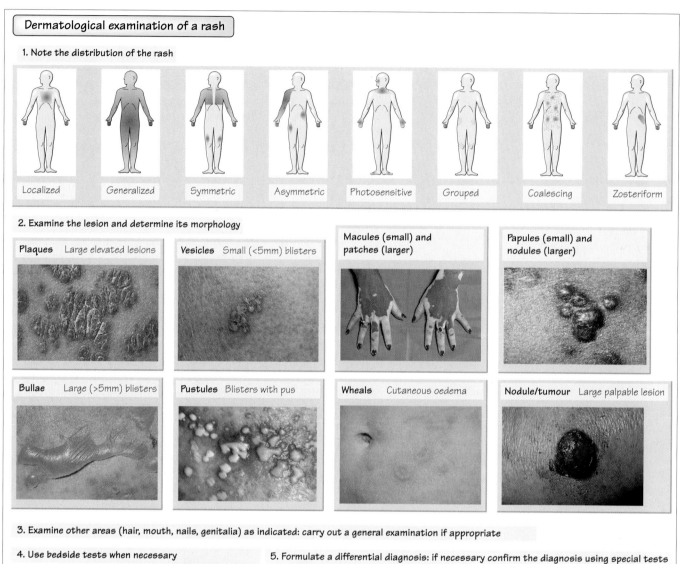

Dermatological examination of a rash

1. Note the distribution of the rash

| Localized | Generalized | Symmetric | Asymmetric | Photosensitive | Grouped | Coalescing | Zosteriform |

2. Examine the lesion and determine its morphology

Plaques Large elevated lesions

Vesicles Small (<5mm) blisters

Macules (small) and patches (larger)

Papules (small) and nodules (larger)

Bullae Large (>5mm) blisters

Pustules Blisters with pus

Wheals Cutaneous oedema

Nodule/tumour Large palpable lesion

3. Examine other areas (hair, mouth, nails, genitalia) as indicated: carry out a general examination if appropriate

4. Use bedside tests when necessary

Wood's light – in fungal infection and erythrasma (as illustrated)

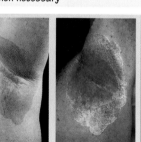

5. Formulate a differential diagnosis: if necessary confirm the diagnosis using special tests

Skin patch tests

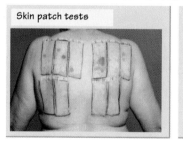

Biopsy Direct immunofluorescence demonstrating (light green) autoantibodies against intercellular desmosomes in pemphigus vulgaris

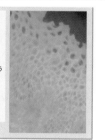

Dermatologists achieve a diagnosis by taking a history (which itself often establishes the diagnosis) and examining the skin.

History

Most patients present with a rash or with a lump/bump. Other symptoms include itch see p. 124), flushing (see p. 55), pain, hair loss, nail changes (see p. 126) and ulceration. It is important to ask about the spatiotemporal characteristics of the presenting symptoms:

- When did the rash/lump appear?
- Where did it spread to?
- When did it ulcerate or bleed?

Determine: age, racial background, occupation, sexual orientation,

Clinical Presentations at a Glance

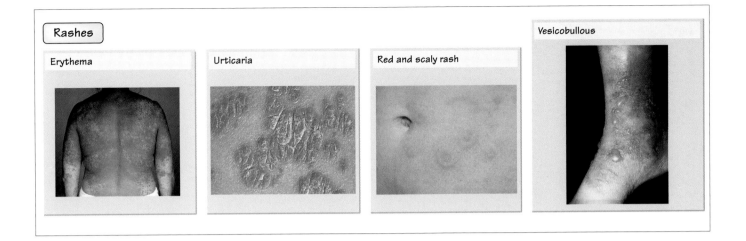

Rashes

Erythema | Urticaria | Red and scaly rash | Vesicobullous

drug history (could a rash represent an adverse drug reaction?), family history (there is a genetic predisposition in eczema, psoriasis and skin cancer), past medical history and current health, associated symptoms (e.g. joints, genitals), sun history (easy burning or tanning, lifelong sun exposure, sunburn, sun beds): sunlight may relieve or exacerbate a rash.

Examination

Skin examination is performed in a good light with the patient lying supine on a couch, using the naked eye first, then a magnifying glass. Undertake a general medical examination (see Chapter 2) when relevant.

- For a rash, ascertain its distribution: asymmetrical (suggests exogenous cause, e.g. local infection), symmetrical (endogenous cause), localized or widespread. Note the morphology: is it an erythema or urticaria, red and scaly (eczematous, psoriasiform or lichenoid), vasculitis, vesicobullous, or erythroderma? Check other sites that may be affected. Complete by examining the scalp, eyes, mouth, hands and nails, breasts, anogenital area and feet. Assess for lymphadenopathy.
- For a lump/bump, note its site, morphology, draining lymph nodes and liver (for distant metastases). Note skin phenotypes that predispose to cancer (fair, freckling, degree and type of moles, iris lentigines). A precise clinical diagnosis is often feasible but the prime objective is to differentiate benign from malignant lesions.

Morphology

Important morphological terms include:
- Macule: flat, no change in surface markings.
- Papule: circumscribed palpable lesion.
- Nodule: palpable mass ≥ 1 cm.
- Vesicles and bullae (blisters): visible accumulations of fluid (vesicles are small, bullae are larger).

Other terms include: telangiectasia, erosion, ulcer, plaque, wheal, comedone, pustule, abscess, cyst, scar, atrophy, purpura and sclerosis.

Special investigations

After physical examination (including urinalysis), the differential diagnosis can be further explored using special investigations:

- Wood's light is ultraviolet radiation of wavelength 360 nm, useful in demonstrating pigmentary diseases, and fungal infections.
- Microbiology: swab for bacteria, scrapings for fungi.
- Biopsy is useful in diagnosing many conditions and to exclude malignancy.
- Patch testing: putative allergens are applied to the skin and the resulting reaction is read at 48 and 96 h.
- Blood tests (e.g. for syphilis, HIV, lupus, iron deficiency).

Dermatological treatment

In the skin a range of pathological processes (inflammation, infection, fibrosis, dysplasia, neoplasia) results in thousands of named diseases, some of which have specific treatments (see individual chapters). Some general principles of management can be outlined.

Supportive treatments

These include:
- Moisturizing the skin and avoiding soap.
- Avoiding the sun, wearing a sunscreen.
- Providing reassurance and psychological support.

Specific treatments

These can be dietary or involve drugs, phototherapy or surgery.
- Diet: essential fatty acids (e.g. greasy fish, evening primrose oil) may be useful in inflammatory dermatoses.
- Drugs may be applied topically or taken orally:
  - topical treatments include emollients and soap substitutes, shampoos, sunscreens, steroids, antibacterials, antifungals, keratolytics, retinoids and cytotoxics
  - systemic treatments include antibacterials, antifungals, antihistamines, anti-inflammatory drugs, e.g. dapsone, antimalarials, retinoids, steroids, etc.
- Phototherapy: ultraviolet B (UVB) and PUVA (psoralens + ultraviolet A), photochemotherapy may be useful in severe dermatoses and mycosis fungoides.
- Surgery is used for diagnosis by biopsy and may be curative for skin cancer.

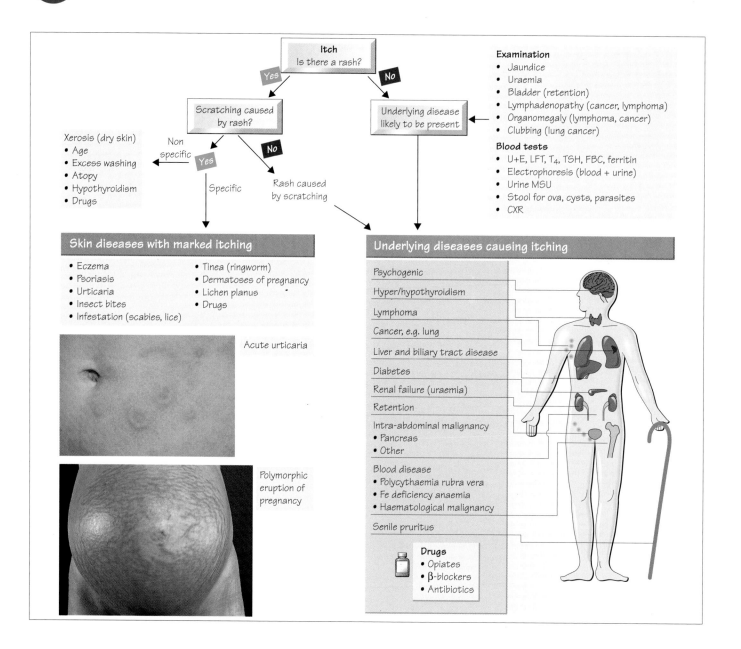

Itch
Is there a rash?

Yes / No

Scratching caused by rash?

Underlying disease likely to be present

Examination
- Jaundice
- Uraemia
- Bladder (retention)
- Lymphadenopathy (cancer, lymphoma)
- Organomegaly (lymphoma, cancer)
- Clubbing (lung cancer)

Blood tests
- U+E, LFT, T_4, TSH, FBC, ferritin
- Electrophoresis (blood + urine)
- Urine MSU
- Stool for ova, cysts, parasites
- CXR

Xerosis (dry skin)
- Age
- Excess washing
- Atopy
- Hypothyroidism
- Drugs

Non specific

Yes / No

Specific

Rash caused by scratching

Skin diseases with marked itching
- Eczema
- Psoriasis
- Urticaria
- Insect bites
- Infestation (scabies, lice)
- Tinea (ringworm)
- Dermatoses of pregnancy
- Lichen planus
- Drugs

Acute urticaria

Polymorphic eruption of pregnancy

Underlying diseases causing itching

Psychogenic

Hyper/hypothyroidism

Lymphoma

Cancer, e.g. lung

Liver and biliary tract disease

Diabetes

Renal failure (uraemia)

Retention

Intra-abdominal malignancy
- Pancreas
- Other

Blood disease
- Polycythaemia rubra vera
- Fe deficiency anaemia
- Haematological malignancy

Senile pruritus

Drugs
- Opiates
- β-blockers
- Antibiotics

Pruritus

Pruritus (itching) may be localized or generalized. Primary skin disease, underlying systemic disease, or rarely a psychological condition must be considered (see figure).

History

Localized pruritus suggests a local cause. Generalized pruritus may relate to dermatological or systemic disease. If a rash is present, determine whether the itching occurred before (suggests underlying systemic disorder, with the signs caused by scratching) or after (suggests underlying skin disease) the rash. Undertake a general assessment including a drug history.

Examination and treatment

Excoriations, eczematization and impetiginization are non-specific secondary signs from scratching. Determine whether there are any signs of a primary dermatosis or underlying illness (see figure). Treatment is for the underlying cause and includes emollients and antihistamines.

Rashes

Distinguish the distribution, the type of rash and the morphology (Chapter 59).

Erythemas

The causes of erythema in the skin are listed in Table 60.1.

Table 60.1 Causes of erythema.

Toxic erythema: drug or viral
Specific viral exanthems
Erythema chronicum migrans—Lyme borreliosis
Erythema multiforme (see p. 430)
Erythema nodosum (see p. 426)
Erythema marginatum—very rare reticular erythema
Still's disease—diurnal angulated macular erythema
Erythema ab igne—from close contact with heat

Table 60.2 Eruptions that may have red scaly patches.

Eczema/dermatitis	Pityriasis versicolor
Psoriasis	Mycosis fungoides
Lichen planus	Solar keratosis
Lichen sclerosus	Bowen's disease
Pityriasis rosea	Paget's disease
Lupus erythematosus	Superficial basal cell carcinoma
Dermatomyositis	Drug eruption
Tinea	

Urticarial lesions

The causes are:
• idiopathic urticaria
• drug eruptions
• prodromal bullous pemphigoid
• Henoch-Schönlein purpura.

Red scaly patches

The causes of red scaly patches are listed in Table 60.2.

Erythroderma

Erythroderma is a widespread confluent erythematous eruption that may develop acutely or insidiously. Causes, complications and treatment are listed in the figure.

Blistering

Blistering is common and examples include acute eczema, herpes, impetigo and insect bites. Some drug eruptions are bullous, e.g. toxic epidermal necrolysis (p. 420), as are some systemic diseases, e.g. por-phyria cutanea tarda and amyloid. Primary bullous disease is discussed on p. 420.

Vasculitis

Vasculitis can be localized to the skin or involve internal organs (Chapter 203 p. 406). Vasculitic manifestations range from erythema, livedo reticularis and urticaria, to palpable purpuric papules, nodules, necrosis and infarction, depending on the calibre of vessel involved, the nature of the inflammatory response and the severity of the vasculitic insult.

Flushing (see Chapter 28)

Skin diseases to consider are rosacea (Chapter 208), urticaria (p. 414 or Chapter 206) and erythromelalgia.

Pustules

Causes of pustules include acne (Chapter 208), rosacea, impetigo and autoimmune blistering diseases.

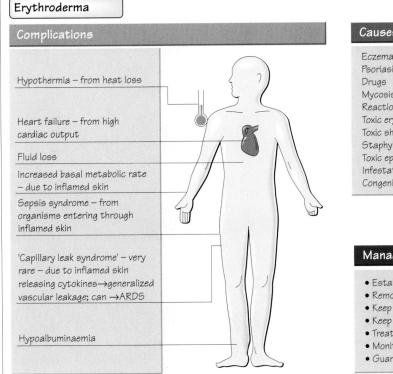

Erythroderma

Complications

Hypothermia – from heat loss

Heart failure – from high cardiac output

Fluid loss

Increased basal metabolic rate – due to inflamed skin

Sepsis syndrome – from organisms entering through inflamed skin

'Capillary leak syndrome' – very rare – due to inflamed skin releasing cytokines→generalized vascular leakage; can →ARDS

Hypoalbuminaemia

Causes of erythroderma

Eczema
Psoriasis
Drugs
Mycosis fungoides (Sézary syndrome)
Reactions to sunlight
Toxic erythema
Toxic shock syndrome
Staphylococcal scalded skin syndrome
Toxic epidermal necrolysis
Infestations (scabies and lice)
Congenital disorders

Management

• Establish diagnosis rapidly
• Remove any non-essential drugs
• Keep warm – may need 'space' blanket
• Keep well hydrated
• Treat infection early
• Monitor vital organs, electrolytes regularly
• Guarded prognosis – 10-15% of severe cases may die

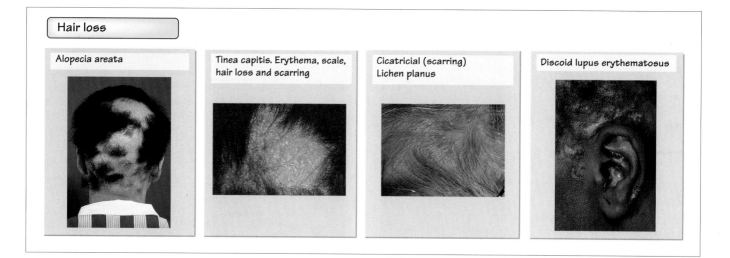

Hair loss

Alopecia areata

Tinea capitis. Erythema, scale, hair loss and scarring

Cicatricial (scarring) Lichen planus

Discoid lupus erythematosus

Alopecia

Alopecia, or hair loss, is common and may be male pattern, localized or generalized. Establish whether there is any underlying disease and whether there is permanent loss of hair as a result of *scarring*.

Clinical features and investigations

The duration of the process, sites affected and the patients general condition (pregnancy, nutrition, health) must be ascertained. On examination elicit local signs (erythema, scarring, pustulosis) and look for signs of a more widespread dermatosis or systemic illness. Helpful investigations include mycology, microbiology, skin biopsy and tests for an underlying systemic illness (full blood count, renal and liver function, iron studies, antibodies for systemic lupus erythematosus [SLE] and syphilis).

• **Diffuse non-scarring alopecia**: the differential diagnosis of diffuse non-scarring alopecia includes systemic illness, thyroid disorders, iron deficiency anaemia, skin diseases such as psoriasis, seborrhoeic dermatitis and alopecia areata, and drugs, such as lithium or cytotoxics.

• **Androgenic alopecia** in men is physiological and consists of focal frontal and vertical loss with eventual confluence of baldness and occipital sparing. In women the picture is of more diffuse thinning. Minoxidil 2–5% lotion may help some cases. In women the antiandrogen cyproterone acetate given with ethinyl oestradiol to regulate the menstrual cycle has some effect.

• **Alopecia areata** refers to focal areas of complete, non-scarring alopecia. Topical or intralesional corticosteroids help. The prognosis is unpredictable, although patients with nail pits or widespread hair loss do worse. Occasionally patients may have or develop another organ-specific autoimmune disease.

• **Scarring alopecia**: the differential diagnosis of scarring alopecia includes infection and inflammatory dermatoses (Table 61.1). Skin biopsy is essential. Diagnosis and treatment must be prompt to save the hair. The principal differential diagnosis is tinea capitis (treat with systemic antifungals), lichen planus (topical/systemic corticosteroids) and lupus erythematosus (topical/systemic steroids and systemic antimalarials).

Table 61.1 Causes of scarring alopecia.

Infections
• Tinea capitis and kerion
• Staphylococcal folliculitis/folliculitis decalvans
• Syphilis
• Herpes simplex and zoster
• Lupus vulgaris (tuberculosis)

Other skin diseases
• Lichen planus
• Lupus erythematosus (especially DLE)
• Sarcoid
• Scleroderma
• Basal cell carcinoma
• Acne keloidalis nuchae (keloid reaction to acne)

Nail disorders

The key points in diagnosing nail disorders are to establish whether the signs point to an underlying disease or to a treatable cause of nail dystrophy. The common nail disorders are:

• **Clubbing**: there are many causes for clubbing (see figure), although in practice lung cancer is the most common, followed by cryptogenic fibrosing alveolitis, cystic fibrosis and inflammatory bowel disease.

• **Dystrophy**: means a misshapen disorganized nail. A very common cause is fungal infection: exclude by examination of clippings. Arterial insufficiency (peripheral vascular disease or severe Raynaud's phenomenon). Psoriasis and trauma are other common causes.

• **Onycholysis**, where the nail plate lifts from the nail bed, occurs commonly in psoriasis, tinea and drug eruptions. Aggressive nail manicure may also be responsible.

• **Nail pits** are found in psoriasis, eczema and alopecia areata.

• **Leukonychia** (white nails) occurs most commonly as thin white bands in young people, in whom it is of no significance. Pathological leukonychia occurs mainly in long-standing systemic disease, such as cirrhosis, diabetes mellitus, cardiac failure and severe anaemia.

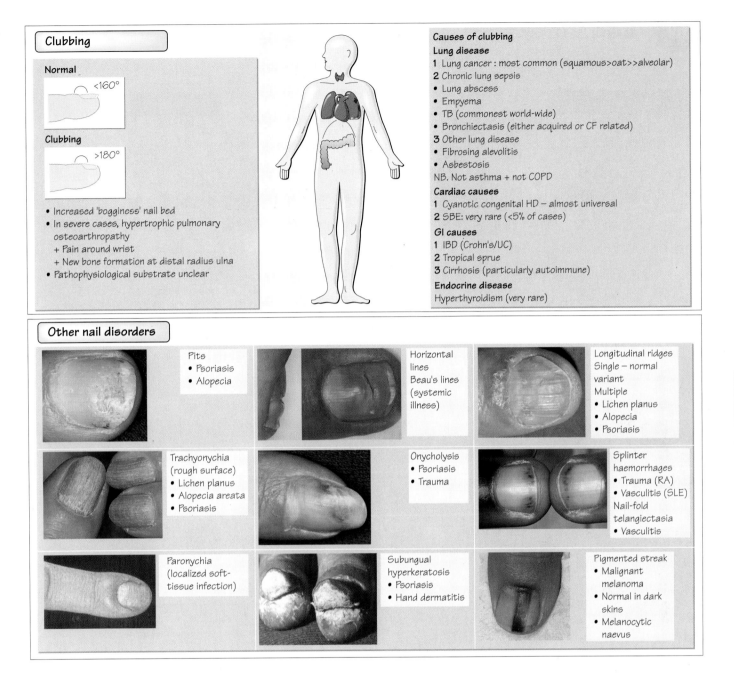

Clubbing

Normal

<160°

Clubbing

>180°

- Increased 'bogginess' nail bed
- In severe cases, hypertrophic pulmonary osteoarthropathy
  + Pain around wrist
  + New bone formation at distal radius ulna
- Pathophysiological substrate unclear

Causes of clubbing
Lung disease
1 Lung cancer : most common (squamous>oat>>alveolar)
2 Chronic lung sepsis
- Lung abscess
- Empyema
- TB (commonest world-wide)
- Bronchiectasis (either acquired or CF related)
3 Other lung disease
- Fibrosing alveolitis
- Asbestosis
NB. Not asthma + not COPD
Cardiac causes
1 Cyanotic congenital HD – almost universal
2 SBE: very rare (<5% of cases)
GI causes
1 IBD (Crohn's/UC)
2 Tropical sprue
3 Cirrhosis (particularly autoimmune)
Endocrine disease
Hyperthyroidism (very rare)

Other nail disorders

Pits
- Psoriasis
- Alopecia

Horizontal lines
Beau's lines (systemic illness)

Longitudinal ridges
Single – normal variant
Multiple
- Lichen planus
- Alopecia
- Psoriasis

Trachyonychia (rough surface)
- Lichen planus
- Alopecia areata
- Psoriasis

Onycholysis
- Psoriasis
- Trauma

Splinter haemorrhages
- Trauma (RA)
- Vasculitis (SLE)
Nail-fold telangiectasia
- Vasculitis

Paronychia (localized soft-tissue infection)

Subungual hyperkeratosis
- Psoriasis
- Hand dermatitis

Pigmented streak
- Malignant melanoma
- Normal in dark skins
- Melanocytic naevus

- **Koilonychia** (spoon-shaped nails) may be associated with local nail dystrophy, or with a dermatosis such as psoriasis or lichen simplex. Rarely it is a sign of iron deficiency.

- **Splinter haemorrhages** occur with trauma, in autoimmune rheumatic disease and endocarditis.

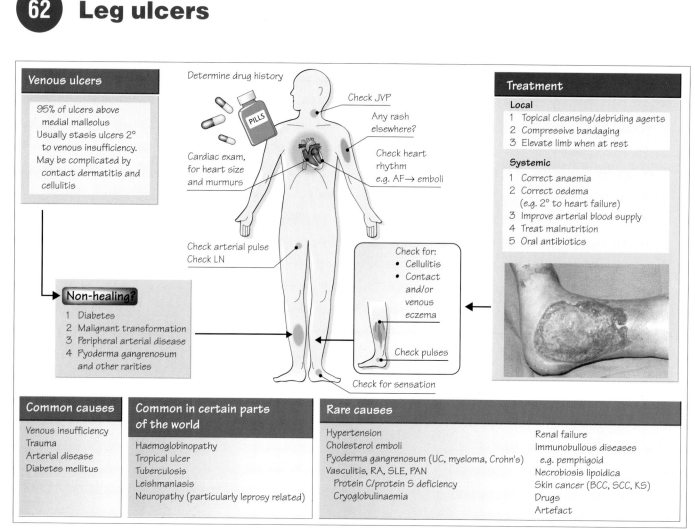

Venous ulcers

95% of ulcers above medial malleolus
Usually stasis ulcers 2° to venous insufficiency.
May be complicated by contact dermatitis and cellulitis

Determine drug history
PILLS
Cardiac exam, for heart size and murmurs
Check JVP
Any rash elsewhere?
Check heart rhythm e.g. AF→ emboli

Check arterial pulse
Check LN

Non-healing?
1 Diabetes
2 Malignant transformation
3 Peripheral arterial disease
4 Pyoderma gangrenosum and other rarities

Check for:
• Cellulitis
• Contact and/or venous eczema
Check pulses

Check for sensation

Treatment
Local
1 Topical cleansing/debriding agents
2 Compressive bandaging
3 Elevate limb when at rest
Systemic
1 Correct anaemia
2 Correct oedema (e.g. 2° to heart failure)
3 Improve arterial blood supply
4 Treat malnutrition
5 Oral antibiotics

Common causes

Venous insufficiency
Trauma
Arterial disease
Diabetes mellitus

Common in certain parts of the world

Haemoglobinopathy
Tropical ulcer
Tuberculosis
Leishmaniasis
Neuropathy (particularly leprosy related)

Rare causes

Hypertension
Cholesterol emboli
Pyoderma gangrenosum (UC, myeloma, Crohn's)
Vasculitis, RA, SLE, PAN
  Protein C/protein S deficiency
  Cryoglobulinaemia

Renal failure
Immunobullous diseases
  e.g. pemphigoid
Necrobiosis lipoidica
Skin cancer (BCC, SCC, KS)
Drugs
Artefact

Most leg ulceration is the result of venous disease, although other causes should always be considered. The common causes for acute deterioration in chronic leg ulcers are infection (cellulitis) and allergic contact dermatitis (resulting from a topical medicament or dressing). All chronic ulcers are at risk of malignant transformation (Marjolin's squamous carcinoma), so regular reassessment, especially in elderly people, should occur.

Clinical features

It is important to determine the duration of ulceration, the degree of associated pain (e.g. whether diabetic neuropathy is present), the presence of associated infection and systemic upset (e.g. sepsis), and whether the patient has diabetes, renal failure, arthritis or a connective tissue disease, a haemoglobinopathy or inflammatory bowel disease. Drugs, particularly when applied locally, may result in hypersensitivity.

Examination

This should be particularly for stasis or contact eczema, venous and arterial insufficiency, inguinal lympadenopathy, and for cellulitis.

Investigations

Investigations should be used in selected cases to determine the arterial blood supply to the leg (Doppler studies and/or angiography), venous drainage (leg and pelvic ultrasonography or phlebography). Skin biopsy (including immunofluorescence) is necessary when the cause is in doubt.

Treatment

Exclude and treat causes other than venous stasis (see figure). Maximize arterial blood supply (e.g. angioplasty), and treat anaemia and infection (systemic antibiotic continued long term), heart failure and malnutrition (protein, iron, vitamin C or zinc deficiency).

Encourage regular exercise and weight loss. Elevate the limb at rest and apply compressive bandaging (non-adherent or paraffin gauze), after using a topical cleansing and/or debriding agent to encourage granulation tissue formation. Other measures include mild-to-moderate potency steroids to non-ulcerated eczematous skin. Beware of contact sensitization to topical applications. If a clean granulating ulcer base can be achieved consider 'pinch' skin grafting.

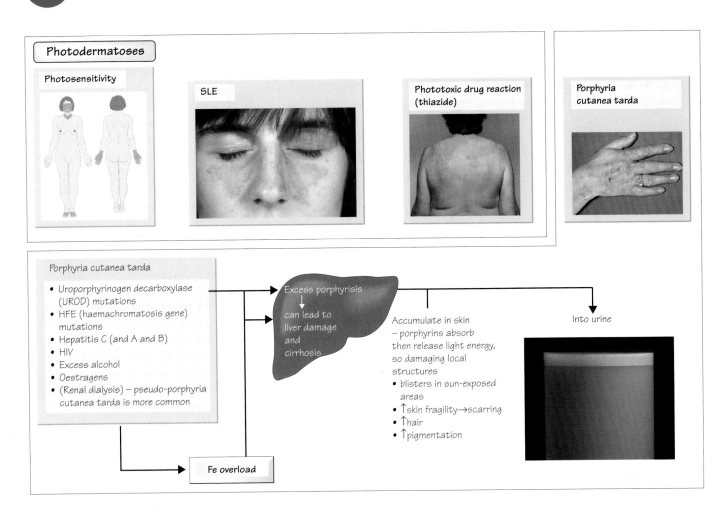

Photodermatoses

Photosensitivity

SLE

Phototoxic drug reaction (thiazide)

Porphyria cutanea tarda

Porphyria cutanea tarda
- Uroporphyrinogen decarboxylase (UROD) mutations
- HFE (haemachromatosis gene) mutations
- Hepatitis C (and A and B)
- HIV
- Excess alcohol
- Oestragens
- (Renal dialysis) – pseudo-porphyria cutanea tarda is more common

Excess porphyrisis can lead to liver damage and cirrhosis

Accumulate in skin – porphyrins absorb then release light energy, so damaging local structures
- blisters in sun-exposed areas
- ↑skin fragility→scarring
- ↑hair
- ↑pigmentation

Into urine

Fe overload

A cardinal clue that an eruption is sunlight related (i.e. a photodermatosis) is its distribution in sun-exposed areas (forehead, cheeks, ears, nose, chin, anterior chest in a 'V' distribution, and hands) with sparing of areas photo-protected by clothes or natural shadows (around the orbit, behind the ears, under the chin). Some primary dermatoses (e.g. psoriasis, acne) can improve with sunlight. Photo-eruptions occur in:
- Atopic eczema (this also sometimes improves with sunlight).
- Systemic lupus erythematosus (see Chapter 204).
- Lichen planus.
- Drug eruptions may be light sensitive. In phototoxic drug eruptions (increased susceptibility to the normal effects of sunlight), sunburn occurs within minutes of sun exposure, e.g. with amiodarone, thiazides or tetracycline. Extracts from many plants can act as topical sensitizers. Photoallergic drug reactions are idiosyncratic inflammatory reactions (resembling contact dermatitis) to (e.g.) phenothiazines and angiotensin-converting enzyme inhibitors.
- Polymorphic light eruption is the most common photodermatosis: it can cause erythema, papules, urticarial weals and plaques usually 4–6 h after (early summer) sun exposure. Topical steroids may help short term. Sun avoidance and sunscreens are essential. Prophylactic PUVA or UVB (before holidays) can be used. Gradual exposure to sunlight results in tolerance, which lasts until the following year.
- Solar urticaria is rare, but is characterized by an immediate urticarial response to sun exposure. It fades in the shade.
- Porphyrias result from deficiencies in the enzymes synthesizing haem. Haem precursors are deposited in the skin, resulting in disease. Porphyria cutanea tarda may be familial or sporadically affect young women (related to alcohol and the contraceptive pill) or middle-aged men (alcoholism). There is an association with hepatitis B/C, HIV and renal dialysis. Skin fragility and photosensitive blistering with scarring occurs on exposed sites, especially the hands. Hypertrichosis occurs on the face. Clinical and/or biochemical liver disease may occur. There is a deficiency of uroporphyrinogen decarboxylase activity and uroporphyrin III is found in urine and faeces. Treatment is avoidance of alcohol, oestrogen and sunlight, venesection and/or low-dose hydroxychloroquine.
- Pellagra (niacin deficiency) may result in a classic triad of symptoms (diarrhoea, dementia and dermatitis). The classic skin sign is a rash around the neck, 'Casal's necklace'.

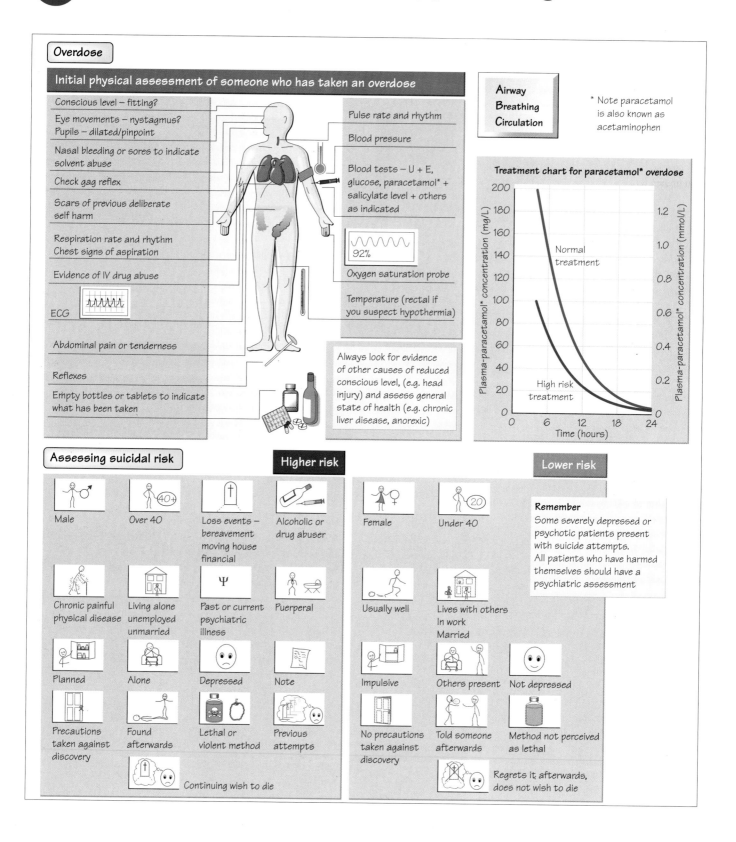

Overdose

Initial physical assessment of someone who has taken an overdose

Conscious level – fitting?

Eye movements – nystagmus?
Pupils – dilated/pinpoint

Nasal bleeding or sores to indicate solvent abuse

Check gag reflex

Scars of previous deliberate self harm

Respiration rate and rhythm
Chest signs of aspiration

Evidence of IV drug abuse

ECG

Abdominal pain or tenderness

Reflexes

Empty bottles or tablets to indicate what has been taken

Pulse rate and rhythm

Blood pressure

Blood tests – U + E, glucose, paracetamol* + salicylate level + others as indicated

92%

Oxygen saturation probe

Temperature (rectal if you suspect hypothermia)

Always look for evidence of other causes of reduced conscious level, (e.g. head injury) and assess general state of health (e.g. chronic liver disease, anorexic)

Airway
Breathing
Circulation

* Note paracetamol is also known as acetaminophen

Treatment chart for paracetamol* overdose

Plasma-paracetamol* concentration (mg/L)

Normal treatment

High risk treatment

Plasma-paracetamol* concentration (mmol/L)

Time (hours)

Assessing suicidal risk

Higher risk

Male | Over 40 | Loss events – bereavement moving house financial | Alcoholic or drug abuser

Chronic painful physical disease | Living alone unemployed unmarried | Past or current psychiatric illness | Puerperal

Planned | Alone | Depressed | Note

Precautions taken against discovery | Found afterwards | Lethal or violent method | Previous attempts

Continuing wish to die

Lower risk

Female | Under 40

Usually well | Lives with others In work Married

Impulsive | Others present | Not depressed

No precautions taken against discovery | Told someone afterwards | Method not perceived as lethal

Regrets it afterwards, does not wish to die

Remember
Some severely depressed or psychotic patients present with suicide attempts.
All patients who have harmed themselves should have a psychiatric assessment

Clinical Presentations at a Glance

Poisoning is a common reason for hospital admission. Most poisonings are deliberate, although some are accidental. Attempted suicide may be the first presentation of psychiatric illness.

History

The key facts to establish are:
- The circumstances of the attempt.
- Psychiatric history (past and present).
- Past medical history.

Important points in the history are what was taken, when, how much and in what circumstances? How do they feel about it now? What was their suicide intent and risk? Psychiatric history should include the presence of current or past psychiatric illness: suicide rates are up to 50-fold higher in psychiatric inpatients. Lifetime suicide risks are:
- 15% in depression
- 30–60% in personality disorder
- 10% in schizophrenia
- 3% in alcoholism.

Anorexia also carries a risk and affects medical treatment. Likewise, medical illness and drug use affects treatment, e.g. liver disease or enzyme-inducing drugs lower the treatment threshold for paracetamol.

Drug information

The national poisons centres can be found in the *British National Formulary* (BNF). They offer invaluable phone advice 24 h a day.

Examination

Overdose patients may be unconscious, fully alert, or anything in between. Assess **a**irway, **b**reathing and **c**irculation. Look for:
- Hypotension.
- Arrhythmias: particularly with antiarrhythmics, tricyclics.
- Respiratory depression: e.g. with opiates.
- Aspiration if vomiting with reduced conscious level (unprotected airway).
- Hypothermia: with barbiturate or phenothiazine.
- Glucose and electrolyte imbalance: should be measured.
- Convulsions and coma: common in severe poisoning with many drugs.

Immediate treatment

- Activated charcoal, which binds poisons in the gastrointestinal tract, preventing absorption, is the treatment of choice for most poisons. It is most effective if used within 2 h, although for drugs that delay gastric emptying or modified release preparations, it is useful for longer or repeated doses. The only common side effect is constipation (give a laxative). It is not useful for lithium, iron or pesticide ingestion.
- Gastric lavage is rarely used nowadays. It is only helpful within 1–2 h, in conscious patients, with non-corrosive toxins.
- Ipecacuanha, which induces vomiting, is not used because it does not prevent absorption.
- Haemodialysis may be needed for severe salicylate, phenobarbital (phenobarbitone), methanol or ethylene glycol poisoning. Haemoperfusion can be used for theophylline and barbiturate poisoning.

Some specific commonly ingested poisons

Paracetamol

For paracetamol, 12 g (24 tablets) is a potentially fatal dose in most patients, whereas 7.5 g may be lethal in high-risk individuals. Symptoms are delayed up to 3 days after the overdose, when nausea, vomiting and abdominal pain, and late fulminant hepatic failure, can occur. Paracetamol is metabolized by liver conjugation: when this pathway is saturated a toxic metabolite is formed, usually inactivated by glutathione. When glutathione stores run out, this metabolite binds to cell proteins, causing cell death. Lower doses are toxic in people on enzyme-inducing drugs (e.g. phenytoin, carbamazepine, rifampicin) and undernourished people (anorexia, alcoholism, starvation).

Management

Activated charcoal. *N*-Acetylcysteine to increase liver glutathione if paracetamol level high 4 h after ingestion, continued, in high-risk individuals, until paracetamol is no longer detected. Oral methionine is given if *N*-acetylcysteine unavailable/allergic. Monitor urea and electrolytes (U&Es), glucose, liver function tests (LFTs) and clotting initially and 24 h after ingestion. In severe overdose, patients may require liver support, including transplantation.

Tricyclic antidepressants

Tricyclic overdosage causes drowsiness, dilated pupils, dry mouth, tachycardia and urinary retention (anticholinergic effects), and hypothermia with hyperreflexia. In severe toxicity, convulsions, coma, respiratory depression, hypotension, arrhythmias and cardiac arrest may occur. Treatment is activated charcoal and monitoring of heart rhythm (continuous ECG); intubate ± ventilation if respiration inadequate, convulsions or arrhythmias (hyperventilation and bicarbonate improve arrhythmias). On recovery, delirium, agitation, and visual and auditory hallucinations are common and respond to diazepam.

Opiates

Opiates cause respiratory depression, pinpoint pupils, and hypotension, vomiting, fits and pulmonary oedema. Naloxone, a specific antidote, is given. The half-life of naloxone is very short (less than opiate), so an intravenous infusion is often needed.

Salicylates

Salicylates cause restlessness, flushing, sweating and hyperventilation. Nausea, vomiting and tinnitus are common. Confusion, coma and convulsions are rare. Cardiac arrest may occur in severe overdose. Electrolyte abnormalities are common, such as hypokalaemic alkalosis (vomiting), respiratory alkalosis (hyperventilation) or a metabolic acidosis (uncoupling of oxidative phosphorylation). Dehydration and hyperpyrexia occur. Glucose control is impaired causing hypo- or hyperglycaemia. A bleeding tendency may develop. Treat with activated charcoal, repeated and intravenous saline. A forced alkaline diuresis is rarely used nowadays. Monitor full blood count (FBC), U+Es, clotting, glucose and gases. Chest X-ray for pulmonary oedema.

Benzodiazepines

In overdose, benzodiazepines cause drowsiness, ataxia, dysarthria and nystagmus. Flumazenil, a specific antidote, is rarely used because it causes fits in those on long-term benzodiazepines, people with epilepsy and when taken with tricyclics.

Alcohol

Alcohol may be taken as part of the attempt, before the attempt, acutely or chronically. Alcoholism affects liver function, and thus affects any drugs or poisons that affect the liver, such as paracetamol. Acute alcohol intoxication depresses conscious level and respiration—even small quantities of alcohol potentiate CNS depressants.

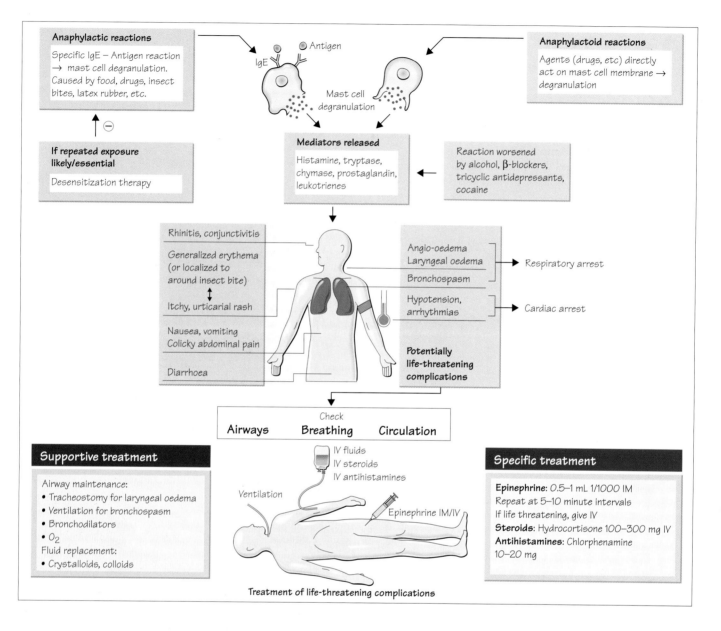

Anaphylactic reactions

Specific IgE – Antigen reaction → mast cell degranulation. Caused by food, drugs, insect bites, latex rubber, etc.

Anaphylactoid reactions

Agents (drugs, etc) directly act on mast cell membrane → degranulation

Antigen

IgE

Mast cell degranulation

If repeated exposure likely/essential

Desensitization therapy

Mediators released

Histamine, tryptase, chymase, prostaglandin, leukotrienes

Reaction worsened by alcohol, β-blockers, tricyclic antidepressants, cocaine

Rhinitis, conjunctivitis

Generalized erythema (or localized to around insect bite)

Itchy, urticarial rash

Nausea, vomiting Colicky abdominal pain

Diarrhoea

Angio-oedema Laryngeal oedema

Bronchospasm

Hypotension, arrhythmias

→ Respiratory arrest

→ Cardiac arrest

Potentially life-threatening complications

Check
Airways   Breathing   Circulation

Supportive treatment

Airway maintenance:
• Tracheostomy for laryngeal oedema
• Ventilation for bronchospasm
• Bronchodilators
• O₂
Fluid replacement:
• Crystalloids, colloids

Ventilation

IV fluids
IV steroids
IV antihistamines

Epinephrine IM/IV

Specific treatment

Epinephrine: 0.5–1 mL 1/1000 IM
Repeat at 5–10 minute intervals
If life threatening, give IV
Steroids: Hydrocortisone 100–300 mg IV
Antihistamines: Chlorphenamine 10–20 mg

Treatment of life-threatening complications

Anaphylaxis is an acute, generalized, life-threatening, allergic reaction, affecting 1 in 10 000 individuals/year and is the cause of 1 in every 2700 hospital admissions.

Mechanism

Anaphylaxis results from the rapid systemic release of large quantities of biologically active mediators from mast cells and basophils, triggered by the interaction of the allergen with specific IgE antibodies bound to cell membranes. Cell activation results in the release of preformed mediators stored in granules (including histamine, tryptase and chymase) and of newly formed mediators (including prostaglandins and leukotrienes). These mediators cause capillary leakage, mucosal oedema, and smooth muscle contraction.

Anaphylactoid reactions result from the non-specific degranulation of mast cells by drugs, chemicals, or other triggers, and do not involve IgE-based sensitivity. These reactions are clinically indistinguishable from anaphylactic reactions. Acutely the discrimination is unnecessary as the management is the same. However, discrimination between IgE-mediated and non-IgE mediated disease may subsequently be important in identifying the precipitating agent.

Clinical features

Patients present with a range of clinical features:
• Feeling of impending doom
• Generalized pruritus
• Erythema and/or urticaria, though some 50% of patients may not experience any rash
• Angioedema
• Bronchospasm
• Laryngeal oedema ± stridor

- Rhinitis
- Conjunctivitis
- Nausea, vomiting, abdominal pain, uterine contractions
- Palpitations, cardiac arrhythmias
- Hypotension
- Cardiorespiratory arrest.

The symptoms are usually of rapid onset, within minutes of exposure, although may be delayed up to several hours. Route of exposure to the triggering agent, as well as quantity of antigen, rate of administration, and coexistent features such as alcohol and exercise, determine the severity of a reaction. Reactions are not always of the same degree of severity, even on exposure to the same allergen.

The immediate symptoms are caused by release of stored histamine. Occasionally the symptoms of anaphylaxis recur after some hours, a *biphasic reaction*, so all individuals should be kept under observation for at least 6 hours after an anaphylactic episode. Late phase reactions are caused by synthesis de novo by the mast cells of leukotrienes, which have similar biological properties to histamine. The late reaction can be blocked by early administration of corticosteroids.

Source of allergen

The commonest causes of anaphylaxis are foods. The majority of food reactions are to peanut (a pea, not a nut!) and to the tree nuts (hazel nut, almond, brazil nut, walnut, cashew, etc.). Peanut-allergic patients often also have allergy to tree nuts as well as other legumes. Peanuts and almonds may be present as a hidden allergen in many different foods. Particular care needs to be taken with oriental food. Shellfish and fish are potent causes of severe allergic reactions, and miniscule levels of exposure may cause severe reactions. Any other food is capable of causing reactions.

Other causes include:
- Stinging insects (bees, bumblebees, wasps, hornets and fire ants) can cause severe reactions.
- Severe reactions to latex are increasing due to the use of latex in healthcare. Most patients with latex allergy, however, have type IV delayed hypersensitivity reactions, mainly against the chemicals in the rubber rather than the rubber proteins, leading to contact dermatitis.
- Many drugs can cause IgE-mediated reactions including penicillins, muscle relaxants (which are all highly cross-reactive) and other anaesthetic agents and biological products such as vaccines. Opiate drugs such as morphine and codeine cause anaphylactoid reactions due to direct degranulation of mast cells; fentanyl does not seem to have this effect. Non-steroidal anti-inflammatory drugs also cause severe reactions through non-IgE mechanisms. Radiocontrast media, particularly non-ionic media, are potent mast cell degranulating agents.
- Exercise, alone or with foods, can trigger anaphylaxis.
- In some cases no cause can be identified despite extensive searching (idiopathic anaphylaxis).

Differential diagnosis

Some clinical features of anaphylaxis are similar to other local or systemic disease. Accurate clinical assessment is essential:
- Shock (see p. 20)
- Airway obstruction: status asthmaticus, acute bacterial epiglottitis, acute foreign body upper airway obstruction
- Mediator release: mastocytosis, carcinoid syndrome

- Recurrent angioedema: inherited and acquired C1 esterase inhibitor deficiency, drug-induced angioedema; idiopathic angioedema.
- Vasovagal syncope
- Factitious anaphylaxis (usually occurring in patients with known anaphylaxis)
- Globus hystericus (characterized by a lack of evidence of airway obstruction, despite protestations of swelling in the throat, and no rash or other symptoms).

Management

Acute management: anaphylaxis is an acute medical emergency, which in the absence of appropriate treatment carries a significant mortality. Resuscitation should follow the normal rules of A (airway) B (breathing) and C (circulation):
- Airway maintenance: look for obstruction (swollen tongue, stridor). Administer high flow oxygen. Consider a tracheotomy if complete airway obstruction likely.
- Check breathing: full resuscitation if not breathing.
- Circulation: check pulse and blood pressure. Patients with excess histamine are usually warm and vasodilated with hypotension. Pulse is rapid. Obtain i.v. access.
- Adrenaline: *early* administration of adrenaline is essential. 0.3–1.0 mL 1/1000 solution i.m., repeat after 5 minutes if no response intervals; further doses may be required. Do not administer subcutaneously (poor absorption). In the hospital setting, i.v. adrenaline may be administered ONLY with appropriate ECG monitoring. It must be given well diluted (10 mL 1/10 000 solution diluted into 100 mL normal saline and administered via an infusion pump).
- Corticosteroids: i.v. hydrocortisone 200 mg (this prevents late reactions).
- Antihistamines: chlorphenamine 10 mg i.v. (this is traditional but not of proven value).
- Fluid replacement: use colloid or crystalloid to restore blood pressure.
- Use nebulized salbutamol for bronchospasm.
- Keep under observation for a minimum of 6 hours before discharge, even if there is rapid recovery.
- Do not discharge without a clear plan for further investigation and follow-up.

Subsequent management: all individuals who have experienced anaphylaxis should be referred to a clinical immunologist or allergist for further investigation to identify the trigger factor and to educate the patient in avoidance and management of subsequent episodes. Consideration should be given to supplying adrenaline for self-injection. In the specific event of bee or wasp venom-induced anaphylaxis, immunotherapy with graded concentrations of allergen is effective in reducing the risk of further reactions.

Prognosis

The natural history and prognosis of anaphylaxis is variable. There are no predictors of the severity of further reactions. Avoidance remains the mainstay. Anxiety is extremely common and needs to be addressed. If the trigger factor cannot be identified or cannot be avoided, recurrence may be common and should be anticipated. Many children will grow out of early food-induced reactions, although peanut sensitivity is usually life-long. Food challenges may be required to prove loss of sensitization.

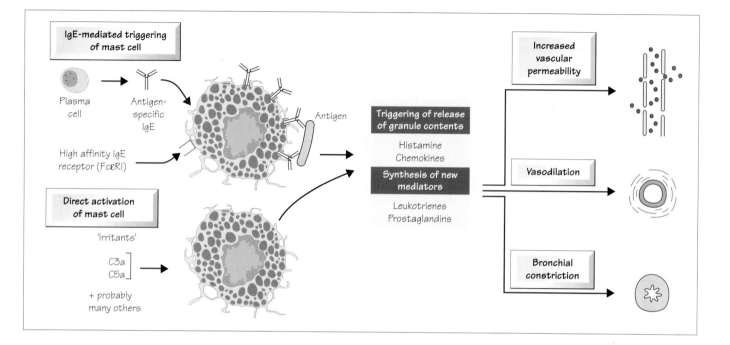

The severity of an allergic reaction depends upon the dose, site of allergen exposure and individual characteristics including medication and previous history. In most the history provides the key to the diagnosis, especially as in non-urgent situations most patients will have few physical signs. Allergic disorders include:
• Summer hayfever (pollen-induced allergic rhinoconjunctivitis)
• Perennial rhinitis
• Allergic asthma (including occupational asthma)
• Allergy to drugs
• Food allergy and food intolerance; oral allergy syndrome
• Allergy to stinging insects
• Allergic skin disorders, e.g. atopic eczema
• Anaphylaxis (acute generalized allergic reaction)
• Urticaria (see p. 414)
• Angioedema.

Inhalant allergy

Allergy to inhalant allergens such as house dust mite, animal danders and pollens (grasses, trees, weeds) will trigger allergic rhinoconjunctivitis, sinusitis and asthma. Typical features include sneezing, blocked and running nose, headache and sinus pain, itchy red eyes often with discharge, with or without asthmatic symptoms. Onset is rapid on exposure, but symptoms may be chronic if exposure cannot be avoided. A good history will usually identify the most likely triggers. Diagnosis is by skin prick test or 'RAST' test (see below). Management is by the use of topical treatments to eye (sodium cromoglicate, nedocromil sodium), the nose (nasal steroid sprays such as beclomethasone, mometasone, triamcinolone, fluticasone), and lung (inhaled bronchodilators such as salbutamol, salmeterol and steroids, beclomethasone, budesonide, fluticasone), accompanied by oral antihistamines (potent non-sedating long-acting antihistamines such as fexofenadine, cetirizine, leveocet-

irizine). For upper airway allergy, desensitization by immunotherapy is possible for patients whose symptoms cannot be controlled on maximal medical therapy.

Food allergy

Food 'allergy' is blamed for a plethora of symptoms, not all of which are related to true, IgE-mediated, food allergy. There is no evidence that irritable bowel symptoms are related to food allergy, although sufferers often complain of bloating with wheat-based products. Excess nasal catarrh is sometimes associated with milk intolerance. Anaphylaxis represents the severe end of the spectrum of disease, but urticaria and angioedema may represent less severe reactions. Eczema is associated with food allergies in children, often to dairy products and wheat, but adult eczema is less commonly helped by dietary manipulation. The oral allergy syndrome is the association of inhalant allergy to birch pollen in association with lip and tongue swelling when eating soft fruits such as peaches, nectarines, apples, almonds and other closely related fruits. This syndrome is rarely associated with anaphylaxis. The allergens are heat labile and destroyed by cooking. Occasionally it may be necessary to undertake an elimination diet with sequential reintroduction of foods to identify foods causing symptoms. Double-blind placebo-controlled challenge is the gold standard for investigation of food-related symptoms.

Angioedema

Angioedema relates to deep tissue swelling, which is usually non-itchy. It may occur alone or with urticaria. Bradykinin is the main trigger. It often presents acutely to accident and emergency and acute medical services. It must be distinguished from systemic allergic reactions. Hereditary angioedema is extremely rare and is due to deficiency of the complement regulatory protein C1 esterase inhibitor (see p. 416).

Acquired angioedema caused by autoantibodies against the inhibitor may very rarely be seen in older patients in association with lymphoma and myeloma or in association with other autoimmune disease such as systemic lupus erythematosus (SLE). The commonest causes of angioedema however are stress, infections, and allergic reactions to foods and drugs. The commonest drugs causing angioedema are angiotensin-converting enzyme inhibitors (ACE-I), which cause angioedema by preventing the breakdown of bradykinin, non-steroidal anti-inflammatory drugs (NSAIDs) and statins (cholesterol-lowering drugs). Many cases, particularly of nocturnal angioedema, do not have an identifiable trigger (idiopathic). Antihistamines are not effective in most cases of angioedema, but tranexamic acid, an anti-fibrinolytic drug, may be valuable in preventing swelling where there is no avoidable trigger identified. Acute attacks usually require treatment with intravenous or oral corticosteroids. Adrenaline should be reserved for angioedema where there is clear laryngeal involvement.

Urticaria

The typical rash in urticaria is that of wheal and flare (nettle-rash), caused by histamine. The rash may be generalized and patients may feel systemically unwell. Presentation to accident and emergency is common. The causes of acute urticaria are stress, infection, allergy, physical (sun, pressure, water, vibration, heat, cold), in association with thyroid disease, haematinic deficiency. However, in many cases there is no identifiable cause. Chronic urticaria, lasting beyond 6 weeks, is rarely associated with allergy. Acute treatment is with high-dose antihistamine given orally (cetirizine 10–20 mg daily) or intravenously (chlorphenamine 10 mg i.v.) and 24–48 hours of oral corticosteroid (prednisolone 20 mg/day). Treatment of chronic urticaria is with antihistamines, and it may be necessary to use larger doses than those normally used. Tricyclic antidepressants such as doxepin are valuable as they have potent anti-H1 and H2 blocking activity. Montelukast may also be helpful. Corticosteroid therapy should be avoided in chronic urticaria apart from emergency management, as the risks of side effects outweigh the benefits.

Investigation of allergic disease

Skin-prick tests are cheap, quick, and are used to support the diagnosis. The patient is exposed to standardized solutions of allergen extract through a skin prick to the forearm. Positive (histamine) and negative (saline) controls are included. A wheal > 2 mm greater than the negative control is a positive test. Testing should be carried out with great caution in patients who have had anaphylaxis. Skin must be normal so this type of testing is inappropriate in patients with eczema.

Antihistamines should be discontinued for 1 week before testing as they abolish the response. Other drugs such as calcium channel blockers (for hypertension) and antidepressant drugs also interfere with the tests.

'RAST' tests measure specific IgE in a blood sample to the putative antigen. This laboratory test is a useful alternative when skin-prick tests are not available, or if a patient is on antihistamines. The results are similar to skin-prick tests for inhalant allergens and nuts, but are not useful for drug allergy, and certain foods with labile allergens (fruits).

67 Cardiac and respiratory arrest

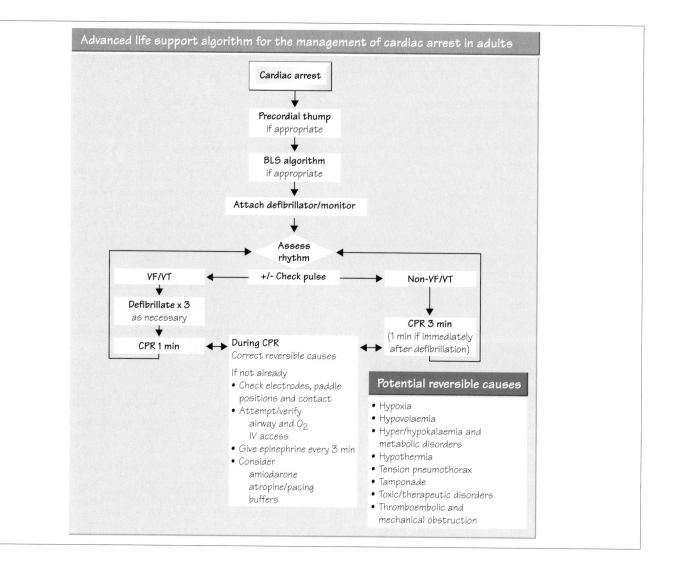

Advanced life support algorithm for the management of cardiac arrest in adults

Cardiac arrest

↓

Precordial thump
if appropriate

↓

BLS algorithm
if appropriate

↓

Attach defibrillator/monitor

↓

Assess rhythm

+/- Check pulse

VF/VT ← → Non-VF/VT

Defibrillate x 3
as necessary

CPR 1 min ↔ **During CPR**
Correct reversible causes

↔ **CPR 3 min**
(1 min if immediately
after defibrillation)

If not already
• Check electrodes, paddle
  positions and contact
• Attempt/verify
  airway and O₂
  IV access
• Give epinephrine every 3 min
• Consider
  amiodarone
  atropine/pacing
  buffers

Potential reversible causes

• Hypoxia
• Hypovolaemia
• Hyper/hypokalaemia and
  metabolic disorders
• Hypothermia
• Tension pneumothorax
• Tamponade
• Toxic/therapeutic disorders
• Thromboembolic and
  mechanical obstruction

Cardiac and respiratory arrests are common in the community and in hospital. The common causes of circulatory failure, 'cardiac arrest' sufficiently severe to cause unconsciousness and compromise life, are:
• **Ventricular arrhythmias**: these can be due to acute coronary occlusions, scar tissue late after a myocardial infarction, heart failure of any aetiology and metabolic disturbance, e.g. hypo- and hyperkalaemia, hypoxaemia, drugs including tricyclic antidepressants, non-sedating antihistamines, major antipsychotics, macrolide antibiotics, etc.
• **Bradyarrhythmias**: due to conducting tissue disease, e.g. complete heart block, during myocardial infarction, following prolonged ventricular arrhythmias or respiratory arrest (see below).
• **Cardiogenic shock**: often caused by large myocardial infarctions or advanced heart failure.

If circulatory failure occurs and QRST complexes are seen on the ECG monitor ('electromechanical dissociation' [EMD]) consider:
• Hypovolaemia: e.g. stab wounds, torrential gastrointestinal or retroperitoneal haemorrhage, e.g. ruptured abdominal aortic aneurysm.
• Pericardial tamponade: stab wounds, recent myocardial infarction

(where it indicates cardiac rupture), malignancy or immediately after cardiac surgery.
• Pulmonary embolus.
• Tension pneumothorax: in people with asthma, in chronic lung diseases, especially chronic obstructive pulmonary disease (COPD), or after trauma.

There are a number of common causes of failure to breathe sufficiently to maintain life—'respiratory arrest':
• Severe lung disease: pneumonia, severe airway obstruction, e.g. asthma, exacerbation of COPD, end-stage COPD, etc.
• Airway obstruction: foreign body, or the tongue in a comatose patient.
• Left ventricular failure.
• Brain injury: stroke, overdose of narcotic drugs (e.g. opiates) or hypnotics, e.g. major tranquillizers, etc.

Many patients present with combined circulatory and respiratory arrest. This usually means that the initial cardiac or respiratory arrest is far advanced, because one inevitably leads to the other.

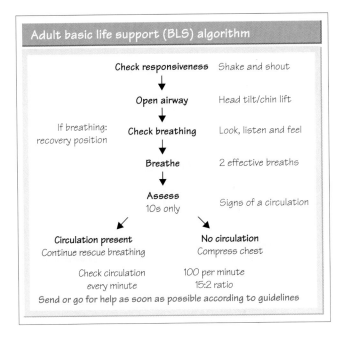

Check responsiveness — Shake and shout

↓

Open airway — Head tilt/chin lift

↓

Check breathing — Look, listen and feel

↓

Breathe — 2 effective breaths

↓

Assess 10s only — Signs of a circulation

If breathing: recovery position

Circulation present
Continue rescue breathing

No circulation
Compress chest

Check circulation every minute

100 per minute
15:2 ratio

Send or go for help as soon as possible according to guidelines

Cardiopulmonary resuscitation

Cardiopulmonary resuscitation (CPR) is the term applied for the immediate treatment of cardiac and/or respiratory arrest. CPR constitutes support both for the circulation and for respiration, and is a generic treatment applicable to most cases of cardiac/respiratory arrest. However, it does not remove the need to make an accurate diagnosis so that specific therapy, when available, can be given early on when it is most likely to be life saving. Establish the diagnosis using all available tools, e.g. the bystander history (nurses, ambulance staff, etc.), finding prescription or street drugs in pockets, physical examination, immediate ECG, chest X-ray, etc.

Key principles underlying CPR

Appropriateness: treatment aims to restore the patient to a high quality life. If this is not possible, consider whether CPR is inappropriate. 'Do not attempt resuscitate' orders (DNAR) (always clearly recorded in the notes) are made on the basis of:
• The chance of immediate CPR success (relates to age, disease)
• The chance of restoring long-term high quality life (relates to pre-existing quality of life)
• Patients' and relatives' wishes, which must be established.

Speed: after total circulatory/respiratory failure irreversible hypoxic brain injury follows within 3–4 min (unless extreme hypothermia is present). Furthermore, cardiac anoxia develops quickly, preventing successful restoration of the circulation. The penalty for incorrect *and/ or late* diagnosis and treatment is the death of the patient!

Summon additional help as soon as possible.

Assess **a**irway, **b**reathing and **c**irculation (ABC) and apply the adult **basic life support** (BLS) algorithm (basic = no equipment available). If victims do not respond to shaking/shouting, turn them on to their back, open and inspect the airway. Remove any obstruction. Determine within 10 s whether breathing is normal:
• Look for chest movement
• Listen at the victim's mouth for breath sounds
• Feel for air on your cheek.

If normal breathing is found, turn him or her into the recovery position and seek help. If only weak respiratory efforts occur, give two slow, effective rescue breaths into the mouth (each of 700–1000 mL), with the nose pinched shut, sufficient to make the chest rise and fall. After two effective breaths (use five or more attempts for this), check the circulation (carotid/femoral pulse if you have been trained to do so). If there is no circulation, start chest compressions, pushing the sternum down 4–5 cm each time, at a rate of 100/min, alternating 15 compressions to two breaths. Chest compressions restore 30% of normal cerebral perfusion. Continue this sequence until movement or breathing occurs or expert help arrives.

Advanced life support

Advanced life support (i.e. equipment is available): apply BLS, attach ECG electrodes and diagnose the heart rhythm:
• Ventricular fibrillation (VF), pulseless ventricular tachycardia (VT) are the common, survivable causes of cardiac arrest. Success rates decline by 7–10% for every minute that defibrillation is delayed. Charge the defibrillator and give three shocks with energies of 200 J, 200 J and 360 J. After successful cardioversion, transient (≥ 10 s) asystole and/ or a weak pulse (myocardial stunning) may occur; accordingly give CPR for 1 min after the three shocks before reevaluating the rhythm. If VF/VT persists, secure the airway (endotracheal tube, laryngeal mask airway [LMA] or a Combi-Tube), ventilate at 12 breaths/min using 100% oxygen. Establish peripheral intravenous access (central access is unsafe during CPR). Give adrenaline (epinephrine) to improve the efficacy of CPR (α-adrenergic actions cause vasoconstriction, increasing myocardial and cerebral perfusion pressures). Refractory VF/VT may respond to further shocks or intravenous amiodarone, lidocaine (lignocaine) or procainamide (never give these drugs in combination). Continue until the circulation is restored, or the decision is made to stop. Give bicarbonate if pH ≥ 7.1, in tricyclic overdose, or if hyperkalaemia is present.
• Asystole is usually lethal. Consider giving atropine. Complete heart block responds to pacing (external or transvenous) and/or isoprenaline. Beware spurious asystole: VF with a low voltage trace, or incorrectly applied electrodes.
• Unremarkable ECG tracing: see EMD above.

Discontinue CPR, after consultation with other team members, when the situation is irrecoverable, based on duration of CPR and whether a stable circulation was ever attained. Pupil dilatation is an unreliable sign of irreversible brain damage.

68 Acute confusional states

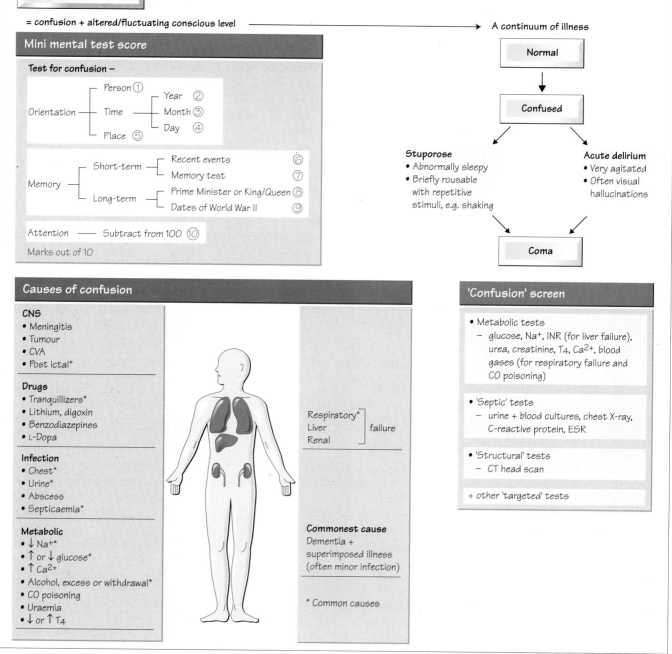

Acute confusional state

= confusion + altered/fluctuating conscious level ———————→ A continuum of illness

Mini mental test score

Test for confusion –

Orientation
- Person ①
- Time
  - Year ②
  - Month ③
  - Day ④
- Place ⑤

Memory
- Short-term
  - Recent events ⑥
  - Memory test ⑦
- Long-term
  - Prime Minister or King/Queen ⑧
  - Dates of World War II ⑨

Attention —— Subtract from 100 ⑩

Marks out of 10

Normal
↓
Confused

Stuporose
- Abnormally sleepy
- Briefly rousable with repetitive stimuli, e.g. shaking

Acute delirium
- Very agitated
- Often visual hallucinations

Coma

Causes of confusion

CNS
- Meningitis
- Tumour
- CVA
- Post ictal*

Drugs
- Tranquillizers*
- Lithium, digoxin
- Benzodiazepines
- L-Dopa

Infection
- Chest*
- Urine*
- Abscess
- Septicaemia*

Metabolic
- ↓ Na+*
- ↑ or ↓ glucose*
- ↑ Ca2+
- Alcohol, excess or withdrawal*
- CO poisoning
- Uraemia
- ↓ or ↑ T4

Respiratory*
Liver   failure
Renal

Commonest cause
Dementia + superimposed illness (often minor infection)

* Common causes

'Confusion' screen

- Metabolic tests
  - glucose, Na+, INR (for liver failure), urea, creatinine, T4, Ca2+, blood gases (for respiratory failure and CO poisoning)

- 'Septic' tests
  - urine + blood cultures, chest X-ray, C-reactive protein, ESR

- 'Structural' tests
  - CT head scan

+ other 'targeted' tests

Acute confusional states are also known as acute brain syndromes and constitute an important but difficult diagnostic and management problem. They comprise those conditions that result in global impairment of cognitive function with variably impaired conscious level. The latter is the key clinical distinguishing feature from dementia (i.e. the chronic brain syndromes).

Syndromic diagnosis

This requires impaired cognition, assessed from the Mini-Mental test score (see figure). Although many patients are floridly confused, not knowing who they are, when it is, where they are, with rambling conversation, unable to concentrate on questions, stopping conversation in mid-sentence, etc., it is important to be alert to more subtle confusional states, e.g. early hepatic encephalopathy, where mild defects in visuospatial ability need to be carefully looked for. It is therefore wise to include specific clinical tests for the major brain areas in the routine examination.

Visual hallucinations are common, although not always readily volunteered. They may induce fear (snakes, spiders), amusement (butterflies) or incredulity (mythical animals, etc.). Most patients have insight. Auditory hallucinations are rare and when present, especially if offensive, raise the possibility of a psychotic illness or, much more rarely, of pathological processes of the temporal lobe.

Impairment of conscious level is an essential aspect of diagnosis —many patients fall 'asleep' in mid-conversation, or have periods of hyperactivity during which their behaviour can be challenging, alternating with periods of sleepiness (e.g. the intoxicated patient). Excitability at night, with daytime sleepiness, is common.

Differential diagnosis of acute confusional states

In the following, conscious level is unimpaired, unlike in confusional states:

• **Dementia** is a common alternative diagnosis; family and friends are an incomparable source of information in establishing the diagnosis. Other chronic amnestic syndromes, e.g. Korsakov's psychosis or chronic bilateral limbic system damage, can be confused with acute brain syndromes.

• **Acute psychosis** results in grossly disordered thought processes, with spontaneous laughing, crying, talking and easy distraction. Thought insertion, control, withdrawal and broadcasting also may occur. Sufferers may believe that they are under the control of external agencies. Auditory hallucinations are common. Delusions (i.e. beliefs alien to cultural norms) are frequent. Early diagnosis and treatment are crucial, because the suicide rate during a first psychotic episode is 10–30%.

• **Expressive dysphasia**, especially if fluent, can occasionally be confused with a confusional state. The key difference is that comprehension is completely normal in pure expressive dysphasia (as tested by one-, two- and three-stage commands) and conscious level is normal.

• **Intellectual retardation** may present as apparent acute cognitive failure.

Causes of acute confusional states

• Confusional states are more likely in those whose brains are already damaged, especially those with dementia, where 'acute-on-chronic confusion' occurs.

• Infections: intracranial sepsis (meningitis or encephalitis) is especially likely to cause confusion with drowsiness/coma, as are other infections associated with a high fever (e.g. pneumococcal pneumonia). In the demented, 'trivial' infections, e.g. urinary tract infections, can underlie confusion.

• Metabolic disarray: hypoglycaemia, or hyperglycaemia, especially when hyperosmolar. Hyponatraemia (often induced by diuretics). These disorders are so common as to mandate immediate glucose and sodium measurement in all confused patients regardless of time of day or night. Hypercalcaemia is not uncommon. Hypothyroidism is frequently considered, but is an exceptionally rare cause of confusion,

except in those with hypothermia, which itself should be excluded in elderly people by rectal temperature measurement. Liver failure is an under-diagnosed cause. Severe uraemia, which is rare, may cause confusion—mild renal failure does not provoke confusion—and alternative pathologies should be sought.

• Hypoxia and/or hypercapnia is a very common cause. Respiratory rate is not a good clue to the presence or absence of respiratory failure. Oxygen saturation measurements should be recorded, although the only reliable assessment of carbon dioxide tension comes from arterial blood gases.

• Hypotension needs to be severe to cause confusion.

• Drug intoxication is the most common cause in accident and emergency departments (A&E) (alcohol, 'street drugs'). Alcohol withdrawal is a potent cause of confusion 1–3 days after admission—a diagnosis easy to miss in those admitted for other reasons on to general surgical or orthopaedic wards. Prescription drugs, such as hypnotics, major tranquillizers, anticonvulsants (e.g. phenytoin), lithium; antiparkinsonian drugs.

• Intracerebral pathology, including strokes, subdural haemorrhages, tumours. Subarachnoid haemorrhage in the absence of localizing signs can cause confusion at any age.

• Epilepsy is usually obvious, but occasionally 'twilight' states from semi-continuous seizures can occur, without visible shaking. Once these conditions are considered, they are often easily diagnosed from the EEG. Unusual behaviour can result from temporal lobe seizures. Very rarely temporal lobe dysfunction can be the consequence of a migraine attack. Post-ictal confusion is a much more difficult diagnosis to make if the appropriate history is not present.

Management

Undiagnosed confusion can rapidly progress to life-threatening illness, so patients should be monitored in high-dependency areas, close to an intensive care unit. A full history and clinical examination usually narrows the differential diagnosis substantially. Blood sugar should be measured immediately. Investigations to exclude metabolic disarray should be performed: electrolytes (particularly Na^+ and Ca^{2+}), renal and liver function tests (including international normalized ratio [INR]). In some, arterial blood gases are needed. A septic screen should be performed (full blood count for white cell count, urine dipstick, blood and urine cultures, chest X-ray, C-reactive protein). If the patient is markedly drowsy without clear cause, computed tomography (CT) of the head should be done, and if this is normal lumbar puncture should be performed. Focal neurology should lead to immediate CT head scan. Treatment is of the underlying cause.

Sedation

Confused patients can be a danger to themselves or others and sedatives may be needed to settle them, such as major tranquillizers, e.g. haloperidol. All tranquillizers depress respiration, so respiratory rate and oxygen saturation *must* be carefully monitored.

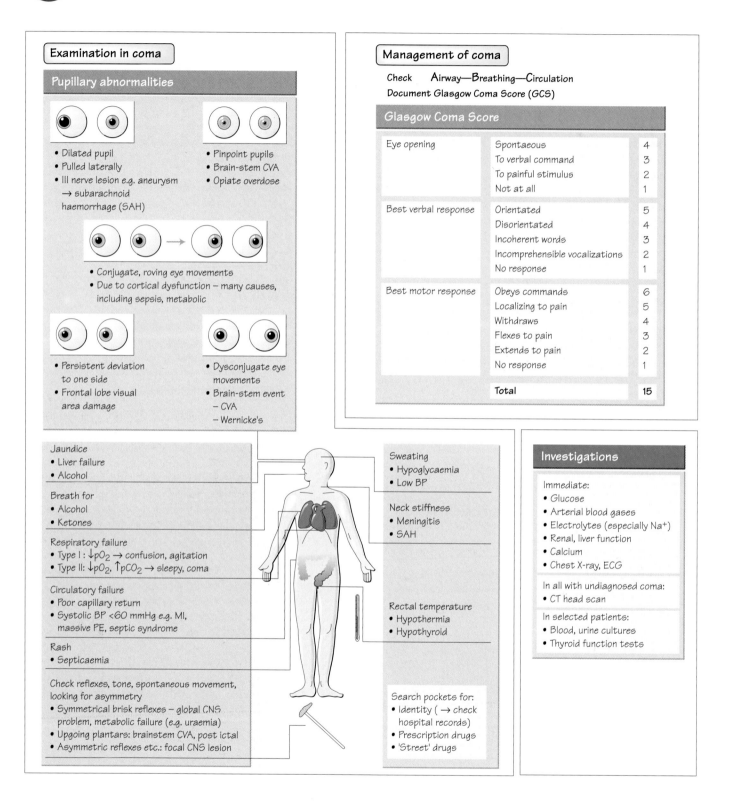

Examination in coma

Pupillary abnormalities

- Dilated pupil
- Pulled laterally
- III nerve lesion e.g. aneurysm → subarachnoid haemorrhage (SAH)

- Pinpoint pupils
- Brain-stem CVA
- Opiate overdose

- Conjugate, roving eye movements
- Due to cortical dysfunction – many causes, including sepsis, metabolic

- Persistent deviation to one side
- Frontal lobe visual area damage

- Dysconjugate eye movements
- Brain-stem event
  – CVA
  – Wernicke's

Jaundice
- Liver failure
- Alcohol

Breath for
- Alcohol
- Ketones

Respiratory failure
- Type I: $\downarrow pO_2$ → confusion, agitation
- Type II: $\downarrow pO_2$, $\uparrow pCO_2$ → sleepy, coma

Circulatory failure
- Poor capillary return
- Systolic BP <60 mmHg e.g. MI, massive PE, septic syndrome

Rash
- Septicaemia

Check reflexes, tone, spontaneous movement, looking for asymmetry
- Symmetrical brisk reflexes – global CNS problem, metabolic failure (e.g. uraemia)
- Upgoing plantars: brainstem CVA, post ictal
- Asymmetric reflexes etc.: focal CNS lesion

Sweating
- Hypoglycaemia
- Low BP

Neck stiffness
- Meningitis
- SAH

Rectal temperature
- Hypothermia
- Hypothyroid

Search pockets for:
- Identity (→ check hospital records)
- Prescription drugs
- 'Street' drugs

Management of coma

Check   Airway—Breathing—Circulation
Document Glasgow Coma Score (GCS)

Glasgow Coma Score

Eye opening	Spontaeous	4
	To verbal command	3
	To painful stimulus	2
	Not at all	1
Best verbal response	Orientated	5
	Disorientated	4
	Incoherent words	3
	Incomprehensible vocalizations	2
	No response	1
Best motor response	Obeys commands	6
	Localizing to pain	5
	Withdraws	4
	Flexes to pain	3
	Extends to pain	2
	No response	1
	Total	**15**

Investigations

Immediate:
- Glucose
- Arterial blood gases
- Electrolytes (especially Na^+)
- Renal, liver function
- Calcium
- Chest X-ray, ECG

In all with undiagnosed coma:
- CT head scan

In selected patients:
- Blood, urine cultures
- Thyroid function tests

Coma is 'the absence of consciousness' and should be distinguished from states such as akinetic mutism, catatonia and the persistent vegetative state.

Approach to coma

Coma is a medical emergency and speedy examination and investigation are vital. The history may be diagnostic but is often unavailable—relatives/friends may provide vital clues. Examination should identify systemic or neurological illness.

General examination of the comatose patient

Check **ABC**—**a**irway, **b**reathing and **c**irculation. Measure blood sugar immediately. Record the Glasgow Coma Score (GCS). An alternative scoring system, one much easier to remember, is the AVPU score (A for 'alert', V for 'reacting to vocal stimuli', P for 'reacting to pain', U for 'unconscious'; which corresponds roughly to a GCS of A = 15, V = 13, P = 8 and U = 3).

Look for evidence of vital organ failure, septic syndromes and poisoning:

Respiratory failure Respiratory rate (high or low) may provide a clue but is unreliable. Cyanosis (confirm by pulse oximetry and blood gases), hypercapnia (metabolic flap).

Cardiovascular failure and shock (see p. 20) Capillary return, blood pressure (heart rate is less reliable). Severe hypotension (systolic BP < 60 mmHg) is needed to impair consciousness.

Liver failure Especially jaundice, signs of chronic liver disease (thin and wasted muscles, bruising, ascites, upper body spider naevi, caput medusa).

Renal failure Is a rare cause of coma and difficult to detect clinically. A palpable bladder and rectal examination (prostatic carcinoma) may provide clues.

Metabolic failure especially:
• Hypoglycaemia: sweating—unreliable in long-standing diabetes.
• Hyperglycaemia: suspect in people known to have diabetes or obese elderly people.
• Acidosis: few clinical clues except deep sighing respiration (Kussmaul's breathing); lactic acidosis; renal failure; diabetic keto-acidosis, urine dipstick shows ketones + + + +.
• Hyponatraemia: usually excess 5% dextrose postsurgery, or chronic diuretic use.
• Hypercalcaemia: known malignancy.
• Hypothyroidism: myxoedema coma.
• Vitamin depletion such as Wernicke's encephalopathy (alcohol abuse, dysconjugate eye movements).

Usually there are no focal neurological signs in metabolic failure although multifocal myoclonus may occur.

Thermoregulatory failure Always measure the rectal temperature.

Septic syndrome Especially if shock is present or vital organs are involved (brain, lung). Examine for a rash (meningococcal or staphylococcal septicaemia). Travel history (malaria).

Drug induced Alcohol (breath), tricyclic overdose (tachycardia, arrhythmias), morphine (needle marks, pinpoint pupils), benzodiazepine or major tranquillizer (empty container).

Neurological examination

Look for signs of meningism (meningitis, encephalitis, subarachnoid haemorrhage)—specifically a stiff neck.

Examine the limbs For lateralizing signs suggestive of focal intracranial pathology: spontaneous movement/tone/reflexes (especially extensor plantar responses), although in coma these may be unreliable localizing signs (hypo- and hyperglycaemia can cause focal signs, e.g. hemiparesis).

Note the breathing pattern Hyper- or hypoventilation may relate to brain-stem dysfunction or metabolic disturbance.

Examine the eyes:
• Fundi for papilloedema.
• Pupil inequality and direct and consensual light reflexes:
  • a *unilateral dilated pupil* suggests nerve III compression from ipsilateral local herniation or mass lesions.
  • *small, unreactive pupils* suggest a brain-stem catastrophe, e.g. pontine haemorrhage or drug overdose.
  • *dilated, unreactive* pupils occur in severe anoxia (poor prognosis).
• Spontaneous eye movements:
  • *roving eye movements* suggest cortical dysfunction but an intact brain stem.
  • *absent oculocephalic* (dolls head) reflexes suggests brain-stem dysfunction, confirmed by caloric testing (ice water into the external auditory canal elicits conjugate gaze deviation towards the side of the stimulus—the oculovestibular reflex, nystagmus, is absent in deep coma).
  • *persistent eye deviation* to one side implies that the lesion is in the ipsilateral frontal eye field (eyes point away from a hemiparesis, intact oculovestibular reflex) or the pons (eyes deviated towards the hemiparesis, impaired oculovestibular reflex).
• Dysconjugate vertical gaze in the resting position (skew deviation) occurs with brain-stem lesions, including compression from raised intracranial pressure as a prelude to coning.

Immediate investigation

This is driven by the clinical context, and includes: blood sugar, blood count, 'routine' biochemistry (sodium, calcium, renal and liver function, including international normalized ratio [INR]), a septic screen (chest X-ray, blood and urine cultures), blood gases, toxicology screen for recreational and therapeutic drugs (e.g. lithium). If the cause is not apparent, early brain imaging (computed tomography) is mandatory.

Management

Good nursing care (e.g. intensive therapy unit or high-dependency unit), careful hydration/feeding and accurate information to relatives (especially regarding prognosis) are all vital.

Causes

• Post-ictal.
• Trauma: usually obvious. Monitor using the GCS.
• Post-anoxic coma after cardiac resuscitation is associated with

stimulus-sensitive generalized myoclonus. If this persists for ≥ 2 days post-arrest, the prognosis is poor.

- Vascular: stroke causes coma if the lesion is:
  - in the posterior cerebral circulation affecting the conscious centres in the brain stem.
  - deep in the diencephalon.
  - in a very large hemispheric (middle cerebral artery) territory, as a result of 'brain shock' (a poorly understood mechanism); brain swelling leading to transtentorial herniation may occur; deep coma has a poor prognosis.
  - cerebral venous sinus thrombosis (see p. 368); coma arises from bilateral infarction of deep brain structures.
  - cerebellar—haemorrhage causes brain-stem compression and coma; ataxia and other cerebellar signs usually precede this; immediate neurosurgical haematoma evacuation can be life saving.
  Stroke management—see p. 366.
- Metabolic: many metabolic derangements can produce coma—the approach depends on the clinical context (see specific chapters). In possible opiate overdose, a therapeutic challenge with naloxone should be performed. Wernicke's encephalopathy should be considered if there has been alcohol abuse or severe vomiting. Give parenteral thiamine.
- Vital organ failure—see specific chapters.
- Infective: always consider bacterial meningitis and viral meningo-encephalitis in unexplained coma. In suspected encephalitis treat early with aciclovir, then confirm the diagnosis.

Related conditions

- 'Locked-in syndrome' is a state of complete motor dysfunction in which the patient is mute and motionless but alert. Vertical eye movements may be the sole surviving voluntary function. Lesions of the pons, including haemorrhage, infarct or central pontine myelinolysis, typically cause this.
- The persistent vegetative state, caused by massive hemispherical damage, is characterized by complete lack of awareness, retained sleep-wake cycles and preserved autonomic reflexes > 1 month after the initial insult.

Diseases and Treatments at a Glance

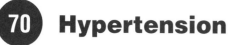

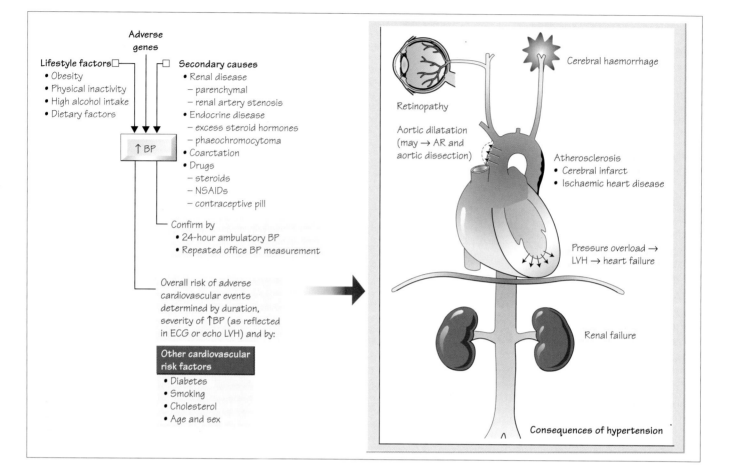

Consequences of hypertension

Definition

Blood pressure (BP) is distributed continuously. The incidence of complications is proportional to BP, so there is no absolute definition of hypertension. Treatment is often beneficial with sustained BPs > 140/90 mmHg.

Incidence

Increases with age. Prevalence of mild hypertension is 2% in those aged 25 years or less, rising to 25% in those in their 50s and 50% in those in their 70s.

Pathophysiology

Most (95%) hypertension is **essential**, a combination of numerous genetic and environmental factors that results in a hypertensive phenotype. **Secondary hypertension**, caused by an identifiable cause, is uncommon (Table 70.1), and suggested by:

- Renal dysfunction.
- Young age (especially 30 years or less).
- Severe treatment-resistant hypertension.
- Hypokalaemia (in the absence of diuretics).

Clinical features

Hypertension is usually asymptomatic, until end-organ damage occurs. Most headaches in hypertension are **not** related to BP. Malignant

Table 70.1 Causes and features of secondary hypertension (mainly endocrine or renal disorders).

High mineralocorticoids	
Hyperaldosteronism	Conn's syndrome
	Adrenal hyperplasia
High glucocorticoids	Cushing's syndrome
	Iatrogenic steroid therapy
High renin:	
Renal artery stenosis	Renal bruit/?small kidney
Small vessel renovascular disease	
Renal parenchymal disease	Multiple pathologies
Coarctation	Radiofemoral delay, systolic murmur
High catecholamines	Phaeochromocytoma

phase hypertension may present with headache and visual loss (papilloedema).

Effects of hypertension

The long-term risk of hypertension is end-organ damage:

- **Cerebrovascular disease**: thrombotic and haemorrhagic stroke.
- **Vascular disease**: coronary artery disease.
- **Left ventricular hypertrophy** (LVH) is a compensatory response

to a chronically elevated BP. It is an independent predictor of early death (sudden cardiac death from ventricular arrhythmias, heart failure, myocardial infarction [MI], cerebrovascular accident [CVA]). Heart failure may relate to LVH (long-standing hypertrophied muscle develops first diastolic and later systolic contractile failure) or to premature coronary disease.

- **Renal failure**: hypertension leads to renovascular damage and glomerular loss.

Investigation

- **Confirm hypertension**: repeated office BP measurement, or ambulatory 24-h recording.
- **Assess for secondary cause**: renal disease (dipstick urine, check creatinine, renal size, non-invasive renal artery imaging by magnetic resonance imaging [MRI]). Exclude coarctation (clinical examination, 'rib notching' on chest X-ray); hypokalaemia (Cushing's and Conn's syndromes, p. 290); phaeochromocytoma (see p. 291).
- **Assess end-organ damage**: ECG, cardiac ultrasonography (for LV hypertrophy), renal function.

Treatment

Treatment removes the excess stroke risk, and halves the excess coronary risk.

Overall approach

Other cardiovascular risk factors must also be addressed, e.g. smoking, diabetes control, cholesterol (statin therapy is often indicated).

Non-pharmacological measures

Lifestyle modification (weight loss, lower salt and alcohol intake, regular exercise) may be sufficient in mild hypertension. Pharmacological therapy if BP too high on several recordings or on 24-h BP monitor.

Pharmacological treatments

Large long-term clinical trials have shown a clear mortality reduction from treating hypertension, principally from fewer strokes, but also from less sudden cardiac death, heart failure and MI. The benefit of treatment relates to the degree of hypertension, i.e. the more severe the hypertension the greater the impact of treatment. However, even mild hypertension benefits from treatment when the risk of end-organ damage is high, or already present (e.g. elderly people, people with diabetes, previous MI, etc.). The risk reduction is related to the lowering of BP. There is **no good evidence that any drug is better than any other**, although individual drugs are particularly suited to some patients:

- **β-Blockers**, e.g. atenolol and metoprolol, reduce heart rate and BP by antagonizing adrenergic signalling. Unequivocal evidence for long-term benefit, especially in coronary disease. Side effects include lethargy, impotence, cold peripheries, exacerbation of diabetes and hyperlipidaemia. Contraindicated in people with asthma, caution in peripheral vascular disease.
- **Diuretics**, e.g. bendrofluazide: safe and effective.

- **Calcium channel antagonists**: vasodilators that lower BP. Nifedipine (possibly amlodipine) causes a reflex tachycardia unless a β-blocker is co-prescribed. Diltiazem and verapamil cause a bradycardia, useful when β-blockers are contraindicated. Side effects: flushing, ankle oedema, worsening heart failure (not amlodipine).
- **Angiotensin-converting enzyme (ACE) inhibitors**, e.g. captopril, enalapril, lisinopril and ramipril, exert antihypertensive effects by blocking the formation of angiotensin II. Mortality data are strong for patients with heart failure, impaired LV function or known coronary artery disease (CAD). May cause profound hypotension or acute renal failure in those with renovascular hypertension, i.e. bilateral renal artery stenosis. Side effects include dry cough (common) and angioedema.
- **Angiotensin II receptor antagonists**, e.g. losartan and valsartan, antagonize the angiotensin II-renin axis. Comparable efficacy to ACE inhibitors, although trial data supporting their use are less comprehensive. Indicated in heart failure or impaired LV function if cough from ACE inhibitor is troublesome. Effects on renal function in renovascular hypertension are similar.
- **α-Antagonists**, e.g. doxazosin. Vasodilators that lower BP by antagonism of α-adrenergic receptors in the peripheral vasculature.
- **Other drugs** include centrally acting agents (e.g. methyldopa, or the newer moxonidine).

Initial treatment is usually with a β-blocker and/or diuretic. Current guidelines reserve ACE inhibitors as second-line agents, although increasing evidence of benefit in cardiovascular disease often results in their use as first-line therapy. If hypertension is not controlled with the optimal dose of one agent, combination therapy with two or more agents is indicated. The choice of antihypertensive therapy is influenced by other disease or risk factors, e.g. patients with coexistent heart failure, stroke or coronary disease gain significant benefit from a β-blocker and ACE inhibitor. β-Blockers should not be given in asthma; instead calcium channel antagonists or ACE inhibitors are commonly used.

Malignant or accelerated hypertension

Rarely, patients present with severe, uncontrolled hypertension (e.g. ≥ 220/120) and headache, confusion ('hypertensive encephalopathy') or acute end-organ damage (cerebral haemorrhage, acute renal failure, aortic dissection or heart failure). **Malignant phase hypertension** is the combination of hypertension, high-grade retinal changes and progressive renal failure—untreated 1 year's mortality rate is ≥ 50%.

Treatment

Admit to hospital as a medical emergency because the risks of end-organ damage and life-threatening complications are high. Oral agents are given, unless the patient is critically unwell (repeated hypertensive seizures, severe LV failure, aortic dissection) when cautious intravenous therapy may be given; however, BP lowering **must** be gradual because sudden falls in BP can precipitate a stroke. Intravenous agents include sodium nitroprusside (a very potent, rapidly acting vasodilator) and labetolol, a β-blocker that also has α-adrenergic antagonist effects.

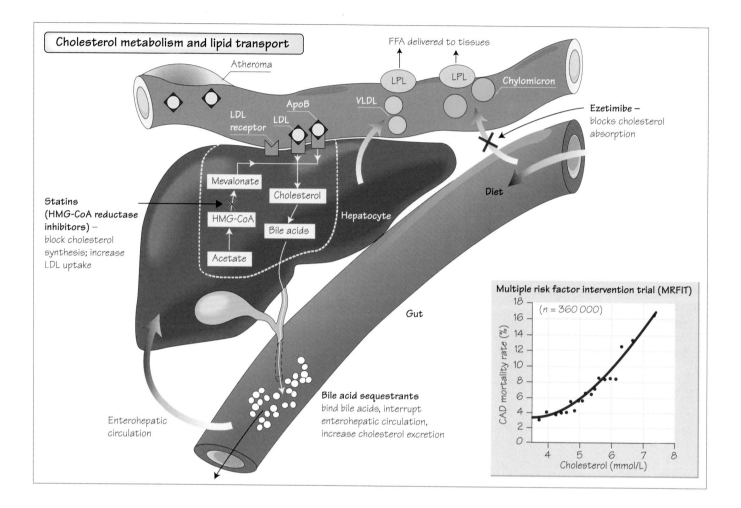

Cholesterol metabolism and lipid transport

FFA delivered to tissues

Atheroma

LPL   LPL   Chylomicron

ApoB   VLDL

LDL receptor   LDL

Ezetimibe – blocks cholesterol absorption

Statins (HMG-CoA reductase inhibitors) – block cholesterol synthesis; increase LDL uptake

Mevalonate

Cholesterol

HMG-CoA

Bile acids

Hepatocyte

Diet

Acetate

Gut

Enterohepatic circulation

Bile acid sequestrants bind bile acids, interrupt enterohepatic circulation, increase cholesterol excretion

Multiple risk factor intervention trial (MRFIT)
($n = 360\,000$)

Definition and incidence

Elevated levels of cholesterol and/or triglycerides. Hypercholesterolaemia is common: $\geq 60\%$ of the UK population have a total cholesterol > 5.2 mmol/L and 3% > 7.5 mmol/L.

Lipid metabolism and lipoproteins

Cholesterol and triglycerides are transported in the bloodstream complexed with phospholipid and proteins (**apoproteins**) in particles called **lipoproteins**. **Apoproteins** act as signalling molecules or enzymes and play very important roles in controlling lipid transport. The different classes of lipoproteins transport lipids between different tissues and are defined by characteristic composition of lipids and apoproteins (Table 71.1). Cholesterol is principally metabolized in the liver. Blood levels are controlled by the balance between blood uptake, cholesterol production (activity of cholesterol biosynthetic pathway) and gastrointestinal excretion (bile acids).

Secondary hyperlipidaemias

Before deciding whether a hyperlipidaemia is primary, diseases producing secondary hyperlipidaemias should be excluded:
- Diabetes
- Hypothyroidism
- Chronic renal failure or nephrotic syndrome
- Chronic liver disease, especially alcoholic
- Chronic biliary obstruction
- Drugs: steroids, oestrogens.

Genetic hyperlipidaemias

Single gene defects in lipid metabolism causing extreme hyperlipidaemias are rare. However, common genetic variability or heterozygote status is a very important determinant of cholesterol levels in the general population.
- **Familial hypercholesterolaemia**: a group of single gene disorders affecting the low-density lipoprotein (LDL) receptor and causing deficient or absent uptake of LDL particles, which therefore accumulate in the bloodstream. Homozygotes (1/1000 000) have extremely high cholesterol levels (10–25 mmol/L) and coronary artery disease (CAD) in their teens or 20 s. Heterozygotes (1/500) have moderately high cholesterol (7–12 mmol/L) and are at risk of premature CAD. Patients may have corneal arcus, xanthelasmas and tendon xanthomas.
- **Polygenetic hypercholesterolaemia** and **familial combined hyperlipidaemia**: inherited conditions (1/300–600) characterized by moderately elevated cholesterol (7–12 mmol/L) with or without high triglycerides, not caused by a single gene disorder, although in some

Table 71.1 Composition and function of lipoproteins and apoproteins.

	Composition	Function	Major apoproteins
Chylomicrons	Rich in triglyceride (85%) Very large particle (200–500 nm) with low density Very little protein (2%)	Transports lipid from the gut to the liver in the postprandial state	**ApoCII**: activator of lipoprotein lipase (LPL) enzyme that breaks down triglycerides for delivery to tissues **ApoE** (see below)
VLDL	Rich in triglyceride Size 50–80 nm	Transports lipid from the liver to the tissues	**ApoCII** (see above) **ApoB$_{100}$** **ApoE**: binds to ApoE receptors on hepatocytes, mediates uptake of lipoprotein remnants after catabolism
LDL	Rich in cholesterol Size 20 nm	Produced by catabolism of VLDL, via IDL. Taken up by liver	**ApoB$_{100}$**: the ligand for the LDL receptor on hepatocytes, mediates uptake of LDL. **ApoE** (see above)
HDL	Smallest (8 nm) and most dense lipoprotein > 50% protein	Carries cholesterol esters back to liver from tissues and other lipoproteins ('reverse cholesterol transport')	**ApoAI**: activates LCAT enzyme that esterifies cholesterol.

inheritance is apparently autosomal dominant. Very important cause of increased atherosclerosis risk in the population. Very high triglycerides may cause pancreatitis.

• **Apoprotein E genotype**: genetic variation in the *ApoE* gene results in different isoforms of the ApoE protein. The *ApoE2* isoform binds less avidly to hepatic receptors, resulting in hyperlipidaemia. *ApoE2* homozygotes are uncommon (1/100) but *ApoE2* heterozygotes (15% of population) appear to have a significantly increased risk of CAD.

• **Lipoprotein lipase deficiency, ApoCII deficiency**: extremely rare. Very elevated chylomicrons, eruptive xanthomas, hepatomegaly and pancreatitis.

Lipids in atherosclerosis

Studies have identified elevated plasma cholesterol as an important risk factor for the development of CAD:

• Total cholesterol > 6.5 mmol/L doubles the risk of lethal CAD: > 7.8 mmol/L increases risk fourfold.

• Reducing total cholesterol by 20% reduces coronary risk by 10%.

• The strongest association is with LDL-cholesterol, whereas high-density lipoprotein (HDL)-cholesterol is protective. LDL : HDL-cholesterol ratio is a useful indicator, a ratio > 4 indicating high risk.

Elevated cholesterol (especially oxidized LDL) damages the endothelium early in atherosclerosis and is taken up into the lipid core of established plaques by macrophages (foam cells). Lowering LDL-cholesterol reduces cholesterol deposition into atherosclerotic plaques and may reverse this process. Crucially, cholesterol lowering stabilizes plaques, reducing the risk of acute plaque rupture.

Lipid lowering and risk factor modification

• **Lipid lowering by diet**: reducing fat intake, especially high cholesterol foods (red meat, eggs, high-fat diet, dairy products) lowers cholesterol by 1 mmol/L and reduces body weight. However, diet alone is *insufficient* in patients with elevated cholesterol and CAD.

• **Lipid-lowering drugs**: current guidelines recommend drug lipid-lowering therapy in patients with, or at risk of, CAD whose total cholesterol remains > 4.8 mmol/L despite dieting.

• **Bile acid sequestrants** ('resins'): e.g. cholestyramine. These lower cholesterol by binding cholesterol in the gastrointestinal tract, interrupting the enterohepatic circulation, so increasing cholesterol excretion. They are distasteful and may have intolerable gastrointestinal side effects. They can be effective and remain useful in familial hypercholesterolaemia.

• **HMG-CoA reductase inhibitors** ('statins'): e.g. simvastatin, pravastatin. These are potent agents that inhibit hydroxymethylglutarylcoenzyme (HMG-CoA) reductase, the rate-limiting enzyme in cholesterol biosynthesis. This increases hepatic cholesterol uptake because reduced intracellular cholesterol biosynthesis increases expression of cell-surface LDL receptors. For this reason, they are less effective in patients with familial hypercholesterolaemia. Statins typically lower LDL-cholesterol 30% or more, and may modestly increase HDL-cholesterol. They have relatively little effect on plasma triglycerides.

Large intervention trials (e.g. 4S, WOSCOPS, CARE, LIPID, Heart Protection Study) show that cholesterol lowering with statins significantly reduces the subsequent incidence of coronary events. The benefits are apparent within months, implying that changes in the composition of atherosclerotic plaques occurs rapidly. Angiographic follow-up studies also show that statins can result in regression of established atheroma.

• **Fibric acid derivatives** ('fibrates'): e.g. bezafibrate, fenofibrate. These agents reduce cholesterol moderately, but also reduce triglycerides and increase HDL-cholesterol. The mechanism of action is complex but involves stimulation of lipoprotein lipase activity (increases chylomicrons and very-low-density lipoprotein [VLDL] catabolism) and increased cholesterol excretion via bile acids. More useful in patients with mixed hyperlipidaemia and/or low HDL.

Multiple risk factor modification

Lipid lowering represents only one aspect of reducing coronary risk, and needs to be considered in the context of the whole coronary risk factor profile for that individual patient. Aggressive lipid lowering is more important in patients who already have an adverse risk factor profile (diabetes, hypertension, smoking) because *multiple risk factors are synergistic in increasing coronary risk*. In contrast, isolated mild hypercholesterolaemia in a patient without other risk factors could be managed by dietary intervention.

72 Acute coronary syndromes

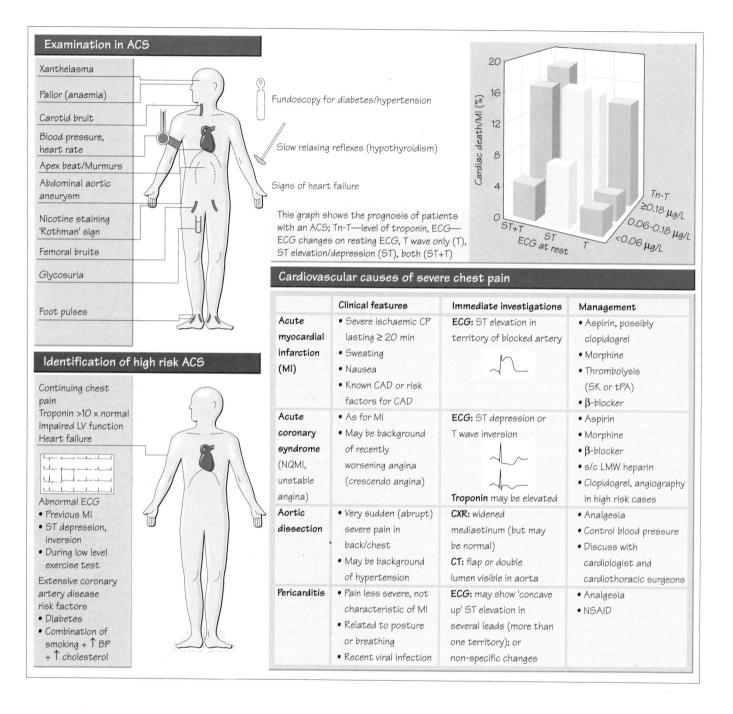

Examination in ACS

- Xanthelasma
- Pallor (anaemia)
- Carotid bruit
- Blood pressure, heart rate
- Apex beat/Murmurs
- Abdominal aortic aneurysm
- Nicotine staining 'Rothman' sign
- Femoral bruits
- Glycosuria
- Foot pulses

Fundoscopy for diabetes/hypertension

Slow relaxing reflexes (hypothyroidism)

Signs of heart failure

This graph shows the prognosis of patients with an ACS; Tn-T—level of troponin, ECG—ECG changes on resting ECG, T wave only (T), ST elevation/depression (ST), both (ST+T)

Identification of high risk ACS

Continuing chest pain
Troponin >10 x normal
Impaired LV function
Heart failure

Abnormal ECG
- Previous MI
- ST depression, inversion
- During low level exercise test

Extensive coronary artery disease risk factors
- Diabetes
- Combination of smoking + ↑ BP + ↑ cholesterol

Cardiovascular causes of severe chest pain

	Clinical features	Immediate investigations	Management
Acute myocardial infarction (MI)	• Severe ischaemic CP lasting ≥ 20 min • Sweating • Nausea • Known CAD or risk factors for CAD	**ECG:** ST elevation in territory of blocked artery	• Aspirin, possibly clopidogrel • Morphine • Thrombolysis (SK or tPA) • β-blocker
Acute coronary syndrome (NQMI, unstable angina)	• As for MI • May be background of recently worsening angina (crescendo angina)	**ECG:** ST depression or T wave inversion **Troponin** may be elevated	• Aspirin • Morphine • β-blocker • s/c LMW heparin • Clopidogrel, angiography in high risk cases
Aortic dissection	• Very sudden (abrupt) severe pain in back/chest • May be background of hypertension	**CXR:** widened mediastinum (but may be normal) **CT:** flap or double lumen visible in aorta	• Analgesia • Control blood pressure • Discuss with cardiologist and cardiothoracic surgeons
Pericarditis	• Pain less severe, not characteristic of MI • Related to posture or breathing • Recent viral infection	**ECG:** may show 'concave up' ST elevation in several leads (more than one territory); or non-specific changes	• Analgesia • NSAID

Acute chest pain is a common presentation, accounting for 10% of medical patients. Management aims to separate out, and treat early, those patients with acute myocardial infarction (AMI) or other high-risk acute coronary syndromes from other life-threatening diagnoses such as aortic dissection from other benign causes of pain such as pericarditis or gastro-oesophageal pain.

General approach

The initial assessment of the patient should enable a diagnosis or differential diagnosis that guides immediate management and enables administration of emergency treatment with as little delay as possible. Rapid clinical assessment by history and examination is combined with simple investigations such as ECG and chest X-ray.

Myocardial ischaemia is presumptively diagnosed when:
- The pain is retrosternal, tight and especially if it is severe. Radiation into the neck, or down the left arm, increases the probability of myocardial ischaemia.
- Pains occurring for > 4 weeks have a strong relationship to exercise. However, in pains present for < 2 weeks, often (surprisingly) there is no/little relationship with effort.

- Pains felt during a previous **unambiguous** episode of myocardial ischaemia are similar to the current pains.
- If multiple episodes of pain are present over several weeks they should each be of short duration (i.e. < 20–30 min).

Physical examination

This is often unrevealing, but may show evidence of risk factors (nicotine-stained hands, cholesterol deposits around the eyes, hypertension, vascular disease elsewhere) or complications (arrhythmias, heart failure), or suggest other diagnoses.

Investigations

The important **investigations** early on in suspected myocardial ischaemia are:
- **ECG**, repeated frequently (i.e. whenever there is pain, and at least daily otherwise).
- **Chest X-ray**, to exclude complicating heart failure and alternative pathologies.
- **Markers** of myocardial necrosis: '**traditional**' cardiac markers (usually creatine kinase [CK], rarely aspartate aminotransferase [AST], lactate dehydrogenase [LDH] and **especially** cardiac-specific troponins).
- **Haemoglobin**.
- **Cholesterol** (on admission, because AMI artefactually lowers cholesterol from days to months afterwards), triglycerides, glucose. Anyone with elevated cholesterol should have his or her thyroid function checked.
- **Renal function**.

Acute MI and acute coronary syndromes

The common pathology underlying AMI, non-Q-wave MI and unstable angina is rupture or erosion of a coronary artery plaque, leading to intra-coronary thrombosis. The resulting clinical syndrome depends on whether the coronary artery has occluded totally (thus producing AMI), or whether it is only partially or transiently (< 20 min at a time) totally occluded (producing a non-Q-wave MI or unstable angina). Damage to the heart can result from the occlusion itself. However, even if the occlusion is not complete, myocardial necrosis can still result from thrombus embolizing down the coronary, infarcting distal tissue.
- **Acute MI** is defined by **ST segment elevation** on the ECG, termed an 'acute MI with ST segment elevation'. This is also called a 'threatened Q-wave MI' because, in the absence of treatment, this syndrome frequently progresses to a Q-wave or full-thickness MI. Therapy aims to prevent this progression and minimize infarction size such that Q-waves do not develop. Management of MI is outlined in Chapter 73.
- **Acute coronary syndromes** include both non-Q-wave MI and unstable angina, a distinction often only made retrospectively.

Both syndromes present with **ST depression and/or T-wave inversion** on the ECG (see Table 72.1) in the setting of ischaemic chest pain. Elevation in traditional cardiac enzymes (e.g. CK two times or more the upper limit of normal) defines non-Q-wave MI as against unstable angina. Acute coronary syndromes include a group of patients at high risk of early (> a few weeks) adverse events (including AMI and death), and are thus medical emergencies requiring immediate treatment and close monitoring on a coronary care unit (CCU). Acute coronary syndromes **do not** benefit from thrombolytic treatment. They do benefit from:
- Immediate aspirin (chewed).
- Analgesia, with morphine if pain is ongoing.
- β-Blocker, given intravenously, in a dose sufficient to reduce the resting heart rate to 45–50 beats/min. Mild heart failure (i.e. crepitations less than one-third of the way up the lungs) is **not** a contraindication to β-blockade.
- Subcutaneous low-molecular-weight heparin (LMW heparin).

Risk stratification of acute coronary syndromes

After immediate medical management, further investigation and treatment are determined by whether a patient is at high risk of further cardiac events. Factors associated with high risk include:
- ST segment depression on the ECG at presentation and/or elevated troponin levels (10 times or more the detectable limit).
- Recurrent episodes of chest pain.
- Diabetes, previous AMI, impaired left ventricular (LV) function, heart failure (even if cardiac ultrasonography shows good LV function).

Patients without these factors, whose chest pain symptoms settle, are mobilized. If they remain pain free, an exercise ECG should be performed. Inducible ischaemia (i.e. > 2-mm ST segment depression or angina) at a low workload (i.e. less than stage II of the Bruce protocol) indicates high risk.

High-risk patients should be given more aggressive antiplatelet drugs (**platelet IIb/IIIa receptor** antagonists or clopidogrel) and undergo early **cardiac catheterization**, because they may have critical coronary lesions amenable to percutaneous intervention (percutaneous transluminal coronary angioplasty [PTCA], usually with intra-coronary stenting), or severe multi-vessel coronary artery disease that requires coronary artery bypass graft surgery (CABG). All patients should have aggressive management of atherogenic risk factors after an acute coronary syndrome:
- Cholesterol reduction: most patients benefit from statin therapy (this should not preclude appropriate dieting and achievement of ideal body mass).
- Blood pressure should be < 140/85 (< 130/80 for patients with diabetes), using non-pharmacological approaches (ideal weight, regular exercise, low salt) and drugs as necessary.
- Long-term antiplatelet agent (aspirin or clopidogrel).
- Most benefit from angiotensin-converting enzyme (ACE) inhibitor therapy, even if LV function is not impaired.

Table 72.1 Quick guide to acute coronary syndromes.

ECG	Troponin	Diagnosis
ST elevation	+ to +++	STEMI
No ST elevation	+	Non-STEMI
usually ST depression	No rise	Unstable angina
or T wave inversion	or trivial rise	or troponin –ve ACS

STEMI = ST elevation myocardial infarction

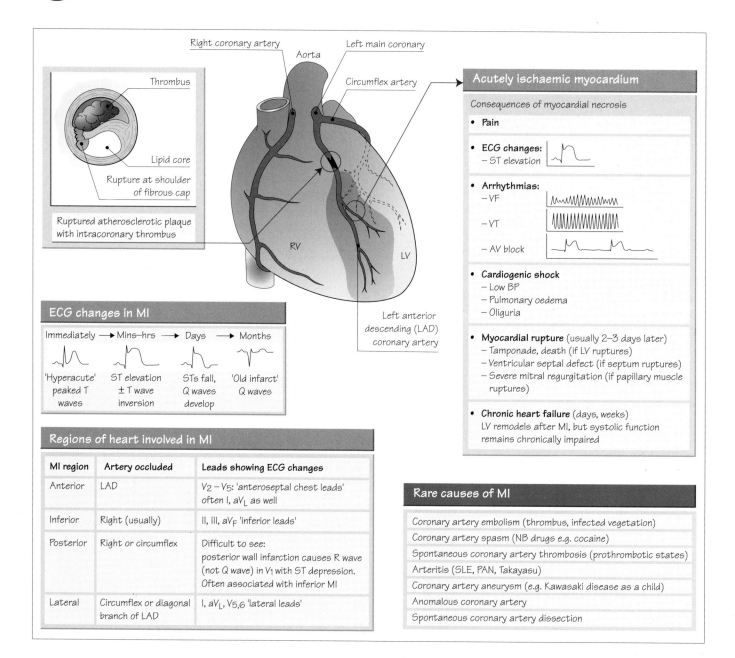

Ruptured atherosclerotic plaque with intracoronary thrombus
- Thrombus
- Lipid core
- Rupture at shoulder of fibrous cap

Right coronary artery · Aorta · Left main coronary · Circumflex artery · Left anterior descending (LAD) coronary artery · RV · LV

Acutely ischaemic myocardium

Consequences of myocardial necrosis

- **Pain**

- **ECG changes:**
  - ST elevation

- **Arrhythmias:**
  - VF
  - VT
  - AV block

- **Cardiogenic shock**
  - Low BP
  - Pulmonary oedema
  - Oliguria

- **Myocardial rupture** (usually 2–3 days later)
  - Tamponade, death (if LV ruptures)
  - Ventricular septal defect (if septum ruptures)
  - Severe mitral regurgitation (if papillary muscle ruptures)

- **Chronic heart failure** (days, weeks)
  LV remodels after MI, but systolic function remains chronically impaired

ECG changes in MI

Immediately → Mins–hrs → Days → Months

| 'Hyperacute' peaked T waves | ST elevation ± T wave inversion | STs fall, Q waves develop | 'Old infarct' Q waves |

Regions of heart involved in MI

MI region	Artery occluded	Leads showing ECG changes
Anterior	LAD	V₂ – V₅: 'anteroseptal chest leads' often I, aV_L as well
Inferior	Right (usually)	II, III, aV_F 'inferior leads'
Posterior	Right or circumflex	Difficult to see: posterior wall infarction causes R wave (not Q wave) in V₁ with ST depression. Often associated with inferior MI
Lateral	Circumflex or diagonal branch of LAD	I, aV_L, V₅,₆ 'lateral leads'

Rare causes of MI

Coronary artery embolism (thrombus, infected vegetation)
Coronary artery spasm (NB drugs e.g. cocaine)
Spontaneous coronary artery thrombosis (prothrombotic states)
Arteritis (SLE, PAN, Takayasu)
Coronary artery aneurysm (e.g. Kawasaki disease as a child)
Anomalous coronary artery
Spontaneous coronary artery dissection

- **Definition**: ischaemic necrosis of the myocardium as a result of acute occlusion of a coronary artery.
- **Incidence**: very common; 250 000 myocardial infarctions (MIs) per year in the UK (one every 2 min); 100 000 deaths.
- **Pathogenesis**: MI occurs when a coronary artery occludes, the myocardium supplied by that artery becomes ischaemic and necrosis occurs over several hours; early restoration of blood flow may abort the infarction and limit necrosis. The overwhelmingly common cause is **atheromatous coronary artery disease**, when an existing coronary atheromatous plaque (not necessarily one severely narrowing the artery) becomes eroded or ruptures, causing a sudden expansion of the plaque

and thrombosis of the coronary artery lumen. Other causes of MI occur very occasionally (see figure).

Clinical features

- **Classic presentation**: severe crushing central chest pain ≥ 20 min, unrelieved by nitrates, associated with sweating, pallor and nausea.
- **Other presentations** include arrhythmia, cardiac arrest or acute heart failure.
- May be atypical in **elderly people** (collapse or confusion) and in those with **diabetes**, who may have no chest pain, and develop worsening of metabolic status or heart failure.

- Most patients have risk factors or known coronary artery disease; 50% have no preceding angina.

Investigations
Initial investigations should quickly establish the diagnosis. The most important is the ECG:
- The diagnostic hallmark of acute MI is ST segment elevation.
- A few patients have bundle branch block.
- Twenty per cent of patients are subsequently shown to have had an MI present with other ECG changes such as ST depression or T-wave inversion. These patients **do not benefit** from thrombolysis, so can safely be treated as a non-ST segment elevation acute coronary syndromes.

Important differential diagnoses to exclude are **acute aortic dissection** (wide mediastinum on chest X-ray, loss of pulses, aortic regurgitation) and **pericarditis** (widespread non-specific changes on the ECG). In general, thrombolysis is more commonly withheld from patients who justify therapy, rather than administered inappropriately to patients with other conditions.

Management
The patient should be moved to a coronary care unit (CCU) for monitoring, **but** initial management **must** not be delayed by waiting for transfer to CCU:
- Opiate analgesia, oxygen by mask.
- Immediate aspirin, chewed not swallowed.
- Thrombolysis, usually with either streptokinase or tissue plasminogen activator (tPA) (other thrombolytics are often equally efficacious).
- In some hospitals, immediate coronary angioplasty/stenting (**primary PCI**) is used as an alternative or adjunct to thrombolysis.
- β-Blocker, intravenously, especially if hypertensive or tachycardic without overt cardiac failure.
- Diuretic if pulmonary oedema.
- Angiotensin-converting enzyme (ACE) inhibitor (day 2 or 3) especially if clinical heart failure, or significantly impaired left ventricular (LV) function (anterior MI, large enzyme release, impaired LV on echocardiography).

Complications
Immediate/hours
- **Ventricular arrhythmias** (tachycardia or fibrillation) usually occur within 24 h or less and are the principal cause of pre-hospital death. Patients should be monitored close to a defibrillator.
- **Failed reperfusion** is the failure of thrombolytic therapy to re-establish blood flow in the occluded artery 90 min after thrombolysis; chest pain continues and ST segment elevation fails to resolve. If untreated, progression to full-thickness Q-wave infarction occurs. Repeat thrombolytic (tPA) and contact cardiologist.
- **'Salvage' percutaneous transluminal angioplasty** (PTCA) may reopen the 'infarct-related' artery and prevent MI completion.

Hours/days
Cardiac rupture into pericardium is uncommon, but typically occurs on days 2–5; cardiac arrest with electromechanical dissociation (EMD; see p. 136) is usually fatal. Re-infarction is common after thrombolysis, because a culprit plaque may cause repeat coronary thrombosis. Give repeat thrombolytic (tPA) and contact a cardiologist. PTCA may reopen artery; treat the underlying culprit lesion. Heart failure with pulmonary oedema results from acute impairment of LV function. Cardiogenic shock occurs when cardiac output is inadequate to maintain arterial BP, resulting from severe impairment of LV function, infarction of right ventricular (RV) (usually in inferior MI) causing inadequate left heart filling or mechanical catastrophe such as:
- **Ventricular septal rupture** (VSD): new loud pansystolic murmur at the lower left sternal edge.
- **Papillary muscle rupture**: severe mitral regurgitation (MR), murmur may not be loud, but severe pulmonary oedema out of proportion to apparent LV damage.

Both require immediate cardiological assessment with a view to early surgical repair.

Days/weeks
- **Thromboembolism** (cerebrovascular accident [CVA], gut or limb ischaemia): may result from mural thrombus forming at the site of the infarct. Unusual now that thrombolysis and heparin widely used. Give warfarin for 3–6 months after large anterior wall MI or if severe LV impairment.
- **Chronic heart failure**: LV remodelling after MI may worsen rather than improve LV function. Treat with ACE inhibitors, diuretics, cautious β-blockade, spironolactone.
- **Ventricular tachycardia**: may occur ≥ 24 h, and implies that the myocardial scar is a substrate for re-entrant circuits. β-Blockers and amiodarone help but, if impaired LV function or collapse, the risk of future sudden cardiac death is significant and justifies automatic defibrillator (AICD) implantation.
- **Dressler's syndrome**: usually self-limiting autoimmune pericarditis several weeks after a full-thickness MI. Occasionally requires steroids, more commonly responds to NSAIDs.

Risk stratification, prognosis and rehabilitation
Long-term outlook after MI is governed largely by the extent of **LV damage**, and the severity of the underlying **coronary artery disease**. Most post-MI deaths are caused by heart failure, sudden cardiac death or further MI. Secondary prophylaxis to prevent further MI and other vascular events comprises:
- Aspirin, β-blockers and ACE inhibitors.
- **Risk factor modification**: stop smoking, reduce cholesterol (diet and statins), treat hypertension and diabetes.
- **Rehabilitation programme** to increase physical exercise, encourage lifestyle changes and provide psychological support.

Risk stratification
After the acute event, patients at high risk (see below) of further cardiac events need to be identified, because they require coronary angiography and consideration for revascularization either by percutaneous intervention (PTCA/stent) or coronary artery bypass graft (CABG), or by more aggressive management of heart failure or arrhythmias.
- Recurrent ischaemia (chest pain): spontaneous or on mobilization.
- Re-infarction or threatened re-infarction (chest pain with recurrent ST elevation).
- Adverse exercise tolerance test (chest pain at low workload, poor haemodynamic response, arrhythmia, ST depression).
- Refractory heart failure.
- Recurrent or refractory arrhythmias > 24 h after the acute MI.

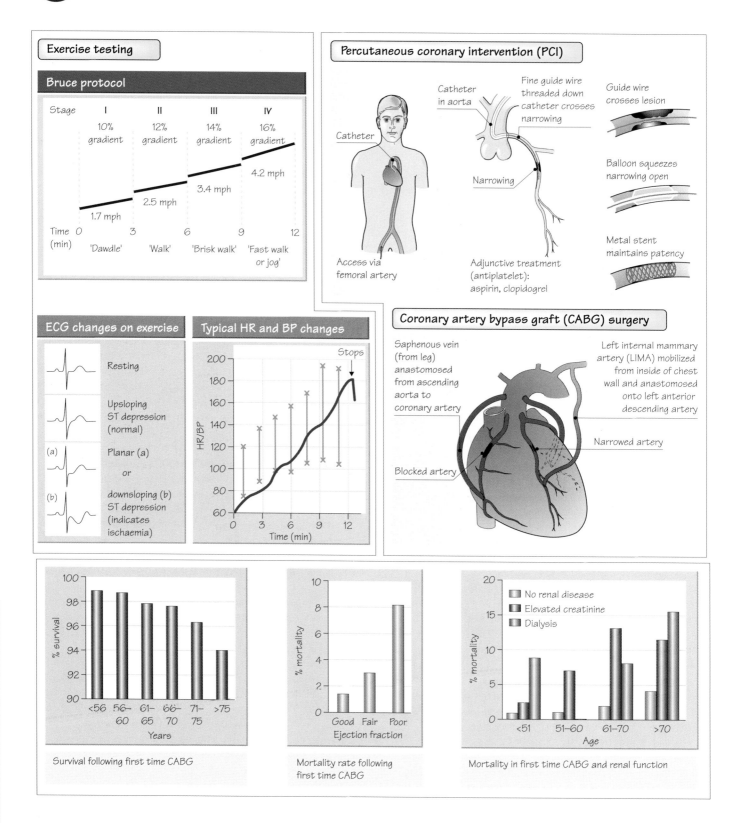

Exercise testing

Bruce protocol

Stage	I	II	III	IV
	10% gradient	12% gradient	14% gradient	16% gradient

4.2 mph

3.4 mph

2.5 mph

1.7 mph

Time (min) 0 — 3 — 6 — 9 — 12

'Dawdle' 'Walk' 'Brisk walk' 'Fast walk or jog'

ECG changes on exercise

Resting

Upsloping ST depression (normal)

(a) Planar (a)

or

(b) downsloping (b) ST depression (indicates ischaemia)

Typical HR and BP changes

Stops

HR/BP axis: 200, 180, 160, 140, 120, 100, 80, 60

Time (min): 0, 3, 6, 9, 12

Percutaneous coronary intervention (PCI)

Catheter

Catheter in aorta

Fine guide wire threaded down catheter crosses narrowing

Guide wire crosses lesion

Narrowing

Balloon squeezes narrowing open

Access via femoral artery

Adjunctive treatment (antiplatelet): aspirin, clopidogrel

Metal stent maintains patency

Coronary artery bypass graft (CABG) surgery

Saphenous vein (from leg) anastomosed from ascending aorta to coronary artery

Left internal mammary artery (LIMA) mobilized from inside of chest wall and anastomosed onto left anterior descending artery

Blocked artery

Narrowed artery

Survival following first time CABG

(% survival: 90–100; Years: <56, 56–60, 61–65, 66–70, 71–75, >75)

Mortality rate following first time CABG

(% mortality: 0–10; Ejection fraction: Good, Fair, Poor)

Mortality in first time CABG and renal function

- No renal disease
- Elevated creatinine
- Dialysis

(% mortality: 0–20; Age: <51, 51–60, 61–70, >70)

Diseases and Treatments at a Glance

Chronic chest pain is common as is coronary artery disease (CAD). The key to managing chronic chest pain is to establish whether symptoms relate to coronary disease and, if they do, the risk of an adverse event occurring.

Diagnosis

Chronic stable angina usually relates to CAD, although other pathologies may be responsible (see Chapter 4). The symptomatology is usually classic: day-to-day symptoms occur with the same amount of effort and are rapidly (< 1 min) relieved by rest/glyceryl trinitrate (GTN). The longer rest/GTN takes to relieve symptoms, the less likely they are to relate to CAD. Effort capacity is decreased by the cold, the wind, on hills or after eating. Symptoms usually comprise a retrosternal chest tightness, which may radiate to the jaw or left arm. Symptoms may be very atypical—the diagnostic clue is the clear provocation with effort and rapid relief by rest, in the presence of appropriate coronary risk factors (age, sex, etc.). Breathlessness, rather than chest pain, may be an 'anginal equivalent' in people with diabetes.

The diagnosis is usually clear from the history alone. If not, exercise testing may help, although occasionally coronary angiography is needed.

Risk stratification

The outlook in chronic angina is worsened by:
- Increasing age.
- Exercise intolerance, especially if caused by chest pain/cardiac dyspnoea.
- Impaired left ventricular (LV) function (e.g. previous myocardial infarction [MI], hypertensive heart disease) or frank heart failure.
- Extensive and severe coronary disease. A non-invasive measure of this can be obtained from the exercise ECG test (or exercise myocardial imaging using radioisotopes). Most patients with angina should therefore undergo periodic exercise ECG tests.
- Symptoms and/or ST depression ≥ 2 mm in stage II of the Bruce protocol (see figure) correlates with a poorer outcome.
- Exercise-induced hypotension likewise suggests extensive CAD.
- Extensive atherogenic risk factors, particularly diabetes.
- Vascular disease elsewhere, e.g. peripheral vascular disease.

Although some patients with few symptoms benefit from revascularization (and can be identified by non-invasive means), many patients can be identified on clinical criteria: 1) Symptomatic angina despite medical therapy. 2) Worsening or unstable angina. 3) Post infarct angina. 4) Heart failure with angina.

These patients should undergo coronary angiography to determine the location and severity of coronary stenosis and whether revascularization will reduce subsequent adverse events.

Treatment

Many patients are managed on medical therapy alone. Action should be taken to improve diet (omega-3 fish oils, fruit, decrease animal fats, low cholesterol), lose weight and exercise (which lessens BP by ± 10 mmHg and cholesterol by 1.0–1.5 mmol/L).
- Stop smoking.
- Treat diabetes and hypertension aggressively (target BP < 140/85).
- **Hypercholesterolaemia** (see Chapter 71). Most patients should be on statin therapy.
- **ACE inhibitors** have anti-atherogenic actions in those at high risk of vascular events.
- **Anti-platelet agents**: aspirin has prognostic benefit. In aspirin allergy/intolerance clopidogrel is used.

Anti-ischaemic therapy
- **Nitrates** are highly effective in relieving angina. Nitrate tolerance develops if they are given throughout the 24 h. A 'nitrate-free' period of 12–14 h/day is needed.
- **β-Blockers** are first-line therapy. They reduce cardiac work, lessen angina and improve prognosis after an MI and in heart failure.
- **Calcium channel blockers**: second-line therapies are used only when β-blockers are contraindicated. They are relatively contraindicated in heart failure. Only those with heart rate-slowing properties (e.g. diltiazem or verapamil, not nifedipine) can be given as monotherapy in angina. Those without any negatively chronotropic action must be given with a β-blocker.

Revascularization in CAD
Patients benefit from revascularization procedures if their symptoms interfere with their lifestyle, or if they fall into a group known to benefit prognostically from coronary artery bypass graft (CABG), i.e. those with stenoses (> 70% luminal narrowing) affecting: 1) All three coronary arteries. 2) The left main coronary artery. 3) The proximal portion of the left anterior descending artery.

Impaired LV function and diabetes magnify the benefit of surgery.

Percutaneous coronary intervention (PCI)
Percutaneous transluminal angioplasty (PTCA) involves passing an angioplasty balloon over a fine guide-wire previously steered down the artery and across the lesion. Inflating the balloon opens the artery up. **Stents** (mesh-like stainless steel tube) are usually inserted to help maintain short- and long-term patency (i.e. to lessen re-stenosis). During PCI, the vessel may **close acutely** if there is an extensive dissection (treated with stenting) or extensive *in situ* thrombus (treated with abciximab, a potent monoclonal antibody drug that blocks platelet action). If the vessel cannot be re-opened, an MI may occur (overall risk is 0.5%). Immediate CABG is only very rarely indicated to prevent this. **Restenosis** can occur 6 weeks to 1 year after PCI. Intimal hyperplasia (the consequence of balloon injury to the vessel wall) impinges on the lumen of the artery sufficient to produce recurrent angina in 10–20% of patients. Further PTCA may establish long-term patency. The introduction of cytotoxic and cytostatic **drug-eluting stents** has partially reduced the problem of in-stent re-stenosis by inhibiting vascular smooth muscle cell growth.

Coronary artery bypass surgery
Coronary surgery is highly effective at relieving anginal symptoms and in some cases improves prognosis (see above). In many patients, angioplasty can be safely used to delay the need for CABG, i.e. PTCA and CABG are complementary rather than competitive treatments. In CABG, bypass grafts are connected from the aorta to the coronary artery distal to the stenosis. Usually this requires stopping the heart and supporting the patient by a cardiopulmonary bypass machine, but it is often possible to apply grafts without stopping the heart—'off-pump surgery'. There are two forms of bypass graft:
- **Vein grafts** (from leg saphenous veins) are easy to use and quick to apply, but have an annual failure rate of $\pm 8\%$.
- **Arterial grafts** are technically more difficult to apply, have much better long-term survival rate, and therefore a better medium-term patient survival. The most commonly used arterial graft is the internal mammary artery, usually applied to the left anterior descending artery.

Elective surgery has a $\pm 1\%$ mortality rate. After surgery anti-atherogenic and anti-platelet measures must continue.

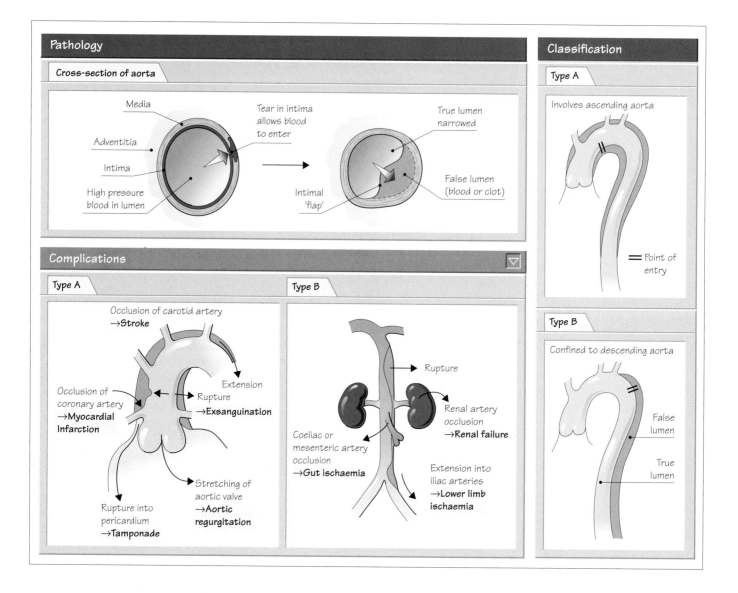

Pathology

Cross-section of aorta

Media
Adventitia
Intima
High pressure blood in lumen
Tear in intima allows blood to enter
Intimal 'flap'
True lumen narrowed
False lumen (blood or clot)

Complications

Type A

Occlusion of carotid artery →**Stroke**
Occlusion of coronary artery →**Myocardial Infarction**
Extension
Rupture →**Exsanguination**
Rupture into pericardium →**Tamponade**
Stretching of aortic valve →**Aortic regurgitation**

Type B

Rupture
Renal artery occlusion →**Renal failure**
Coeliac or mesenteric artery occlusion →**Gut ischaemia**
Extension into iliac arteries →**Lower limb ischaemia**

Classification

Type A

Involves ascending aorta

Point of entry

Type B

Confined to descending aorta

False lumen
True lumen

Aortic dissection affects 1/40 000 of the population per year and consists of a tear in the intima of the thoracic aorta, causing bleeding into the aortic wall, and raising a flap; this then propagates distal to the original tear, interrupting vital organ blood supply. Aortic rupture may occur.

Aetiology
- Hypertension.
- Atherosclerosis.
- Marfan's syndrome predisposes to aortic aneurysm formation, dissection and rupture.

Pathology
High blood pressure, stretched connective tissues and the presence of diseased intima (atherosclerosis) result in sudden tearing of the intima. Blood enters the layer between the intima and media, and high pressure causes the blood to track longitudinally along the aorta, forwards and

backwards from the point of entry, forming a false lumen. Blood in the false lumen may clot, or remain liquid with some flow. Dissections are classified into one of two types, depending on whether the ascending aorta is involved:
- **Type A**: point of intimal tearing is in the ascending aorta. The dissection usually tracks distally to involve the descending aorta and proximally to disrupt the aortic valve apparatus and into the pericardium.
- **Type B**: point of intimal tearing is in the descending aorta, typically just beyond the origin of the left subclavian artery. It is rare for the tear to propagate proximally.

Clinical features
The clinical presentation is extremely variable because of the diverse consequences and complications of aortic dissection. Symptoms arise from the stripping of the intima away from the aortic wall (presentation symptoms) and from either the interruption of the blood supply to vital organs or rupture. The most common presentation is with abrupt onset

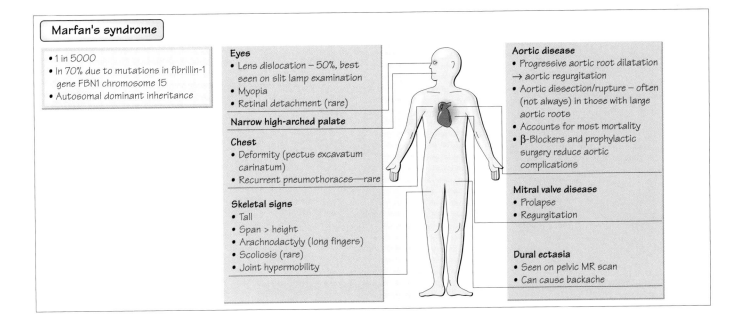

of extremely severe pain felt in the chest or back (interscapular), particularly in a middle-aged hypertensive man. The complications of dissection are:
- **Rupture**: catastrophic pain, hypotension and collapse. Often fatal, but may be contained as BP falls. Occurs retroperitoneally, in the mediastinum or into the left (although never the right) pleural space.
- **Pericardial tamponade**: rupture of a type A dissection backwards into the pericardium results in haemopericardium and pericardial tamponade, the clinical features of which are hypotension (pulsus paradoxus) and a raised jugular venous pressure (JVP) (Kussmaul's sign).
- **Aortic regurgitation**: involvement of aortic root disrupts the aortic valve ring, causing the valve to leak. Early diastolic murmur.
- **Aortic side branch occlusion**: the false lumen compresses the origin of arterial branches as they arise from the aorta. Any branch, at any point along the ascending, descending and abdominal aorta, can be involved. This can lead to a myocardial infarction (MI) (only patients with inferior infarction are seen, because left main coronary dissection is lethal), stroke, upper or lower limb ischaemia, paraparesis caused by spinal artery occlusion, renal failure or gut ischaemia.
- **Extension**: initial dissection may extend along the aorta, typically causing further pain in the direction of the extension.

Investigations
- **ECG**: principally to exclude MI. May show left ventricular (LV) hypertrophy from long-standing hypertension.
- **Chest X-ray**: may show widened mediastinum as a result of haemo-mediastinum, or a pleural effusion, caused by aortic rupture into the (usually left) pleural space.
- **CT scan**: in most hospitals this is the imaging technique of choice. Its use should **never** be delayed. Cross-sectional images of aorta show flap, true and false lumina when contrast is given.
- **Echocardiography** rarely shows the dissection flap, but may show complications such as haemopericardium and aortic regurgitation.
- **Transoesophageal echocardiography** (TOE) is very sensitive in

imaging both the ascending and the descending aorta. A specialized echo probe is passed down the oesophagus, and positioned behind the heart, allowing imaging of the great vessels and heart, unimpeded by ribs or lungs. Images of a high quality are obtained. The procedure requires a highly skilled operator and is invasive, and patients require sedation; because it may transiently increase the blood pressure, thus provoking extension of the dissection, it should be carried out only in cardiothoracic centres with access to immediate surgery.

Management
Aortic dissection is a medical emergency and should be treated with the very highest priority. In both type A and B, the immediate concern is to lower the blood pressure to less than 100 mmHg systolic to prevent further dissection or rupture, using opiate analgesia and intravenous β-blocker. Those with hypotension due to bleeding should be resuscitated to maintain a modest BP only. Specific treatment depends on the site of origination of the flap:
- **Type A dissection**: the risk of catastrophic complications, particularly rupture into the pericardium, is extremely high, with an **hourly** mortality rate of ± 2%. Patients should be transferred by blue light/air ambulance to a cardiothoracic centre immediately, whatever the time of day, for immediate surgery to replace the aortic root, with or without a concomitant aortic valve procedure.
- **Type B**: Surgery is high risk and therefore not indicated as first-line treatment. Aggressive BP control is indicated, aiming for a systolic BP of < 100 mmHg. Surgery is reserved for life-threatening complications, such as threatened rupture. A false lumen may clot and stabilize.

Prognosis
Type A dissection has a very high immediate mortality, but if the patient does not have life-threatening complications (e.g. stroke, paraplegia) the outlook after successful surgery is good. The immediate outlook for type B dissection is better, although there are late complications, including aneurysm formation and rupture.

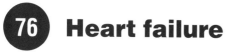

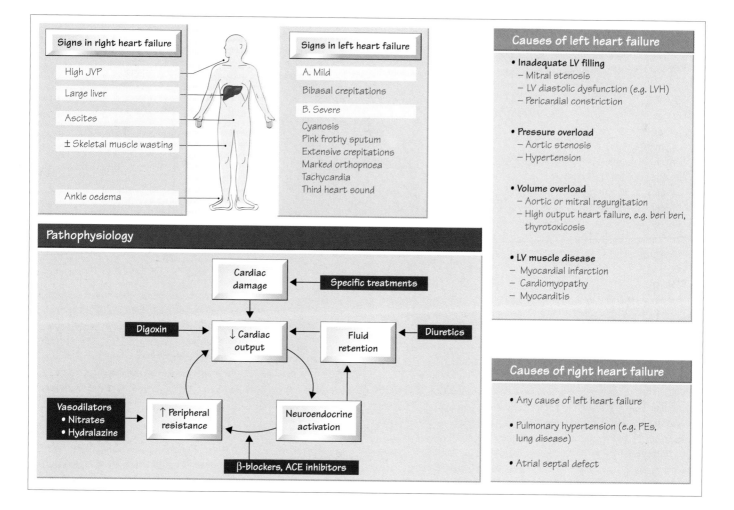

Signs in right heart failure

High JVP

Large liver

Ascites

± Skeletal muscle wasting

Ankle oedema

Signs in left heart failure

A. Mild

Bibasal crepitations

B. Severe

Cyanosis
Pink frothy sputum
Extensive crepitations
Marked orthopnoea
Tachycardia
Third heart sound

Causes of left heart failure

• **Inadequate LV filling**
  – Mitral stenosis
  – LV diastolic dysfunction (e.g. LVH)
  – Pericardial constriction

• **Pressure overload**
  – Aortic stenosis
  – Hypertension

• **Volume overload**
  – Aortic or mitral regurgitation
  – High output heart failure, e.g. beri beri, thyrotoxicosis

• **LV muscle disease**
  – Myocardial infarction
  – Cardiomyopathy
  – Myocarditis

Pathophysiology

Cardiac damage → Specific treatments

Digoxin → ↓ Cardiac output ← Fluid retention ← Diuretics

Vasodilators
• Nitrates
• Hydralazine → ↑ Peripheral resistance ← Neuroendocrine activation

β-blockers, ACE inhibitors

Causes of right heart failure

• Any cause of left heart failure

• Pulmonary hypertension (e.g. PEs, lung disease)

• Atrial septal defect

Cardiac failure is the clinical syndrome resulting from the inability to maintain an adequate cardiac output; it has characteristic clinical and pathophysiological consequences. It affects 1–2% of those aged ≥ 65 years and 10% of those aged ≥ 75 years. The prognosis is poor; in severe heart failure, ≥ 50% die within 3 years.

Pathophysiology

Heart failure is a **syndrome** because, despite many different causes, once present the symptoms, signs and pathophysiology are similar. An inadequate cardiac output stimulates compensatory mechanisms resembling the response to hypovolaemia. Initially beneficial, these in turn become maladaptive:

• **Neurohormonal activation** occurs with increases in vasoconstrictors (renin, angiotensin II, catecholamines) provoking salt and water retention and increasing cardiac afterload. These decrease left ventricular (LV) emptying and depress cardiac output further, producing greater neuroendocrine activation, so increasing afterload, etc., resulting in a vicious downward spiral.

• **Ventricular dilatation**: impaired systolic function (reduced ejection fraction) and fluid retention increase ventricular volume (dilatation). A dilated heart is mechanically inefficient ('law of Laplace'). If energy

supply is limited (e.g. coronary disease) this may lead to further contractile failure and neuroendocrine activation.

Classification

Classification of various heart failure syndromes groups common features dominating the clinical syndrome together. This may be useful in diagnosis.

• **Acute heart failure** is largely synonymous with left heart failure and results from a sudden failure to maintain cardiac output. There is insufficient time for compensatory mechanisms to develop and the clinical picture is dominated by acute pulmonary oedema.

• **Chronic heart failure** (CHF) is largely synonymous with **right heart failure**. Cardiac output declines gradually, symptoms and signs are less florid, and features relating to compensatory mechanisms dominate. Confusingly both left and right heart failure commonly coexist, usually because chronic left heart failure results in secondary pulmonary hypertension and right heart failure. Chronic biventricular failure is termed 'congestive cardiac failure'.

Symptoms and signs

• **Left heart failure**: breathlessness, worse when lying down (orthop-

Diseases and Treatments at a Glance

Table 76.1 New York Heart Association classification.

NYHA class	Breathlessness
I	None
II	On strenuous exercise
III	On moderate effort
IV	At rest

noea), especially in the middle of the night (paroxysmal nocturnal dyspnoea [PND]). Signs comprise tachypnoea, tachycardia, third heart sound ('gallop rhythm') and bibasilar inspiratory pulmonary crepitations. Elevation of the jugular venous pressure (JVP) and peripheral oedema may **not** occur.

• **Right heart failure**: fluid retention in the legs, in severe cases ascites. Signs comprise raised JVP and peripheral oedema.

• **Chronic heart failure**: in long-standing CHF the heart enlarges (cardiomegaly and secondary mitral/tricuspid regurgitation). Skeletal muscle loss ('cardiac cachexia') may be substantial and responsible for fatigue, tiredness and weakness. The New York Heart Association (NYHA) classification grades severity (Table 76.1).

Aetiology

Underlying diseases that damage or overload the pumping ability of the heart result in cardiac failure (see figure).

Provoking/exacerbating factors

It is vital to consider whether there are contributory factors:

• Arrhythmias (e.g. atrial fibrillation).

• Drug issues (non-compliance, fluid retaining drugs, e.g. non-steroidal anti-inflammatory drugs [NSAIDs]).

• Anaemia.

• Infection, e.g. pneumonia, urinary tract infection.

• Thyroid disease.

Investigations

These detect causes, assess severity and monitor treatment:

• **Echocardiography**: essential simple, non-invasive tool useful in diagnosing aetiology, severity and ruling out important valvar heart disease.

• **ECG**: old MI, LV hypertrophy (LVH, e.g. hypertension, aortic stenosis). A normal ECG makes CHF very unlikely. Arrhythmias, e.g. atrial fibrillation (AF).

• **Chest X-ray**: large heart, pulmonary congestion (Kerley B lines) or pulmonary oedema.

• **Biochemistry**: electrolytes, renal function and haematology (anaemia). Thyroid function.

• **Nuclear isotope scanning**: useful for accurate measurement of ejection fraction (isotope ventriculography or multiple-gated acquisition scans [MUGA]) or the presence of hibernating myocardium (living heart muscle, currently not contracting as a result of a tight coronary stenosis in the nutrient artery, which will contract if the blood flow is improved by percutaneous coronary intervention [PCI] or coronary artery bypass graft [CABG]).

• **Cardiac catheterization**: in all unexplained heart failure to exclude critical coronary artery disease, or to assess CAD severity and treatment options in those with known ischaemic heart disease (IHD).

• **24-h ECG** recording to investigate arrhythmias.

Treatment

• **General measures**: treat the underlying cause and any arrhythmias.

Reduce salt and water intake, monitor treatment by daily weights. Treat hypertension and CAD risk factors vigorously.

• **Diuretics** are the mainstay of symptomatic treatment. The dose should be sufficient largely to remove pulmonary and/or peripheral oedema. Principal side effect is hypokalaemia (give K$^+$ supplements or sparing diuretic, e.g. amiloride). **Spironolactone**, a potassium-sparing diuretic (aldosterone antagonism), improves prognosis in severe CHF.

• **ACE inhibitors** block conversion of angiotensin I to II, interrupting the maladaptive neuroendocrine response, vasodilating and lowering blood pressure. Several large randomized controlled trials show they improve symptoms, quality of life and prognosis in overt heart failure or impaired LV function. May provoke renal failure in bilateral renal artery stenosis (check U&Es). The most common other side effect is a persistent dry cough in 15%.

• **Angiotensin II receptor antagonists**, e.g. losartan, block angiotensin II by direct antagonism of its receptor. Similar effects and benefits as angiotensin-converting enzyme (ACE) inhibitors.

• **β-Blockers**, e.g. bisoprolol, metoprolol and carvedilol, previously felt to be contraindicated in heart failure. However, high circulating catecholamines and down-regulation of adrenergic receptors are detrimental in heart failure. β-Blockers (started **only in stable patients**, at very low doses, increased slowly) reverse these abnormalities and improve functional status and prognosis. Reduce both pump failure and arrhythmic sudden deaths.

• **Digoxin** has a positive inotropic effect in sinus rhythm and results in symptomatic improvement and a reduction in hospital admissions, although it has no mortality benefit.

• **Multisite ventricular pacing**: in advanced heart failure, not infrequently, 'dyscoordinate' ventricular contraction occurs. This means that, instead of the physiological situation, where the conducting tissue ensures that all parts of the ventricle contract fairly simultaneously, different parts of the ventricle contract at different times. This leads to a loss of cardiac output, as blood can move around the ventricle, as one segment contracts against a segment yet to contract, rather than contribute to cardiac output. This condition is suspected by finding a broad QRS complex on the standard ECG, and confirmed by measuring the difference between the onset of the QRS complex to pulmonary and aortic blood ejection (easily done from the cardiac ultrasound). Patients with dyscoordinate contraction benefit from complex pacemakers: in addition to the standard atrial lead, leads are place in the apex of the right ventricle and the lateral wall of the left ventricle (via the coronary sinus). This two ventricular leads allow simultaneous activation of two widely separated parts of the ventricle, so minimising dyscoordinate contraction and maximising cardiac output. Cardiac resynchronisation therapy CRT improves symptoms and lowers mortality. It can be combined with implantable defibrillator therapy (see below).

Complications

• **Thromboembolism**: the risk of venous clot (deep venous thrombosis or DVT and pulmonary embolism or PE) and of systemic emboli is high, especially in severe CHF. It may be reduced by warfarin.

• **AF** commonly complicates CHF, when it can provoke a dramatic deterioration. Rate control (digoxin/β-blocker) and warfarin are indicated.

• **Progressive pump failure** may respond to increasing doses of diuretics. Heart transplantation is an option in selected patients.

• **Ventricular arrhythmias** are common, may cause syncope or **sudden cardiac death** (25–50% of deaths in CHF). In those successfully resuscitated, amiodarone, β-blockers and implantable defibrillators have a role. ICDs also have a prophylactic role in a few.

77 Aortic valve disease

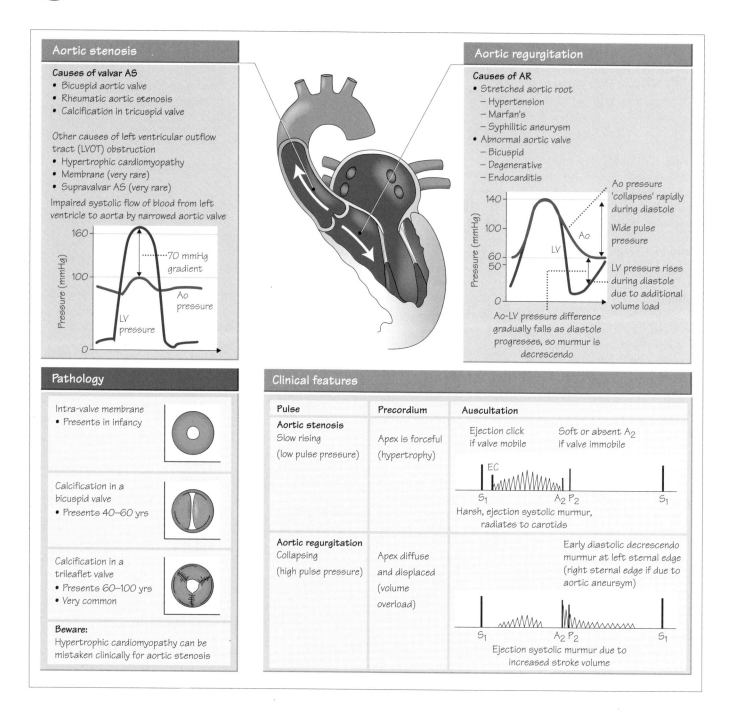

Aortic stenosis

Causes of valvar AS
- Bicuspid aortic valve
- Rheumatic aortic stenosis
- Calcification in tricuspid valve

Other causes of left ventricular outflow tract (LVOT) obstruction
- Hypertrophic cardiomyopathy
- Membrane (very rare)
- Supravalvar AS (very rare)

Impaired systolic flow of blood from left ventricle to aorta by narrowed aortic valve

Aortic regurgitation

Causes of AR
- Stretched aortic root
  - Hypertension
  - Marfan's
  - Syphilitic aneurysm
- Abnormal aortic valve
  - Bicuspid
  - Degenerative
  - Endocarditis

Ao pressure 'collapses' rapidly during diastole

Wide pulse pressure

LV pressure rises during diastole due to additional volume load

Ao-LV pressure difference gradually falls as diastole progresses, so murmur is decrescendo

Pathology

Intra-valve membrane
- Presents in infancy

Calcification in a bicuspid valve
- Presents 40–60 yrs

Calcification in a trileaflet valve
- Presents 60–100 yrs
- Very common

Beware:
Hypertrophic cardiomyopathy can be mistaken clinically for aortic stenosis

Clinical features

Pulse	Precordium	Auscultation
Aortic stenosis Slow rising (low pulse pressure)	Apex is forceful (hypertrophy)	Ejection click if valve mobile / Soft or absent A2 if valve immobile. Harsh, ejection systolic murmur, radiates to carotids
Aortic regurgitation Collapsing (high pulse pressure)	Apex diffuse and displaced (volume overload)	Early diastolic decrescendo murmur at left sternal edge (right sternal edge if due to aortic aneursym). Ejection systolic murmur due to increased stroke volume

Aortic stenosis

There are three causes of aortic stenosis:

1 Congenital aortic stenosis: this is very rare, and may be the result of a bicuspid valve, or a subaortic membrane, constricting the left ventricular (LV) outflow tract.

2 Premature calcification of a congenitally **bicuspid aortic valve**: patients typically develop symptoms from age 40 years onwards.

3 Calcific aortic stenosis of a normal valve: this is an exceptionally common valve lesion, occurring from age 65 years onwards. At aged 80

years, about 10% of the population have aortic stenosis. Calcification occurs earlier in those with renal failure or hypercholesterolaemia, where it can be found in those aged 20 years.

Symptoms

There is a classic triad of symptoms associated with aortic stenosis. All are exertional and progressive:
- **Effort dyspnoea**.
- **Effort angina**.

- **Effort dizziness or syncope.**
- **Sudden cardiac death**: this is the 'non-classic' fourth symptom of aortic stenosis, and is very rare in those without any of the above symptoms, but becomes increasingly likely as other symptoms develop. It is for this reason that asymptomatic patients are followed up, whereas symptomatic patients undergo valve replacement surgery.

Angina at rest is caused by concomitant coronary disease, not aortic stenosis. Syncope at rest is usually the result of atrioventricular (AV) block (e.g. complete heart block) because concomitant conducting tissue disease is very common.

Signs

Ejection systolic murmur, which is often harsh and loud. The area where the murmur is heard loudest varies. Usually it is the middle of the left sternal edge, sometimes in the 'aortic' area (second right intercostal space), and occasionally in the 'mitral' area, i.e. at the apex (fifth intercostal space, midclavicular line). The murmur often radiates into the carotids. Slow rising pulse, absent second heart sound and signs of LV hypertrophy (LVH) indicate severity. Signs of complicating heart failure may also be present.

Investigation

Echocardiography allows assessment of LV function, valve structure (e.g. bicuspid or tricuspid, calcified or not) and severity of stenosis. Stenosis severity is usually quoted as the peak velocity of blood (determined from the Doppler ultrasonic probe) through the valve (values of 3.5 m/s indicate that the aortic stenosis may be sufficiently severe to cause symptoms). This peak velocity can be used to estimate the (instantaneous) pressure drop over the valve (making a number of assumptions), using the formula:

$$\text{Pressure drop (mmHg)} = 4 \times (\text{Peak velocity})^2$$

Occasionally, the valve area is estimated, especially if LV function is poor. Cardiac catheterization is now rarely used to measure valve function, but is commonly used once the decision to proceed with surgery has been made, to determine whether there is coronary disease that may need bypass grafting at the same time. A chest X-ray is not useful in making the diagnosis, although it is if complicating heart failure is suspected. An ECG may show LVH, and occasionally conducting tissue disease (calcium from the valve 'burrows' down into the interventricular septum, interfering with electrical impulse propagation).

Treatment

Anti-endocarditis advice: in the absence of symptoms, medical therapy monitors LV function and the severity of the stenosis. When symptoms occur or the left ventricle deteriorates, there is a high risk of deterioration as a result of heart failure or sudden death, and valve replacement within 2 months is indicated.

Aortic regurgitation

There are two pathologies that give rise to aortic regurgitation (AR). They can be usually distinguished echocardiographically:

1 Disease processes affecting the aortic valve (including rheumatic heart disease, endocarditis, SLE). Calcific aortic stenosis is often associated with significant AR.

2 Diseases resulting in dilatation of the aortic root and thus the aortic valve ring (including aortic aneurysm caused by hypertension, Marfan's syndrome, ankylosing spondylitis or syphilis, or the rarer annulo-ectasia, which is idiopathic dilatation of the aortic root). Aortic dissection disrupts the aortic root, causing acute AR.

Symptoms

With gradual-onset AR, even if the leak is severe, symptoms are often mild or absent. If the leak worsens, or if LV decompensation occurs, exertional dyspnoea can develop, which when severe may happen at rest.

Signs

Collapsing pulse with volume-overloaded left ventricle (hyperdynamic apex beat). The diastolic BP, which relates directly to how much blood has leaked back from the aorta into the left ventricle, is a good guide to the severity of chronic AR (low diastolic BP = severe AR). Wide pulse pressure may cause:
- Corrigan's sign (visible carotid pulsations)
- de Musset's sign (head bobbing)
- Quinke's sign (nail-bed pulsations)
- Pistol shot femorals (also known as Traube's phenomenon; auscultation over the femoral arteries reveals a loud sound during systole, likened to a pistol shot, due to the large forward stroke volume)
- Duroziez's murmur, a to-and-fro murmur heard when the femoral artery is auscultated, and slight pressure placed on the stethoscope, relates to the large forward and then backward flow in the aorta from the AR.

An early diastolic murmur is heard along the left sternal edge (with the patient leaning forward in end-expiration), unless the AR is caused by an aortic root aneurysm, when the murmur is loudest along the right sternal edge. The murmur may be surprisingly loud in mild AR, and is often quiet in very severe AR, or if the lesion is acute as, for example, in endocarditis.

Investigation

Echocardiography is useful for monitoring LV function, determining whether the regurgitation is the result of a valve or aortic root problem, and determining its severity. Although the aortic root diameter can be measured, if there is substantial enlargement, computed tomography (CT) or magnetic resonance imaging (MRI) of the thoracic aorta is needed to determine how much of the aortic arch (and descending aorta) is enlarged. Chest X-ray may show an enlarged heart, or aortic aneurysm. ECG usually shows LVH. Coronary angiography is useful to assess for concomitant coronary disease once surgery has been decided on.

Treatment

Angiotensin-converting enzyme inhibitors (possibly other vasodilators such as calcium channel blockers) and diuretics may maintain LV function for many years in the face of significant AR. Increasing LV dimensions and symptoms are indications for AV replacement. If AR is the result of dilatation of the aortic root, valve and root replacements are necessary.

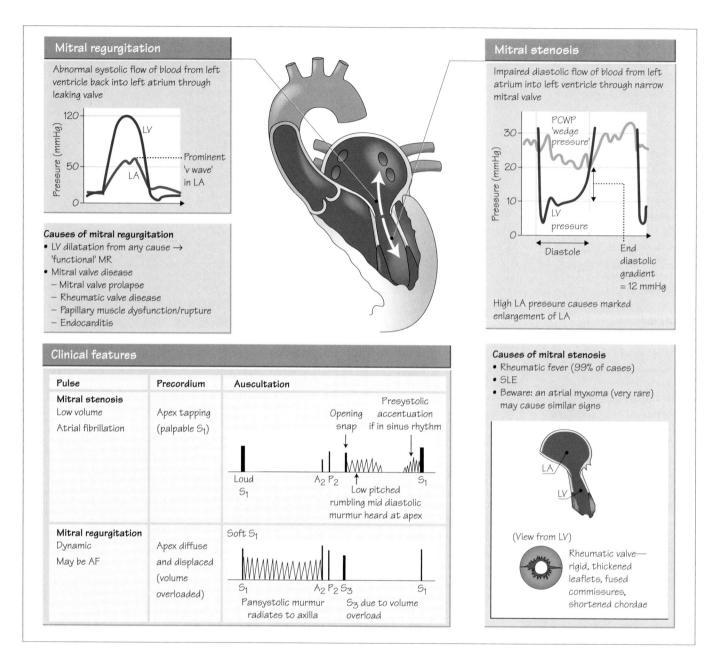

Mitral stenosis

Although on a worldwide basis mitral stenosis (MS) is still very common, this is now a relatively rare lesion in the developed world, because of the decline in the incidence of rheumatic valve disease. In practice, all mitral stenosis relates to previous rheumatic fever.

Symptoms

Half of those diagnosed have documented/remembered childhood rheumatic fever. Symptomatic MS develops within a few years in deprived communities, but may take decades in the West. Typically there is the gradual onset of progressive exertional dyspnoea, as a

result of chronic heart failure, in those aged 40–50 years. Sudden and severe symptoms occur with the onset of atrial fibrillation (AF). MS with AF is a very potent substrate for systemic thromboemboli (e.g. a stroke) that are sometimes the first manifestation of the lesion.

Signs

- Female > male.
- Mitral facies (malar flush).
- May be signs of chronic heart failure (CHF): elevated jugular venous pressure (JVP), oedema.
- Usually atrial fibrillation AF.

- Right ventricular (RV) 'heave' if secondary pulmonary hypertension.
- 'Tapping' apex beat (palpable S1), which is undisplaced in the absence of significant mitral regurgitation.
- Low-pitched, rumbling, mid-diastolic murmur, best heard with the bell in left lateral position.
- Opening snap (rigid valve opening) precedes murmur.

Investigations

Echocardiography confirms the diagnosis and follows disease progression. The valve may be 'rheumatic' (thickened and distorted). The velocity of the blood flow during diastole through the mitral valve can be measured using the Doppler probe. In normal individuals this starts high, then declines rapidly as diastole proceeds; a much slower velocity decline is found in MS, and the severity of MS can be deduced from the rate of velocity decline ('the pressure half-time'). Pulmonary hypertension can also often be diagnosed from Doppler measurements of regurgitant blood through the tricuspid valve. Concomitant mitral regurgitation and aortic valve disease likewise can be diagnosed and followed up. ECG may show left atrial enlargement (when in sinus rhythm) or AF. In pulmonary hypertension, a dominant R wave may appear in chest lead V1. Chest X-ray may show left atrial enlargement (cardiomegaly, 'splayed' tracheal bifurcation).

Treatment

- **Medical therapy** (with diuretics, digoxin and warfarin) maintains good functional status for decades. The only indication for surgery is symptoms not controlled by drugs.
- **Surgical treatment**: there are two approaches:
- **Mitral valvotomy**: this can be carried out percutaneously in some, using a balloon, or at thoracotomy (often made over the left lung, so as to gain easy access to the valve through the left atrium)
- **Mitral valve replacement**: this is a common operation. Usually a mechanical valve (rather than biological one) is used because warfarin is already indicated on account of the AF.

Differential diagnosis of mitral stenosis

Very rarely, similar symptoms and signs are caused by an atrial myxoma, a benign tumour, usually found in the left atrium attached to the interatrial septum, which grows sufficient to impede mitral diastolic blood flow. It causes episodic or progressive breathlessness, and occasionally fever, weight loss with an elevated erythrocyte sedimentation rate (ESR). Cardiac ultrasonography is diagnostic. Immediate surgery is usually curative.

Mitral prolapse

In mitral valve prolapse (MVP) (Barlow's syndrome), the mitral valve is larger than usual and/or the chordae attached to the mitral valve are too long. As a consequence of this, a component of the mitral valve 'prolapses' back into the left atrium during ventricular systole. There may or may not be mitral regurgitation (MR; see below). In MVP without MR, the usual signs are of a 'click', heard in early mid-systole. The 'click' of MVP can be a rather intermittent phenomenon. There is some controversy about whether MVP without MR causes symptoms: most cardiologists feel that it probably does not. MVP with MR predisposes to bacterial endocarditis (see Chapter 82).

Mitral regurgitation

Mitral regurgitation is an extremely common valve lesion. Like aortic regurgitation (AR), there are two underlying pathologies:
- Those caused by **intrinsic valve disease** (e.g. myxomatous degeneration, rheumatic heart disease, infective endocarditis), disease of the valve-related apparatus (e.g. chordal rupture, as in some cases of floppy mitral valve) or of the papillary muscles (e.g. dysfunction/rupture resulting from ischaemia/infarction, usually of the circumflex artery)
- **Secondary** (also termed 'functional') caused by stretching of the valve ring when the left ventricle is dilated, as in many cases of left heart failure. The MR murmur may become dramatically quieter as the heart failure responds to treatment.

Symptoms

Patients are often asymptomatic for many years, unless the lesion has occurred/progressed over a very short time span. Unfortunately, during this asymptomatic period left ventricular (LV) function may be permanently damaged. Symptoms when they occur are those of heart failure, such as breathlessness, effort intolerance and fatigue.

Signs

- Displaced, diffuse apex resulting from volume overload.
- Loud pansystolic murmur at apex.
- Functional MR may not be pansystolic.
- The murmur radiates up the left ventricular outflow tract (i.e. is heard along the left sternal edge/aortic area) in posterior leaflet mitral valve prolapse, and is heard in the back in anterior mitral valve leaflet prolapse.

Investigation

Echocardiography can be helpful in establishing both the presence of mitral regurgitation and its mechanism. Often, transthoracic echocardiography (TTE) provides a good estimate of the severity of the mitral regurgitation, but this is not always true, and sometimes transoesophageal echocardiography (TOE) is needed to determine severity more accurately. This is particularly true if an artificial mitral valve is present (i.e. previous mitral valve replacement). Cardiac ultrasonography is also useful in monitoring LV function, although this can easily be overestimated. Chest X-ray is useful for diagnosing heart failure. ECG often shows LV hypertrophy, and may show AF.

Treatment

Initially medical therapy with diuretics and angiotensin-converting enzyme inhibitors are used; they can control symptoms and maintain systolic function of LV for years in the face of severe MR. In intrinsic valve disease, when are symptoms intrusive, or if the LV enlarges progressively, surgery is indicated. Prognosis after mitral valve repair is better than after mitral valve replacement.

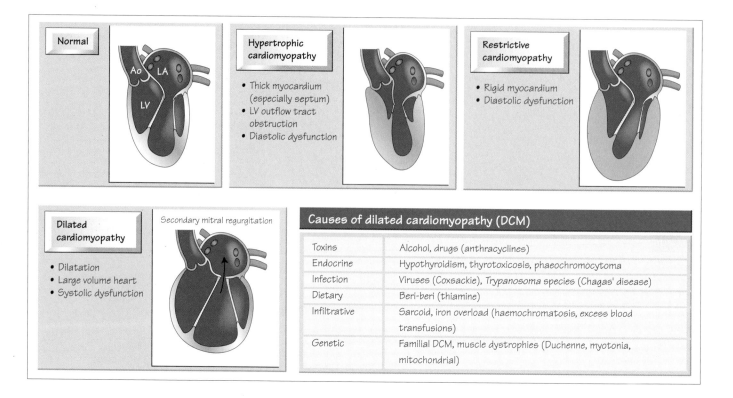

Causes of dilated cardiomyopathy (DCM)

Toxins	Alcohol, drugs (anthracyclines)
Endocrine	Hypothyroidism, thyrotoxicosis, phaeochromocytoma
Infection	Viruses (Coxsackie), *Trypanosoma* species (Chagas' disease)
Dietary	Beri-beri (thiamine)
Infiltrative	Sarcoid, iron overload (haemochromatosis, excess blood transfusions)
Genetic	Familial DCM, muscle dystrophies (Duchenne, myotonia, mitochondrial)

Cardiomyopathies are **primary heart muscle diseases**. They are uncommon but not rare, e.g. dilated cardiomyopathy underlies 5–10% of heart failure. Cardiomyopathies are classified according to the echocardiographic findings.

Dilated cardiomyopathy

Dilated cardiomyopathy (DCM) causes left ventricular (LV) (and often right ventricular [RV]) enlargement, and often massive and global hypokinesia (rather than regional, which would suggest coronary artery disease [CAD]). Clinically, LV or congestive cardiac failure occurs, often severe and progressive, with displacement of the apex beat and prominent S3. Functional mitral regurgitation (MR) and atrial fibrillation (AF) are common. There is a high risk of thromboembolism. The chest X-ray shows a large heart. Several illnesses can cause **secondary DCM**, the most common of which is **excess alcohol**. 'Idiopathic' or 'primary' DCM is a diagnosis of exclusion. One-third of cases have a family history, suggesting a significant genetic contribution. **Treatment** is standard heart failure therapy. **Cardiac transplantation** is an important option for younger patients with severe refractory heart failure.

Hypertrophic cardiomyopathy

Hypertrophic cardiomyopathy (HCM) is a genetic disease characterized by asymmetrical hypertrophy of the LV myocardium, especially the septum. The myocardial structure is abnormal (**myocyte disarray** and **interstitial fibrosis**). Gross hypertrophy results in a small LV cavity, diastolic dysfunction and secondary MR. Septal hypertrophy results in dynamic LV outflow tract obstruction. Often asymptomatic, but severe, hypertrophy and outflow tract obstruction may cause exer-

tion breathlessness, chest pain or dizziness. The greatest risk is of collapse or sudden death as a result of ventricular arrhythmias, which may be unheralded and occur in otherwise fit patients. HCM is most commonly caused by mutations in genes encoding a variety of contractile proteins including myosin, actin, troponins, and myosin binding protein C. Different mutations in different genes are associated with variations in the phenotype, including the age of onset, severity of hypertrophy and risk of sudden death from arrhythmias. Treatment is:
• **β-Blockers** or **calcium channel antagonists** are used to treat exertional symptoms.
• **Amiodarone** is used in those at high risk of ventricular tachycardia. Implantable defibrillators (ICDs) may be justified in patients with high risk and/or a strong family history of sudden death.
• **Genetic counselling** and **screening** of asymptomatic family members by echocardiography are important aspects of management.

Restrictive cardiomyopathy

Restrictive cardiomyopathy (RCM) results in a rigid, stiff and thickened myocardium, usually as a result of myocardial infiltration by abnormal materials or of fibrosis. It causes congestive cardiac failure resulting from diastolic dysfunction, which is manifest predominantly as RV failure. These are rare. The most common is amyloid (primary amyloid AL type, e.g. multiple myeloma/paraproteinaemia or in secondary amyloid AA type, e.g. chronic inflammatory conditions). Other causes include sarcoid, scleroderma, endomyocardial fibrosis and hypereosinophilic syndromes. RCM is usually refractory to treatment. Symptomatic cardiac amyloid has a very poor prognosis. Treatment is usually limited to diuretics to reduce features of right heart failure.

Diseases and Treatments at a Glance

80 Pericardial disease

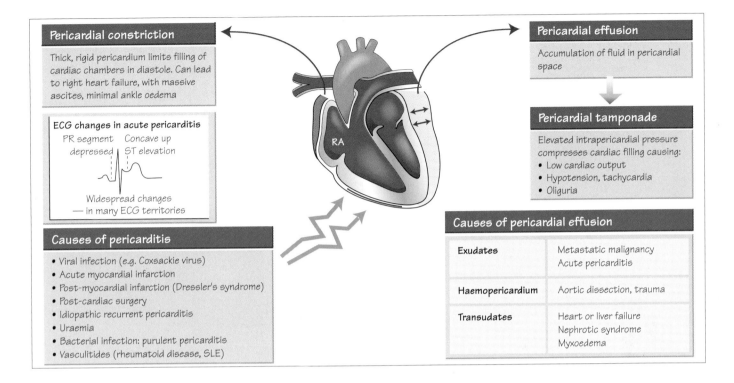

Pericardial constriction

Thick, rigid pericardium limits filling of cardiac chambers in diastole. Can lead to right heart failure, with massive ascites, minimal ankle oedema

ECG changes in acute pericarditis

PR segment depressed | Concave up ST elevation

Widespread changes — in many ECG territories

Causes of pericarditis

- Viral infection (e.g. Coxsackie virus)
- Acute myocardial infarction
- Post-myocardial infarction (Dressler's syndrome)
- Post-cardiac surgery
- Idiopathic recurrent pericarditis
- Uraemia
- Bacterial infection: purulent pericarditis
- Vasculitides (rheumatoid disease, SLE)

Pericardial effusion

Accumulation of fluid in pericardial space

Pericardial tamponade

Elevated intrapericardial pressure compresses cardiac filling causing:
- Low cardiac output
- Hypotension, tachycardia
- Oliguria

Causes of pericardial effusion

Exudates	Metastatic malignancy Acute pericarditis
Haemopericardium	Aortic dissection, trauma
Transudates	Heart or liver failure Nephrotic syndrome Myxoedema

Pericardial disease presents as one of four syndromes. **Pericarditis** describes inflammation of the pericardium, either acute or chronic. The accumulation of fluid within the pericardial space, **pericardial effusion**, can result in **pericardial tamponade**. Chronic or recurrent pericarditis may result in fibrosis of the pericardium, adherence of the visceral and parietal layers and **pericardial constriction**.

Acute pericarditis

Pleuritic chest pain, often positional, classically relieved by sitting forwards. Many patients experience only a dull central ache without any specific features. A **pericardial rub** may be heard, often only in one position or on inspiration. There may be fever or systemic features. ECG shows **ST segment elevation** that is **concave upwards**, typically **affecting leads in multiple territories**, not one territory as in myocardial infarction (MI). Echocardiography may demonstrate a small pericardial effusion. Specific tests may demonstrate the cause. NSAIDs reduce the pain and inflammation.

Pericardial effusion

Pericardial effusion refers to the accumulation of fluid within the pericardial space. The effusion is categorized according to the protein content of the fluid into **transudates** (high protein), **exudates** (low protein) or bloody (**haemopericardium**). Occasionally the effusion is **purulent** as a result of bacterial infection. **Cardiac tamponade** is caused by accumulation of a pericardial effusion to the point where elevated intrapericardial pressures compromise cardiac filling. Slowly enlarging pericardial effusions allow the pericardium to stretch to accommodate the fluid; they may be very large (> 1 L) before tamponade occurs. Rapidly growing effusions cause tamponade early on (the pericardium does not comply). A pericardial rub does **not** exclude tamponade.

Clinical features and treatment of cardiac tamponade

- Low output state (tachycardia, low BP, cold peripheries, oliguria).
- Greatly elevated jugular venous pressure (JVP) (Kussmaul's sign: JVP increases further rather than falls with inspiration).
- Pulsus paradoxus: BP falls with inspiration. Radial pulse may disappear in severe tamponade. Quiet heart sounds, *no* gallop.
- Large 'globular' heart on chest X-ray, but no pulmonary congestion. Echocardiography confirms the presence of large pericardial effusions and evidence of tamponade (diastolic collapse of the atrium early on, and of the right ventricle in advanced cases). A simple pericardial effusion without haemodynamic compromise does not need drainage. In contrast, pericardial tamponade is a medical emergency requiring immediate percutaneous or surgical drainage.

Constrictive pericarditis

Acute, chronic or relapsing pericarditis (often caused by tuberculosis or radiotherapy) may cause pericardial fibrosis sufficient to constrict the heart, impede cardiac filling and decrease cardiac output. Progressive **exertional dyspnoea**, peripheral **oedema** and **ascites** occur.

A greatly elevated JVP; and pericardial knock (loud diastolic heart sound) are seen. CT/MRI suggests, and cardiac catheterization proves the diagnosis. Diuretics relieve symptoms. Surgery may help.

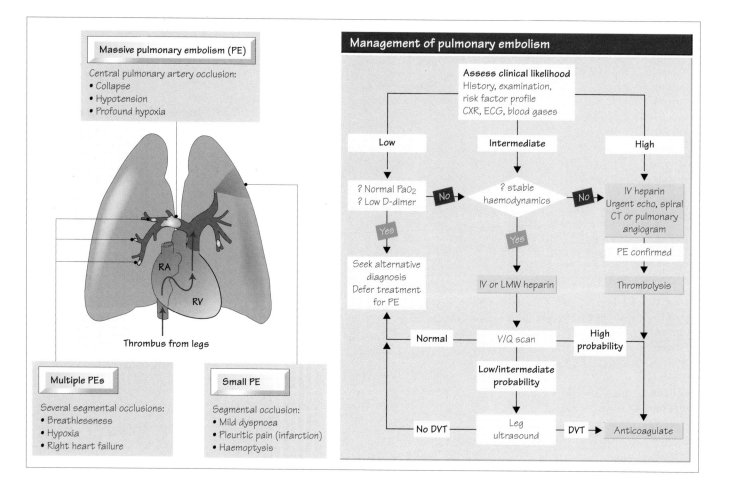

Definition

Pulmonary embolisms (PEs) result when thrombi (often from the deep veins of the thigh or pelvis) embolize via the right heart into the pulmonary arteries.

Risk factors

Predisposing factors are found in 90% of patients and are an important clue to diagnosis. They comprise:

- Surgery less than 12 weeks ago.
- Immobilization for more than 3 days in the last 4 weeks.
- Previous deep venous thrombosis (DVT)/PE or family history.
- Lower limb fracture.
- Malignancy.
- Postpartum.

Clinical features

The clinical presentation of PE can be varied, so a high degree of clinical suspicion is required. PEs cause hypoxia from ventilation–perfusion mismatch, interrupt pulmonary blood flow, causing pulmonary infarcts (so inflaming the pleura) and lowering cardiac output; these features are responsible for the **three distinct clinical syndromes** with which pulmonary thromboembolic disease present:

1 Pleurisy and/or haemoptysis: small or moderate-sized PEs cause pulmonary infarction. *Dyspnoea is absent or minor*.

2 Dyspnoea with hypoxia in the absence of other causes, this suggests a moderate or large PE or repeated PEs over a period of time. There may be signs of cardiopulmonary disturbance (tachycardia, tachypnoea, elevated jugular venous pressure (JVP), left parasternal lift from acute right heart strain). *Pleurisy/haemoptysis is often absent*.

3 Circulatory collapse: large or massive PE. Typically a high-risk patient (e.g. post-surgery) with unheralded collapse or unexplained clinical deterioration, and with hypotension, tachycardia and hypoxia.

Investigations

An assessment of the likelihood of PE, based on clinical, blood gas and chest X-ray parameters remains central to the diagnosis of PE, and directs early therapy. Later therapy is guided by more specific tests, e.g. ventilation-perfusion ($\dot{V}/\dot{Q}$) scans, although these often suggest rather than confirm the diagnosis.

- **Chest X-ray**: excludes other conditions, e.g. pneumonia, pneumothorax, pulmonary oedema. In PE, the chest X-ray abnormalities are minimal/minor in relation to the degree of cardiorespiratory compromise.
- **Arterial blood gases**: haemodynamically significant PE causes ventilation–perfusion mismatching and hypoxia. Compensatory hyper-

ventilation results in a reduced Pa_{CO_2}. The alveolar–arterial gradient is increased (see p. 176). **In hypoxaemia with a normal/near normal chest X-ray, always consider the diagnosis of PE.**

• **ECG**: abnormalities are common, but are usually non-specific and not diagnostically useful, e.g. sinus tachycardia, minor ST and T-wave abnormalities (especially in V1–3). In large or massive PE, the more classic ECG features of acute right ventricular (RV) strain (S1, Q3, T3), right bundle-branch block (RBBB) or AF may occur.

• **D-dimers** are cross-linked fibrin degradation products. A normal D-dimer level implies a very low probability of PE. High D-dimers are found in many conditions (e.g. recent surgery, malignancy and inflammatory states) including PE.

• **Echocardiography** occasionally detects large thrombi in the pulmonary artery, or the right atrium or ventricle. More commonly, echocardiography shows right heart dilatation and strain (i.e. poor systolic contractile function).

• **Ventilation–perfusion scanning**: isotope $\dot{V}/\dot{Q}$ scanning relies on the fact that a significant PE results in regional hypoperfusion of a segment or lobe of the lung without a corresponding defect in ventilation. To simplify the procedure, a normal chest X-ray is sometimes used as a surrogate to imply normal ventilation. Widely used, but significant diagnostic limitations:

  • **Strengths**: a **high probability scan** or a **normal scan** is diagnostically powerful (> 95%), especially in the setting of high or low clinical suspicion.
  • **Limitations**: 75% of scans are in the low or intermediate categories, which are less useful in confirming or excluding the diagnosis. Even a high-probability $\dot{V}/\dot{Q}$ scan fails to detect > 50% of PEs.

• **Pulmonary angiography**: historically the 'gold standard' investigation for the diagnosis of PE. Invasive, costly. Useful when rapid diagnosis critical, e.g. in critical illness.

• **CT and MRI**: spiral CT and MRI allows imaging of the pulmonary arteries to detect thrombi with high sensitivity and specificity. Increasingly replacing $\dot{V}/\dot{Q}$ scanning and invasive pulmonary angiography.

Treatment (Table 81.1)

• **Oxygen**: should be given to all patients with suspected PE.
• **Heparin**: heparin should be administered when there is clinical suspicion of PE, while investigations are completed. Intravenous heparin for large or massive PE, or subcutaneous low-molecular-weight heparin in small or moderate PE.
• **Thrombolysis**: streptokinase or tissue plasminogen activator (tPA) dissolves thrombi. Indicated for confirmed PE with hypotension, severe hypoxia or other evidence of marked haemodynamic compromise.
• **Warfarin**: initial treatment with heparin should be followed by oral anticoagulation with warfarin once the diagnosis of PE is confirmed, aiming for an international normalized ratio (INR) of 2.5–3.0. If there is a remediable underlying cause (e.g. surgery, immobility), anticoagulation for 6 weeks is adequate. If not, the incidence of recurrent PE is high, so anticoagulation should be continued for longer, often indefinitely.

Table 81.1 Management of pulmonary embolism.

Small PE	Subcutaneous heparin if PE suspected. Warfarin after confirmation of diagnosis with $\dot{V}/\dot{Q}$ scans
Large or massive PE	Immediate high-dose O_2; intravenous heparin and intravenous fluids if chest X-ray and ECG exclude MI/pulmonary oedema
	Consider echocardiography, spiral CT or pulmonary angiography if clinical conditions and local availability allow
	If haemodynamic compromise or deterioration, thrombolysis with tPA, then continued intravenous heparin
	For massive PE, surgical embolectomy is an alternative if immediately available
Multiple chronic PE	Warfarin. Refer for cardiological assessment

MI, myocardial infarction; PE, pulmonary embolism; tPA, tissue plasminogen activator.

Chronic thromboembolic disease

Although the usual mode of presentation of PE is with an acute illness, occasionally patients present with a more chronic picture. The typical history is of several months' progressive breathlessness, markedly limiting the time of presentation. The physical signs are of cyanosis with marked pulmonary hypertension (left parasternal lift, raised jugular venous pressure [JVP], sometimes peripheral oedema). Investigations show marked hypoxaemia; ventilation-perfusion scanning is usually floridly abnormal and CT often shows large thrombi in the central pulmonary arteries. Echocardiography allows determination of the pulmonary artery pressure often = 70–80 mmHg. Treatment is problematic. Much thrombus is endothelialized and does not regress on standard anticoagulant therapy. In a few selected patients surgical pulmonary thromboembolectomy has a role, although the operative mortality rate of > 10% restricts this to highly selected cases.

Thrombophilia

Rare disorders of blood coagulation predispose to thromboembolism, and should be considered in those:

• Aged < 40 with no other risk factor.
• First-degree relative with a history of venous thromboembolism.
• Previous episodes of venous thromboembolism.

Deficiencies of proteins S, protein C or antithrombin III are the most common of these rare disorders (see p. 346). Other procoagulant states include lupus anticoagulant (anticardiolipin antibodies) and homocystinuria. More common are genetic polymorphisms in genes encoding clotting proteins—these increase thromboembolic risk, e.g. factor V Leiden.

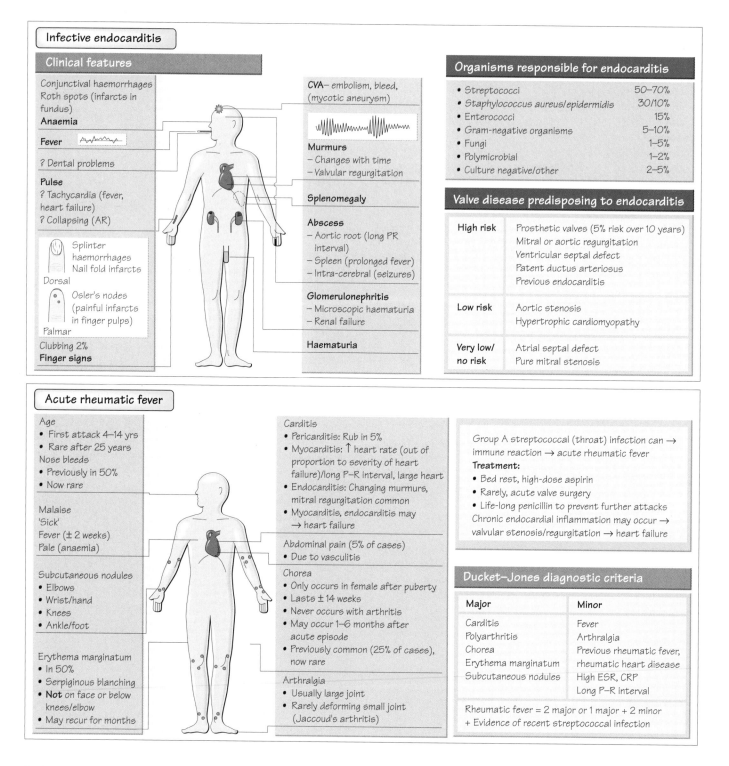

Infective endocarditis

Infection of the lining of the heart, usually heart valves, which are commonly **diseased** or **prosthetic**; 3000 cases/year in the UK.

Aetiology and pathogenesis

Blood-borne organisms settle on a heart valve. Fibrin deposits together with micro-organisms form **vegetations** on a valve leaflet or cusp. The clinical manifestations are from valve damage (heart failure), embolization of infected material from the heart (abscesses, infarction of vital organs) or the immune response to chronic infection (renal failure). The most common source of infection is the **mouth** after dental procedures or a tooth abscess. **Skin infections** (*Staphylococcus aureus*) and the gastrointestinal tract are also common sources. **Intravenous drug abusers** are at risk of tricuspid valve endocarditis and infection with unusual organisms (coliforms, fungi, etc.). **Prosthetic valves** are at high risk of infection: < 3/12 after surgery from skin-related organisms (e.g. *Staph. epidermidis, Staph. aureus*), and later the same organisms as native valves.

Clinical features

Presentation is typically **non-specific**, so a high clinical suspicion is required. Duration of symptoms before diagnosis is often weeks or months.

• **Systemic features** are common, especially with low virulence organisms, e.g. *Streptococcus viridans*. Fatigue, fever, anaemia or weight loss. A common and surprising symptom is back pain of obscure origin.

• **Valve destruction** by infection causes valvular regurgitation, not stenosis, leading to heart failure, new or changing heart murmur; 99% of endocarditis patients have a murmur.

• **Systemic complications** result from 'seeding' of infection caused by bacteraemia or embolism of infected vegetation fragments, leading to new infection or abscess formation at distant sites, and/or manifestations of thromboembolism:

  • Cerebrovascular accident (CVA) from embolism, or haemorrhage resulting from ruptured mycotic aneurysm
  • Finger/toe gangrene caused by embolism ± vasculitis
  • Renal or splenic abscess or infarction
  • Mesenteric embolism (ischaemic bowel and an acute abdomen).

• **Acute renal failure** may occur from immune complex disease, haemodynamic upset (acute heart failure), damage during cardiac surgery, and nephrotoxic antibiotics. Close monitoring of renal function throughout the illness is mandatory.

The physical examination often only reveals evidence of fever (temperature), mild weight loss, murmurs and sometimes complicating heart failure. Rarely (< 2%) clubbing is found. Splinter haemorrhages are more common (50%). More substantial hand infarcts (Osler's nodes) are very rare but pathognomonic. Splenomegaly is common. Dipstick haematuria is almost universal.

Investigations

• **Blood tests**: the most important investigation is **blood culture**, three sets of which detect bacterial endocarditis in 97% of cases.

  • Systemic inflammatory markers: erythrocyte sedimentation rate (ESR), C-reactive protein (CRP) are usually elevated
  • Anaemia of chronic disease, elevated white cell count
  • Urine dipstick and microscopy (haematuria).

• **Echocardiography** is important, but only rarely makes the diagnosis, and **can never exclude endocarditis**. Echocardiography is more important in assessing the degree and consequences of valvular damage and guiding subsequent management.

• **Transoesophageal echocardiography** is useful when transthoracic images are unclear or with prosthetic valves, because higher resolution allows more detailed imaging. It is also useful in assessing complications of endocarditis (abscess formation or acute valvular destruction) before surgery.

Treatment and prognosis

Antibiotic therapy is the mainstay of treatment, based on blood culture findings and organism sensitivities. This requires close collaboration with microbiologists. Antibiotics are usually **intravenous**, often in **drug combinations** in order to attain best antibacterial killing and tissue penetration. Treatment commonly continues for 4 or 6 weeks. **Surgery** to remove and replace the infected valve is sometimes indicated for:

• Severe valvular destruction causing heart failure.
• Abscess formation.
• Failure to eradicate infection despite prolonged antibiotic therapy.
• Prosthetic valve endocarditis.

Prognosis is variable, but overall mortality rate is 10–20%.

Antibiotic prophylaxis to prevent infective endocarditis

Patients with known valvular disease or prosthetic valves should have antibiotics before undergoing procedures that provoke bacteraemia (*dental procedures involving the gums* and other invasive procedures, e.g. lower gastrointestinal endoscopy). Further details are found in the *British National Formulary*.

Myocarditis

Myocarditis is inflammation of the heart muscle caused by:

• **Viral infections**, e.g. Coxsackie, mumps and influenza. Subclinical infection is common in HIV infection.
• **Bacterial infection** may occur in severe septicaemia, although other features dominate the clinical picture.
• **Radiation exposure**: much commoner before targeted beam therapy.
• **Autoimmune disease**: the commoner myocarditis on a worldwide basis is rheumatic fever (see figure).
• **Toxin damage** such as from diphtheria infection.

The clinical features depend on the severity and duration of the inflammation. In **acute myocarditis** the dominant feature is acute heart failure. The patient may be severely unwell, breathless, in a low output state. The clue that myocarditis is present is that the tachycardia is out of proportion to the severity of the heart failure. A particularly distressing manifestation of acute myocarditis is **sudden cardiac death**, which may be more prevalent in athletic sufferers. In **chronic myocarditis**, e.g. South American trypanosomiasis (*Trypanosoma cruzii*) infection, patients may present with chronic heart failure. Investigations:

• **Echocardiography** shows impaired systolic contractile function, and in chronic processes dilatation of the left ventricle and atrium.
• **Cardiac enzymes** are elevated and, unlike myocardial infarction (MI), often stay high for many days or weeks before declining.
• **Inflammatory markers**: CRP and ESR are usually high.
• **Serological tests** may reveal the responsible organism.

Treatment and prognosis

There is rarely any specific treatment. Standard anti-heart-failure therapy is given (see Chapter 76). The prognosis in acute severe myocarditis is good provided that life can be maintained; this may require circulatory support with an implantable left ventricular (LV) assist device. In refractory cases cardiac transplantation should be considered.

Pericarditis (see Chapter 80)

Rheumatic fever (see figure)

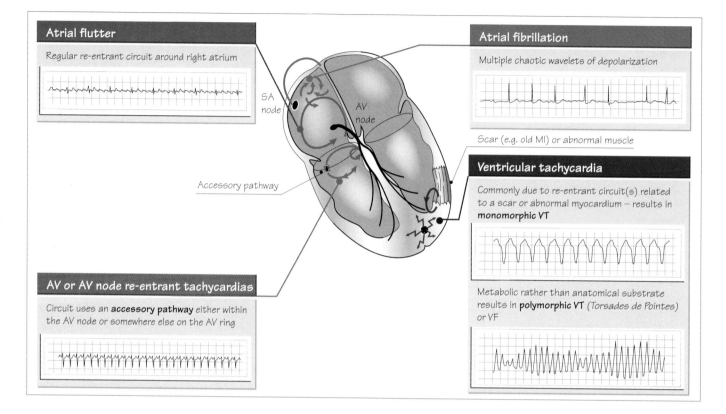

Arrhythmias are abnormal heartbeats, either fast (tachyarrhythmias) or slow (bradyarrhythmias). Minor arrhythmias are universal. The most common sustained arrhythmia, atrial fibrillation, occurs in 1% of those aged 50 or more, and 10% of the over-80s. Sudden cardiac death is often the result of arrhythmias (usually VT and VF) and causes 15–40% of deaths in coronary artery disease (CAD) or heart failure.

Clinical features

Arrhythmias may be asymptomatic, cause intermittent minor palpitation, or be the cause of blackouts, severe cardiovascular compromise or cardiac arrest. **Palpitation** is the symptom that describes an abnormal awareness of the heartbeat; however, it does not necessarily mean that the heart rhythm is abnormal.

Key facts for understanding arrhythmias

The heartbeat is controlled by the fastest pacemaker focus. During a tachyarrhythmia, the normal sinus node depolarizations are 'suppressed' by the faster depolarizations of the abnormal focus. The surface ECG is a 'superimposed' graph of both atrial and ventricular activity. Atrial and ventricular activity are not necessarily linked during arrhythmias, so atrial and ventricular activity need to be considered separately. Arrhythmias are categorized according to where the initial depolarization originates:

• **Supraventricular arrhythmias** originate in the atria or around the atrioventricular (AV) node.
• **Ventricular arrhythmias** originate in the ventricles.

In the normal heart, the **only** communication between the atria and ventricles is the AV node, so the ventricular rate during arrhythmias arising in the atria is governed not just by the arrhythmia itself, but by conduction through the AV node. The normal AV node acts as a 'turnstile', because it conducts depolarizations slowly and is refractory for a relatively long period after each depolarization. Abnormal additional conducting pathways between the atria and ventricles ('accessory pathways') are common, and in some people may allow depolarizations to spread from atria to ventricles, or from ventricles to atria, without necessarily passing fully through the AV node. This allows re-entry circuits to be set up, and in some circumstances bypasses the normal 'safety valve' of the AV node.

Supraventricular tachyarrhythmias (SVT)
AV-reciprocating tachycardias (paroxysmal SVT)
Pathogenesis

A re-entrant circuit is set up by the presence of an accessory pathway, an additional conducting pathway:

• Between the atria and ventricles, causing AV re-entrant tachycardia (AVRT). This additional pathway may be seen in the ECG during normal sinus rhythm (see below).
• Between the atrium and the AV node to form a complete circuit within the AV node: this is the most common additional pathway and underlies AV nodal re-entrant tachycardia (AVNRT).

ECG diagnosis

Regular, narrow QRS complex tachycardia, usually at a rate of 150–200 beats/min. Regular P waves may be visible interspersed between the QRS complexes.

Clinical features
Usually presents as recurrent attacks of rapid palpitation, lasting from a few minutes to hours or even days.

Treatment
Slowing conduction through the AV node may stop the tachycardia:
- **Vagotonic manoeuvres** that increase vagal tone, e.g. Valsalva manoeuvre, swallowing cold drinks or carotid sinus massage; patients may discover these themselves.
- **Drug treatment** slows or blocks conduction in the AV node.
  - **Intravenous adenosine** transiently (≤ 4 s) blocks AV node conduction, terminating any tachycardia using the AV node as part of the circuit (i.e. both AVRT and AVNRT), so restoring sinus rhythm.
  - **β-Blockers, verapamil or flecainide** is an alternative, useful as long-term oral prophylaxis or intermittent therapy.
- **Radiofrequency ablation** is the treatment of choice if symptoms are severe enough for long-term medication. During an electrophysiological study, applying radiofrequency energy through a catheter destroys the accessory pathway. Successful ablation cures the patient.

Accessory pathways, pre-excitation and the Wolff–Parkinson–White (WPW) syndrome
An accessory pathway, which conducts atrial depolarizations directly into the ventricular myocardium, bypassing the AV node, characterizes the WPW syndrome: **pre-excitation, AV reciprocating tachycardias** (see above) and **pre-excited AF** may occur.
- **Pre-excitation**: atrial impulses are propagated more quickly to the ventricle by the accessory pathway than by the normal AV node. The part of the myocardium into which the accessory pathway is inserted depolarizes earlier (i.e. is **pre-excited**) than the part of the ventricle depolarized by the normally conducted beat. This **shortens the PR interval**. Electrical activity propagates slowly from the pre-excited ventricular myocardium by myocyte-to-myocyte transmission, not through specialized conducting tissue, so slurring the first part of the QRS complex (δ wave).
- **Atrial fibrillation (AF)**: normally the AV node acts as a 'safety valve' preventing an over-rapid ventricular response in AF. Some accessory pathways conduct impulses more frequently than the normal AV node, allowing AF to be conducted to the ventricles at ≤ 250 beats/min, shortening diastole, impairing ventricular filling and lessening cardiac output, so that haemodynamic collapse or ventricular fibrillation ('sudden cardiac death') occurs. The ECG in 'pre-excited' AF has very abnormal, wide QRS complexes, because ventricular depolarization is largely from the impulse conducted down the accessory pathway. Pre-excited AF is treated with immediate DC cardioversion. As a result of the tendency for fast pre-excited AF, all patients with WPW **must** have formal electrophysiological studies to ascertain the conducting potential of the accessory pathway. If it is high then the pathway is ablated.

Atrial fibrillation (AF)
Pathophysiology
The atria depolarize spontaneously in a rapid (frequently > 300/min), uncoordinated fashion, bombarding the AV node continuously with electrical impulses. Conduction to the ventricles is limited by AV node refractoriness (often to < 200 beats/min) and occurs unpredictably, causing a completely irregular ventricular response.

ECG diagnosis
The QRS rate is usually fast and irregularly irregular. No P waves are visible; the baseline may be flat or show fast, small depolarizations. The key diagnostic feature is that no other cardiac rhythm is **truly irregularly irregular**.

Clinical features
There are many causes of AF:
- **Cardiac**; 1) Ischaemic heart disease 2) Hypertensive heart disease (left ventricular hypertrophy) 3) Mitral valve disease (especially mitral stenosis) 4) Pericarditis 5) Cardiomyopathy, heart failure (any cause)
- **Metabolic**; 1) Thyrotoxicosis 2) Alcohol (acute or chronic)
- **Pulmonary**; 1) Pulmonary embolism 2) Pneumonia 3) Chronic obstructive pulmonary disease 4) Cor pulmonale.

In some no cause is found—idiopathic or 'lone AF'. AF incidence increases with age. The pulse rate is usually fast (90 to > 150) and irregular. The patient may be asymptomatic, experience rapid palpitations, or be breathless from heart failure.

Treatment
- **Rate control**: decrease the ventricular rate by decreasing conduction through the AV node using digoxin, β-blockers or certain calcium channel antagonists. AF itself continues. Most patients require digoxin (which slows the ventricular response to AF at rest, but not during exercise) and β-blockers (to slow the ventricular rate during exercise).
- **Reversion back to sinus rhythm**: drugs (amiodarone, flecainide or sotalol) can convert AF back to sinus rhythm and/or prevent further episodes of AF. Direct current (DC) cardioversion under anaesthesia/deep sedation can be effective in restoring sinus rhythm provided that AF has been present < 1 year, and the heart is not that abnormal.
- **Anticoagulation**: systemic thromboembolism (stroke, embolic occlusion of a limb or visceral artery) is a significant risk in AF persisting for 2 days or more. This arises from thrombus in the left atrium. The risk is especially high in those with structural cardiac disease (especially mitral stenosis), large left atria (≥ 40 mm) or in those aged 65 years or over. In persistent AF, patients are **anticoagulated** with warfarin (target international normalized ratio [INR] = 2.5–3.0).

Atrial flutter
Pathophysiology
The atria depolarize in a rapid coordinated fashion, as a result of a macro-re-entry circuit moving anticlockwise around the right atrium. Atrial depolarizations occur at a rate of 300/min; conduction to the ventricles is limited to every second, third or fourth depolarization, because of AV node refractoriness.

ECG diagnosis
The QRS rate is exactly 150/min if alternate flutter waves are conducted ('atrial flutter with 2-1 block'), or can be other divisibles of the flutter rate, e.g. 100 (3-1), 75 (4-1), sometimes varying every few beats. Continuous sawtooth 'flutter waves' are visible instead of P waves, most obviously in leads II, III, aVf and V1. **If a regular tachycardia has a constant rate of exactly 150/min**, always think of atrial flutter, even if flutter waves are not obvious—they may be obscured by the QRS/T waves.

Clinical features
The pulse rate is usually 150 and regular. The patient may be asymptomatic, experience rapid palpitation or breathlessness, or be in heart failure. The incidence and causes of atrial flutter are similar to those of AF; these two arrhythmias commonly occur in the same patient.

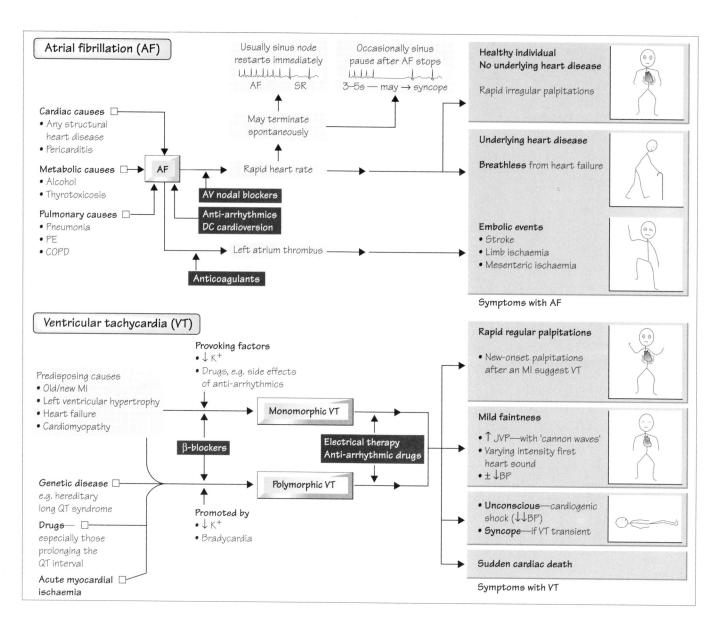

Symptoms with AF

Symptoms with VT

Treatment

Similar to AF. As atrial flutter is the result of a macro-re-entry circuit, *radiofrequency ablation* of the critical part of the circuit in the right atrium may be curative. It is indicated if drug therapy fails or in patients (e.g. young) in whom long-term drug treatment is not a good option.

Ventricular tachycardias (VTs)
Pathogenesis

Rapid depolarizations arise in the ventricular myocardium, as a result of:

• **Re-entrant circuit(s)** in an anatomically abnormal substrate such as myocardial infarction scar tissue. The ECG shows **monomorphic VT**.

• Abnormal **triggered activity** in ventricular myocardium, resulting from electrophysiological/metabolic disturbances that often prolong the QT interval, such as acute ischaemia and drugs. The ECG shows **polymorphic VT**.

The most powerful stimulus to VT is myocardial damage, e.g. in heart failure VT is common. For each 10% decrease in ejection fraction, the chance of an arrhythic death occuring increases by 65%. If patients

with impaired LV function develop syncope, unless there is clear evidence for an alternative diagnosis, VT should be strongly suspected.

ECG diagnosis

The QRS complexes are broad with an abnormal shape. VT should **always be suspected** when patients known to have heart disease (especially recent or remote MI) present with a regular tachycardia with broad QRS complexes:

• In monomorphic VT, the QRS morphology is uniform; typically the rate is 120–190 beats/min. There may be evidence of independent atrial activity, i.e. dissociated P waves.

• Polymorphic VT (see Table 83.1) is less regular, more chaotic, sometimes with a characteristic phasic variation in the QRS morphology— 'torsades de pointes'. Polymorphic VT is inherently unstable and often degenerates early on into ventricular fibrillation (VF).

Clinical features

The pulse rate is fast, may be weak, or there may be no pulse palpable. The patient may be in acute cardiac failure, be severely compromised,

Causes of sudden death

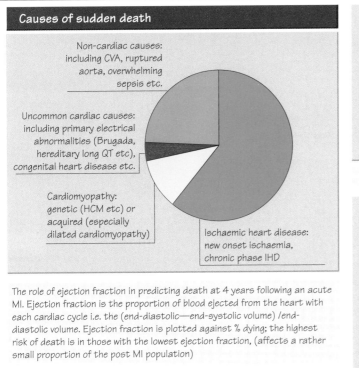

Non-cardiac causes: including CVA, ruptured aorta, overwhelming sepsis etc.

Uncommon cardiac causes: including primary electrical abnormalities (Brugada, hereditary long QT etc), congenital heart disease etc.

Cardiomyopathy: genetic (HCM etc) or acquired (especially dilated cardiomyopathy)

Ischaemic heart disease: new onset ischaemia, chronic phase IHD

The role of ejection fraction in predicting death at 4 years following an acute MI. Ejection fraction is the proportion of blood ejected from the heart with each cardiac cycle i.e. the (end-diastolic—end-systolic volume) /end-diastolic volume. Ejection fraction is plotted against % dying; the highest risk of death is in those with the lowest ejection fraction, (affects a rather small proportion of the post MI population)

Reproduced with permission of The European Society of Cardiology

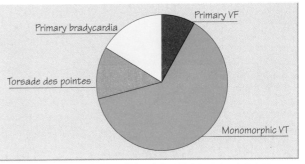

Arrhythmias underlying sudden cardiac death

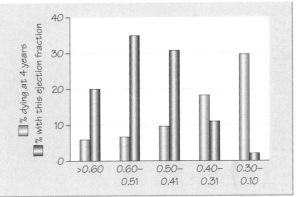

Table 83.1 Causes of polymorphic ventricular tachycardia.

Acute ischaemia
Drugs (cause prolongation of the QT interval):
 Quinidine, Sotalol, amiodarone, Tricyclic antidepressants,
 Antihistamines
Hypokalaemia
Hypomagnesaemia
Hypocalcaemia
Bradycardias (any cause)
Congenital QT prolongation syndromes (ion channel mutations)
 Jervell–Lange–Nielsen syndrome, Romano–Ward syndrome

suffer cardiac arrest (pulseless VT), or be relatively well, except for rapid palpitation or breathlessness. A good clinical state to a patient **does not exclude VT**, and the risk of haemodynamic deterioration remains.

Treatment
This is of individual episode:

- **Pulseless VT, or impending cardiovascular collapse**: DC cardioversion, either immediate or after urgent anaesthesia/sedation.
- **Haemodynamically stable VT**: intravenous lidocaine (lignocaine) or drugs such as amiodarone. **Never** use multiple drug combinations. If drugs are unsuccessful, use DC cardioversion.
- **Polymorphic VT**: DC cardioversion, intravenous magnesium, correction of the underlying metabolic or electrophysiological abnormality. Slow heart rates prolong the QT interval and may worsen polymorphic VT. Increasing the heart rate by pacing often prevents or dramatically reduces the incidence of polymorphic VT.

Prevention of future episodes
- **Long-term drug therapy**: β-blockers, amiodarone, ACE inhibitors and spironolactone to improve LV function and maintain K^+.
- **Revascularization (CABG or PCI)**: for severe coronary disease.
- **Implantable defibrillators (ICDs)**: monitor the cardiac rhythm and deliver antitachycardic therapy (overdrive pacing and/or intracardiac shocks) if VT or VF is detected. Indicated for survivors of cardiac arrest, and in symptomatic VT with impaired LV function.

Ventricular fibrillation (see Chapter 67)

Diseases and Treatments at a Glance

84 Bradyarrhythmias

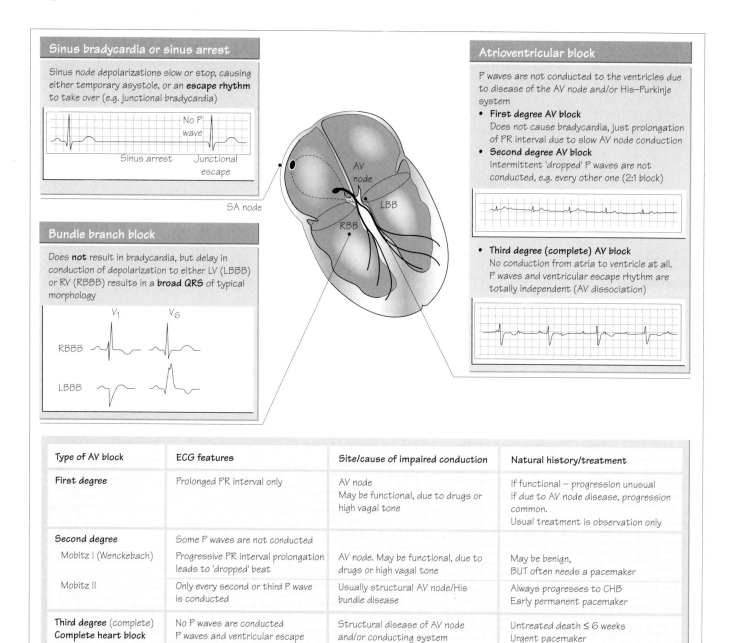

Sinus bradycardia or sinus arrest

Sinus node depolarizations slow or stop, causing either temporary asystole, or an **escape rhythm** to take over (e.g. junctional bradycardia)

Sinus arrest   Junctional escape
No P wave

SA node

Bundle branch block

Does **not** result in bradycardia, but delay in conduction of depolarization to either LV (LBBB) or RV (RBBB) results in a **broad QRS** of typical morphology

V_1 V_6
RBBB
LBBB

Atrioventricular block

P waves are not conducted to the ventricles due to disease of the AV node and/or His–Purkinje system
- **First degree AV block**
  Does not cause bradycardia, just prolongation of PR interval due to slow AV node conduction
- **Second degree AV block**
  Intermittent 'dropped' P waves are not conducted, e.g. every other one (2:1 block)

- **Third degree (complete) AV block**
  No conduction from atria to ventricle at all. P waves and ventricular escape rhythm are totally independent (AV dissociation)

AV node
LBB
RBB

Type of AV block	ECG features	Site/cause of impaired conduction	Natural history/treatment
First degree	Prolonged PR interval only	AV node May be functional, due to drugs or high vagal tone	If functional – progression unusual If due to AV node disease, progression common. Usual treatment is observation only
Second degree Mobitz I (Wenckebach)	Some P waves are not conducted Progressive PR interval prolongation leads to 'dropped' beat	AV node. May be functional, due to drugs or high vagal tone	May be benign, BUT often needs a pacemaker
Mobitz II	Only every second or third P wave is conducted	Usually structural AV node/His bundle disease	Always progresses to CHB Early permanent pacemaker
Third degree (complete) **Complete heart block (CHB)**	No P waves are conducted P waves and ventricular escape rhythm are completely independent (AV dissociation)	Structural disease of AV node and/or conducting system	Untreated death ≤ 6 weeks Urgent pacemaker Immediate pacemaker if any history of syncope, or heart rate <35 bpm

Definition
Bradyarrhythmias are abnormally slow heartbeats (< 60/min).

Clinical features
Mild or transient bradyarrhythmias may be asymptomatic or even physiological, e.g. sinus bradycardia during sleep or in a healthy athlete. Symptomatic bradycardias commonly cause dizziness or syncope, or less commonly fatigue or heart failure. Palpitations are not a feature of bradyarrhythmias.

The classic syncopal episode caused by a bradyarrhythmia is a **Stokes–Adams attack**. The characteristics are:
- Sudden onset without warning (within a few seconds).
- Immediate collapse with loss of consciousness.
- Pale and still 'as if dead'.
- Duration a few seconds to 1 or 2 min.
- Rapid recovery back to normal, only transient disorientation at most for few minutes and no focal neurological symptoms or signs.

Diseases and Treatments at a Glance

Aetiology

Bradyarrhythmias arise either from the failure of the sinoatrial (SA) node to provide regular depolarizations (**sinoatrial disease**), or by failure of the conducting system to convey the depolarizations into the ventricles (**atrioventricular [AV] block** or **complete heart block**). The total absence of any depolarizations (**asystole**) is usually prevented for more than a few seconds by the emergence of an **escape rhythm**, arising from the next most active intrinsic cardiac pacemaker. When the sinus node stops, this is usually the AV node (**junctional escape rhythm**); when AV conduction is blocked, a **ventricular escape rhythm** arises either from the conducting tissues or from the ventricular myocardium itself. The 'lower' (i.e. further away from the SA node) the escape rhythm, the slower it is.

Sinoatrial node disease

Dysfunction of the sinus node that manifests either as inappropriate **sinus bradycardia** or by periods of **sinus arrest**. May be one aspect of the *sick sinus syndrome*, where patients experience both episodes of bradyarrhythmias and episodes of atrial tachyarrhythmias such as atrial fibrillation (AF). The bradycardias in SA disease may be exacerbated by drugs used to control tachyarrhythmias, such as β-blockers or digoxin. Another manifestation of SA node disease is 'fainting' (syncope) or feeling faint ('pre-syncope'), occurring at the moment that an episode of AF stops—the usual mechanism for this is a prolonged sinus pause before the intrinsic SA node pacemaker starts up (see p. 170).

Atrioventricular block

Disease of either the AV node and/or the conducting system results in failure of transmission of the P waves to the ventricles. AV block is classified according to the extent of the failure of transmission, seen on the ECG, and this is broadly related to the site and extent of the disease in the AV node/His-Purkinje system (see figure). The signs depend on the type of AV block. First-degree block is difficult to detect clinically: the first heart sound may be quiet. Second degree usually has a heart rate of < 40 beats/min. In third-degree block the atria, which beat independently of the ventricles, occasionally contract on a closed tricuspid valve. Blood cannot leave the atria for the ventricle and instead will be propelled into the neck veins, seen as a prominent jugular venous pressure (JVP) pulsation—'cannon' waves.

Investigations

Distinguishing Stokes–Adams attacks from other causes of dizziness or syncope (e.g. vasovagal episode, seizure, transient ischaemic attack [TIA]) is often difficult. The clinical history and additional information from a witness are extremely important, and may be the only information on which to base management decisions.

The diagnostic investigation is an ECG during an attack—this is often not possible to obtain:

- **12-lead ECG**: may show circumstantial evidence of bradyarrhythmias, e.g. first-degree AV block or bundle branch block (BBB). The risk of intermittent complete heart block (CHB) is increased by extensive conducting tissue disease. The left bundle is a much larger structure than the right bundle; thus, isolated left BBB is more likely to give rise to intermittent CHB than right BBB. However, extensive conducting tissue disease on the 12-lead ECG is only a guide that symptoms arise from CHB, e.g. patients with ischaemic heart disease (IHD) and extensive conducting tissue disease may black out either from CHB or ventricular tachycardia.
- **24-h ECG recording (Holter monitor)** is commonly used to detect the occurrence of both tachyarrhythmias and bradyarrhythmias, but is often not useful unless the patient experiences a typical episode during the recording. Furthermore, minor rhythm disturbances are commonly detected on Holter monitors and may not necessarily be related to the symptoms.

Treatment

Minor arrhythmias that do not cause symptoms do not require specific treatment. SA disease requires treatment only if symptomatic or if a potentially exacerbating medication cannot be stopped. First-degree AV block, BBB and Wenckebach block do not require treatment. However, higher degrees of AV block (Mobitz II and complete) should always be treated even if not symptomatic, because there is a high risk of future syncope or even of sudden death.

- **Pacemaker implantation** is the preferred treatment for symptomatic bradyarrhythmias. A permanent pacemaker is a small electronic device that generates regular pulses to depolarize the heart through an electrode inserted into the right side of the heart through the venous system. A **single-chamber pacemaker** has an electrode in either the right ventricle or the right atrium. A **dual-chamber pacemaker** paces both the atrium and the ventricle through two electrodes, and can pace the ventricle synchronously after each P wave that is sensed in the atrium. This provides a close approximation to the physiological depolarization of the heart, and allows the heart beat to change rate in track with the sinus node.
- **Pacemaker nomenclature**: first letter—chamber paced (V, ventricle; A, atrium; D, both); second—chamber sensed (V, A or 0 for none); third letter—pacemaker response to the detection cardiac electrical activity (I, inhibited, T, triggered, D, both). Fourth letter for whether the pacemaker stimulates quicker on physical activity is the letter R, for rate responsive (e.g. VVI-R).

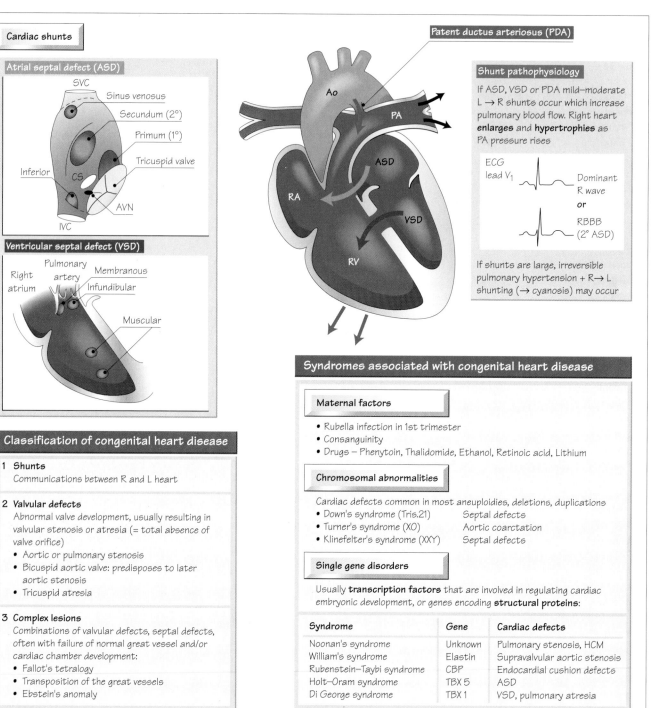

Cardiac shunts

Atrial septal defect (ASD)

SVC
Sinus venosus
Secundum (2°)
Primum (1°)
Tricuspid valve
Inferior
CS
AVN
IVC

Ventricular septal defect (VSD)

Right atrium
Pulmonary artery
Membranous
Infundibular
Muscular

Patent ductus arteriosus (PDA)

Ao
PA
ASD
RA
VSD
RV

Shunt pathophysiology

If ASD, VSD or PDA mild–moderate L → R shunts occur which increase pulmonary blood flow. Right heart **enlarges** and **hypertrophies** as PA pressure rises

ECG lead V₁ — Dominant R wave
or
RBBB (2° ASD)

If shunts are large, irreversible pulmonary hypertension + R→ L shunting (→ cyanosis) may occur

Classification of congenital heart disease

1 Shunts
Communications between R and L heart

2 Valvular defects
Abnormal valve development, usually resulting in valvular stenosis or atresia (= total absence of valve orifice)
• Aortic or pulmonary stenosis
• Bicuspid aortic valve: predisposes to later aortic stenosis
• Tricuspid atresia

3 Complex lesions
Combinations of valvular defects, septal defects, often with failure of normal great vessel and/or cardiac chamber development:
• Fallot's tetralogy
• Transposition of the great vessels
• Ebstein's anomaly

Syndromes associated with congenital heart disease

Maternal factors

• Rubella infection in 1st trimester
• Consanguinity
• Drugs – Phenytoin, Thalidomide, Ethanol, Retinoic acid, Lithium

Chromosomal abnormalities

Cardiac defects common in most aneuploidies, deletions, duplications
• Down's syndrome (Tris.21)   Septal defects
• Turner's syndrome (XO)   Aortic coarctation
• Klinefelter's syndrome (XXY)   Septal defects

Single gene disorders

Usually **transcription factors** that are involved in regulating cardiac embryonic development, or genes encoding **structural proteins**:

Syndrome	Gene	Cardiac defects
Noonan's syndrome	Unknown	Pulmonary stenosis, HCM
William's syndrome	Elastin	Supravalvular aortic stenosis
Rubenstein–Taybi syndrome	CBP	Endocardial cushion defects
Holt–Oram syndrome	TBX 5	ASD
Di George syndrome	TBX 1	VSD, pulmonary atresia

Definition: abnormal embryological cardiac development, or persistence of some parts of the fetal circulation after birth resulting in structural cardiac defects. The conditions discussed here (along with congenital aortic and pulmonary stenosis) account for 80% of congenital heart disease (CHD). The **incidence** of major defects is 8/1000 live births. Minor defects are more common, e.g. bicuspid aortic valve affects 2%.

Classification (see figure)

Ventricular septal defect (VSD)

Twenty-five per cent of CHD. A defect in the interventricular septum allows systolic blood flow from left to right ventricle.
• **Small defects** produce high-velocity jets and a loud murmur (Maladie de Roger) that is not of haemodynamic significance.

- **Large defects** may have a quiet murmur and a large left to right shunt. Untreated, this may cause pulmonary hypertension and Eisenmenger's syndrome. **Treatment** is surgical closure before pulmonary hypertension develops.

There is a high risk of endocarditis (especially small defects), so antibiotic prophylaxis is essential.

Atrial septal defect (ASD)

Ten per cent of CHD. A defect in the interatrial septum allowing shunting of blood from left to right atrium.
- **Secundum ASD**: 70%.
- **Primum ASD**: 30% often involve the atrioventricular (AV) valves with mitral or tricuspid regurgitation. May be associated with other defects including VSD.

Left-to-right shunting increases pulmonary blood flow, producing a systolic pulmonary flow murmur, wide fixed splitting of the second heart sound and right ventricular hypertrophy. ECG shows right bundle branch block (RBBB) with right axis deviation and right ventricular hypertrophy (RVH; secundum) or left axis deviation with RVH (primum). Supraventricular tachycardias, e.g. atrial fibrillation, are common. ASDs may be undetected until adult life when they present with exertional dyspnoea and fatigue. The **diagnosis** is confirmed by transoesophageal cardiac ultrasonography. **Treatment** is closure of the defect, either by surgery or by percutaneous closure device.

Patent ductus arteriosus

Fifteen per cent of CHD. The ductus arteriosus fails to close after birth, resulting in left-to-right shunting from the aorta to pulmonary artery and a continuous (machinery) murmur. A large duct with significant shunt leads to left ventricular hypertrophy (LVH) and heart failure, or pulmonary hypertension and Eisenmenger's syndrome. Duct endocarditis is a significant long-term risk.
- **Treatment**: in neonates, indomethacin blockade of prostaglandin production may provoke duct closure. Ducts remaining open require surgical ligation or percutaneous closure (coil or umbrella devices).

Eisenmenger's syndrome

This describes **irreversible pulmonary hypertension** (from the high pulmonary blood flow of large left-to-right shunts) **with shunt reversal** (from left to right to right to left) resulting from the high right-sided heart pressures. Patients experience worsening symptoms with breathlessness; there is cyanosis, **clubbing** and signs of severe pulmonary hypertension. Surgical closure of left-to-right shunts must be undertaken before Eisenmenger's syndrome develops; the only surgical treatment for established Eisenmenger's syndrome is heart–lung transplantation.

Coarctation of the aorta

Five per cent of CHD. A developmentally hypoplastic segment of the aorta causes narrowing of the aorta and a significant pressure gradient, usually (98%) immediately distal to the origin of the left subclavian artery. Sixty per cent also have a bicuspid aortic valve. Blood flow to the lower body is maintained by an increase in collateral flow (which may be huge) via the mammary arteries and intercostal arteries. Usually presents as (upper limb) hypertension with absent or weak femoral pulses and radial–femoral delay. Features of LVH and palpable collaterals around the scapulae. There may be signs of bicuspid aortic valve and systolic murmur from the coarctation. The **diagnosis** is by echocardiography, computed tomography or magnetic resonance imaging. **Treatment** is surgical correction of the narrowing, preferably in older childhood (allows a sufficient increase in aortic calibre). Percutaneous dilatation using a balloon is sometimes a viable alternative.

Complex CHD

In complex CHD there are abnormal relationships of the arteries, ventricles and great vessels, abnormalities of chamber development, often with septal defects, and/or valvular lesions.

Fallot's tetralogy

The most common 'complex' CHD; 10% of CHD. A combination of VSD with right-to-left shunt, due to:
- **Pulmonary stenosis**, either infundibular or valvar.
- **Right ventricular overload** and hypertrophy
- **Dextro position** of the aorta so that it overrides the VSD.

There is cyanosis, clubbing, signs of RVH and a pulmonary systolic murmur (the large VSD does not generate a murmur). Children with Fallot's tetralogy experience exertional breathlessness, dizziness and growth retardation. Squatting kinks the femoral arteries, increases systemic resistance and reduces the right-to-left shunt. **Surgery** aims to:
- Totally **correct the defects**, if the pulmonary arteries are large enough.
- Alternatively, **pulmonary blood flow is increased** using systemic to pulmonary artery shunts:
  - **Blalock–Taussig** shunt: subclavian artery to pulmonary artery
  - **Waterston** shunt: ascending aorta to right pulmonary artery
  - **Potts'** shunt: descending aorta to left pulmonary artery.

Ebstein's anomaly

The tricuspid valve is displaced downwards into the right ventricle, resulting in a very small RV cavity and a very large right atrium. There is tricuspid regurgitation and usually an ASD. Twenty per cent have accessory pathways (Wolff–Parkinson–White syndrome).

Transposition of the great arteries

There is ventriculo-arterial discordance: the aorta arises from the right ventricle and the pulmonary artery from the left ventricle. In isolation, this is incompatible with life (totally separate pulmonary and systemic circulations); an associated ASD usually allows shunting. Surgical treatments include:
- **Balloon septostomy** (Rashkind): increases shunting and reduces cyanosis.
- **Interatrial shunt** (Mustard or Senning operation): directs systemic venous return from the right atrium across the ASD into the morphological left ventricle; pulmonary venous return passes in the opposite direction and into the aorta.
- **Arterial 'switch' operation** totally corrects the defect by reconnecting aorta to left ventricle and pulmonary artery to right ventricle.
- **Congenitally corrected transposition**: the right and left ventricles and AV valves are interchanged (venous return drains via the right atrium into a morphological left ventricle, which ejects blood into the pulmonary artery). Usually well tolerated in childhood but heart failure in adult life (the morphological right ventricle cannot sustain systemic pressures long term).

Lung volumes

Normal lung volumes and the changes which occur in obstructive and restrictive ventilatory defects

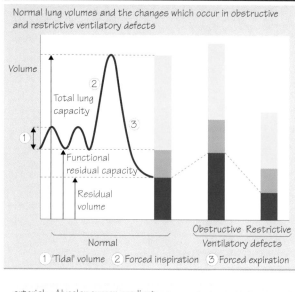

Volume

Total lung capacity

② Functional residual capacity

Residual volume

Obstructive Restrictive

Normal Ventilatory defects

① 'Tidal' volume ② Forced inspiration ③ Forced expiration

arterial – Alveolar oxygen gradient

$$a - A \text{ gradient} = P_{Alveoli}O_2 - P_{arterial}O_2$$
$$P_{Alveoli}O_2 = P_{Inspired}O_2 - 1.2 \times P_{arterial}CO_2 \quad] \text{ from ABG}$$

- Normal < 2 kPa
- ↑Gradient in $\dot{V}/\dot{Q}$ mismatch, shunting, diffuse lung disease
- Normal gradient in hypoventilation, low inspired O_2

Simple spirometry

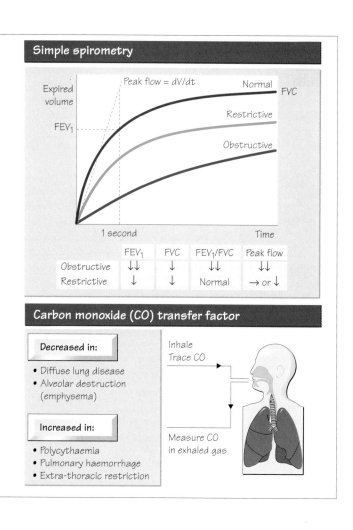

Peak flow = dV/dt Normal FVC

Expired volume

FEV₁

Restrictive

Obstructive

1 second Time

	FEV_1	FVC	FEV_1/FVC	Peak flow
Obstructive	↓↓	↓	↓↓	↓↓
Restrictive	↓	↓	Normal	→ or ↓

Carbon monoxide (CO) transfer factor

Decreased in:

- Diffuse lung disease
- Alveolar destruction (emphysema)

Increased in:

- Polycythaemia
- Pulmonary haemorrhage
- Extra-thoracic restriction

Inhale Trace CO

Measure CO in exhaled gas

Definitions

Spirometric tests of airway function are simple, cheap and reproducible:

- **Forced expiratory volume in 1 second** (FEV_1).
- **Forced vital capacity** (FVC) is the total volume of air expelled by a forced expiration after maximal inspiration.
- **FEV_1/FVC ratio** (%) is the percentage of FVC exhaled in 1 s during forced expiration. These measures allow for the classification of lung diseases into restrictive or obstructive. In obstructive disease the ratio is less than 70% and in restrictive there is reduction of both FEV_1 and FVC with a normal or high ratio.
- **Peak expiratory flow rate** (PEFR): fastest flow rate attained at the start of a forced expiration after maximal inspiration. Useful for monitoring changes in airflow obstruction.
- **Reversibility testing**: measurement of airway function before and after an inhaled bronchodilator. An improvement of ≥ 20% and 300 mL represents a positive test.

Lung volumes

Total lung capacity (TLC) is measured by dilution of an inert gas such as helium or in an enclosed box (total body plethysmograph):

- TLC: the total amount of gas in the lungs at maximal inspiration.

Residual volume (RV) is the amount of gas left in the lung after maximal expiration and is derived from the TLC and vital capacity (VC).

- Functional residual capacity (FRC): the amount of gas left in the lung at end expiration during tidal breathing, derived by helium dilution during tidal breathing.

Tests of gas exchange

- Carbon monoxide (CO) transfer factor (K_{CO}): measured by inhalation of a trace of CO, which is avidly taken up by haemoglobin. Assesses the size and efficiency of the gas-exchanging area.
- Pulse oximetry: measured by the light absorbance by haemoglobin, used to assess hypoxaemia and in particular the response to oxygen therapy. CO_2 is not measured.
- Blood gas analysis (see respiratory failure).

Other investigations

- **Flow–volume loops** are useful for diagnosing large airway obstruction within the thorax or extra-thoracic airway obstruction.
- **Tests of respiratory muscles**: muscle power is measured by breathing against a closed orifice or by a sniff. Maximal inspiratory pressure is measured at FRC and expiratory pressure at TLC. Values < 60 cmH_2O are abnormal.

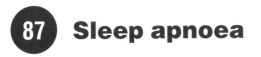

87 Sleep apnoea

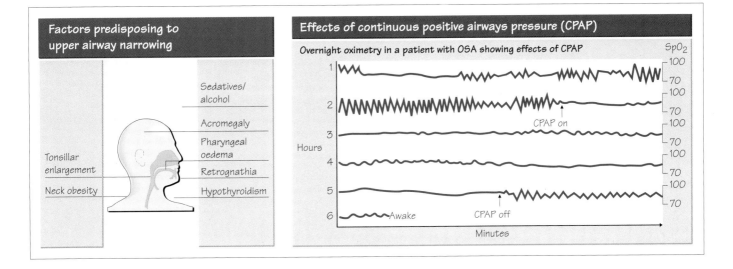

Factors predisposing to upper airway narrowing

- Sedatives/alcohol
- Acromegaly
- Pharyngeal oedema
- Retrognathia
- Hypothyroidism
- Tonsillar enlargement
- Neck obesity

Effects of continuous positive airways pressure (CPAP)

Overnight oximetry in a patient with OSA showing effects of CPAP

CPAP on

CPAP off

Awake

Hours

Minutes

SpO₂

Sleep apnoea may relate to conditions disturbing the control of breathing, although most relates to obstruction to the upper airways—obstructive sleep apnoea (OSA). Pathological episodes of nocturnal apnoea often occur during rapid eye movement (REM) sleep in:
- Brain-stem disease, either as a result of hypnotics or as a pre-terminal event in many conditions.
- Motor weakness, most commonly motor neuron disease, occasionally from previous poliomyelitis.
- OSA (see below).
- Chronic obstructive airway disease (COAD).

Apnoea leads to hypoxaemia, sometimes profound, arousal and waking. Frequent episodes disturb sleep, resulting in daytime sleepiness. Severe sleep apnoea may lead to nocturnal arrhythmias (and death) or right-sided heart failure.

Obstructive sleep apnoea

A syndrome of upper airway collapse leading to sleep disruption which results in symptoms, usually of daytime sleepiness. It is very common: 5% of middle-aged adult men are affected. More common in men but increasingly recognized in women.

Aetiology

OSA is caused by upper airway narrowing and obstruction due to reduction in muscle tone during sleep. Arousal from sleep results. Sleep fragmentation causes the predominant symptom of excessive daytime sleepiness. Factors leading to upper airway narrowing predispose to OSA:
- Neck obesity, retrognathia and tonsillar enlargement.
- Endocrine abnormalities, including acromegaly, amyloidosis and hypothyroidism predispose to upper airway obstruction by enlarged tissues around the oropharynx.
- Neuromuscular disease or myopathy.

- Alcohol, sedatives and sleep deprivation worsen the effects of an anatomically narrow airway.

Clinical features

Classic symptoms are snoring in association with excessive daytime sleepiness. A partner may describe clearly the episodes of obstruction with apnoea, terminating with a sudden loud gasp. Sleepiness may impair performance at work and there is a sevenfold increased risk of motor accidents. Potential symptoms are of morning headache, poor concentration and impotence. Examination reveals factors predisposing to upper airway narrowing (see above).

Investigation

Overnight sleep studies including video and pulse oximetry confirm the diagnosis. Apnoea typically decreases oxygen saturation by $\geq 4\%$; such episodes may occur many times each hour (see figure). Full polysomnography studies include measurement of EEG, airflow, ribcage and abdominal movement, as well as recordings of snoring and continuous oximetry. Endocrine or neurophysiology studies are occasionally appropriate.

Treatment and prognosis

Avoid alcohol and sedatives. Treat any underlying illness.
- **Severe cases**: continuous positive airway pressure (CPAP) delivered overnight by a tight-fitting nasal mask splints the upper airway open, prevents obstruction and arousal, and results in rapid improvement in symptoms.
- **Milder cases**: weight loss and/or mandibular advancement devices may be sufficient.
- **Surgery**: tonsillectomy may be curative, particularly in young patients with significant tonsillar enlargement. Palatal surgery may help but, if unsuccessful, can make future application of CPAP difficult.

Effective treatment results in rapid improvement of symptoms.

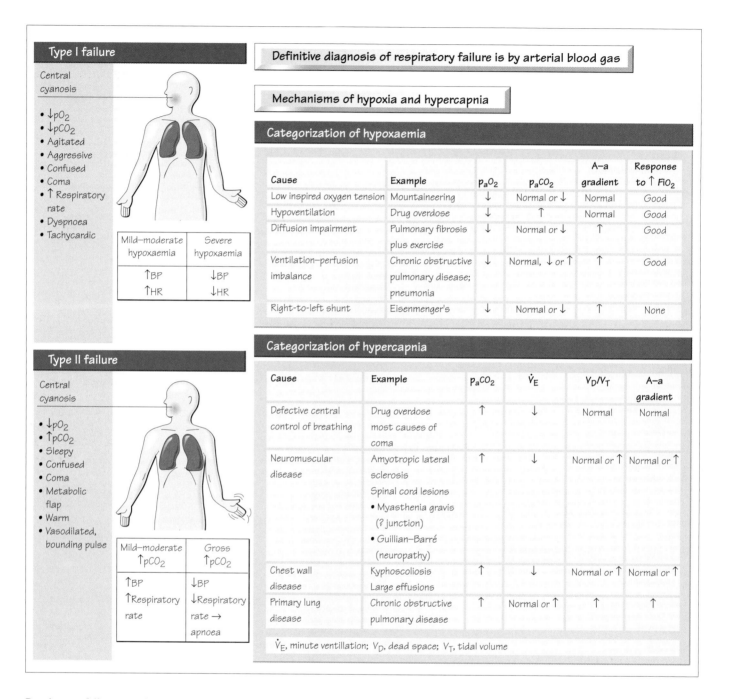

Type I failure

Central cyanosis

- $\downarrow pO_2$
- $\downarrow pCO_2$
- Agitated
- Aggressive
- Confused
- Coma
- $\uparrow$ Respiratory rate
- Dyspnoea
- Tachycardic

Mild–moderate hypoxaemia	Severe hypoxaemia
$\uparrow$BP	$\downarrow$BP
$\uparrow$HR	$\downarrow$HR

Type II failure

Central cyanosis

- $\downarrow pO_2$
- $\uparrow pCO_2$
- Sleepy
- Confused
- Coma
- Metabolic flap
- Warm
- Vasodilated, bounding pulse

Mild–moderate $\uparrow$pCO_2	Gross $\uparrow$pCO_2
$\uparrow$BP	$\downarrow$BP
$\uparrow$Respiratory rate	$\downarrow$Respiratory rate $\rightarrow$ apnoea

Definitive diagnosis of respiratory failure is by arterial blood gas

Mechanisms of hypoxia and hypercapnia

Categorization of hypoxaemia

Cause	Example	p_aO_2	p_aCO_2	A–a gradient	Response to $\uparrow$ FiO_2
Low inspired oxygen tension	Mountaineering	$\downarrow$	Normal or $\downarrow$	Normal	Good
Hypoventilation	Drug overdose	$\downarrow$	$\uparrow$	Normal	Good
Diffusion impairment	Pulmonary fibrosis plus exercise	$\downarrow$	Normal or $\downarrow$	$\uparrow$	Good
Ventilation–perfusion imbalance	Chronic obstructive pulmonary disease; pneumonia	$\downarrow$	Normal, $\downarrow$ or $\uparrow$	$\uparrow$	Good
Right-to-left shunt	Eisenmenger's	$\downarrow$	Normal or $\downarrow$	$\uparrow$	None

Categorization of hypercapnia

Cause	Example	p_aCO_2	$\dot{V}_E$	V_D/V_T	A–a gradient
Defective central control of breathing	Drug overdose most causes of coma	$\uparrow$	$\downarrow$	Normal	Normal
Neuromuscular disease	Amyotropic lateral sclerosis Spinal cord lesions • Myasthenia gravis (? junction) • Guillian–Barré (neuropathy)	$\uparrow$	$\downarrow$	Normal or $\uparrow$	Normal or $\uparrow$
Chest wall disease	Kyphoscoliosis Large effusions	$\uparrow$	$\downarrow$	Normal or $\uparrow$	Normal or $\uparrow$
Primary lung disease	Chronic obstructive pulmonary disease	$\uparrow$	Normal or $\uparrow$	$\uparrow$	$\uparrow$

$\dot{V}_E$, minute ventillation; V_D, dead space; V_T, tidal volume

Respiratory failure may be acute, chronic or acute-on-chronic (for example a patient with an exacerbation of COPD and pre-existing hypoxia). Abnormal levels of arterial oxygen ($PaO_2 < 8$ kPa) or carbon dioxide ($PaCO_2 > 6.7$ kPa) are used to define the presence of respiratory failure, which is thus divided into:
- Hypoxaemic (type I): failure of oxygenation
- Hypercapnic (type II): failure of ventilation to remove CO_2

Generally hypercapnic failure is the result of a disorder with respiratory muscles ('pump failure'), whereas hypoxaemic failure is usually due to pulmonary pathology. However, type II respiratory failure often supersedes type I failure as the patient becomes exhausted.

What is the A-a gradient?

Alveolar O_2 and CO_2 levels are interdependent and a high alveolar partial pressure of carbon dioxide results in a lower partial pressure of oxygen. The alveolar arterial oxygen gradient (A-a gradient) is calculated from the alveolar gas equation and is a measure of ventilation and perfusion mismatch (reflecting the severity of lung disease).

$$A\text{-a gradient} = FiO_2 \text{ (atmospheric pressure} - \text{water pressure)} - PaO_2 - 1.25(PCO_2)$$
$$= 0.21 (101 \text{ kPa} - 6.3 \text{ kPa}) - PaO_2 - 1.25(PCO_2)$$
$$= 19.9 \text{ kPa} - PaO_2 - 1.25(PCO_2) \text{ (on air } - 21\% \text{ oxygen)}$$

Normal A-a gradient is 2–4 kPa, it increases with age and at FiO_2 > 0.28 (FiO_2 = fraction of O_2 in inspired air). Certain disease processes also increase the A-a gradient (see figure); measuring the A-a gradient is thus helpful in ruling in or out these diseases in patients with respiratory failure.

Causes of hypoxaemia

- Shunt: lung is perfused but not ventilated (the opposite of dead space). Right to left shunt leads to hypoxaemia that does not respond to 100% oxygen.
- Ventilation/perfusion mismatch ($\dot{V}/\dot{Q}$ mismatch): **this is by far the commonest form**, even in diseases like pulmonary fibrosis where one might expect diffusion block. Poorly ventilated alveoli contribute to hypoxaemia, which is overcome by an increase in FiO_2.
- Diffusion block (uncommon): a thickened interstitium between alveolus and capillary. Only important during exercise when erythrocytes have insufficient time to equilibrate for gas exchange.
- Low FiO_2 at altitude.
- Hypoventilation: ventilation is inversely proportional to $PaCO_2$. The interdependence of PaO_2 and $PaCO_2$ thus leads to hypoxaemia in hypoventilation.

All causes of hypoxaemia other than true shunts improve with an increase in FiO_2.

Causes of hypercapnia

This is a failure of ventilation, which may be caused by CNS, neuromuscular, chest wall or primary lung diseases. There is either insufficient respiratory drive or ineffective (↑ dead space) ventilation.

Symptoms and signs of respiratory failure (see figure)

Treatment of respiratory failure

It is important to establish whether the onset of respiratory failure is acute, chronic or acute-on-chronic and the underlying aetiology. Patients need to be appropriately monitored in a critical care area. Ideally monitoring should include respiratory rate, continuous ECG, oximetry, arterial line (blood pressure, arterial blood gas analysis) and GCS. Although, as discussed below, one can treat the consequences of respiratory failure (hypoxaemia and hypercapnia) the **cornerstone of management is treating the underlying disease process**. This is considered in the following chapters on specific respiratory diseases.

Hypoxaemia
Oxygen therapy
Oxygen may be delivered by variable or fixed performance devices.

Variable performance devices Air is entrained during breathing whilst oxygen is delivered from a reservoir. The latter may be the nasopharynx, mask or reservoir bag. The FiO_2 delivered to the lungs therefore depends on the oxygen flow rate, the patient's inspiratory flow, respiratory rate and the amount of air entrained. Examples include: nasal cannula, facemasks and non-rebreathing masks with reservoir bags.
- **Nasal cannulae**: oxygen flow rates up to 4 L/minute (higher rates dry

nasal mucosa). Nasopharynx acts as reservoir. FiO_2 varies between breaths for given flow rate depending on patient's respiration, delivers between 24 and 34%.
- **Facemask**: flow rates must exceed 5 L/minute to stop rebreathing of CO_2. Mask provides additional reservoir to oro/nasopharynx. FiO_2 can be 50–60% at 15 L/minute.
- **Non-rebreathing masks**: these have a reservoir bag, which should be full before placing on the patient. A one-way valve stops exhaled air entering the oxygen reservoir. High flow rates 10–15 L/minute provide FiO_2 > 60% (often approaching 100%).

Fixed performance devices Are independent of the patient's pattern of breathing and use the Venturi principle to entrain air into the mask, exceeding inspiratory flow and thus deliver a fixed oxygen concentration. Typically colour coded and deliver 24%, 28%, 31%, 35%, 40%, 60% FiO_2 for a prescribed flow rate.
- **Continuous positive airway pressure (CPAP)**: uses a tight-fitting mask and a flow generator to delivery a positive pressure throughout the respiratory cycle (5–15 cmH$_2$O). This increases functional residual capacity, thereby recruiting more alveoli and improving oxygenation.
- **Intubation and mechanical ventilation**: may be required if hypoxia does not respond to treating the underlying disease, oxygen therapy and/or CPAP.

What is adequate oxygenation?
Generally one should aim for oxygen saturations exceeding 90% as this puts the patient on the flat part of the oxygen dissociation curve. Further increases in PaO_2 will have only small effects on oxygen delivery (as almost all oxygen in blood is bound to haemoglobin). However, caution should be exercised about relying too much on oxygen saturations alone. Despite adequate oxygen the patient may continue to deteriorate and require invasive ventilation. Furthermore oximetry gives no information on the patient's CO_2 or pH. Some patients (e.g. many with COPD) with chronic hypoxia depend on hypoxaemia rather than hypercapnia to drive respiration, and oxygen therapy may remove this drive and stop them breathing (whilst initially being well oxygenated!). It is essential to continue to monitor patients when supplemental oxygen is prescribed and ideally an arterial blood gas should be performed.

Hypercapnia
Any sedative drugs should be reversed (opiates, benzodiazepines). If hypercapnia and respiratory acidosis persist, despite treating the underlying condition, artificial ventilation should be considered. Non-invasive ventilation is now widely available and can be delivered via nasal, face, full face or helmet interfaces. It is not a substitute for invasive ventilation, which should be adopted if this method fails.

Indications for intubation and mechanical ventilation in respiratory failure
- Apnoea
- ↑ Acidosis, $PaCO_2$
- PaO_2 < 8 kPa despite FiO_2 > 0.5 (+/– CPAP)
- GCS < 8
- Unable to clear pulmonary secretions by conventional methods
- Tiring; ↑ respiratory rate, tachycardia, dyskinetic respiratory pattern.

89 **Basic chest Xray interpretation**

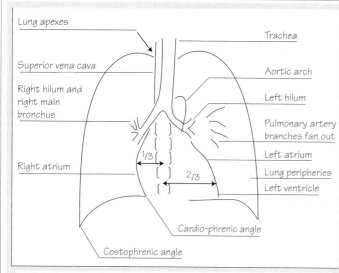

Structure seen in the normal chest Xray. An abnormality may be obvious, but if not, check the apexes (lung cancer or tuberculosis are commonly restricted to this area), the bases (small pleural effusions can easily be missed), behind the mediastinal contents) for, amongst others, signs of left lower lobe collapse (the sail sign). If the patient is genuinely in respiratory failure (confirmed by blood gases), and the chest Xray is normal, think of: 1) Pulmonary emboli (common) – a cardiac ultrasound may help early management (expect some right heart dilatation and decrease in function); 2) Pneumocystis carinii pneumonia (rare in the UK) – reviewing the history may help; 3) Early pneumonia; 4) Early ARDS – for 3&4 repeating the CXR after a few hours may help (treat empirically in the mean time)

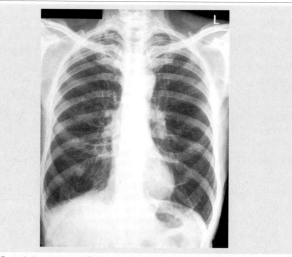

Typical chest Xray in COPD; the lungs are hyperinflated. There are several radiological signs for this; counting the posterior ribs (i.e. the ribs just as they leave the spinal column) – normal is 8-9, so ≥10 is abnormal. Alternatively, count the number of the last rib that can be seen crossing the diaphragm. The 8th rib can be seen here, ≥7 is abnormal. The diaphragms are flat, and the heart shadow is 'thin'. BEWARE that though COPD can be strongly suggested from the CXR, it cannot really be diagnosed from the CXR. Always confirm the presence of COPD by lung function tests, and its functional impact by, among other tests, blood gases. As pneumothoraces are common in COPD these should always be looked for (they can 'hide' in the lung apexes); as cigarette smoking is almost universal, always look for radiological evidence of lung cancer in these patients

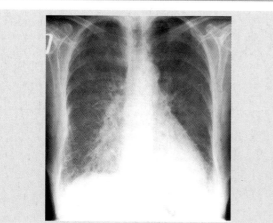

A CXR from a patient with left heart failure (=pulmonary oedema). There are a number of characteristic findings: 1) the heart is enlarged (the normal cardio-thoracic ratio is ≤50%; 2) there is interstitial pulmonary oedema ('fuzzy' shadows), especially in the mid and lower zones (where the pulmonary venous pressure is highest – provided the patient has been upright!); 3) the upper lobe veins, which are usually smaller than the lower lobe ones, have become enlarged (upper lobe venous diversion, otherwise known as pulmonary venous imbalance). There is fluid in the lymphatics, seen as Kerley B lines (short horizontal lines 1-2 cm in length, extending horizontally from the lower outer lung fields; heart failure is the commonest cause, though malignancy and infection rarely can underlie them); 4) there are small bilateral pleural effusions (shadowing at both lung bases). The shape of the heart usually gives no clues as to the cause of the heart failure; occasionally, enlargement of the left atrium (seen as 1) great splaying of the left and right bronchi to ≥ 90°, 2) a large 3rd bulge down the left heart border – the aorta is the 1st, the pulmonary artery the 2nd, and the ventricle the 4th – leads one to suspect mitral valve disease

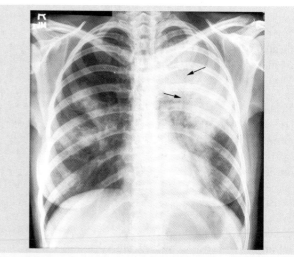

A CXR from a patient with pneumococcal pneumonia. There is extensive shadowing of the left upper zone, within which an air bronchogram (arrows) is seen. An air bronchogram is a pathognomonic sign of consolidation – and by far the commonest cause of consolidation is an infective process. There is also some patchy shadowing in the right mid zone. Respiratory failure is unusual in otherwise well patients who develop pneumonia, but can occur if the infection is severe, or if there is underlying lung disease, such as COPD (which the CXR may underestimate. BEWARE also that patients immobile from septic processes can also develop pulmonary emboli, which can contribute to hypoxaemia. Clinical deterioration in a patient known to have pneumonia may relate to worsening of the infective process, but also may be due to PEs

Xray images from *The Hands-on Guide to Imaging* by Howlett and Ayers

Diseases and Treatments at a Glance

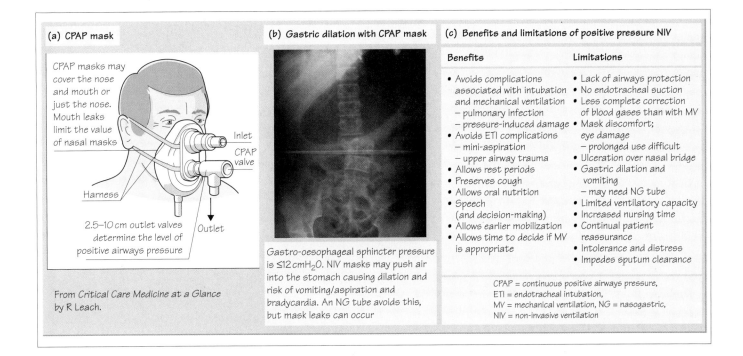

(a) CPAP mask

CPAP masks may cover the nose and mouth or just the nose. Mouth leaks limit the value of nasal masks

Inlet
CPAP valve

Harness

2.5–10 cm outlet valves determine the level of positive airways pressure

Outlet

From *Critical Care Medicine at a Glance* by R Leach.

(b) Gastric dilation with CPAP mask

Gastro-oesophageal sphincter pressure is ≤12 cmH$_2$O. NIV masks may push air into the stomach causing dilation and risk of vomiting/aspiration and bradycardia. An NG tube avoids this, but mask leaks can occur

(c) Benefits and limitations of positive pressure NIV

Benefits	Limitations
• Avoids complications associated with intubation and mechanical ventilation – pulmonary infection – pressure-induced damage • Avoids ETI complications – mini-aspiration – upper airway trauma • Allows rest periods • Preserves cough • Allows oral nutrition • Speech (and decision-making) • Allows earlier mobilization • Allows time to decide if MV is appropriate	• Lack of airways protection • No endotracheal suction • Less complete correction of blood gases than with MV • Mask discomfort; eye damage – prolonged use difficult • Ulceration over nasal bridge • Gastric dilation and vomiting – may need NG tube • Limited ventilatory capacity • Increased nursing time • Continual patient reassurance • Intolerance and distress • Impedes sputum clearance

CPAP = continuous positive airways pressure,
ETI = endotracheal intubation,
MV = mechanical ventilation, NG = nasogastric,
NIV = non-invasive ventilation

Non-invasive ventilation (NIV) is provided by machines that support ventilation and assist gas exchange without the need for endotracheal intubation (ETI). It is most successful in alert, cooperative, self-ventilating, haemodynamically stable patients who are able to protect and clear their airways.

Indications include respiratory support during acute (e.g. COPD exacerbation) or chronic (e.g. neuromuscular disease) respiratory failure, when ETI is considered inappropriate (e.g. end-stage respiratory disease) and to aid weaning from mechanical ventilation.

Individual NIV techniques deliver varying degrees of ventilatory support and/or alveolar recruitment with corresponding reductions in the work of breathing (WoB) and/or improvements in oxygenation.

1 Negative pressure ventilation (NPV) was originally developed to support victims of poliomyelitis-induced respiratory paralysis. Patients were placed in **tank ventilators** sealed at the neck. Lowering tank pressures expanded the chest causing inspiration. Expiration was passive. However, these 'iron lungs' were limited by difficulties with nursing access, poor CO$_2$ clearance and secretion retention which caused airways obstruction or pneumonia. NPV has largely been superseded by the development of positive pressure ventilators, which are particularly successful in the management of acute respiratory failure. NPV is now rarely used except in patients with chronic hypoventilation (e.g. kyphoscoliosis) or as part of rehabilitation programmes (e.g. spinal injury). Current NPV techniques include (i) **jacket (cuirass) ventilators**, which only produce a negative pressure around the chest but leaks often limit effectiveness, and (ii) **rocking beds**, which utilize gravity to enhance diaphragmatic movement.

2 Positive pressure NIV is delivered through tight-fitting nasal or full facemasks (figure a). Figure (c) lists potential benefits and disadvantages.

• **Nasal intermittent positive pressure ventilation** (NIPPV): de-livers inspiratory pressure support (PS; ~10–30 cmH$_2$O), for a prescribed inspiratory time, adjusted according to the patient's requirements. It augments tidal volume (V$_T$), clears CO$_2$ and reduces WoB. Modern NIV ventilators also provide adjustable positive end-expiratory pressure (PEEP). NIPPV is effective in chronic respiratory failure, primary alveolar hypoventilation, nocturnal hypoventilation, and in some patients with acute exacerbations of COPD or acute hypercapnic respiratory failure who are tiring and cannot maintain WoB. Successful use requires well-trained staff, gradual introduction to a cooperative patient and careful synchronization of breathing with the ventilator.

• **Continuous positive airways pressure** (CPAP): typically ~5–10 cmH$_2$O is maintained throughout inspiration and expiration by a flow generator. Resulting alveolar recruitment due to reinflation of collapsed or oedematous lung reduces $\dot{V}/\dot{Q}$ mismatch and improves oxygenation. Increased functional residual capacity (FRC) reduces WoB by moving the lung pressure–volume relationship into the steep part of the curve, making the lungs easier to inflate (i.e. increased compliance). CPAP is most successful when initiated early in diseases that respond to modest airways pressures (e.g. cardiogenic pulmonary oedema, pneumonia). It also helps prevent upper airways collapse in obstructive sleep apnoea. Both CPAP and PEEP may aid ventilation or weaning of COPD or asthma patients who are intubated or have tracheostomies by preventing small airways collapse and reducing gas trapping. A nasogastric tube prevents gastric distension and reduces the risk of aspiration (figure b).

• **Bilevel positive pressure ventilation** (BIPAP): delivers two levels of CPAP whilst allowing spontaneous respiration. The higher pressure augments alveolar ventilation and CO$_2$ clearance; the lower pressure maintains alveolar recruitment.

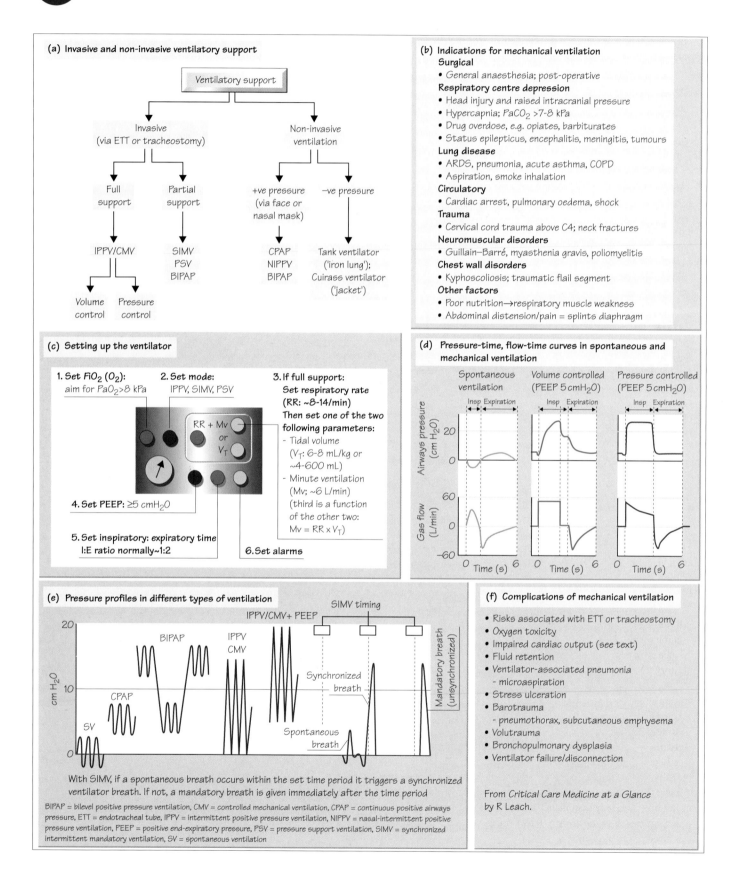

(a) Invasive and non-invasive ventilatory support

Ventilatory support

- Invasive (via ETT or tracheostomy)
  - Full support
    - IPPV/CMV
      - Volume control
      - Pressure control
  - Partial support
    - SIMV
    - PSV
    - BIPAP
- Non-invasive ventilation
  - +ve pressure (via face or nasal mask)
    - CPAP
    - NIPPV
    - BIPAP
  - −ve pressure
    - Tank ventilator ('iron lung'); Cuirass ventilator ('jacket')

(b) Indications for mechanical ventilation

Surgical
- General anaesthesia; post-operative

Respiratory centre depression
- Head injury and raised intracranial pressure
- Hypercapnia; $PaCO_2$ >7-8 kPa
- Drug overdose, e.g. opiates, barbiturates
- Status epilepticus, encephalitis, meningitis, tumours

Lung disease
- ARDS, pneumonia, acute asthma, COPD
- Aspiration, smoke inhalation

Circulatory
- Cardiac arrest, pulmonary oedema, shock

Trauma
- Cervical cord trauma above C4; neck fractures

Neuromuscular disorders
- Guillain–Barré, myasthenia gravis, poliomyelitis

Chest wall disorders
- Kyphoscoliosis; traumatic flail segment

Other factors
- Poor nutrition→respiratory muscle weakness
- Abdominal distension/pain = splints diaphragm

(c) Setting up the ventilator

1. Set FiO_2 (O_2):
   aim for PaO_2 >8 kPa
2. Set mode:
   IPPV, SIMV, PSV

RR + Mv or V_T

4. Set PEEP: ≥5 cmH₂0

5. Set inspiratory: expiratory time
   I:E ratio normally~1:2

3. If full support:
   Set respiratory rate
   (RR: ~8-14/min)
   Then set one of the two
   following parameters:
   - Tidal volume
     (V_T: 6-8 mL/kg or
     ~4-600 mL)
   - Minute ventilation
     (Mv; ~6 L/min)
     (third is a function
     of the other two:
     Mv = RR x V_T)

6. Set alarms

(d) Pressure-time, flow-time curves in spontaneous and mechanical ventilation

Spontaneous ventilation | Volume controlled (PEEP 5 cmH₂0) | Pressure controlled (PEEP 5 cmH₂0)

Airways pressure (cm H₂0): 20, 0
Gas flow (L/min): 60, 0, −60
Time (s): 0 ... 6

(e) Pressure profiles in different types of ventilation

cm H₂0: 20, 10, 0

SV | CPAP | BIPAP | IPPV CMV | IPPV/CMV+ PEEP | SIMV timing

Mandatory breath (unsynchronized)

Synchronized breath

Spontaneous breath

With SIMV, if a spontaneous breath occurs within the set time period it triggers a synchronized ventilator breath. If not, a mandatory breath is given immediately after the time period

BIPAP = bilevel positive pressure ventilation, CMV = controlled mechanical ventilation, CPAP = continuous positive airways pressure, ETT = endotracheal tube, IPPV = intermittent positive pressure ventilation, NIPPV = nasal-intermittent positive pressure ventilation, PEEP = positive end-expiratory pressure, PSV = pressure support ventilation, SIMV = synchronized intermittent mandatory ventilation, SV = spontaneous ventilation

(f) Complications of mechanical ventilation

- Risks associated with ETT or tracheostomy
- Oxygen toxicity
- Impaired cardiac output (see text)
- Fluid retention
- Ventilator-associated pneumonia
  - microaspiration
- Stress ulceration
- Barotrauma
  - pneumothorax, subcutaneous emphysema
- Volutrauma
- Bronchopulmonary dysplasia
- Ventilator failure/disconnection

From *Critical Care Medicine at a Glance*
by R Leach.

During critical illness, ventilatory support (figure a) may be required to maintain gas exchange and reduce the work of breathing (WoB). Mechanical ventilation (MV) is usually delivered through an endotracheal tube or tracheostomy and provides complete or partial respiratory support. Non-invasive ventilation (NIV) aids spontaneous ventilation and avoids the need for endotracheal intubation.

Indications for MV (figure b)

Outside the operating theatre, the main indication for MV is respiratory failure. However, its value in the support of other organs, especially during shock or cardiac failure, is increasingly being recognized. Apart from in acute emergencies (e.g. cardiac arrest), the difficult decision is when and whether to ventilate a progressively deteriorating patient. There are no simple guidelines. However, hypoxaemia ($PO_2 < 8$ kPa on $FiO_2 > 0.4$), hypercapnia ($PCO_2 > 7.5$ kPa), respiratory/metabolic acidosis (pH < 7.2) and physical factors (e.g. confusion, exhaustion, poor cough) usually indicate the need for MV. Trends in these variables are often more helpful than absolute values. MV should only be considered when there is a reasonable chance of survival. In terminal illness, support may be limited to NIV, after appropriate discussion with the patient and/or relatives.

Ventilator set-up (figure c)

Typical initial adult intermittent positive pressure ventilation (IPPV) settings would be: tidal volume (V_T) ~6–8 mL/kg; respiratory frequency (f) ~8–14 breaths/min; and minute ventilation ($M_V = V_T \times f$) ~ 6 L/min. FiO_2 and M_V are adjusted to maintain $PaO_2 > 8$ kPa and $PaCO_2 < 7$ kPa, respectively, but acceptable values depend on individual disease processes. Initially PEEP is set at 3–5 cmH$_2$O and the inspiratory : expiratory time (I : E ratio) at ~1 : 2.

Mode of ventilation (figure e)

Mode of ventilation describes whether a breath is: (i) fully or partially supported; (ii) volume or pressure controlled; (iii) mandatory (delivered by the ventilator regardless of patient respiratory effort); or (iv) spontaneously triggered (figures a and e). The duration of a breath may be fixed (i.e. timed) or variable (i.e. dependent on tidal volume delivery). Modern ventilators with microprocessor controls provide considerable flexibility, allowing a change from mandatory, full support modes to partial support modes that minimize sedation requirements and allow patients to be conscious but comfortable.

- **Full (mandatory) support modes** (e.g. IPPV, controlled mechanical ventilation (CMV)) are uncomfortable and may require sedation as no allowance is made for spontaneous respiration. They are used in severe respiratory disease, in circulatory instability or when respiratory drive is absent. Volume- and pressure-controlled ventilatory (VCV, PCV) modes are available but the pattern of gas flow in PCV achieves optimal gas exchange.

   Volume-controlled IPPV/CMV (figure d) is often used postoperatively. Each breath is delivered at a preset volume over a fixed time. Airway pressure varies with lung compliance.

   Pressure-controlled IPPV/CMV (figure d) delivers a preset pressure and there is no direct control of tidal volume, which depends on inspiratory time, lung compliance and airways resistance. PCV protects lungs by limiting peak inspiratory pressures (PIPs) and encourages alveolar recruitment.

- **Partial support modes** reinforce spontaneous ventilation and are preferred when possible, to allow a reduction in sedation. Breaths are initiated by the patient and detected by sensitive flow/pressure triggers in the ventilator, which then provides inspiratory support.

   Assist control: the ventilator delivers a breath when triggered by inspiratory effort or independently if the patient does not breathe within a certain time.

   Synchronized intermittent mandatory ventilation (SIMV) delivers a set number of mechanically imposed breaths to achieve a minimum minute ventilation but allows pressure-supported spontaneous breathing. Imposed breaths are reduced as the patient becomes ventilator independent during weaning.

   Pressure support: a preset pressure supports every spontaneous breath. The rate is dependent on the patient. Gradual pressure reductions make it a comfortable and effective mode of weaning.

- **Positive end-expiratory pressure (PEEP)** describes a positive pressure, maintained throughout expiration, that increases functional residual capacity (i.e. alveolar recruitment), prevents alveolar collapse at end-expiration, reduces $\dot{V}/\dot{Q}$ mismatch and decreases alveolar oedema by increasing lymphatic drainage. PEEP improves oxygenation and oxygen delivery for any given mode of ventilation, provided that the cardiac output (CO) is not significantly reduced by the associated increase in intrathoracic pressure (IP).

Physiological responses to MV

1 Cardiovascular effects are due to increased IP and alveolar overdistension. Increased IP has two effects on the heart.

   (i) **Right ventricular (RV) preload reduction** is due to increased right atrial pressure, which reduces venous return and RV cardiac output. However, fluid infusion rapidly restores venous return and CO.

   (ii) **Left ventricular (LV) afterload reduction** is due to reduced LV transmural pressure, which decreases LV work. In the normal heart, any beneficial effect of LV afterload reduction is offset by reduced venous return. However, in the failing heart, CO is relatively insensitive to preload changes but very sensitive to afterload reduction. Consequently, MV may increase CO in heart failure, a useful therapeutic effect.

   The overall response to raised IP depends on the state of the heart, vasomotor tone and fluid status (e.g. hypovolaemia). MV also increases lung volumes. Overinflated alveoli compress alveolar blood vessels, increasing pulmonary vascular resistance and causing pulmonary hypertension. Subsequent RV distension displaces the septum into the LV cavity, reducing LV filling and CO, an effect known as interventricular dependence.

2 Respiratory effects: MV reduces WoB, which increases the proportion of CO going to other potentially ischaemic organs. Re-expansion of collapsed lung segments also improves oxygenation. Unfortunately, supine position, reduced surfactant production and ventilation of poorly perfused lung increases $\dot{V}/\dot{Q}$ mismatch.

3 Fluid retention is due to antidiuretic hormone secretion.

Complications of MV (figure f)

A number of complications may arise. '**Barotrauma**' refers to pressure-induced lung damage (e.g. pneumothorax). High PIP (> 35 cmH$_2$O) due to reduced lung compliance (e.g. ARDS) may cause airways disruption and interstitial gas formation. '**Volutrauma**' describes damage to healthy alveoli due to overdistension during recruitment of diseased lung. '**Protective**' ventilation strategies use low tidal volumes (~ 6 mL/kg) to avoid volutrauma, keep PIP < 35 cmH$_2$O and maintain alveolar recruitment with PEEP > 5 cmH$_2$O.

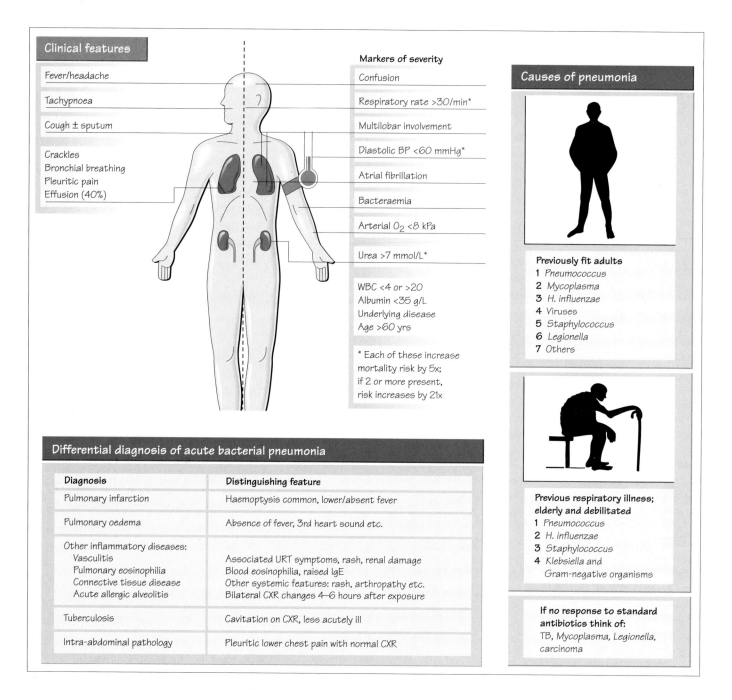

Clinical features

Fever/headache

Tachypnoea

Cough ± sputum

Crackles
Bronchial breathing
Pleuritic pain
Effusion (40%)

Markers of severity

Confusion

Respiratory rate >30/min*

Multilobar involvement

Diastolic BP <60 mmHg*

Atrial fibrillation

Bacteraemia

Arterial O₂ <8 kPa

Urea >7 mmol/L*

WBC <4 or >20
Albumin <35 g/L
Underlying disease
Age >60 yrs

* Each of these increase
mortality risk by 5x;
if 2 or more present,
risk increases by 21x

Causes of pneumonia

Previously fit adults
1 Pneumococcus
2 Mycoplasma
3 H. influenzae
4 Viruses
5 Staphylococcus
6 Legionella
7 Others

**Previous respiratory illness;
elderly and debilitated**
1 Pneumococcus
2 H. influenzae
3 Staphylococcus
4 Klebsiella and
   Gram-negative organisms

**If no response to standard
antibiotics think of:**
TB, Mycoplasma, Legionella,
carcinoma

Differential diagnosis of acute bacterial pneumonia

Diagnosis	Distinguishing feature
Pulmonary infarction	Haemoptysis common, lower/absent fever
Pulmonary oedema	Absence of fever, 3rd heart sound etc.

Other inflammatory diseases:
  Vasculitis
  Pulmonary eosinophilia
  Connective tissue disease
  Acute allergic alveolitis
	
	Associated URT symptoms, rash, renal damage
	Blood eosinophilia, raised IgE
	Other systemic features: rash, arthropathy etc.
	Bilateral CXR changes 4–6 hours after exposure

Tuberculosis	Cavitation on CXR, less acutely ill
Intra-abdominal pathology	Pleuritic lower chest pain with normal CXR

Pneumonia is an acute infective respiratory illness causing radiological shadowing. It is classified according to the setting in which it is acquired, because this influences the likely microbial pathogens and therefore the best empirical treatment:
- Community acquired.
- Hospital acquired (nosocomial).
- Aspiration pneumonia.
- Pneumonia in immunocompromised individuals.

Community-acquired pneumonia
Epidemiology and pathophysiology
Very common. Community incidence is 1–3/1000 in adults. A quarter of cases require hospital admission. M = F, although Legionnaire's disease is more common in males. Pneumonia tends to occur at the extremes of age, but it remains an important cause of morbidity and even mortality in young adults.

Infection occurs by droplet spread. Organisms multiply in the lung

Pathogen	% cases	Specific features
Streptococcus pneumoniae	60–75	Commonest in winter months
		Lobar involvement >> bronchopneumonic pattern
		Rapid onset, high fever, herpes labialis, vomiting. Mortality 5–10%
Mycoplasma pneumoniae	5–18	Mainly in autumn. Epidemics every 3–4 years
		Complications (20%): myocarditis, meningo-encephalitis, rash,
		haemolytic anaemia (cold haemagglutinin)
Haemophilus influenzae	4–5	Bronchopneumonia. Usually underlying lung disease
Legionella	2–5	Commonest in autumn in previously healthy individuals, from contaminated
		air conditioning. Key features: confusion, hepatitis, renal impairment, $\downarrow$Na$^+$
Chlamydia psittaci	2	From infected birds. Protracted illness. 50% hepato-splenomegaly
Staphylococcus aureus	1–5	During influenza A epidemics. Rapid progression and high mortality (30%)
		Cavitation in 50%, pleural effusion/empyema in 15%, pneumothorax
Gram-negative pneumonia	10	Underlying illness, often chronic. Increased chance in nosocomial infections.
		Often severe pneumonia, with septic shock. Klebsiella, Pseudomonas, E. coli
Influenza	5–8	Preceding myalgia + severe prostration. Epidemic
Other	2–8	

Confusion

Urea (>7 mmol/L)

Respiratory rate (>30/min)

Blood pressure (DBP <60 mmHg)

Interpretation
- 2 CURB criteria = severe pneumonia
- No CURB criteria = non-severe pneumonia
- One CURB criterion use clinical judgement and age (>60 years)/ hypoxia (pO_2 <8 kPa) to decide whether to treat with cefuroxime

and, if local defence mechanisms are overcome, pneumonia develops. Tobacco smoke impairs local defences by depressing ciliary function. The causes of pneumonia are listed in the figure.

Clinical features

Fever and cough (initially non-productive) are common symptoms. Chest pain and breathlessness may also occur. Systemic features (more common but not specific to atypical pneumonia) include headache, confusion, myalgia and malaise. A prolonged prodrome is more specific to the atypical organisms. Examination may reveal local signs of consolidation and crackles over the affected lobe. Tachypnoea, hypotension, confusion and cyanosis all suggest severe disease.

Differential diagnosis of pneumonia (see figure)

Investigations aim to:
- **Confirm diagnosis**: this is usually done radiologically using a plain chest X-ray.
- **Define cause**: microbiological diagnosis is achieved by diagnostic Gram stain, by growing the organism, by demonstrating a characteristic antigen from the organism or serologically (or other diagnostic blood test). All these tests have advantages and disadvantages and a combined approach may be necessary.
- **Assess severity**: see markers of severity in figure.
- **Identify complications**: complications can be detected by chest X-ray, computed tomography and bronchoscopy, and include pleural effusion and empyema, lobar collapse (sputum retention), pneumothorax (in cavitating pneumonia) and organizing pneumonia.
- **Exclude cancer**: bronchoscopy should be considered in all people aged ≥ 50 years who smoke presenting with pneumonia, to exclude underlying lung cancer.

Management and prognosis

General supportive measures: intravenous fluid, oxygen and physiotherapy.

Antibiotic therapy: severe pneumonia—intravenous cephalosporin (e.g. cefuroxime) and macrolide (erythromycin/clarithromycin). In less severe cases, ampicillin is substituted for the cephalosporin and in mild cases, amoxicillin alone is adequate.

The outcome is generally good. Mortality is higher in the elderly. Overall mortality is 5% but increases to 20% if hospital admission is required and 50% if intensive care is needed. Following improvement, particularly in smokers, radiological resolution should be confirmed to exclude underlying pulmonary abnormality, including lung cancer.

Hospital-acquired pneumonia

This is pneumonia occurring ≥ 2 days after admission to hospital. Infection before this is classified as community acquired.
- Causative organisms predominantly Gram-negative.
- Broad-spectrum antibiotics necessary.
- High mortality associated with co-morbid factors.

Epidemiology and aetiopathogenesis

This is more common in elderly people, complicates 2–5% of all hospital admissions and accounts for 10–15% of hospital-acquired infections.

Several factors predispose patients to the development of pneumonia in hospital—principally increased aspiration risk, reduced host defences and lung/skin instrumentation breaching the normal defences. Although those organisms that cause community-acquired pneumonia also cause infections in hospital, Gram-negative bacteria, *Staphylococcus aureus* and anaerobic organisms are far more likely to be found. Patients with underlying lung disease who develop postoperative pneumonia are still most likely to have pneumococcal or haemophilus infection.

Clinical features and investigation

These are as for community-acquired pneumonia. The severity of illness is often greater as a result of the presence of underlying disease.

Management
- **General supportive treatment**: oxygen, fluids and physiotherapy.

- **Specific antibiotic treatment** needs to cover Gram-negative organisms which are resistant to the antibiotics given in community-acquired pneumonia. Antibiotics for nosocomial pneumonia:
  - Third-generation cephalosporin (e.g. cefotaxime) + aminoglycoside.
  - Thienamycin (imipenem, meropenem).
  - Anti-pseudomonal penicillin (piperacillin/tazobactam).
  - Consider anti-staphylococcal ± methicillin-resistant *Staph. aureus* (MRSA) cover (flucloxacillin/vancomycin).

The prognosis depends on the causative organism and underlying disease severity. Pneumonia is often the cause of death in elderly hospital patients. In ventilated patients in intensive care, pseudomonas pneumonia has a 50% mortality rate.

Lung abscess

A lung abscess is localized infection of the lung parenchyma with associated cavitation caused by necrosis. It is an uncommon problem occurring mainly in elderly people.
- Certain specific pneumonic agents are more likely to cavitate: *Staphylococcus aureus*, *Klebsiella* spp. and anaerobic infection.
- Aspirated gastric contents, typically in those who have lost consciousness, with bulbar palsy or have problems with alcohol. Infected sinuses also predispose to anaerobic infection.
- Intravenous drug abusers with right-sided endocarditis develop multiple lung abscesses.
- Tuberculosis (TB) also causes cavitation, although the presentation is generally less acute.

Clinical features

These are of severe infection with fever and systemic upset. Large amounts of purulent and offensive sputum are produced if an abscess drains into an airway. Rapid weight loss and finger clubbing occur, and make the distinction from cavitating bronchial carcinoma important. Localized clinical signs in the chest may be minimal or there may be signs of consolidation and a pleural rub if there is pleural inflammation.

Investigations

These are as for pneumonia to confirm the diagnosis, the cause and assess the severity of the illness. By definition, the chest X-ray will show signs of cavitation, although this must be distinguished from the cavitation found in cancer, TB, vasculitis (Wegener's granulomatosis) and other rarer causes.

Management and prognosis

Prolonged (6 weeks) antibiotics, e.g. amoxicillin, or cefuroxime if unwell, and metronidazole to cover *Klebsiella* spp. and anaerobes are usually adequate. Drainage of the abscess usually occurs via the airway and this may be encouraged at bronchoscopy, which will also exclude an underlying obstructing lesion. Percutaneous drainage is not employed because there is a risk of introducing infection into the pleural cavity.

With adequate drainage and appropriate antibiotics, the prognosis is generally very good.

Pneumonia in the immunocompromised
Definition and epidemiology

Pneumonia occurring in patients with deficiency of cellular or humoral immune mechanisms. The incidence is increasing as a result of the use of immunosuppressive drugs (transplantations, vasculitis), chemotherapy (malignancy) and HIV infection. Effective antiretroviral treatment and prophylaxis against *Pneumocystis carinii* has significantly reduced the incidence of pulmonary infections complicating HIV (see p. 300).

Pathophysiology

Pulmonary infection is normally prevented by a combination of mechanical elements (epiglottis, cough and gag reflexes, and the mucociliary escalator) and specific immunological mechanisms (macrophage/neutrophils, antibodies produced by B lymphocytes, and cellular immunity effected by T lymphocytes). Defects in any of these mechanisms lead to increased risk of infection. Infection with multiple organisms is common. Infections associated with immunosuppression are:
- **Neutropenia**: Gram-negative bacteria, *Staphylococcus aureus*, fungi (*Candida*, *Aspergillus* spp.).
- **Reduced immunoglobulins**: bacteria (pneumococci, *Haemophilus influenzae*).
- **T-cell defects**: bacteria (pneumococci, *H. influenzae*, *Staph. aureus*), fungi (*Candida*, *Pneumocystis* spp.), viruses (herpes group CMV, adenovirus), and mycobacteria.

Clinical features and investigations

The diagnosis may be clear with fever, cough and breathlessness with focal clinical signs—symptoms that suggest bacterial infection. Symptoms are often more vague when infection is with opportunistic organisms. Onset may be over several weeks and fever may be absent. A high index of suspicion is necessary in patients known to be immunosuppressed.
- Investigation of the underlying immunological defect may be necessary. Full blood count, Ig levels and other tests including HIV.
- Plain chest X-ray may reveal focal changes. Computed tomography may reveal alternative pathology but cannot provide a microbiological diagnosis.
- Standard microbiological investigation includes culture of sputum, blood and pleural fluid. If doubt exists, bronchoalveolar lavage may be necessary, but this has risks and should be reserved for those in whom initial investigation does not achieve a diagnosis. In those who fail to improve or where diagnostic doubt remains, lung biopsy may be necessary.
- At all stages in investigation, close liaison with microbiologists is necessary because specific culture techniques are necessary to identify likely organisms, particularly mycobacteria, viruses and fungi. DNA amplification techniques are used increasingly, particularly for diagnosis of viral infection.

Management and prognosis

A microbial diagnosis is often not known before treatment is started. In general, broad-spectrum antibacterial agents are necessary while the results of cultures are awaited. Combinations should cover Gram-negative bacteria, including *Pseudomonas* spp. and staphylococci. A combination of anti-pseudomonal penicillin or third-generation cephalosporin with an aminoglycoside is often used as empirical treatment. Treatment can subsequently be changed according to the results of microbiological investigation. Treatment for viral and fungal infections will include specific antiviral and antifungal agents such as ganciclovir and amphotericin.

Infections often progress rapidly in immunocompromised patients. Achieving an accurate diagnosis to guide treatment is therefore important. Despite full supportive treatment and antibiotics, pulmonary infection in these patients accounts for up to 50 or 60% of the mortality.

93 Upper respiratory tract infection

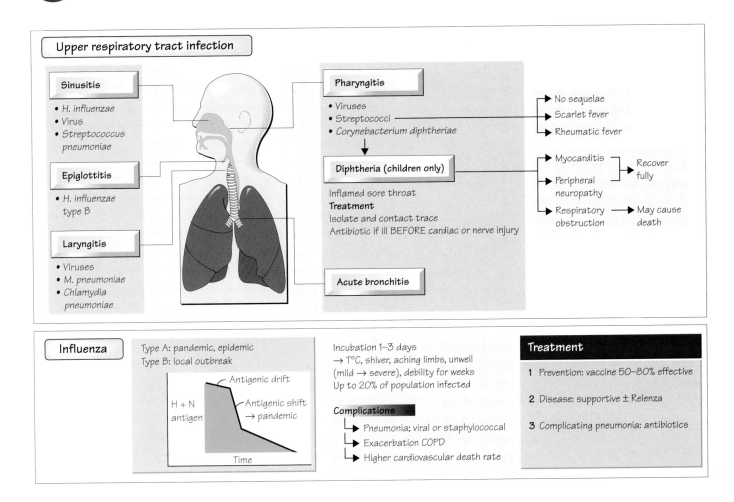

Table 93.1 The common causes of upper respiratory tract infection, their features and management.

	Cause	Features	Investigation	Management	Prognosis
Common cold (coryza)	Viruses	Sneezing, nasal blockage and discharge	None	Symptomatic	Remits in days
Pharyngitis (all ages)	Viral; occasionally streptococcal	Fever, sore throat	Throat swab ASO titre	Antibiotics if bacterial; surgery if abscess develops	Remits in 1 week if viral
Laryngitis (adults)	Viral; occasionally pneumococci or *Haemophilus* spp.	Fever, hoarse voice	Throat swab	Antibiotics, humidification	Remits in about 1 week
Epiglottitis (children)	*Haemophilus influenzae* (occasional pneumococci)	Fever, sore throat, stridor, upper airway obstruction	Throat swab blood cultures, lateral neck X-ray	IV antibiotics, humidification, facilities for intubation Prevention by HIB vaccination	Slow improvement with treatment, risk of death from airway obstruction
Bronchitis (all ages)	Viral; occasional pneumococci or *Haemophilus* spp.	Dry cough, retrosternal soreness, wheeze; sputum if bacterial	Sputum culture	Usually resolves but antibiotics often given	Improves over a week
Sinusitis (all ages)	Various bacteria 15% viral	Headache, facial pain, nasal congestion	None; sinus X-ray if severe	Antibiotics; decongestants may help; sinus washout or surgery if persistent	Remits if acute; chronic problems are common

Diseases and Treatments at a Glance

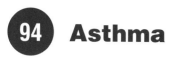

94 Asthma

Asthma

Asthma is an inflammatory condition causing reversible airway obstruction and symptoms of:

- Cough
- Wheeze   } All, or
- Chest tightness } any one
- Breathlessness

Symptoms respond to β2 agonists

Consider underlying disease when asthma bad, adult onset, abnormal laboratory tests or CXR.
1 Allergic bronchopulmonary aspergillosis
2 Churg–Strauss
3 Bronchiectasis

Peak flow chart showing classical morning dipping

(Peak flow rate axis: 100, 200, 300, 400, 500; x-axis: am pm am pm am pm)

	I. Intrinsic	II. Extrinsic

- Adults
- Fewer have ↑ IgE or +ve skin tests

- Children
- Atopic ↑ IgE
- +ve skin tests

Triggers (may be multifactorial)

Drugs
- Aspirin
- β–blockers

Allergens
- Dust mite
- Cat/dog dander
- Pollens

Occupational
- Isocyanates
- Drugs/enzymes
- Wood resin
- Dyes

Environment
- Cold air
- Exercise
- Emotion

Clinical features

❶ Air entry
- Normal   ⎤
- Wheezy   ⎥ ↑ Severe attack
- Silent   ⎦

❷ ↑ Respiratory rate
Use of accessory muscles of respiration
- Sternocleidomastoid
- Pectorals
Intercostal recession

❸ ↑ Heart rate

❹ ↓ Ability to talk

❺ Deviated trachea if tension pneumothorax

❻ Cyanosis

❼ Clammy, sweating

❽ Confused

} In life-threatening attacks

Obligate investigations in all severe asthma

- CXR (every severe attack)
- ABG (repeated as long as sick)

In between attacks	Moderate	Severe	Life threatening
Normal exam Normal lung function tests	PEFR <65% predicted ↓ Admit to hospital	PEFR <50% Pulse rate >110 Respiratory rate >25 Can't complete sentences Wheezy chest Alert → mild confusion	PEFR <33% Bradychardia Exhaustion Can't talk at all Silent chest Confusion → coma
pO2	↓	↓↓	↓↓↓
pCO2	↓	→	↑
pH	Ⓝ or ↑	Ⓝ	↓
			Alert ITU

Pulsus paradoxus

Arterial pressure (mmHg)
Expiration Inspiration

- Normal <5 mmHg
- Moderate 5–10 mmHg
- Severe 10–20 mmHg
- Life threatening >20 mmHg

NB Large paradox may also arise from tension pneumothorax or from pericardial tamponade

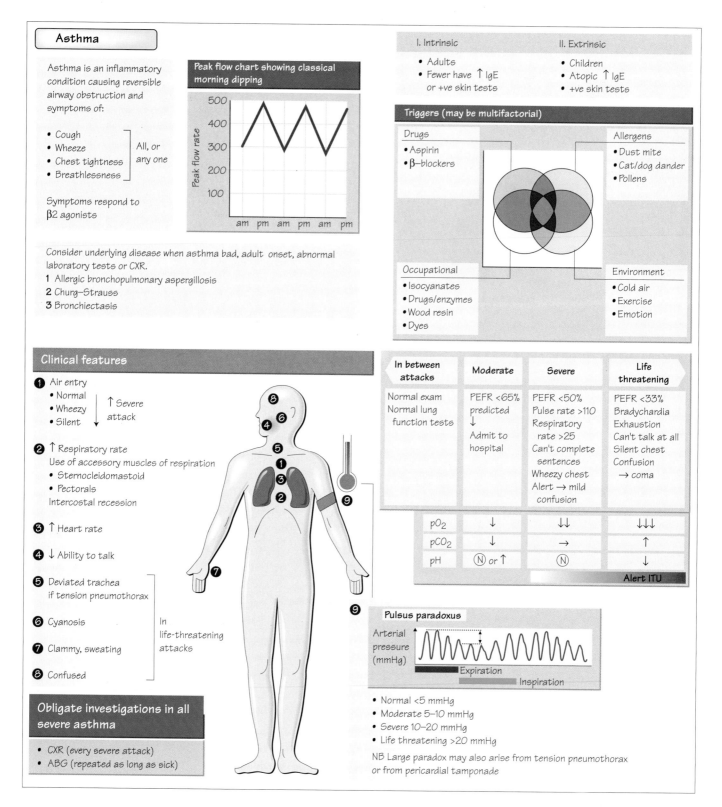

Diseases and Treatments at a Glance

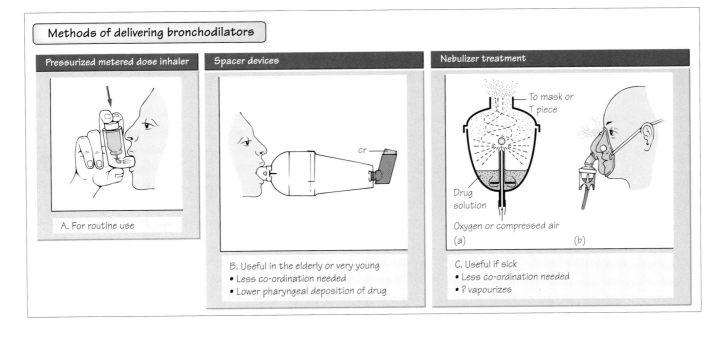

Methods of delivering bronchodilators

Pressurized metered dose inhaler

A. For routine use

Spacer devices

cr

B. Useful in the elderly or very young
• Less co-ordination needed
• Lower pharyngeal deposition of drug

Nebulizer treatment

To mask or
T piece

Drug
solution

Oxygen or compressed air
(a)   (b)

C. Useful if sick
• Less co-ordination needed
• ? vapourizes

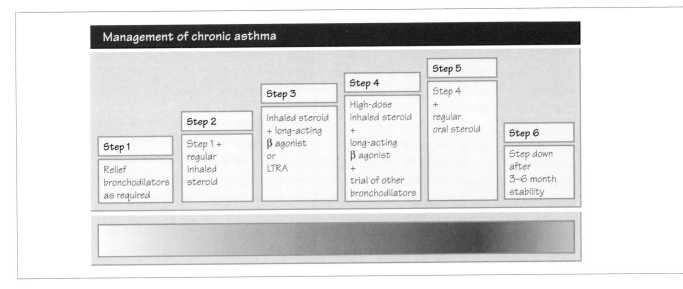

Management of chronic asthma

Step 1
Relief bronchodilators as required

Step 2
Step 1 + regular inhaled steroid

Step 3
Inhaled steroid + long-acting β agonist or LTRA

Step 4
High-dose inhaled steroid + long-acting β agonist + trial of other bronchodilators

Step 5
Step 4 + regular oral steroid

Step 6
Step down after 3–6 month stability

Definition

There is no universally accepted definition. Asthma is present if a combination of cough, wheeze or breathlessness with **variable** airflow obstruction is present.

Epidemiology

Asthma is the single most important cause of respiratory disease morbidity and causes 2000 deaths/year in the UK. The prevalence, currently 10–15%, is increasing in Western societies. The incidence of wheeze is highest in childhood (one in three children wheeze and one in seven schoolchildren have a diagnosis of asthma). Asthma is classified as:

• **Extrinsic**: childhood asthma, associated with atopy (atopy = familial allergic diathesis, manifest as childhood eczema and hay fever). Often remits by teenage years, although it may recur during adult life.

• **Intrinsic**: develops in later life, is less likely to be caused by allergy, may be more progressive and does not respond as well to treatment.

• **Occupational**, when it relates to industrial/work place allergens (e.g. photocopier material, etc.).

Aetiology

Genetics

Asthma runs in families in association with atopy. Genetic studies show linkage to the high-affinity IgE receptor and the T-helper (Th2) cytokine genes (chromosome 5).

Environmental factors

Specific bronchial stimuli include house-dust mite, pollen and cat dander; 3% of the population is sensitive to aspirin.

• **Occupational exposure** to irritants or sensitizers is an important cause of work-related asthma.

• **Non-specific stimuli**: viral infections, cold air, exercise or emotional stress may also precipitate wheeze. High atmospheric levels of ozone

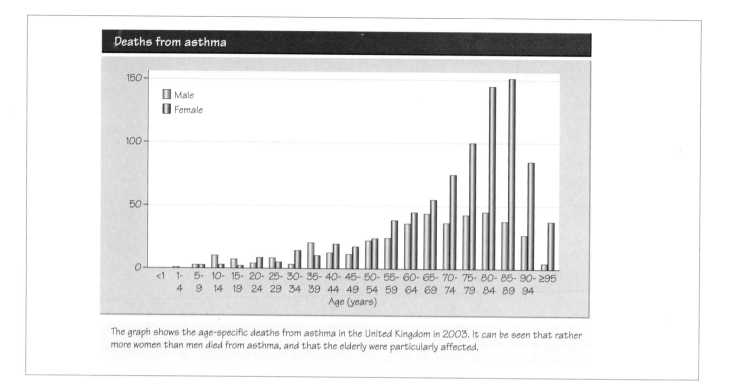

Deaths from asthma

The graph shows the age-specific deaths from asthma in the United Kingdom in 2003. It can be seen that rather more women than men died from asthma, and that the elderly were particularly affected.

(e.g. as found during a thunder storm) or particulate matter predispose to exacerbations of pre-existing asthma.

• **Other environmental factors**, including dietary ones (high Na^+, low Mg^{2+}), falling childhood infections (partly as the result of immunization) and increased environmental load of allergens (dust mite) are responsible for increasing prevalence.

Pathology

Airway remodelling occurs with smooth muscle hypertrophy and fibrosis. Histology shows inflammatory cell infiltrate (particularly eosinophils) in airway walls.

Clinical features

Asthma presents with symptoms of cough, wheeze and breathlessness, which vary over time. An obvious trigger such as exercise or allergen exposure may be present. Examination may be normal or may reveal expiratory wheeze.

Investigations

Lung function tests may show airflow obstruction or may be normal. Serial peak flow measurements are useful in making the diagnosis, and often show a classic pattern of morning dipping. In people with known asthma, peak flow measurements are useful markers of severity.

Management

The objective of treatment is to keep patients free of symptoms on the minimum therapy.

• **Patient education** is vital for successful management, particularly explanation of the triggers, use and role of medication, and how to detect and react to a deterioration. All patients should be given a written self-management plan.

• **Avoidance of environmental triggers or allergens** is important, especially of cigarette smoke.

• **Chronic asthma**: a stepped care approach is recommended (see figure).

• **Acute asthma**: oxygen, systemic corticosteroids, inhaled beta-agonists, anticholinergics and theophyllines if necessary.

Prognosis

Asthma is a chronic disease requiring maintenance treatment. If asthma is not adequately treated with inhaled corticosteroids, lung function is liable to deteriorate over time and airflow obstruction may become irreversible. Risk factors for death from asthma include poor treatment compliance, intensive therapy unit (ITU) admissions and hospital admission despite steroid treatment.

95 Chronic obstructive pulmonary disease

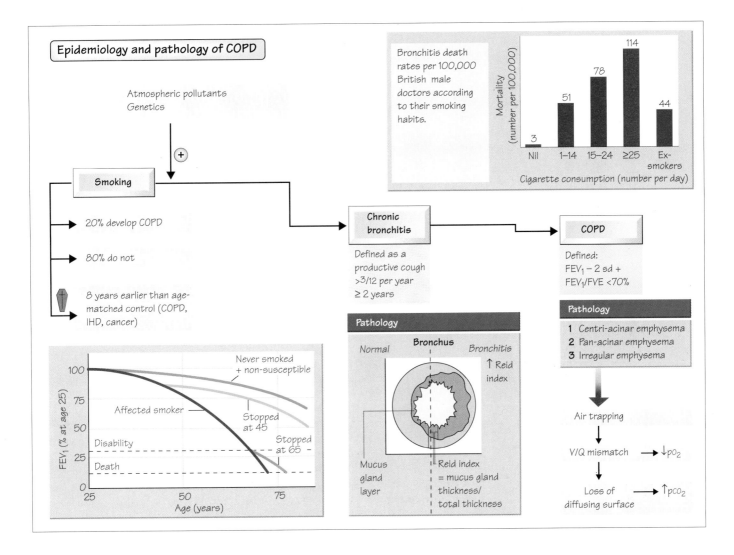

Epidemiology and pathology of COPD

Atmospheric pollutants
Genetics

Smoking

20% develop COPD

80% do not

8 years earlier than age-matched control (COPD, IHD, cancer)

Bronchitis death rates per 100,000 British male doctors according to their smoking habits.

Chronic bronchitis

Defined as a productive cough >3/12 per year ≥ 2 years

COPD

Defined:
$FEV_1 - 2$ sd +
$FEV_1/FVE <70\%$

Pathology

1 Centri-acinar emphysema
2 Pan-acinar emphysema
3 Irregular emphysema

Air trapping

V/Q mismatch → ↓po_2

Loss of diffusing surface → ↑pco_2

Pathology

Normal — Bronchus — Bronchitis

↑ Reid index

Mucus gland layer

Reid index = mucus gland thickness/ total thickness

Definition
Chronic obstructive pulmonary disease (COPD) and chronic obstructive airway disease (COAD) are interchangeable terms. A chronic, slowly progressive disorder characterized by fixed or partially reversible airway obstruction, unlike the reversible airway obstruction seen in asthma (see p. 188).

Epidemiology
COPD is a major public health problem from which 30 000 people die/year in the UK (5.1% of all deaths). The prevalence is ≥ 900 000. Rates are higher in industrialized countries, in inner city areas, among lower income groups and in elderly people. Rates have plateaued in men but are still rising in women.

Aetiology
• **Environmental factors**: cigarette smoking is the major cause, with additional risk from atmospheric pollutants in the workplace or in the inner city. Some patients have chronic, undiagnosed and untreated asthma.

• **Genetics**: α_1-antitrypsin deficiency predisposes to early development of COPD.

Pathology
Smoking causes bronchial mucus gland hypertrophy and increased mucus production, leading to a productive cough. In chronic bronchitis ('productive cough' > 3 months/year for > 2 years) the early changes are in the small airways. In addition, destruction of lung tissue with dilatation of the distal airspaces (emphysema) occurs, leading to loss of elastic recoil, hyperinflation, gas trapping and an increase in the work of breathing, causing breathlessness. As the disease progresses CO_2 levels rise and the drive to respiration switches from CO_2 to hypoxaemia. If supplementary oxygen removes hypoxaemia, the drive to respiration may also be removed, provoking respiratory failure.

Clinical features
Slowly progressing symptoms of cough and shortness of breath over several years in a smoker or ex-smoker suggests the diagnosis. Severity

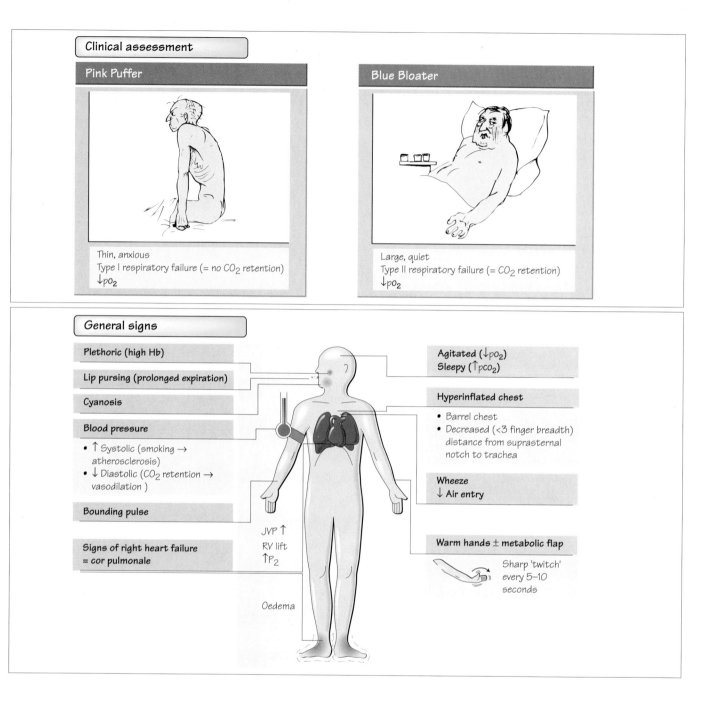

Clinical assessment

Pink Puffer

Thin, anxious
Type I respiratory failure (= no CO_2 retention)
↓po_2

Blue Bloater

Large, quiet
Type II respiratory failure (= CO_2 retention)
↓po_2

General signs

Plethoric (high Hb)

Lip pursing (prolonged expiration)

Cyanosis

Blood pressure

- ↑ Systolic (smoking →
  atherosclerosis)
- ↓ Diastolic (CO_2 retention →
  vasodilation)

Bounding pulse

Signs of right heart failure
= cor pulmonale

JVP ↑
RV lift
↑P_2

Oedema

Agitated (↓po_2)
Sleepy (↑pco_2)

Hyperinflated chest

- Barrel chest
- Decreased (<3 finger breadth)
  distance from suprasternal
  notch to trachea

Wheeze
↓ Air entry

Warm hands ± metabolic flap

Sharp 'twitch'
every 5–10
seconds

is defined according to the degree of airflow obstruction (forced expiratory volume in 1 s [FEV_1], see p. 176):
- Mild disease: FEV_1 50–80% of age/sex predicted—cough, minimal dyspnoea, normal examination.
- Moderate disease: FEV_1 30–49%—cough, breathless on moderate exertion, wheeze, hyperinflation and reduced air entry.
- Severe disease: FEV_1 < 30%—cough, breathless on minimal exertion; signs of moderate COPD and possibly of respiratory failure and cor pulmonale.

Investigations

- **Pulmonary function tests** show airflow obstruction and reduced gas transfer as a result of destruction of lung tissue. Total lung capacity may be normal, or increased as a result of gas trapping. Twenty per cent

of patients derive benefit from bronchodilators. Response to bronchodilator treatment is not predicted by reversibility testing, which is therefore not recommended.
- **Chest X-ray** may be normal but, in emphysema, will reveal hyperinflation with loss of lung markings and a small heart.
- **Computed tomography** may confirm emphysematous bullae.
- **Blood gases** should be analysed if there is any suspicion of respiratory failure. In chronic hypoxaemia the haemoglobin may be increased.

Management

- **Smoking cessation** is a priority.
- **Bronchodilators** (β-agonists or anticholinergics) are used in the 20–40% who benefit. In severe disease up to 10% of patients derive more benefit if high doses are delivered by nebulizer rather than metered dose

Diseases and Treatments at a Glance

The COPD escalator

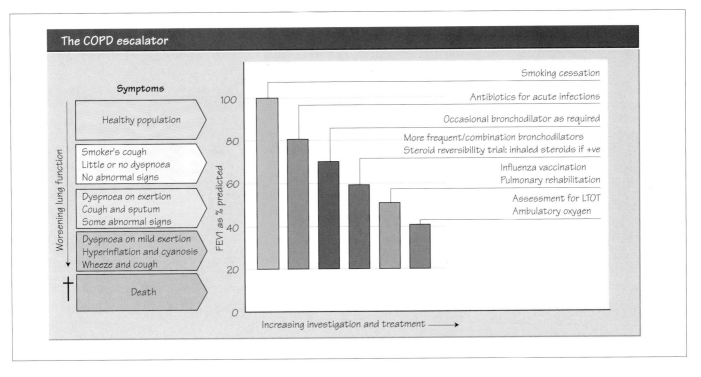

Symptoms

Worsening lung function →

- Healthy population
- Smoker's cough
  Little or no dyspnoea
  No abnormal signs
- Dyspnoea on exertion
  Cough and sputum
  Some abnormal signs
- Dyspnoea on mild exertion
  Hyperinflation and cyanosis
  Wheeze and cough
- † Death

FEV1 as % predicted (0–100)

Increasing investigation and treatment →

- Smoking cessation
- Antibiotics for acute infections
- Occasional bronchodilator as required
- More frequent/combination bronchodilators
  Steroid reversibility trial: inhaled steroids if +ve
- Influenza vaccination
  Pulmonary rehabilitation
- Assessment for LTOT
  Ambulatory oxygen

Investigation of COPD

1 Lung function tests + arterial blood gases
2 CXR to exclude other (smoking-related) pathology
3 ± CT scan

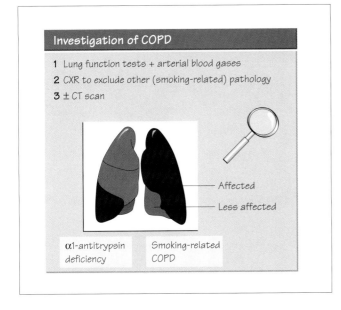

— Affected
— Less affected

| α1-antitrypsin deficiency | Smoking-related COPD |

---

inhaler. A 2-week trial of oral steroids should be considered to determine reversibility (from serial peak flow or spirometry) of airway obstruction if a diagnosis of untreated asthma is suspected.

- Long-term **oxygen therapy** for > 16 h daily prolongs life in patients with chronic respiratory failure (i.e. those with a Pao_2 of 7.3 kPa and FEV_1 of 1.5 L).
- In an acute exacerbation, treatment may need to be increased. **Antibiotics** have not been shown to improve outcome, although short-course antibiotics shorten symptom duration of purulent sputum and respiratory deterioration. **Oral steroids** improve recovery from acute exacerbations. Long-term **inhaled steroids** reduce the frequency of exacerbations in those with moderate + disease and should be used in those with an $FEV_1 < 50\%$ and at least one exacerbation per year.
- **Pulmonary rehabilitation** (especially exercise training) produces significant symptomatic benefit in patients with moderate-to-severe disease.
- **Resection of large bullae** enables adjacent areas of lung to re-inflate. **Lung volume reduction surgery** may also produce improvement by improving elastic recoil and so maintaining airway patency. Selection of patients is important—currently there are no clear criteria. **Lung transplantation** is very rarely used.

Prognosis

This is variable. With continued smoking, decline in lung function will be more rapid than after smoking cessation. Long-term oxygen therapy is the only treatment shown to improve life expectancy.

96 Bronchiectasis

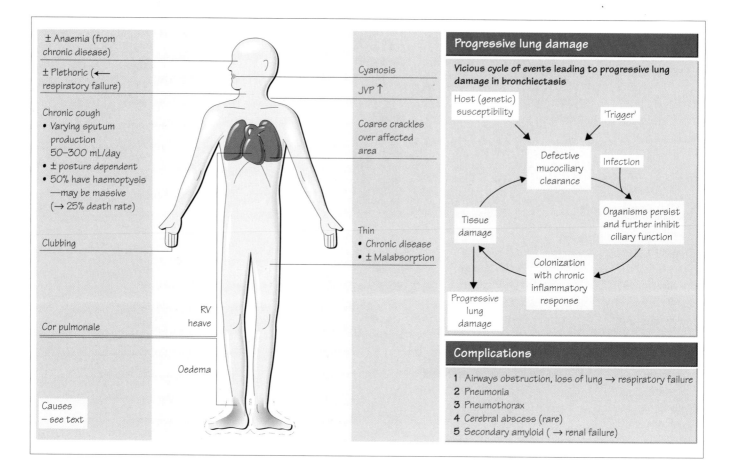

Progressive lung damage

Vicious cycle of events leading to progressive lung damage in bronchiectasis

Host (genetic) susceptibility

'Trigger'

Defective mucociliary clearance

Infection

Organisms persist and further inhibit ciliary function

Tissue damage

Colonization with chronic inflammatory response

Progressive lung damage

Complications

1 Airways obstruction, loss of lung → respiratory failure
2 Pneumonia
3 Pneumothorax
4 Cerebral abscess (rare)
5 Secondary amyloid (→ renal failure)

± Anaemia (from chronic disease)

± Plethoric (← respiratory failure)

Chronic cough
• Varying sputum production 50–300 mL/day
• ± posture dependent
• 50% have haemoptysis —may be massive (→ 25% death rate)

Clubbing

Cor pulmonale

Causes – see text

Cyanosis

JVP ↑

Coarse crackles over affected area

Thin
• Chronic disease
• ± Malabsorption

RV heave

Oedema

Definition and epidemiology

A disease characterized by bronchial wall dilatation, often with super-added pulmonary infection. The incidence is unknown. Prevalence is 1/1000 and falling (less childhood whooping cough and tuberculosis [TB]). The disease has generally been less severe since the introduction of antibiotic therapy.

Aetiology

This depends on the distribution:
• **Localized bronchiectasis** follows severe pneumonia, or occurs distal to endobronchial (foreign body or tumour) or extra-bronchial obstruction (tuberculous hilar nodes—Brock's syndrome).
• **Generalized bronchiectasis**: cystic fibrosis (see p. 196), ciliary dyskinesia (Kartagener's syndrome), Young's syndrome (mucus abnormality) and immune defects (immunoglobulin or complement deficiency, chronic granulomatous disease) cause persistent infection and bronchial wall damage, as do immune complexes (allergic bronchopulmonary aspergillosis, rheumatoid arthritis, inflammatory bowel disease). Underlying pulmonary fibrosis can lead to traction on bronchial walls causing traction bronchiectasis. Rare disease associations are yellow nail syndrome, α_1-antitrypsin deficiency and Marfan's syndrome. (See Table 96.1.)

Pathophysiology

Retention of bronchial secretions occurs and lung infection results, which is not cleared so the lungs become colonized. In addition, certain bacteria further reduce sputum clearance (e.g. *Pseudomonas aeruginosa*). A 'vicious cycle' is set up and the chronic inflammatory response in the airways leads to tissue damage and bronchial wall dilatation (see figure).

Clinical features

These are extremely variable. Some patients have no symptoms or signs. The classic symptoms are of chronic cough and production of large volumes of mucopurulent sputum. Unpleasant breath ('foetor') is common. Haemoptysis occurs in 50% of patients at some stage; 30–40% of patients have associated chronic sinusitis.
• Anaemia, from chronic illness (see p. 338), or polycythaemia, from respiratory failure in late disease, may occur.
• Clubbing is found in severe disease.
• Cyanosis and signs of cor pulmonale are present at a late stage in generalized disease.
• Crackles are present in affected areas, particularly during exacerbations and a significant number of patients have airflow obstruction with wheeze.

Diseases and Treatments at a Glance

Table 96.1 Diseases associated with bronchiectasis.

	General clinical features	Frequency
Cystic fibrosis	Due to malfunction of the gene coding for the CF transmembrane conductance regulator (CFTR) protein. Usually diagnosed at a young age; lung disease often dominates the clinical pictures. Malabsorption very common; cirrhosis, azoospermia, etc.	1 in 400 (Scotland) 1 in 2000–4000 (most white populations) 1 in 15 000–20 000 (African-Americans) 1 in 30 000–100 000 (Asians)
Kartegener's syndrome	Due to mutation in gene coding for dynein protein, resulting in ciliary dysmotility, resulting in sinusitis, situs inversus, infertility in men	1 in 30 000–70 000
Young's syndrome	Triad of bronchiectasis, rhinosinusitis and decreased fertility (obstructive azoospermia) due to abnormally viscous mucus	Rare 15–40% of men with obstructive azoospermia
Immune defects	IgA deficiency: repeated respiratory tract infections, 25% develop autoimmune conditions (e.g. RA, SLE, coeliac disease) IgM deficiency: recurrent infancy/childhood infections with encapsulated organisms. Later on, autoimmune illnesses and malignancy	1 in 600 (Europe) 1 in 250 (Nigeria) 1 in 4000
Allergic bronchopulmonary aspergillosis	Usually complicates long-standing asthma, leading to worsening of asthma symptoms, transient pulmonary infiltrates on CXR often with eosinophilia	ABPA occurs in 10% of those with long-standing asthma
Rheumatoid arthritis	Bronchiectasis can occur before overt arthritis, though more common during overt RA	Clinically relevant bronchiectasis in 1–3% of RA sufferers; occult occurrence in 30%
α1 antitrypsin deficiency	Chest disease, especially in smokers, at a young age. Symptomatic liver disease (cirrhosis) occurs at a young age	1 in 3000–5000
Marfans syndrome	Family history of premature sudden cardiac death, due to aortic dissection; aortic root enlargement ± dissection; tall, joint hypermobility, lens dislocation.	1 in 5000–10 000 Bronchiectasis is a rare complication

Other symptoms and signs relate to the underlying cause (e.g. sinusitis, infertility and dextrocardia in Kartagener's syndrome; bronchial carcinoma, etc.).

Complications

The complications are all uncommon.
- Respiratory failure.
- Brain abscess from haematogenous spread of the infection.
- Amyloid, with renal failure in longstanding severe disease (see p. 261).

Investigations

Diagnosis

- **The chest X-ray** usually shows ring shadows or 'tram lines', representing thickened bronchial walls, although normal in 10%.
- **High-resolution computed tomography (HRCT) chest scan** will confirm the diagnosis. The typical finding is the 'signet ring' sign—a thick-walled bronchus larger than the adjacent blood vessel.
- **Investigation of the cause**: immunoglobulin estimation, aspergillus precipitins and IgE and relevant tests for cystic fibrosis. CT and/or bronchoscopy can demonstrate localized bronchial obstruction.
- **Saccharin test**: if ciliary abnormalities are suspected the time taken for saccharin placed in the nose to reach the taste buds is measured. If prolonged, electron microscopy of cilia confirms the diagnosis.
- **Lung function testing**: may reveal airflow obstruction, which is often reversible.
- **Blood gases**: in severe disease if respiratory failure is suspected.
- **Sputum microscopy and culture**: common bacterial pathogens include *Haemophilus* spp., pneumococci and *Pseudomonas* spp. Atypical organisms, including mycobacteria and fungi, may also cause infection and these should be specifically sought.

Management

- **Physiotherapy**: patients should perform twice daily postural drainage themselves to remove secretions. Supervised physiotherapy is useful during exacerbations.
- **Bronchodilators**: β-agonists, anticholinergics and inhaled steroids are used if reversibility has been demonstrated by formal testing.

Specific treatments

- Immunoglobulin replacement in hypogammaglobulinaemia reduces infections.
- Inhaled α_1-antitrypsin has not been shown to benefit deficient patients.
- **Antibiotics**: in high doses are used for infective exacerbations, guided by sensitivity from sputum cultures. Some patients with frequent exacerbations benefit from continuous/rotating antibiotic courses. *Pseudomonas* infection requires the simultaneous use of two antibiotics from different generic groups for a prolonged (≥ 14 days) course.
- **Oxygen**: for symptom relief in hypoxic patients. Patients with chronic hypoxia and cor pulmonale should be prescribed long-term oxygen therapy.
- **Surgery**: resection of localized disease is sometimes effective in single lobar involvement and to control bleeding in massive haemoptysis, but it is not useful in widespread disease. Lung transplantation should be considered in young patients with severely impaired lung function ($FEV_1 < 30\%$ predicted).

Prognosis

Some patients have few symptoms and lead a normal life with normal life expectancy. Patients with cystic fibrosis or the ciliary dyskinesias that lead to generalized disease tend to progress into respiratory failure.

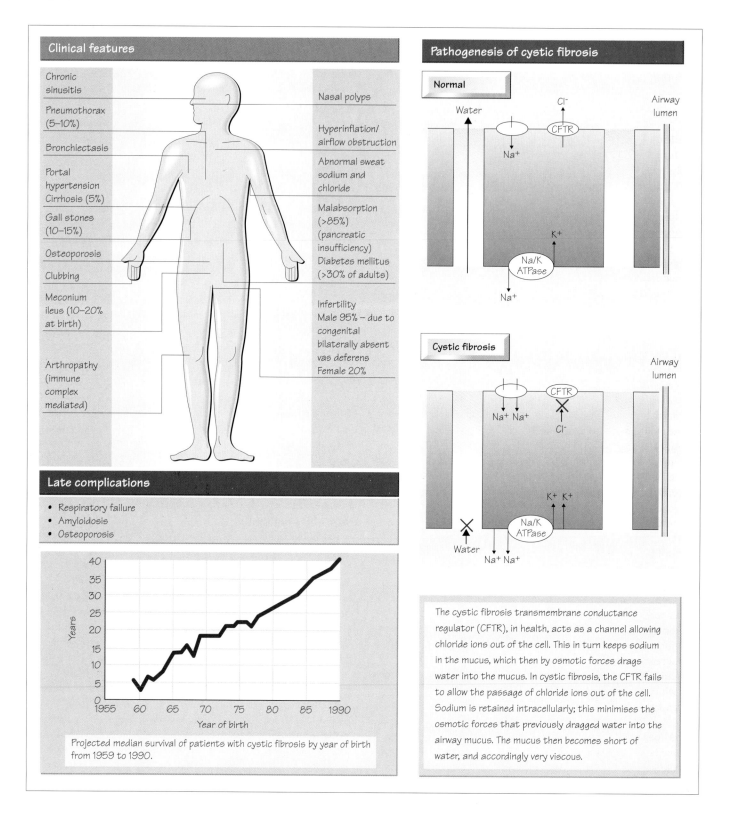

Clinical features

Chronic sinusitis

Pneumothorax (5–10%)

Bronchiectasis

Portal hypertension
Cirrhosis (5%)

Gall stones (10–15%)

Osteoporosis

Clubbing

Meconium ileus (10–20% at birth)

Arthropathy (immune complex mediated)

Nasal polyps

Hyperinflation/airflow obstruction

Abnormal sweat sodium and chloride

Malabsorption (>85%) (pancreatic insufficiency)

Diabetes mellitus (>30% of adults)

Infertility
Male 95% – due to congenital bilaterally absent vas deferens
Female 20%

Late complications

- Respiratory failure
- Amyloidosis
- Osteoporosis

Projected median survival of patients with cystic fibrosis by year of birth from 1959 to 1990.

Pathogenesis of cystic fibrosis

Normal

Cystic fibrosis

The cystic fibrosis transmembrane conductance regulator (CFTR), in health, acts as a channel allowing chloride ions out of the cell. This in turn keeps sodium in the mucus, which then by osmotic forces drags water into the mucus. In cystic fibrosis, the CFTR fails to allow the passage of chloride ions out of the cell. Sodium is retained intracellularly; this minimises the osmotic forces that previously dragged water into the airway mucus. The mucus then becomes short of water, and accordingly very viscous.

Definition

Cystic fibrosis (CF) is a multi-system genetic disease leading to recurrent respiratory infections, pancreatic insufficiency, and abnormal sweat sodium and chloride concentrations.

Epidemiology

CF is the most common autosomal recessive condition in white people: carrier frequency 1 in 25–30 and incidence of 1 in 4000 live births. The incidence is 1 in 20 000 in African–Caribbeans and 1 in 100 000 in Asians.

Aetiology

The abnormal gene is found on the long arm of chromosome 7 and encodes the cystic fibrosis transmembrane conductance regulator (CFTR), a cellular chloride channel that regulates movement of salt and water across membranes. Though there are more than 800 known mutations of the gene; the DF508 mutation accounts for 70% of cases in Europeans and causes more severe disease with pancreatic insufficiency. Generally, the genetic mutation correlates only weakly with disease severity. Genetic screening is available for several of the common mutations. Functionally, the defective channel excretes less chloride into the airway lumen and has a threefold increase in sodium absorption. Water follows sodium uptake, making airway secretions more 'sticky'.

Pathophysiology

The abnormal CFTR results in high concentrations of sodium chloride in sweat and in other secretions, which leads to an increase in the viscosity of bronchial mucus and secretions from the pancreas, liver and reproductive tract. In the lung, mucus clearance is reduced and this predisposes to infection. DNA released from infecting bacteria increases viscosity and exacerbates the problem. Recurrent infection eventually leads to generalized bronchiectasis. Pancreatic secretions are water depleted and therefore more viscid. This leads to reduced secretion of pancreatic enzymes and also local damage to pancreatic tissue, including islet cells. This further worsens secretory function and also results in diabetes mellitus.

Clinical features

• **Pulmonary features**: the lungs are normal at birth but recurrent infections in childhood lead to early onset bronchiectasis, initially in the upper lobes, and a progressive decline in lung function with airflow obstruction, hyperinflation and breathlessness. In the later stages, respiratory failure, clubbing and cor pulmonale are common. Less severe mutations may result in bronchiectasis presenting in adulthood.
• **Pancreatic features**: pancreatic dysfunction leads to steatorrhoea, malnutrition and deficiency of fat-soluble vitamins. Diabetes is common with increasing age, occurring in more than one-third of patients by their late teens.

Investigations

• **Sweat test**: this is the routine diagnostic test of choice. Sweat sodium and chloride levels are both elevated above 60 mmol/L.
• **Genetic testing**: polymerase chain reaction (PCR) on blood is useful if the genetic mutation is known. Screening using PCR looking for the most common mutations will identify over 90% of cases.

• **Radiology**: early on, the chest X-ray reveals upper lobe bronchiectasis, although later this becomes more diffuse. If there is doubt, computed tomography will confirm this.
• **Lung function tests**: these reveal airflow obstruction with increased residual volume. There is often significant reversibility and this should be assessed. On average, lung function deteriorates by about 3% per year. Lung function impairment correlates well with mortality in late disease.
• **Sputum microbiology**: infection with common respiratory pathogens occurs with increased frequency. Most patients eventually become colonized with *Pseudomonas aeruginosa* which requires more intensive treatment. *Burkholderia cepacia* has also been found with increasing frequency and is important because transmission between patients occurs and it can lead to rapid decline in lung function. Segregation of affected individuals may be necessary. Other important respiratory pathogens include atypical mycobacteria and methicillin-resistant *Staphylococcus aureus* (MRSA).
• **Other routine tests**: full blood count (FBC), urea and electrolytes (U&Es), liver function test (LFT), glucose, glycosylated haemoglobin (HbA1c), glucose tolerance test for diabetes. Abdominal ultrasonography for portal hypertension. Tests for malabsorption (see p. 224).

Management

Patients require regular review in specialist units.
• **Lung disease**: this is managed as for bronchiectasis with regular physiotherapy, bronchodilators and aggressive treatment of infection with antibiotics. Resistant organisms such as *Pseudomonas* spp. require prolonged treatment with at least two antibiotics. Indwelling central venous lines may be required if regular courses of antibiotics are required, and patients or relatives can be trained to administer these at home.
• **Recombinant DNase** is used to improve sputum viscosity and aid clearance by breaking down bacterial DNA in sputum. One-third to a half of patients demonstrate improved lung function with this treatment.
• **Influenza immunization** as for all patients with severe lung disease.
• **Nutrition**: nutritional supplements to provide high-calorific intake are often required and may require feeding enterostomy for overnight supplements in severe disease. Pancreatic enzymes are taken by mouth to improve digestion and reduce malabsorption. Fat-soluble vitamin supplements are also given, and insulin for diabetes.
• **Lung transplantation**: patients with an $FEV_1 \leq 30\%$ predicted should be considered for lung or heart-lung transplantation. Survival after transplantation is approximately 55% at 5 years.
• **Gene therapy**: so far, this has not proved a clinically effective treatment. CFTR can be transfected into respiratory epithelium, but currently only at low levels insufficient to reverse the abnormality in airway secretions. In the future, it is hoped that gene therapy may provide a cure for the disease.

Prognosis

Early diagnosis, improved nutrition and effective treatment of respiratory infections have all led to an improved prognosis. Currently median survival is until age 30 years. Patients diagnosed currently have a better prognosis, with 85% anticipated to survive to age 50 years.

Sarcoidosis and other granulomatous lung diseases

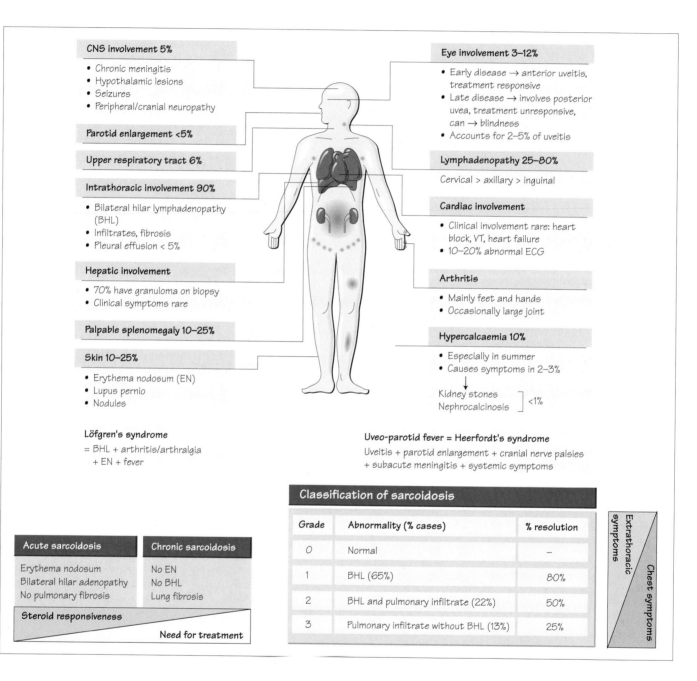

CNS involvement 5%
- Chronic meningitis
- Hypothalamic lesions
- Seizures
- Peripheral/cranial neuropathy

Parotid enlargement <5%

Upper respiratory tract 6%

Intrathoracic involvement 90%
- Bilateral hilar lymphadenopathy (BHL)
- Infiltrates, fibrosis
- Pleural effusion < 5%

Hepatic involvement
- 70% have granuloma on biopsy
- Clinical symptoms rare

Palpable splenomegaly 10–25%

Skin 10–25%
- Erythema nodosum (EN)
- Lupus pernio
- Nodules

Löfgren's syndrome
= BHL + arthritis/arthralgia
+ EN + fever

Eye involvement 3–12%
- Early disease → anterior uveitis, treatment responsive
- Late disease → involves posterior uvea, treatment unresponsive, can → blindness
- Accounts for 2–5% of uveitis

Lymphadenopathy 25–80%
Cervical > axillary > inguinal

Cardiac involvement
- Clinical involvement rare: heart block, VT, heart failure
- 10–20% abnormal ECG

Arthritis
- Mainly feet and hands
- Occasionally large joint

Hypercalcaemia 10%
- Especially in summer
- Causes symptoms in 2–3%
  ↓
Kidney stones
Nephrocalcinosis   ] <1%

Uveo-parotid fever = Heerfordt's syndrome
Uveitis + parotid enlargement + cranial nerve palsies
+ subacute meningitis + systemic symptoms

Classification of sarcoidosis

Grade	Abnormality (% cases)	% resolution
0	Normal	–
1	BHL (65%)	80%
2	BHL and pulmonary infiltrate (22%)	50%
3	Pulmonary infiltrate without BHL (13%)	25%

Acute sarcoidosis	Chronic sarcoidosis
Erythema nodosum	No EN
Bilateral hilar adenopathy	No BHL
No pulmonary fibrosis	Lung fibrosis

Steroid responsiveness

Need for treatment

Extrathoracic symptoms / Chest symptoms

Sarcoidosis
Definition

A multi-system disease of unknown aetiology characterized by the presence of non-caseating granulomas in the affected organs. It may relate to dust inhalation and a significant genetic contribution is suggested by an increased incidence in monozygotic twins. Association with the human leukocyte antigen HLA-B8 has been demonstrated, particularly with the combination of arthritis and erythema nodosum. There is no evidence that the disease is the result of tuberculosis (TB).

Epidemiology

Females > males. Usually presents in early adult life. Incidence in the UK is 5/100 000. The clinical pattern of sarcoidosis is racially determined, in part caused by the ethnic variation in HLA-B8 incidence. Sarcoid is 15 times more common in African–Caribbeans.

Pathophysiology

The organs most commonly involved are the: skin, eyes (see p. 112) and respiratory tract. The cause is unknown but the pathological lesion is

Diseases and Treatments at a Glance

Table 98.1 Clinical features of sarcoidosis in different ethnic groups.

Clinical feature	White	Black	Asian
Abnormal chest X-ray	34	7	10
Respiratory symptoms	25	57	55
Systemic symptoms	5	57	55
Erythema nodosum	20	8.5	17
Eye symptoms	7	12	3
Superficial lymphadenopathy	3	34	17

the non-caseating granuloma. In the lung, a lymphocytic alveolitis is present initially. Subsequent T-lymphocyte-stimulated recruitment of macrophages occurs and these organize into granulomas, which mediate inflammation and long-term damage. A syndrome clinically and histologically indistinguishable from sarcoidosis is found occasionally in patients with underlying malignancy. This should be considered when sarcoidosis presents in older patients.

Clinical features

This is a multi-system disease and features depend on the organs involved. Intra-thoracic involvement is most common. There are two typical patterns:

1 Acute presentation with erythema nodosum, arthralgia and bilateral hilar lymphadenopathy is most common and carries a good prognosis (80% resolution in 1 year).

2 Chronic presentation with slowly progressive breathlessness has a worse prognosis and is associated with progressive pulmonary fibrosis.

Investigations

- **Laboratory tests**: full blood count (FBC) may show lymphopenia in active disease. Thrombocytopenia is described. Erythrocyte sedimentation rate (ESR) is raised in active disease. Serum and urinary calcium are raised in 10%, more commonly so in the summer months, as a result of abnormal vitamin D metabolism. Hypercalcaemia can progress to nephrocalcinosis. Immunoglobulins are diffusely raised in active disease. Serum angiotensin-converting enzyme (ACE) levels are raised in two-thirds of cases, although this is not specific for sarcoidosis.
- **Chest X-ray** findings are traditionally divided into stages that influence prognosis.
- **High-resolution CT (HRCT)** reveals typical findings of mediastinal nodal disease. Pulmonary parenchymal changes include nodules in a bronchovascular, subpleural and fissural distribution.
- **Pulmonary function tests** are often normal. In fibrotic disease, reduced lung volumes and gas transfer are typical. Obstructive pulmonary function with gas trapping may be found.
- **The Kveim test** involved intradermal injection of a preparation of splenic tissue from a patient with sarcoidosis and subsequent skin biopsy. It is no longer used because of concerns over the risk of transmitting infection. Tuberculin tests are negative in two-thirds of patients.
- **Histology** is the best diagnostic test and a tissue diagnosis should always be sought if there is diagnostic doubt. Transbronchial biopsy is positive in 80%.

Management

- **No treatment**: sarcoidosis with a good prognosis (erythema nodosum and bilateral hilar lymphadenopathy [BHL]) requires no treatment. Non-steroidal anti-inflammatory drugs are used for pain.
- **Oral steroids** are used in symptomatic pulmonary disease, cardiac and neurological sarcoid. Patients with pulmonary disease and radio-

logical changes which persist for longer than 6 months have a better long-term outcome if given oral steroids (prednisolone 30–40 mg daily, discontinued after a month if no improvement) for 6 months. Other immunosuppressive drugs have been used with some reported benefit.

- **Topical steroids** for uveitis. Sometimes oral prednisolone is needed.
- **Chloroquine** can be useful in cutaneous and progressive pulmonary disease.

Prognosis

This is worse with older age of onset, more widespread disease and in African–Caribbeans. Two-thirds of white and one-third of black patients recover with no treatment. Fewer than 3% of patients die from sarcoidosis.

Beryllium disease

Beryllium is a heavy metal used in the manufacture of fluorescent lighting tubes. Lung disease resulting from exposure is rare.

- **Acute exposure** to fumes leads to an alveolitis, but industry precautions should prevent this occurring.
- **Chronic low-level exposure** can lead to a systemic disease similar to sarcoidosis. Non-caseating granulomas appear in the skin or lungs. Radiologically, there may be nodularity in the lung fields and bilateral hilar lymphadenopathy. The pulmonary abnormality progresses to fibrosis with small lung volumes, impaired gas transfer and respiratory failure. Early treatment with corticosteroids can result in improved lung function. Workers who have been exposed to beryllium undergo regular screening with chest X-rays to detect development of asymptomatic pulmonary disease. They should of course report the development of respiratory symptoms.

Histiocytosis X (Langerhans' cell histiocytosis)
Epidemiology

This is a rare multi-system disorder of unknown aetiology occurring more often in males and usually presenting in early adult life. The vast majority of patients are smokers.

Pathophysiology and investigation

Initially there is infiltration of lung tissue with eosinophils and Langerhans' cells. This progresses to granuloma formation, which breaks down to form cystic areas, particularly in the upper zones. Ultimately pulmonary fibrosis develops. Pneumothorax is common. The diagnosis can be made radiologically. The plain X-ray and HRCT show diffuse nodularity with cyst formation in the characteristic distribution. Lung volume is often well preserved. Pulmonary function tests often reveal a restrictive defect with high residual volume and normal total lung capacity as a result of gas trapping.

Clinical features

Most patients are breathless but 25% are asymptomatic with an abnormal X-ray. Spontaneous pneumothorax is the presenting feature in 10%.

Management

Smoking cessation is essential and complete resolution with no additional treatment is possible. A variety of immunosuppressive regimens have been used. Oral corticosteroids remain the mainstay of treatment in patients with symptomatic disease. Long-term survival is commonly reported.

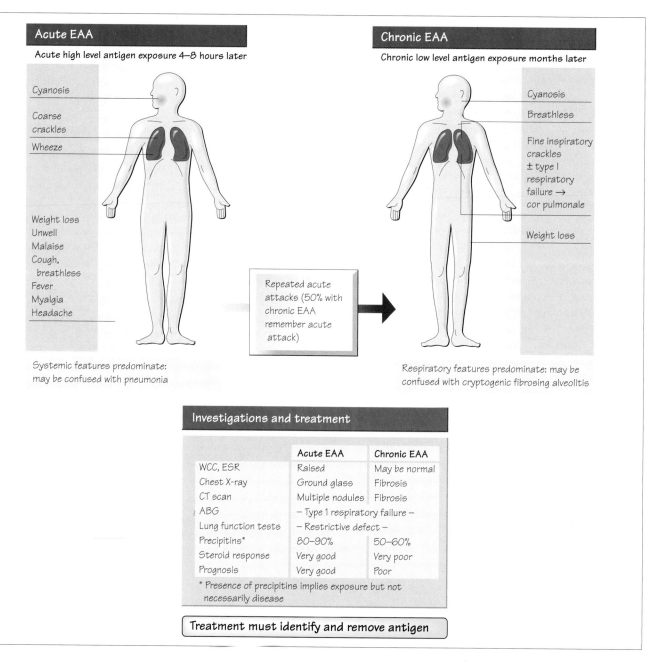

Acute EAA

Acute high level antigen exposure 4–8 hours later

- Cyanosis
- Coarse crackles
- Wheeze

- Weight loss
- Unwell
- Malaise
- Cough, breathless
- Fever
- Myalgia
- Headache

Systemic features predominate: may be confused with pneumonia

Repeated acute attacks (50% with chronic EAA remember acute attack)

Chronic EAA

Chronic low level antigen exposure months later

- Cyanosis
- Breathless
- Fine inspiratory crackles ± type I respiratory failure → cor pulmonale
- Weight loss

Respiratory features predominate: may be confused with cryptogenic fibrosing alveolitis

Investigations and treatment

	Acute EAA	Chronic EAA
WCC, ESR	Raised	May be normal
Chest X-ray	Ground glass	Fibrosis
CT scan	Multiple nodules	Fibrosis
ABG	– Type 1 respiratory failure –	
Lung function tests	– Restrictive defect –	
Precipitins*	80–90%	50–60%
Steroid response	Very good	Very poor
Prognosis	Very good	Poor

* Presence of precipitins implies exposure but not necessarily disease

Treatment must identify and remove antigen

Definition

A condition caused by hypersensitivity to inhaled organic dusts, leading to an inflammatory reaction in the distal airspaces.

Epidemiology

Uncommon: 1–2 per 100 000 in the UK. Mainly in middle-aged people.

Aetiology

Inhalation of a number of antigens may result in a pulmonary inflammatory response. For some causes, see Table 99.1.

Pathophysiology

Extrinsic allergic alveolitis (EAA) is a granulomatous reaction to a variety of organic dusts, including animal proteins (particularly from birds) and microbial spores.

- Occupational or environmental exposure to these dusts results in an immunological response, with inflammatory cell (neutrophil and lymphocyte) activation in the bronchioles extending distally into the alveoli. Accumulation of giant cells leads to granuloma formation in a bronchocentric distribution.
- Progressive fibrosis results if there is persistent inflammatory cell

Table 99.1 Some causes of extrinsic allergic alveolitis—there are many other reported causes.

Disease	Cause	Agent
Farmer's lung	Mouldy hay	Thermophilic actinomycetes
Bird fancier's lung	Pigeon, budgerigar, poultry	Bloom/excreta
Wood worker's lung	Wood	Wood dust
Byssinosis	Cotton dust	? agent
Suberosis	Cork dust	*Penicillium frequentens*
Humidifier fever	Air humidification units	Variety of agents
Malt worker's lung	Whisky maltings	*Aspergillus clavatus*
Coffee worker's lung	Coffee bean dust	Coffee

activation. The formation of granulomas implies that T-cell activation is involved in the pathogenesis of EAA. The presence of IgG serum precipitins implies exposure to an antigenic dust with the formation of immune complexes, but does not relate to the pathology in the lung.

Clinical features

EAA may present as acute or chronic alveolitis:
• **Acute allergic alveolitis**: 4–8 h after exposure to high doses of antigen, systemic features of fever, myalgia and headache develop, with cough and breathlessness. Persistent exposure over weeks can produce considerable weight loss. Examination reveals inspiratory crackles and squeaks.
• **Chronic allergic alveolitis**: presents with progressive exertional breathlessness as a result of pulmonary fibrosis. Prolonged low-level antigen exposure is the cause and there may be a history of acute episodes. Examination reveals inspiratory crackles typical of pulmonary fibrosis.

Investigations

• **Laboratory tests**: in acute alveolitis, a neutrophil leukocytosis may be present. The presence of circulating precipitating antibodies implies antigen exposure but not necessarily disease.
• **Chest X-ray** reveals subtle diffuse ground-glass change with small nodules, which can be confirmed by **high-resolution CT** (HRCT). In chronic alveolitis, fibrosis, typically in mid and upper zones, is present on the chest X-ray and HRCT.
• **Pulmonary function testing**: shows a restrictive pattern in both acute and chronic disease with impaired gas transfer. Respiratory failure with hypoxaemia may be present in severe acute or chronic fibrotic disease.

The combination of symptoms, radiology, pulmonary function abnormality and the relevant exposure (presence of precipitins) is usually sufficient for a diagnosis. If doubt remains, lung biopsy may be necessary.

Management

This is aimed at optimizing lung function and preventing the development of pulmonary fibrosis. The key is antigen avoidance or reduction of exposure by the use of respiratory protection equipment. Oral corticosteroids (prednisolone 40–60 mg daily for 3–6 months) accelerate the rate of recovery, but do not improve long-term outcome. They should be reserved for patients with acute alveolitis or significant respiratory compromise.

Prognosis

• **Acute disease**: usually full recovery after cessation of exposure.
• **Chronic disease**: progressive and permanent lung damage may occur.

100 Fibrosing alveolitis

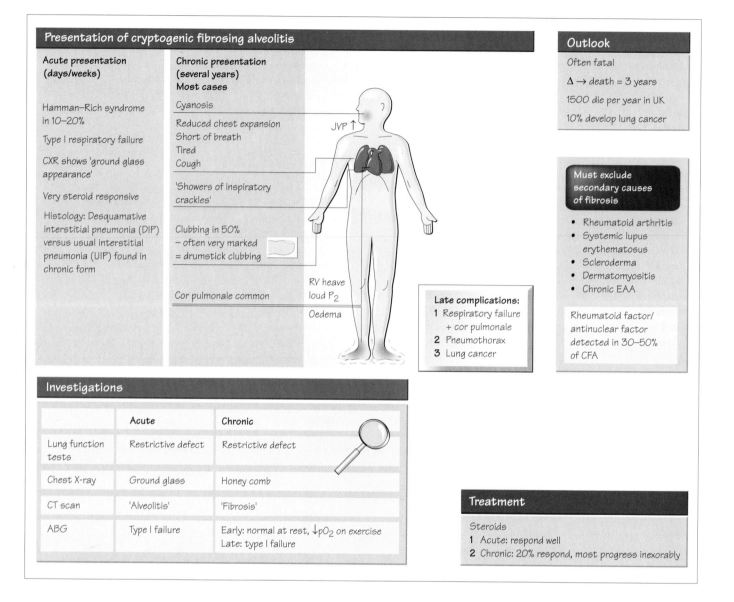

Presentation of cryptogenic fibrosing alveolitis

Acute presentation (days/weeks)

Hamman–Rich syndrome in 10–20%

Type I respiratory failure

CXR shows 'ground glass appearance'

Very steroid responsive

Histology: Desquamative interstitial pneumonia (DIP) versus usual interstitial pneumonia (UIP) found in chronic form

Cor pulmonale common

Chronic presentation (several years) Most cases

Cyanosis

Reduced chest expansion
Short of breath
Tired
Cough

'Showers of inspiratory crackles'

Clubbing in 50%
– often very marked
= drumstick clubbing

JVP ↑

RV heave
loud P₂

Oedema

Late complications:
1 Respiratory failure + cor pulmonale
2 Pneumothorax
3 Lung cancer

Outlook

Often fatal

$\Delta \rightarrow$ death = 3 years

1500 die per year in UK

10% develop lung cancer

Must exclude secondary causes of fibrosis

- Rheumatoid arthritis
- Systemic lupus erythematosus
- Scleroderma
- Dermatomyositis
- Chronic EAA

Rheumatoid factor/ antinuclear factor detected in 30–50% of CFA

Investigations

	Acute	Chronic
Lung function tests	Restrictive defect	Restrictive defect
Chest X-ray	Ground glass	Honey comb
CT scan	'Alveolitis'	'Fibrosis'
ABG	Type I failure	Early: normal at rest, ↓pO₂ on exercise Late: type I failure

Treatment

Steroids
1 Acute: respond well
2 Chronic: 20% respond, most progress inexorably

Definition

A condition involving inflammation and fibrosis of the distal airspaces, defined histologically. The combination of clinical features, restrictive pulmonary function and typical radiological changes suggests the diagnosis, often making a tissue diagnosis redundant.

Aetiology

Unknown, but as an identical disease can be caused by several agents, including asbestos, hard metals, drugs and radiation. This suggests that an inhaled or environmental agent is responsible. A number of auto-immune diseases are also associated with pulmonary fibrosis. A few cases are familial, suggesting genetic influence.

Epidemiology

More frequent with increasing age. Prevalence is increasing and is currently 20/100 000. CFA is more common in males. The median survival

from diagnosis is only 3 years despite intervention. In some individuals, lung function may remain stable for many months.

Pathology

Histologically, alveolar walls become progressively thickened as a result of organizing inflammatory cell infiltrate with proliferation of fibroblasts. Two types are recognized:

1 Usual interstitial pneumonia where inflammatory cells are present in the airspaces and fibrosis leads to contraction of lung tissue and honeycombing.

2 Desquamative interstitial pneumonia in which the predominant infiltrate is mononuclear cell and fibrosis less prominent.

Lung volume is reduced, diffusion impaired and respiratory failure eventually develops.

There is an increased risk of lung cancer (occurs in 10% of patients).

Clinical features

Gradual onset of breathlessness is typical. Cough is very common and is usually non-productive. In 5%, pulmonary fibrosis is an incidental finding and no symptoms are present. Examination reveals clubbing in 50%. Showers of fine, late, inspiratory crackles are present on auscultation. Respiratory distress, cyanosis and signs of cor pulmonale may develop. The Hamman-Rich syndrome is a predominantly inflammatory alveolitis of acute onset and more frequently shows a better response to treatment.

Investigations

• **Laboratory tests**: routine blood tests are normal. Blood gases may show hypoxaemia. Weakly positive titres of antinuclear antibodies and rheumatoid factor are present in a quarter.
• **Pulmonary function tests** show reduction in all lung volumes with impaired gas transfer. Gas transfer, total lung capacity and alveolar volume are used as markers of disease progression. Change in FVC in the 6 months following diagnosis is useful in predicting prognosis. A < 10% change predicts stable disease with a good prognosis and > 10% fall in FVC suggests deteriorating disease with a poor prognosis.
• **Chest X-ray** may show diffuse predominantly basal and peripheral ground-glass change with loss of definition of the heart borders and hemidiaphragms. This may progress to reticulonodular changes and honeycombing.
• **HRCT** reveals subpleural reticulation, ground-glass change, again with progression to honeycombing and traction bronchiectasis.

• **Histological** examination may show typical cellular infiltrate or fibrosis. The changes are patchy and transbronchial biopsy may therefore be inadequate.

Frequently the combination of clinical features and radiological changes is sufficient for the diagnosis to be made.

Management

Oral corticosteroids are the mainstay of treatment. High doses (40–60 mg prednisolone) are often used in patients with severe disease and an acute presentation. In less acutely unwell patients a lower dose (20 mg prednisolone on alternate days) may be used to reduce treatment side effects. A number of additional immunosuppressive drugs have been used to reduce the required steroid dose. The best of these appears to be azathioprine at a dose of 2 mg/kg. A response in terms of improved lung function is seen in 10–20%, with improvement in symptoms in more. Recent reports of improvement in lung function with interferon treatment have unfortunately not been reproduced in clinical trials.

For advanced disease, supportive treatment is required. Long-term oxygen for the relief of breathlessness, diuretics for fluid retention in cor pulmonale and antibiotics for infection may all be useful. In young patients with advanced unresponsive disease, lung transplantation should be considered.

Prognosis

The 5-year survival rate is only 50%. Current treatment has not influenced this figure. In the UK, 1500 people die annually from fibrosing alveolitis.

Causes of pulmonary eosinophilia

Common

- Asthma
- ABPA
- Drugs
- Parasites

Rare

- Churg–Strauss
- Chronic eosinophilic pneumonia
- Polyarteritis nodosa
- Hodgkin's disease

Löffler's syndrome

= eosinophilia + transient CXR infiltrate lasting 4–6 weeks
Often related to

- Drugs
- Parasitic worms

Pulmonary eosinophilia

Disease	Features	Investigations	Treatment
Acute eosinophilic pneumonia	Fever, dry cough, dyspnoea, myalgia, chest pain Crackles or wheeze	Eosinophilia Segmental infiltrates; peripheral ground glass on CT Restrictive lung function	Prednisolone 30–40 mg/day Reduce rapidly following improvement
Chronic eosinophilic pneumonia	Cough, fever, dyspnoea, weight loss	Eosinophilia Bilateral peripheral infiltrates Restrictive lung function	Prednisolone 30–40 mg/day Reduce slowly over 6 months
Hypereosinophilic syndrome	Cough, malaise Cardiac failure (myocardial infiltration)	Eosinophilia $<20 \times 10^9$/L CXR; pulmonary infiltrates and effusions	Prednisolone 30–60 mg/day May require long-term treatment Anticoagulants
Churg–Strauss syndrome	Asthma, sinusitis, multi-system involvement	Eosinophilia, raised IgE ↑ pANCA in 50% Pulmonary infiltrates Pleural effusion in up to 30% Vasculitis on biopsy	Prednisolone 40–60 mg/day reducing over a year Other immunosuppressives in severe disease

Immunologically mediated lung disease

Disease	Features	Investigations	Treatment
Goodpasture's syndrome	Pulmonary haemorrhage (breathless, haemoptysis) Renal failure	Anti-GBM antibody positive ↑ANCA (in some) Pulmonary infiltrates Renal failure — diagnostic renal biopsy	Plasma exchange Prednisolone Other immunosuppressives in severe disease Renal replacement if necessary
Wegener's granulomatosis	Nose bleeds, sinusitis, cough, haemoptysis, dyspnoea, malaise, weight loss Multi-system involvement	Anaemia, leucocytosis, renal failure Active urine sediment Pulmonary nodules (may cavitate) ↑cANCA in almost all cases Biopsy shows necrotizing granulomatous vasculitis	Prednisolone 40–60 mg/day Cyclophosphamide Renal replacement if necessary

Pulmonary eosinophilia

This is a group of rare diseases, mainly of unknown aetiology, which cause chest X-ray abnormalities associated with a raised eosinophil count in peripheral blood. Diseases included in this category include: 1) Acute eosinophilic pneumonia 2) Chronic eosinophilic pneumonia 3) Hypereosinophilic syndrome 4) Churg–Strauss syndrome.

Other diseases that cause pulmonary disease in association with eosinophilia are: 1) Asthma 2) Fungal diseases (including allergic bronchopulmonary aspergillosis [ABPA]) 3) Parasitic infection (e.g. to the filarial parasite Wuchereria bancrofti) 4) Drug reactions (see p. 210) 5) Polyarteritis nodosa 6) Hodgkin's disease.

Epidemiology and prognosis

• **Acute and chronic eosinophilic pneumonia** are more common in women; peak incidence is 40–50 years. Fifty per cent of patients have asthma. Eosinophilic pneumonia responds well to treatment and recurrence is uncommon. Chronic disease responds less well to treatment and recurrence may require long-term steroid treatment.

• **Hypereosinophilic syndrome** is very rare, is usually of unknown cause (although it occurs more often in the tropics where it may relate to parasitic infection) and often responds poorly to treatment. Complicating cardiac failure can occur and carries a poor prognosis.

• **Churg–Strauss syndrome** is a rare form of pulmonary vasculitis (incidence about 1 per million) affecting small and medium-sized vessels. It occurs in patients with asthma. Antineutrophil cytoplasmic antibody (ANCA) is commonly positive. Untreated vasculitis has a poor prognosis (renal involvement). Vasculitis often responds well to treatment and relapse is unusual.

Vasculitis without eosinophilia

Several vasculitides affect the lung without provoking eosinophilia:

• **Rheumatoid arthritis**: pleural disease (thickening, effusion) is the most common manifestation. Localized nodules or more diffuse fibrosing alveolitis can occur. Extensive nodular fibrosis, called Caplan's syndrome, occurs in those with pneumoconiosis.

• **Systemic lupus erythematosus**: pleural inflammation ('pleurisy') is very common. Fibrosing alveolitis occurs but is rare.

• **Wegener's granulomatosis**: see below.

Wegener's granulomatosis

General features

• WG is a multi-system vasculitis (see Table 101.1), involving small and medium-sized vessels, associated with the antineutrophil cytoplasmic antibody (ANCA).

• The aetiology is unknown, but may involve an infectious agent.

• Prevalence is about 1 per 100 000. Men and women are equally affected (i.e. 600 in the UK).

• > 90% of WG first seek attention due to symptoms arising from the upper or lower respiratory tract.

Upper airways

• Nasal/sinus disease → congestion and nose bleed. Nasal septum perforation → saddle nose, occurs in up to 30%.

• Subglottic stenosis occurs in 20% → breathlessness (which may be severe), voice change and cough. The diagnosis of subglottic stenosis is suggested by flow-volume loops): this responds very poorly to systemic

Table 101.1 Profile of organ involvement and during the course of the disease in Wegener's granulomatosis.

	Involvement at presentation %	Involvement during the disease course %
Upper airways	73	92
Lower airways	48	85
Kidneys	20	80
Joint	32	67
Eye	15	52
Skin	13	46
Nerve	1	20

Data from the article by Carol A Langford, Gary S Hoffman. Wegener's granulomatosis *Thorax* 1999; 54: 629–637.

therapy; it may respond to mechanical dilatation with local injection of corticosteroids.

Lower airways

• Parenchymal disease—2/3 of those with parenchymal involvement have symptoms, 1/3 only have asymptomatic CXR abnormalities.

• Variable changes: bilateral nodular infiltrates, cavitatary disease, and pulmonary haemorrhage.

• 15% have inflammation/stenosis of endobronchial airways → cough, wheezing, breathlessness, haemoptysis, or lung collapse.

• Major cause of morbidity, but rare cause of mortality.

Renal disease

Glomerulonephritis: may rapidly progress to renal failure with no/few symptoms. Renal failure is common (affecting up to 40–50%), and end-stage renal failure requiring dialysis occurs in some 10%. GN detected by dipstick testing of urine (red cells, casts, ↑ creatinine). Common cause of death.

Other features

• Eye disease: many possible manifestations, including (epi)scleritis, conjunctivitis, anterior or posterior uveitis, and optic neuritis. Some 8% of patients develop permanent visual loss.

• 15% have mononeuritis multiplex. 8% have CNS involvement.

Diagnosis

The diagnosis is made from a biopsy showing a necrotizing vasculitis, with granuloma formation in a clinically relevant setting. Antibodies against neutrophil cytoplasm are found, in two staining patterns:

• **Cytoplasmic ANCA (cANCA)**: the antigen is proteinase-3 (PR3), a 2-kDa serine proteinase found in the azurophilic granules of neutrophils. cANCA is found in 70–90% of WG. Though cANCA has a high specificity and sensitivity for WG, it should not be relied on in isolation from the clinical situation and appropriate histology, as many patients with WG do not have cANCA. In some patients, cANCA titre relates to disease activity, though in many it does not.

• **Perinuclear ANCA (pANCA)**: the antigen is usually myeloperoxidase (MPO). Found in 5–10% of WG, but also many other conditions, so it has a low sensitivity and specificity for the diagnosis of WG.

Treatment and prognosis

Untreated WG has a very high mortality. Treatment with cyclophosphamide and prednisolone dramatically reduces morbidity and mortality: 75% achieve complete disease remission, and the 2-year survival rate is 80%.

Drug-related side effects (sepsis from immunosuppression, late malignancy) are common. *Pneumocystis carinii* pneumonia is so common as to justify septrin prophylaxis.

Other immunologically mediated disease of the lung

• **Goodpasture's syndrome**: results from immune attack by an antibody against the lung and renal glomerular basement membrane (GBM). Pulmonary haemorrhage (causing anaemia, haemoptysis and respiratory failure) occurs usually some days to months before acute renal failure. Anti-GBM antibodies are found, and less frequently a positive ANCA. Treatment is with immunosuppression and plasma exchange.

• **Idiopathic pulmonary haemosiderosis** is a similar disease to Goodpasture's (though renal involvement is uncommon) occurring in young children (> 7 years).

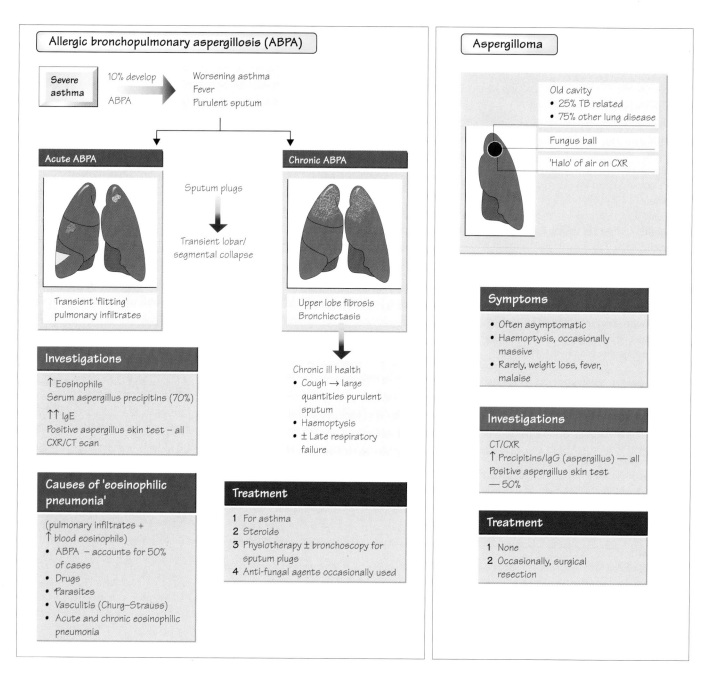

Allergic bronchopulmonary aspergillosis (ABPA)

| Severe asthma | 10% develop ABPA | → | Worsening asthma
Fever
Purulent sputum |

Acute ABPA

Transient 'flitting' pulmonary infiltrates

Sputum plugs
↓
Transient lobar/segmental collapse

Chronic ABPA

Upper lobe fibrosis
Bronchiectasis

Chronic ill health
- Cough → large quantities purulent sputum
- Haemoptysis
- ± Late respiratory failure

Investigations

↑ Eosinophils
Serum aspergillus precipitins (70%)
↑↑ IgE
Positive aspergillus skin test – all
CXR/CT scan

Causes of 'eosinophilic pneumonia'

(pulmonary infiltrates + ↑ blood eosinophils)
- ABPA – accounts for 50% of cases
- Drugs
- Parasites
- Vasculitis (Churg–Strauss)
- Acute and chronic eosinophilic pneumonia

Treatment

1 For asthma
2 Steroids
3 Physiotherapy ± bronchoscopy for sputum plugs
4 Anti-fungal agents occasionally used

Aspergilloma

Old cavity
- 25% TB related
- 75% other lung disease

Fungus ball

'Halo' of air on CXR

Symptoms

- Often asymptomatic
- Haemoptysis, occasionally massive
- Rarely, weight loss, fever, malaise

Investigations

CT/CXR
↑ Precipitins/IgG (aspergillus) — all
Positive aspergillus skin test — 50%

Treatment

1 None
2 Occasionally, surgical resection

Fungal infections

Fungal lung infection develops in the immunologically incompetent and in those with chronic lung disease. Infection is usually localized in the immune competent, but those with immune deficiencies develop invasive fungal pneumonia, which has a very high mortality, caused by *Pneumocystis* spp. (see p. 300), *Aspergillus* spp. (see below), *Candida* spp. (see p. 302) and cryptococcosis (see p. 302).

Aspergillosis

Aspergillus fumigatus is the most important human pathogen and dis-

ease occurs in immunosuppressed individuals and in those with underlying lung disease. There are three pathologies in lung disease: allergy, colonization and invasion (Table 102.1).

Asthma

Some patients with asthma are allergic to *Aspergillus* spp. Asthma attacks occur when fungal spores are inhaled. They have positive skin tests, but such positive reactions are not associated with worse disease, unless allergic bronchopulmonary aspergillosis (ABPA) is also present.

Table 102.1 Pathologies of aspergillus lung disease.

Allergic	Asthma
	Bronchopulmonary aspergillosis (ABPA)
	Allergic aspergillus sinusitis
	Allergic alveolitis
	(Bronchocentric granulomatosis)
Colonizing	Aspergilloma
Invasive	Invasive aspergillus pneumonia

Allergic bronchopulmonary aspergillosis

Epidemiology, aetiology and pathophysiology

This uncommon complication of asthma is found in 10% of difficult asthma cases and underlies some 50% of UK pulmonary eosinophilia. Inhalation of aspergillus spores leads to an IgG- and IgE-mediated hypersensitivity immune reaction, which in turn leads to dense eosinophilic infiltration of lung tissue, mucus plugging and distal collapse. A chronic inflammatory response in the airway wall causes tissue destruction and bronchiectasis. It is not clear why only some patients with asthma develop ABPA, but a genetic predisposition has been suggested.

Clinical features

ABPA patients are usually people with known asthma. Symptoms are of deteriorating asthma with purulent sputum, fever and breathlessness. Transient infiltrates on the chest X-ray occur. In chronic bronchiectatic disease, copious purulent sputum production and haemoptysis are present.

Investigation

ABPA should be considered in people with asthma who have an abnormal chest X-ray and high blood eosinophil count.
- **Skin tests**: a positive skin test to *Aspergillus* spp. (or raised serum-specific IgE) is required for diagnosis.
- **Blood tests**: the eosinophil count is raised, particularly in acute episodes. Total serum IgE is markedly elevated. Precipitating antibodies (IgG) are present in 70%.
- **Sputum examination**: fungal hyphae may be present in the sputum.
- **Chest X-ray**: transient ('flitting') perihilar infiltrates are present during acute attacks. Lobar or segmental collapse may occur as a result of bronchial occlusion. In chronic disease upper lobe contraction, fibrosis and bronchiectasis may occur.

Management and prognosis

Oral corticosteroids (prednisolone) are the mainstay of treatment. They improve asthma control and reduce growth of *Aspergillus* spp. Inhaled steroids do not affect *Aspergillus* spp. but are used, along with bronchodilators, as part of the overall treatment of asthma. Physiotherapy and sometimes bronchoscopy are necessary for removal of mucus plugs. The antifungal agent itraconazole may reduce the dose of steroids required. ABPA usually progresses to bronchiectasis.

Aspergillus sinusitis

Sinusitis unresponsive to medical treatment in patients with nasal polyps has been found occasionally to be caused by *Aspergillus* spp., and may coexist with ABPA. The histology and immunology are identical to ABPA.

Allergic alveolitis caused by *Aspergillus* spp.

This rare disease found in malt workers is caused by *A. clavatus* from mouldy barley. The pathology, clinical features and management are as for extrinsic allergic alveolitis of any cause (see p. 200).

Aspergilloma

Definition

A mycetoma or fungus ball is a collection of fungus.

Aetiology and pathogenesis

The causative organism is *A. fumigatus* in the UK and *A. niger* in the USA. Spores seed a pre-existing lung cavity, often (25%) as a result of previous TB, and thus in the apex of the lung. Twenty per cent of cases are multiple. Spores germinate and a ball of fungus grows to fill the cavity. An immunological reaction to this process occurs. Precipitating antibodies (IgG) are universally present and a positive skin test to *Aspergillus* spp. is found in 50%.

Clinical features

Often asymptomatic and found incidentally on a chest X-ray. The most common symptom is haemoptysis, occurring in 75%, occasionally massive, requiring embolization or surgery. Rarely, systemic features of weight loss, fever and malaise occur. Symptoms of the underlying lung disease are often present.

Investigation

The combination of the radiological features (a dense opacity with surrounding halo or crescent) and the presence of precipitating antibodies suggest the diagnosis. In patients with severe underlying lung disease, a CT scan will define the mycetoma more clearly.

Management and prognosis

Antifungal therapy is ineffective. Corticosteroids have been used for systemic symptoms but increase the risk of invasion (see below). In fit patients with systemic symptoms or significant haemoptysis, surgical resection of the mycetoma or a whole lobe is used. Ten per cent cause no problems and resolve. Death occasionally occurs as a result of massive haemoptysis. Invasive disease worsens outcome.

Aspergillus pneumonia (see p. 303 Infectious diseases)

Other fungal lung infections

Histoplasmosis

Histoplasma capsulatum is found worldwide and particularly so in the USA, in soil contaminated by bird and bat droppings. Histoplasmosis is not found in the UK. Infection usually causes no symptoms but may lead to a febrile illness with cough, chest pain and dyspnoea, followed by resolution. 10% of cases become chronic. In the acute illness, there are bilateral chest X-ray infiltrates with enlarged mediastinal lymph nodes. Calcification of multiple pulmonary nodules can occur sometimes with cavitation. Diagnosis is either made by culture of blood or biopsy specimens or by serological tests, which usually become positive within 3 weeks of acute infection. Treatment is with amphotericin in severe disease. Itraconazole has been used for chronic disease.

Candida spp. (see p. 303)

Cryptococcosis (see p. 303)

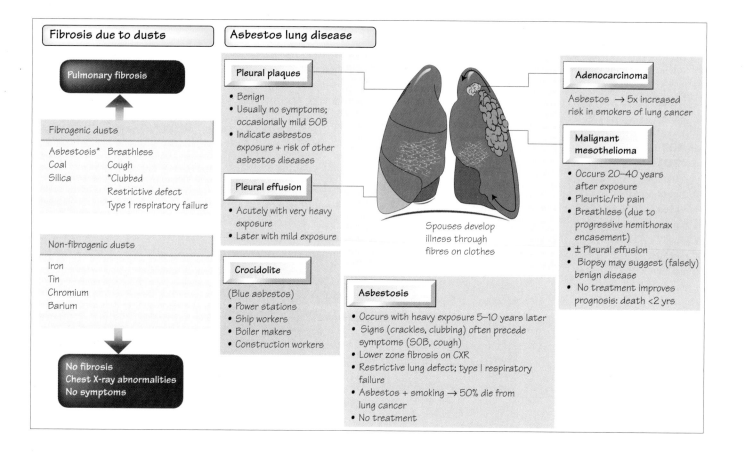

Fibrosis due to dusts

Pulmonary fibrosis

Fibrogenic dusts

Asbestosis*	Breathless
Coal	Cough
Silica	*Clubbed
	Restrictive defect
	Type 1 respiratory failure

Non-fibrogenic dusts

Iron
Tin
Chromium
Barium

No fibrosis
Chest X-ray abnormalities
No symptoms

Asbestos lung disease

Pleural plaques
- Benign
- Usually no symptoms; occasionally mild SOB
- Indicate asbestos exposure + risk of other asbestos diseases

Pleural effusion
- Acutely with very heavy exposure
- Later with mild exposure

Crocidolite
(Blue asbestos)
- Power stations
- Ship workers
- Boiler makers
- Construction workers

Spouses develop illness through fibres on clothes

Asbestosis
- Occurs with heavy exposure 5–10 years later
- Signs (crackles, clubbing) often precede symptoms (SOB, cough)
- Lower zone fibrosis on CXR
- Restrictive lung defect; type I respiratory failure
- Asbestos + smoking → 50% die from lung cancer
- No treatment

Adenocarcinoma
Asbestos → 5x increased risk in smokers of lung cancer

Malignant mesothelioma
- Occurs 20–40 years after exposure
- Pleuritic/rib pain
- Breathless (due to progressive hemithorax encasement)
- ± Pleural effusion
- Biopsy may suggest (falsely) benign disease
- No treatment improves prognosis: death <2 yrs

Inhalation of dusts may lead to pulmonary fibrosis or asthma (see p. 188).

Dust inhalation diseases

- **Fibrogenic dusts** (asbestos, coal and silica) can impair pulmonary function.
- **Non-fibrogenic dusts** (iron, tin, chromium and barium) lead to a nodular appearance on a chest X-ray but do not impair lung function.
- **Organic dusts** can cause extrinsic allergic alveolitis (see p. 200).

Asbestosis

Asbestosis is lung fibrosis resulting from asbestos exposure.

Epidemiology

Asbestos-related diseases are industrial diseases (men > women), found in those exposed to blue asbestos (crocidolite). The greater the asbestos exposure, the higher the asbestosis and mesothelioma rates. Symptoms occur decades after exposure. Rates for asbestos-related diseases will increase for some years because effective legal regulation occurred relatively recently and there is often a long delay between exposure and development of disease.

Pathology

Asbestos fibres are small and penetrate distally into the lung. Fibres are engulfed by macrophages that release cytokines, so producing an inflammatory reaction, which leads to progressive fibrosis, mainly in the lower lobes. Pleural plaques are usually also present. Cigarette smoke acts synergistically with asbestos to increase pulmonary fibrosis and lung cancer rates.

Clinical features

Occupational exposure is usually present. Typical symptoms are:
- Progressive breathlessness.
- Cough.

Clinical signs are of bibasal end-inspiratory crackles, and finger clubbing in 50%. Haemoptysis suggests the development of lung cancer.

Investigations

- **Chest X-ray** reveals symmetrical basal parenchymal changes, and 75% have pleural plaques.
- **High-resolution computed tomography** (HRCT) may be abnormal when the chest X-ray is normal and reveals subpleural changes progressing to honeycombing. Beneath areas of pleural fibrosis, nodular areas of collapse may develop (rounded atelectasis, Blesovsky's syndrome) which on chest X-ray appear as a mass. HRCT distinguishes these appearances from those of carcinoma.
- **Pulmonary function tests** reveal a restrictive defect with reduced lung volumes and gas transfer. Blood gases show respiratory failure in end-stage disease.

Management

- **Prevention**: risk of progression increases with cumulative dose. Prevention by reduction of exposure has reduced the incidence and severity of disease.
- **Treatment**: no treatment works.
- **Prognosis**: 20% of patients with asbestosis die from the disease and 50% from an associated malignancy (lung cancer or mesothelioma).
- **Medicolegal advice**: all patients with asbestosis (and any asbestos injury caused as a result of employment) should be advised that they can make a claim for damages against the employer responsible for the asbestos exposure and should take legal advice.

Other asbestos-related diseases: mesothelioma

A malignant growth arising in the pleura or occasionally in the peritoneum or pericardium. More common in males. Incidence increasing (predicted peak 2010–2020). Develops 20–40 years after exposure as a local mass often associated with pleural effusion (> 80%), which progressively encases the lung and hemithorax. Histological distinction from benign pleural disease can be difficult even with large biopsies and special staining techniques.

Clinical features

Breathlessness caused by pleural effusion is usual at presentation. Local tumour effects include severe pain due to chest wall invasion, and worsening breathlessness as a result of encasement of the lung.

Investigations

- **Chest X-ray** may reveal pleural nodularity or effusion, and pleural plaques.
- **CT** appearances suggestive of malignancy include pleural nodularity, thickening > 1 cm and extension of pleural thickening over the mediastinal pleural surfaces.
- **Pleural aspiration** shows blood-stained fluid (30%). Cytology is often negative. Closed pleural biopsy is positive in 50%. Thoracoscopic biopsy is positive in 90%.

Management

No treatment has been shown to improve outcome. Surgery may be tried in early disease and can be combined with chemo-radiotherapy but without evidence of improved outcome. Treatment is symptomatic: pleural aspiration for effusion causing breathlessness, often combined with pleurodesis (see p. 27). Tumour invasion at aspiration sites is common and is prevented by local radiotherapy. Chemotherapy in the context of a clinical trial should be considered for all patients with good performance status.

Prognosis

Relentless progression occurs with increasing symptoms. Median survival is 12–18 months.

Pleural plaques, pleural thickening and pleural effusion

- **Pleural plaques** are an incidental finding on chest X-ray, implying asbestos exposure and therefore increased risk of other asbestos-related diseases. In themselves they are a benign problem and of no clinical consequence. They occur in 50% of asbestos-exposed people.
- **Diffuse pleural thickening** occurs in 5% of asbestos workers exposed to high doses, and may cause symptoms as a result of restriction of chest wall movement. Lung function tests reveal reduced lung volumes. Such high level exposure increases the risk of other asbestos-related diseases.
- **Pleural effusion** occurs either at the time of high-level exposure or early after exposure. A blood-stained exudative effusion is typical. Resolution is normal but some patients are left with pleural thickening.

Coal worker's pneumoconiosis
Definition, epidemiology and aetiopathogenesis

Now a rare lung disease, presenting in elderly men, caused by inhalation of coal dust. Inhalation of small particles (0.5–7 μm) that are toxic to macrophages initiates the process. Total dose of exposure correlates with disease severity. There are three forms:

1 Simple coal worker's pneumoconiosis (CWP): inhaled dust is enveloped by inflammatory cells resulting in small nodules. Simple CWP produces no symptoms.

2 Complicated CWP: aggregates of small nodules lead to larger nodules > 1 cm in diameter. Surrounding emphysema develops. Cavitation of nodules may occur (termed 'progressive massive fibrosis'). Complicated CWP causes progressive breathlessness. Cough with black sputum (melanoptysis) may occur, as may cor pulmonale.

3 Caplan's syndrome: large nodules may develop in coal workers with positive rheumatoid factor.

Management

- **Diagnosis** is by chest X-ray (small or large nodules) and pulmonary function tests in complicated CWP (reduced lung volumes with airflow obstruction). There is no specific treatment. Avoidance of exposure has reduced the incidence. Disability from CWP is compensatable.
- **Prognosis**: as a result of control of dust levels, severe disease is rare. Respiratory failure develops in patients with progressive massive fibrosis.

Silicosis

A rare restrictive fibrotic lung disease caused by inhalation of silicon dioxide (quartz) particles. Inflammation and damage to local and hilar lymph node structures occur. There are two forms:

1 Acute silicosis results from high-level exposure and causes rapidly progressive breathlessness with death within months.

2 Lower level exposure causes more slowly progressive symptoms and **predisposes to tuberculosis** (TB).

Chest X-ray shows small (1–3 mm) nodules mainly in the upper zones and larger nodules later in the disease. 'Egg shell' calcification of hilar lymph nodes is pathognomonic. Management involves reducing dust levels, the use of respiratory protection and regular screening for TB. With avoidance of exposure, prognosis is usually good. Progressive disease or acute silicosis results in death from respiratory failure.

Radiological features

Lung disease	Typical pattern
Pulmonary fibrosis	Diffuse bilateral infiltrates Usually predominantly basal
Pulmonary eosinophilia	Bilateral sub-pleural opacities Predominantly basal in 50%
Organizing pneumonia (BOOP)	Patchy bilateral opacities Asymmetrical distribution May aggregate and form nodules Variation in distribution over time
Non-cardiogenic pulmonary oedema (ARDS)	Diffuse bilateral alveolar shadowing
Alveolar haemorrhage	Diffuse alveolar shadows
Pleural disease	Effusion ± pleural thickening Occasional pericardial effusion

Drug effects

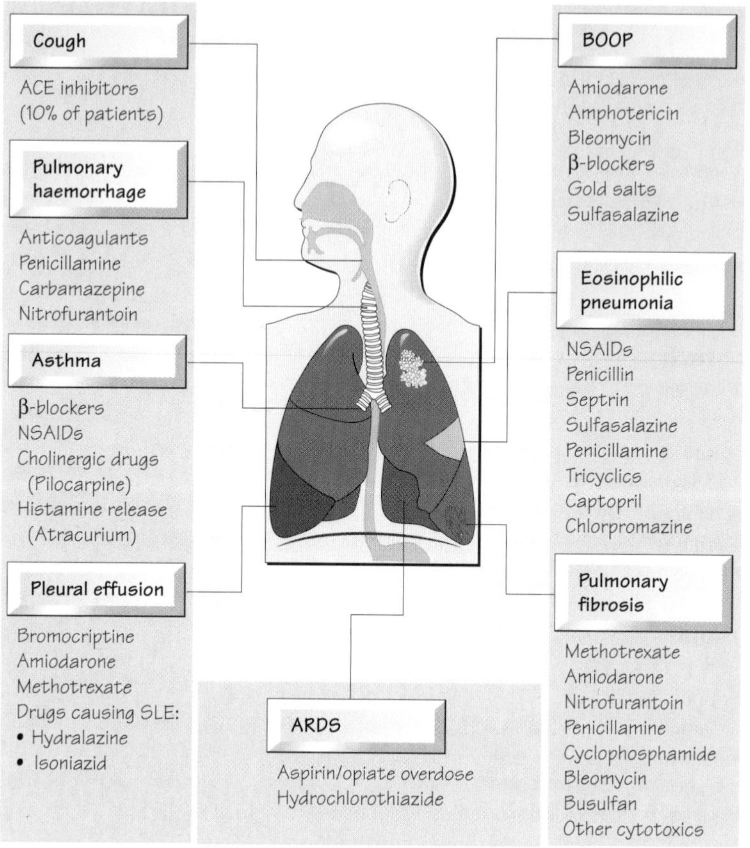

Cough

ACE inhibitors
(10% of patients)

Pulmonary haemorrhage

Anticoagulants
Penicillamine
Carbamazepine
Nitrofurantoin

Asthma

β-blockers
NSAIDs
Cholinergic drugs
(Pilocarpine)
Histamine release
(Atracurium)

Pleural effusion

Bromocriptine
Amiodarone
Methotrexate
Drugs causing SLE:
• Hydralazine
• Isoniazid

ARDS

Aspirin/opiate overdose
Hydrochlorothiazide

BOOP

Amiodarone
Amphotericin
Bleomycin
β-blockers
Gold salts
Sulfasalazine

Eosinophilic pneumonia

NSAIDs
Penicillin
Septrin
Sulfasalazine
Penicillamine
Tricyclics
Captopril
Chlorpromazine

Pulmonary fibrosis

Methotrexate
Amiodarone
Nitrofurantoin
Penicillamine
Cyclophosphamide
Bleomycin
Busulfan
Other cytotoxics

The effects of drugs on the lung are extremely variable. The figure shows common drug effects on the lung and their major causes. It is by no means exhaustive: virtually any lung disease may be drug related and thus drugs as the cause should always enter the differential diagnosis.

Clinical features

These depend on the nature of the resulting lung disease. Some symptoms relate to a predictable pharmacological effect (asthma caused by β-blockers). Others may be dose related (amiodarone) or idiosyncratic. For patients on drugs commonly associated with pulmonary side effects (amiodarone, cytotoxic chemotherapeutic agents), baseline pulmonary function tests are helpful to determine whether new symptoms relate to new lung abnormalities.

Investigations and management

Radiological features (see figure)

Investigations

These are driven according to the nature of the respiratory symptoms. A detailed drug history, including current and previous treatment, should always be sought in any patient with respiratory symptoms. In patients with suspected pulmonary drug toxicity, diagnosis should be based on:
• The likelihood of drug reaction to the drug(s) being taken and exclusion of alternative pathology; this may involve bronchial lavage or biopsy techniques to look for infection or confirm lung pathology.
• Consideration of which drug is responsible. If a drug reaction is confirmed, this will usually result in withdrawal of the agent concerned. Often no specific treatment is necessary. The consequences of stopping treatment need to be weighed against the likely adverse effects of continuation. Alternative treatment may need to be given to replace the effects of the drug being withdrawn.
• **Reporting to the Committee on Safety of Medicines (CSM):** all patients with drug-induced lung disease should be reported to the CSM.

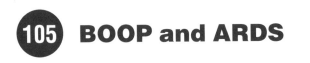

105 BOOP and ARDS

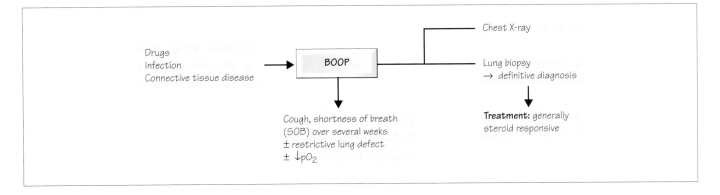

Bronchiolitis obliterans organizing pneumonia

Epidemiology

This rare disease, also known as cryptogenic organizing pneumonia (COP), is of unknown aetiology but may present after infection or drug treatment, or as part of a connective tissue disease. Preponderance in the spring suggests an inhaled agent in some instances. There is no sex difference and no obvious geographical variation.

Pathophysiology

This is a histological diagnosis. Bronchiolitis obliterans organizing pneumonia (BOOP) is a specific way in which the lung may respond to an inflammatory stimulus. The histology reveals the changes of a pneumonitis with organization of inflammatory cells into granulation tissue. The disease originates in the alveoli with a variable amount of extension into the airways.

Clinical features

BOOP presents with systemic upset, usually over a period of a few weeks. Cough and breathlessness are present in the majority. Fever and weight loss are common. Crackles are often present.

Investigations

The chest X-ray and CT show infiltrates which are often multi-focal. The erythrocyte sedimentation rate (ESR) is almost invariably raised and the eosinophil count is normal. Pulmonary function tests may be normal or show a restrictive defect with impaired gas transfer. In severe disease, blood gases may reveal hypoxaemia. Transbronchial biopsy may be helpful but samples are often inadequate. Open lung biopsy is diagnostic.

Management

If a causative drug can be identified, this should be discontinued. Oral corticosteroids will achieve a rapid improvement in symptoms over days in most patients. Radiological changes resolve over months and the steroid course should be reduced over an extended period, as relapse is common. Relapse is likely to respond well to further steroid courses.

Acute respiratory distress syndrome

Acute respiratory distress syndrome (ARDS) is a relatively common complication of conditions that activate inflammatory mediators (Table 105.1), resulting in diffuse lung injury, damaged pulmonary vasculature and non-cardiogenic pulmonary oedema. After several days, the inflamed lungs may fibrose, which can interfere with long-term lung function. Key points are:

• ARDS usually occurs in patients already 'sick' for other reasons. Often multiple pathologies underlie ARDS, e.g. sepsis with hypotension, etc.
• Impaired gas exchange occurs, causing breathlessness and central cyanosis. The first indication of ARDS is usually unexplained breathlessness in an already sick patient. Signs include tachycardia, cyanosis (often with confusion and/or agitation), and inspiratory crackles throughout the lung fields.
• Chest X-ray may initially be fairly unremarkable, but later shows diffuse 'patchy' infiltrates, which can progress to a 'white-out'. The differential diagnosis includes pneumonia, heart failure and interstitial lung diseases. CT scanning may help differentiate these if doubt exists.
• Intravascular capillary obstruction occurs, causing pulmonary hypertension.
• Treatment involves removing the cause (e.g. sepsis), supporting gas exchange (ventilation, which may be difficult, as the lungs are 'stiff') and other failing organs, and minimizing pulmonary oedema (keeping the patient 'dry' without provoking renal failure).
• Mortality is high at around 30–60%.

Table 105.1 Causes of ARDS.

Sepsis, especially if shock present
Hypotension, especially if prolonged, or with trauma
Blood transfusion, especially if massive
The systemic inflammatory response syndrome (SIRS) (see p. 296)
Disseminated intravascular coagulation
Obstetric causes; amniotic fluid embolism, pre-eclampsia
Adverse drug reaction (both prescribed and 'street' drugs e.g. heroin)
Chemical lung injury e.g. toxic gas inhalation, gastric aspiration
High-altitude-related lung injury

Diseases and Treatments at a Glance

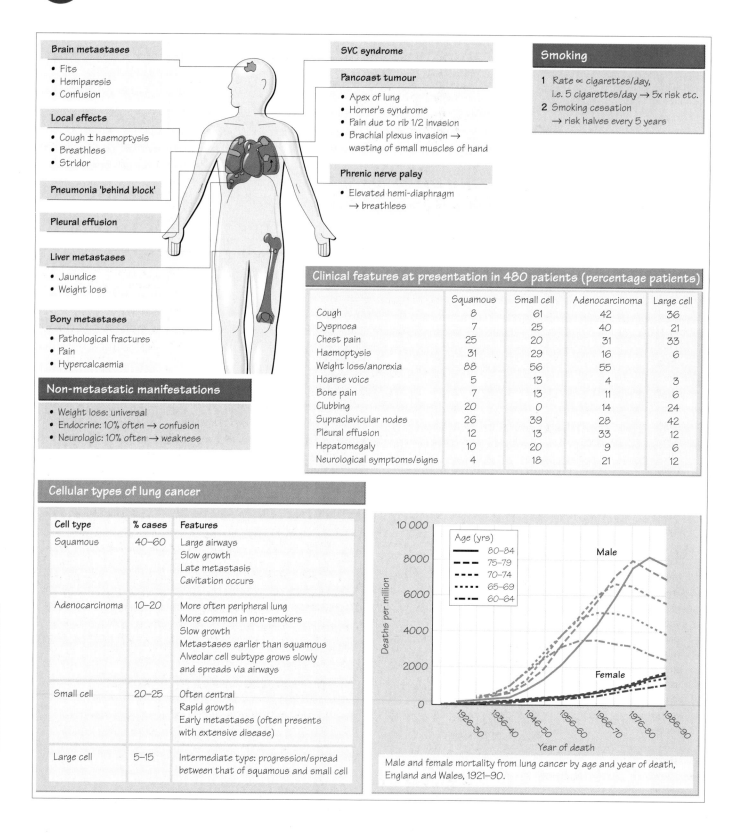

Brain metastases

- Fits
- Hemiparesis
- Confusion

Local effects

- Cough ± haemoptysis
- Breathless
- Stridor

Pneumonia 'behind block'

Pleural effusion

Liver metastases

- Jaundice
- Weight loss

Bony metastases

- Pathological fractures
- Pain
- Hypercalcaemia

SVC syndrome

Pancoast tumour

- Apex of lung
- Horner's syndrome
- Pain due to rib 1/2 invasion
- Brachial plexus invasion →
  wasting of small muscles of hand

Phrenic nerve palsy

- Elevated hemi-diaphragm
  → breathless

Smoking

1. Rate ∝ cigarettes/day,
   i.e. 5 cigarettes/day → 5x risk etc.
2. Smoking cessation
   → risk halves every 5 years

Non-metastatic manifestations

- Weight loss: universal
- Endocrine: 10% often → confusion
- Neurologic: 10% often → weakness

Clinical features at presentation in 480 patients (percentage patients)

	Squamous	Small cell	Adenocarcinoma	Large cell
Cough	8	61	42	36
Dyspnoea	7	25	40	21
Chest pain	25	20	31	33
Haemoptysis	31	29	16	6
Weight loss/anorexia	88	56	55	
Hoarse voice	5	13	4	3
Bone pain	7	13	11	6
Clubbing	20	0	14	24
Supraclavicular nodes	26	39	28	42
Pleural effusion	12	13	33	12
Hepatomegaly	10	20	9	6
Neurological symptoms/signs	4	18	21	12

Cellular types of lung cancer

Cell type	% cases	Features
Squamous	40–60	Large airways Slow growth Late metastasis Cavitation occurs
Adenocarcinoma	10–20	More often peripheral lung More common in non-smokers Slow growth Metastases earlier than squamous Alveolar cell subtype grows slowly and spreads via airways
Small cell	20–25	Often central Rapid growth Early metastases (often presents with extensive disease)
Large cell	5–15	Intermediate type: progression/spread between that of squamous and small cell

Male and female mortality from lung cancer by age and year of death, England and Wales, 1921–90.

Epidemiology

Nearly all primary lung tumours are malignant. Lung cancer is the most common malignancy in the western world, occurring in 1 in 13 men and 1 in 20 women, with 35 000 cases/year in the UK. Most (60–65%) occur in men and are the result of cigarette smoking. Women now smoke more and accordingly their lung cancer rates are rising.

Aetiology

• **Tobacco** causes 85% of lung cancers (not adenocarcinoma). Cancer is rare in never-smokers. The more cigarettes smoked and the higher the tar content, the higher the cancer rates. After smoking cessation, lung cancer risk only falls back to that of never-smokers over the next 40 years.
• **Other risk factors**: passive smoking, occupational exposure to asbestos, silica and nickel; pulmonary fibrosis. Genetic factors play a part.

Clinical features

New or persistent respiratory symptoms in a current or ex-smoker should always raise the suspicion of lung cancer. Symptoms may be absent, non-specific (40%—lack of energy, anorexia and weight loss), as a result of the primary cancer, caused by local spread, distant metastases or non-metastatic manifestations.
• **Effects of the primary**: cough ($\geq 50\%$). Breathlessness resulting from bronchial obstruction, lobar collapse or pleural effusion. Haemoptysis ($\geq 35\%$). Fixed wheeze or stridor suggests large airway narrowing.
• **Effects of local spread**: local pain from chest wall involvement. Apical (Pancoast's) tumours invade the brachial plexus (pain radiating down the arm) and cause Horner's syndrome (see p. 99). Mediastinal invasion causes recurrent laryngeal nerve palsy (hoarseness), superior vena cava (SVC) obstruction, phrenic nerve palsy (breathlessness) and oesophageal compression (dysphagia).
• **Effects of distant metastases**: metastases occur in bone (pain or hypercalcaemia), liver (asymptomatic, capsular pain) or brain (headache, confusion, seizures).
• **Non-metastatic manifestations**: endocrine—syndrome of inappropriate release of antidiuretic hormone (SIADH) (hyponatraemia especially with small-cell lung cancer, see p. 250), hypercalcaemia (parathyroid hormone-related peptide in 6% of squamous carcinoma). Ectopic adrenocorticotrophic hormone (ACTH) secretion in 30% of small-cell tumours, although Cushing's syndrome rarely has time to develop. Gynaecomastia in $\leq 1\%$ of squamous carcinoma.
• **Neurological symptoms**: usually relate to metastases—non-metastatic manifestations include the Lambert-Eaton myasthenic syndrome with small-cell cancer (see p. 361). Cerebellar degeneration, peripheral neuropathy, encephalopathy, mixed and sensory neuropathies all occur relatively infrequently.
• **Finger clubbing**: mainly in squamous carcinoma. Advanced clubbing is associated with hypertrophic pulmonary osteoarthropathy (HPOA) which presents with pain and swelling in the long bones.
• **Other symptoms**: dermatomyositis and the nephrotic syndrome rarely occur.

Investigations

These should confirm the diagnosis, the cell type and stage the disease to determine treatment.
• **Chest X-ray** is usually abnormal by the time symptoms develop.
• **Paraneoplastic syndromes**: diagnosed from the full blood count, urea & electrolytes, and calcium.
• **Lung function tests**: low FEV_1 precludes surgery and percutaneous biopsy.

• **Bronchoscopy or percutaneous biopsy**: bronchoscopy produces diagnostic histology in 70% of central lung cancers. For peripheral tumours, a CT/ultrasound-guided percutaneous approach is used. If the radiological features are highly suggestive of carcinoma, excision biopsy is preferable. If lymph node or liver metastases are present, biopsy of these is preferable.
• **Sputum cytology** is only used when invasive procedures are inappropriate (poor pulmonary function, co-morbid factors).

Staging investigations

For non-small cell cancer
• **Thoracic CT**: to include the common sites for metastases—the liver and adrenal glands (4%). Small mediastinal nodes < 1 cm are not malignant in 25% and, unless 'on-table' mediastinoscopic staging is positive, should not preclude surgery.
• **Isotope bone scanning** for bony metastases (bone pain or hypercalcaemia).
• **Brain CT**: for neurological disease.
• **Positron emission tomography (PET) scanning**: can reveal nodal or distant metastases not revealed by other staging methods and should be used to confirm localized disease in all patients prior to radical treatment (surgery or CHART; see below).

Staging for small-cell lung cancer differs, as metastases are often present at presentation. **Limited disease**: confined to one hemithorax and the ipsilateral supraclavicular fossa. **Extensive disease**: all other patients—70% of cases.

Management

• **Surgery** offers the best chance of cure, but < 25% are operable and only 25% of these (5% of all patients) are alive at 5 years. Perioperative mortality rate is 3% for lobectomy and 6% for pneumonectomy.
• **Radical radiotherapy** is used for inoperable non-small cell lung cancer. Radical treatment is suitable for anatomically localized disease, and cures only a few. Recent studies have shown better results than once-daily conventional radiotherapy with multiple daily radiotherapy doses of continuous hyperfractionated accelerated radiotherapy (CHART).
• **Palliative radiotherapy** for haemoptysis, cough, breathlessness or local pain. Brain metastases are treated with steroids and radiotherapy.
• **Chemotherapy** is used for small-cell lung cancer, because surgery is **never appropriate** with this histology. Response occurs in 60–85%—survival gain is approximately 4 months. Only 10% of patients survive 2 years. In limited disease, radiotherapy after chemotherapy reduces local recurrence rates from 75% to 30%. Chemotherapy is recommended in non-small cell lung cancer for fit patients with metastatic disease.
• **Endobronchial treatments** such as cryotherapy, laser treatment or the use of stents can provide rapid relief of symptoms in patients with significant symptomatic endobronchial disease.
• **Palliative care**: opiates are crucially helpful for pain and dyspnoea. Steroids help non-specific symptoms and improve appetite. Support from carers, family and palliative care specialists is extremely important.

Prognosis

This depends partly on cell type. Overall survival rate at 1 year is 20% and at 5 years is 6%. Even after apparently successful surgical resection, the 5-year survival rate is only 40–50%. Median survival in small-cell disease without treatment is 2–3 months and, with extensive disease at presentation, survival is 4 weeks without treatment.

Food poisoning and gastrointestinal infections

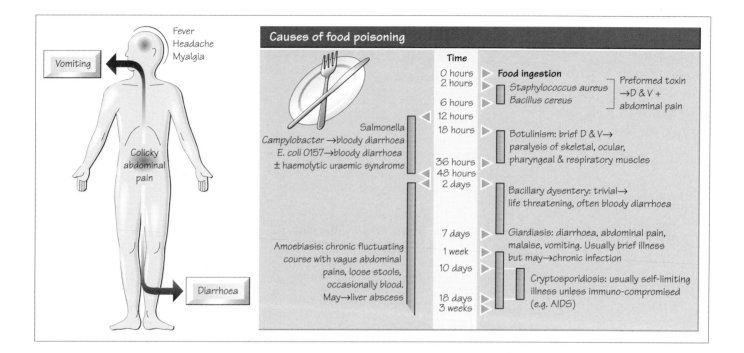

Acute gastroenteritis

Acute gastroenteritis or food poisoning is a more common occurrence now than in previous decades. In many circumstances the diagnosis is empirical and based on history rather than positive cultures. Causes include:
- **Common**: Culture negative (viral), *Campylobacter* spp., *Salmonella* spp., cholera (developing countries).
- **Uncommon**: *Shigella* spp.
- **Rare but important**: *Escherichia coli* 0157, *Staphylococcus aureus*, *Vibrio para-haemolyticus* and *Clostridium botulinum*.

Clinical features

Symptoms are usually of sudden onset. There may be a history of travel or suspect food, and other individuals may also be affected: diarrhoea and vomiting, abdominal pain and fever, headache, myalgia.

Investigations

Most cases settle spontaneously and do not require investigation. In patients sufficiently ill to warrant admission to hospital, investigations should be considered, including stool and blood cultures, full blood count (FBC), electrolytes and plain abdominal radiology.

Management and prognosis

Mild cases require no more than to encourage oral rehydration. More severe cases may require intravenous fluids. Antibiotics are indicated in septicaemia (i.e. fever, positive blood cultures). Ciprofloxacin is a good first-line agent, active against the common bacterial pathogens (*Salmonella*, *Shigella* and *Campylobacter* spp.). If diarrhoea persists for more than 3 weeks, sigmoidoscopy, rectal biopsy and referral to a gastroenterology clinic should be considered. The common causes include hypolactasia, post-infective irritable bowel, giardiasis. Consideration should be given to the presence of an unrelated underlying GI pathology (colitis, coeliac disease).

Chronic infections
Giardiasis

Infection with *Giardia lamblia* may cause a persistent infection. Making a positive diagnosis on culture may prove difficult (even with culture of duodenal aspirates). Empirical treatment with tinidazole or metronidazole is effective.

Tuberculosis (TB)

Gastrointestinal TB is a rare but important diagnosis. The diagnosis should be considered in patients from developing countries who have chronic abdominal symptoms. There are a number of possible clinical presentations:
- **Ileocaecal tuberculosis**, which mimics Crohn's disease (fever, abdominal pain, weight loss and diarrhoea). The chest X-ray is usually normal and TB is not found elsewhere in the body.
- **Tuberculous peritonitis**: exudative ascites. May require peritoneal biopsy to make the diagnosis.
- **Mesenteric lymphadenopathy**, which may cause right iliac fossa pain and subacute obstructive symptoms. Lymph nodes elsewhere (cervical, mediastinal and peritoneal) are also usually affected.

Treatment is the same as for pulmonary TB.

Amoebiasis

Infection with *Entamoeba histolytica* may cause a variety of clinical presentations: asymptomatic excretion of cysts is the most common finding, amoebic dysentery, non-dysenteric colonic disease and invasive disease/hepatic abscess also can occur.

The diagnosis may be made by microscopy of hot stool, histology of colonic biopsies or serology. Treatment is with metronidazole followed by diloxanide furoate.

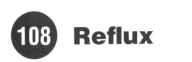

Reflux

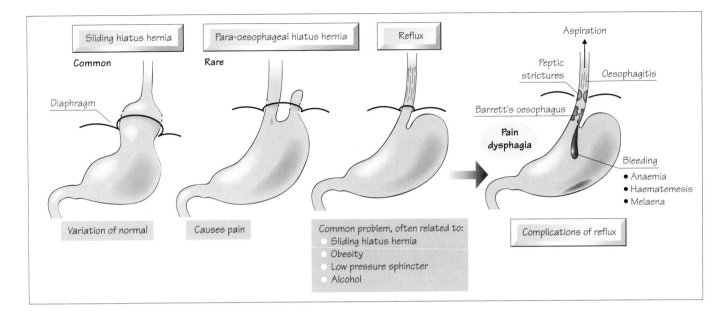

Sliding hiatus hernia — Common — Variation of normal

Para-oesophageal hiatus hernia — Rare — Causes pain

Reflux — Common problem, often related to:
- Sliding hiatus hernia
- Obesity
- Low pressure sphincter
- Alcohol

Diaphragm

Aspiration

Peptic strictures — Oesophagitis

Barrett's oesophagus

Pain dysphagia

Bleeding
- Anaemia
- Haematemesis
- Melaena

Complications of reflux

Incidence

Symptoms of gastro-oesophageal reflux are very common in the western world (20–40% of the population). Symptom severity does not correlate well with the extent of oesophagitis.

Pathophysiology

- **A hiatal hernia** is herniation of the proximal stomach into the chest, caused by a congenital defect in the diaphragm or an acquired abnormality.
- **Gastro-oesophageal reflux** mainly results from lifestyle factors. Obesity increases intra-abdominal pressure. Smoking, stress and dietary factors (e.g. fatty foods, pastry, alcohol, chocolate) all reduce the pressure in the lower oesophageal sphincter and promote reflux.

Clinical features

Symptomatic reflux is diagnosed on the basis of a good clinical history and many patients will have unremarkable investigations

- **Heartburn**: reflux most commonly presents with heartburn and occasionally nausea (see p. 36). Effortless regurgitation and belching will often be present and the symptoms may have a marked postural element.
- **Chest pain** may be the presenting symptoms and results from reflux-precipitated oesophageal spasm. This may be indistinguishable from angina. Cardiac pain should be excluded (often by exercise testing) before the upper gastrointestinal tract is investigated.
- **Transient dysphagia** may be experienced in severe oesophagitis. More persistent dysphagia with regurgitation or vomiting suggests the development of a secondary complication such as a peptic oesophageal stricture or even carcinoma.

Investigations

- **Upper gastrointestinal endoscopy** may be useful in reflux. In many this is normal **or** it may demonstrate oesophagitis. Barrett's epithelium is present in up to 15% of patients with reflux symptoms. This is potentially a pre-malignant condition, predisposing to lower third oesophageal

adenocarcinoma. The incidence of cancer in patients with Barrett's is now recognized to be lower than initially feared (0.4%) but regular surveillance endoscopy and oesophageal biopsies to identify dysplasia may still be deemed appropriate in some instances.

- **Barium swallow/meal** may provide information complementary to endoscopy. In patients with dysphagia, motility disorders such as diffuse oesophageal spasm and achalasia are better demonstrated radiologically. Similarly the size and nature of a hiatal hernia are underestimated by endoscopy.
- **24-h oesophageal manometry and pH recording**: patients with persistent and troublesome symptoms may benefit from manometry and pH recording, which is used to select those patients who might benefit from anti-reflux surgery.

Management and prognosis

- **Lifestyle changes**: most patients with reflux symptoms will experience a significant improvement by:
  - Stopping smoking and limiting chocolate, coffee and alcohol intake.
  - **Maintaining a reasonable body mass index**
  - Eating regular meals (especially breakfast) and avoiding late night eating.
  - Raising the head end of the bed.
- **Antacids**: over-the-counter antacids (often with an alginate) are used intermittently by many reflux sufferers.
- **H_2-receptor antagonists**.
- **Proton pump inhibitors**, e.g. omeprazole, lansoprazole, are the most potent treatment for reflux symptoms and are often used as a therapeutic trial.
- **Pro-kinetics**: patients with more reflux than dyspepsia may be better treated with a pro-kinetic agent (e.g. domperidone).
- **Surgery**: anti-reflux surgery is beneficial in those whose symptoms are resistant to medical therapy, who have unacceptable side effects on proton pump inhibitors (usually diarrhoea), or those with a rolling hiatal hernia and a high risk of incarceration/volvulus.

Diseases and Treatments at a Glance

109 Peptic ulcer disease

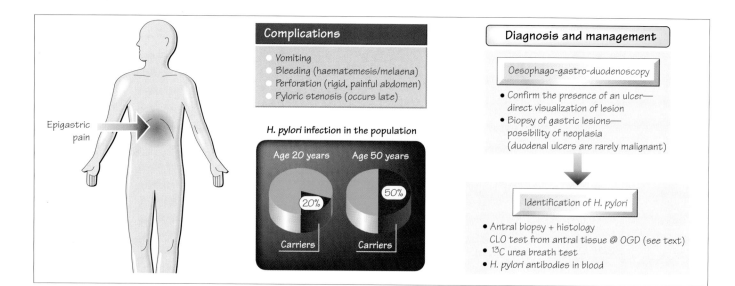

Complications
- Vomiting
- Bleeding (haematemesis/melaena)
- Perforation (rigid, painful abdomen)
- Pyloric stenosis (occurs late)

H. pylori infection in the population

Age 20 years — 20% Carriers

Age 50 years — 50% Carriers

Diagnosis and management

Oesophago-gastro-duodenoscopy

- Confirm the presence of an ulcer—direct visualization of lesion
- Biopsy of gastric lesions—possibility of neoplasia (duodenal ulcers are rarely malignant)

Identification of H. pylori

- Antral biopsy + histology
  CLO test from antral tissue @ OGD (see text)
- ^{13}C urea breath test
- H. pylori antibodies in blood

Epigastric pain

Peptic ulceration of the upper GI tract may occur in either the duodenum or the stomach.

Duodenal ulcer

Duodenal ulceration usually occurs secondary to states of high gastric acid output (c.f. gastric ulcer below).

Incidence

The incidence of duodenal ulcer is declining in line with improvement in living standards, although it still affects 10–15% in certain populations. *Helicobacter pylori* carriage and non-steroidal anti-inflammatory drug (NSAID) use are the major risk factors.

Clinical features

- **Gastrointestinal haemorrhage** is now the most common presentation of peptic ulceration (see p. 38).
- **Dyspepsia**: abdominal pain has historically been considered to be the classic symptom of a duodenal ulcer but many patients presenting with acute gastrointestinal bleeding deny indigestion symptoms.
- **Vomiting** may be the presenting feature if long-standing duodenal ulceration results in pyloric stenosis.
- **Perforation** with peritonitis is occasionally a presenting or complicating feature.

Investigations

- **Endoscopy** is the first line investigation for patients with dyspepsia and for upper gastrointestinal bleeding (for diagnosis and endoscopic therapy in bleeding).
- **Testing for *Helicobacter pylori***: various tests allow the identification of this organism that is characteristically very difficult to culture:
  - Histology of antral biopsy.
  - CLO test for bacterial urease, from endoscopically obtained antral tissue: *H. pylori* secretes urease, which hydrolyses urea to NH_3 and CO_2; *in vitro* urea is added and NH_3 detected by the colour change of a pH-sensitive indicator.
  - ^{13}C-labelled urea breath test: radiolabelled urea is ingested and the

$^{13}CO_2$ produced by hydrolysis is absorbed, excreted in the lungs and detected in the breath.
  - Measurement of *H. pylori* antibodies in blood.

  Detection of *H. pylori* alone is not sufficient for a diagnosis of duodenal ulceration, because 20% (aged 20 years) to 50% (aged 50 years) of the population are carriers.

Gastric ulcer

Although there is some overlap between duodenal and gastric ulcers, the latter commonly occur in circumstances of impaired mucosal defence (e.g. NSAID use). Gastric cancer is more common than duodenal cancer and caution should be exercised as to whether or not a newly identified gastric ulcer might be malignant.

Clinical features

The clinical presentation is similar to duodenal ulcers although, given the reduced acid secretion, dyspepsia is possibly less common.

Investigations

- **Endoscopy**: as newly identified gastric ulcers may represent early gastric cancer, biopsy of the ulcer edge and interval re-endoscopy after 6 weeks of medical therapy are mandatory.

Management and prognosis

- **Medical therapy** results in ulcer healing after 4–6 weeks, either with a H_2-receptor antagonist or proton pump inhibitor. Non-steroidal anti-inflammatory drugs should be stopped **and where possible avoided thereafter**.
- **_H. pylori_ eradication**: ulcer recurrence is common without eradication of *H. pylori*. Eradication regimens consisting of high doses of a proton pump inhibitor in combination with two different antibiotics are 70–80% successful. Success should be documented using the ^{13}C-labelled urea breath test. In failed eradication, re-endoscopy with culture of organisms for antibiotic sensitivity is occasionally indicated.
- **Surgery** is required in those with perforation and recurrent or persistent bleeding. Elective surgery is an infrequent option for persistent ulceration and/or intolerance of medical therapy.

Diseases and Treatments at a Glance

110 Diverticular disease

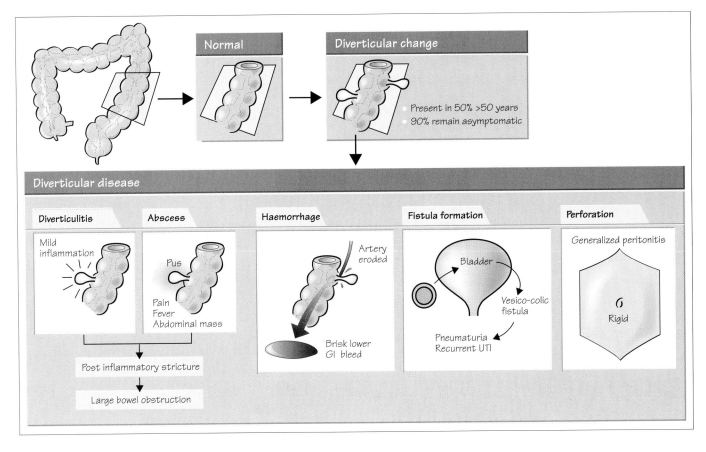

Normal

Diverticular change
- Present in 50% >50 years
- 90% remain asymptomatic

Diverticular disease

Diverticulitis
- Mild inflammation

Abscess
- Pus
- Pain
- Fever
- Abdominal mass

Post inflammatory stricture

Large bowel obstruction

Haemorrhage
- Artery eroded
- Brisk lower GI bleed

Fistula formation
- Bladder
- Vesico-colic fistula
- Pneumaturia Recurrent UTI

Perforation
- Generalized peritonitis
- Rigid

Diverticulosis represents a degenerative change in the colon resulting in the formation of out-pouches or pockets of colonic mucosa extruding through the muscular wall of the bowel. In many elderly people this may be asymptomatic and the terms 'diverticular change' or 'diverticulosis' may be more appropriate than the more commonly used term diverticulitis.

Incidence
The prevalence increases with age and is 5% at 40 years rising to 50% at 80 years.

Pathophysiology
There may be an underlying genetic predisposition to diverticular disease but it is best considered as an acquired condition.

Clinical features
Diverticular change itself is asymptomatic and it is the common complications that lead to symptomatic presentation.
- **Diverticulitis**: an associated inflammation of the colon—often related to infection resulting from impaction of faeces within a diverticulum. This may evolve into a **diverticular abscess** with abdominal pain, fever and a left-sided abdominal mass
- **Colonic bleeding**: this is a frequent presentation of diverticular disease, possibly because diverticula form at the point of maximal weakness in the colon, i.e. at the point where blood vessels penetrate the muscle coat.

- **Repeated infective episodes** may result in the formation of either a **diverticular stricture** presenting with symptoms of colonic obstruction or a **colovesical fistula** presenting with recurrent urinary tract infections or the characteristic symptom of pneumaturia.

Investigations
- **Barium enema** or **colonoscopy**: asymptomatic diverticular change may be demonstrated by either barium enema or colonoscopy.
- **Abdominal computed tomography** is the best way to demonstrate abscesses. Colovesical fistulae require a high index of suspicion (recurrent urinary tract infections, pneumaturia, etc.), but may be identified on barium contrast radiology.

Management and prognosis
The management of diverticular disease is often conservative, though surgery is occasionally required.
- **Avoidance of symptomatic constipation** may reduce the risk of complications.
- **Treatment of complications**: acute diverticulitis requires intravenous fluids, antibiotics and analgesics. Diverticular abscess may require drainage in addition to the above. Bleeding usually settles with supportive treatment.
- **Surgery**: this is usually reserved for complicated diverticular disease (i.e. bleeding, abscess, stricture).

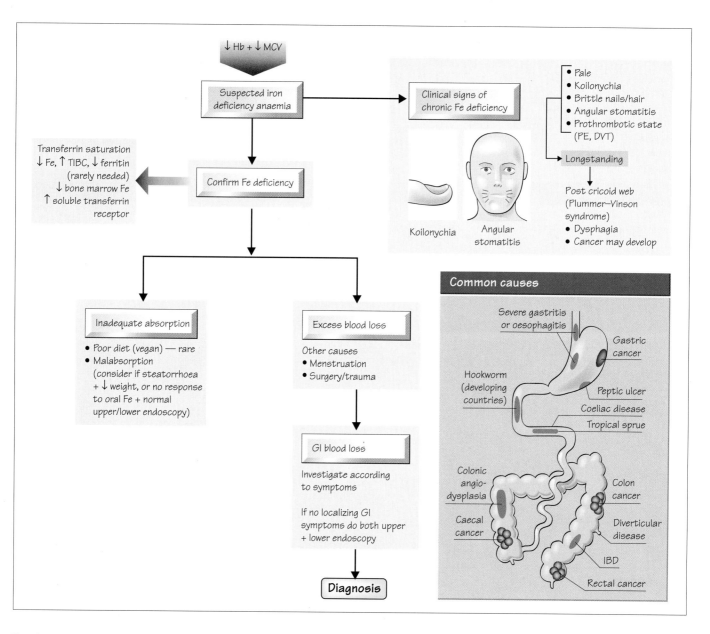

Iron is absorbed in the proximal small intestine. There is no physiological route of iron excretion in humans. Hence there are two potential reasons for iron deficiency.

1 Reduced iron absorption from the gastrointestinal (GI) tract, as a result of mucosal disease (coeliac disease), duodenal bypass (polyagastrectomy) or rarely dietary deficiency.

2 Chronic blood loss, the most common cause, resulting from: a) Menstrual bleeding (pre-menopausal women) b) GI neoplasia (colonic adenomatous polyps, caecal/gastric carcinoma) c) Intestinal angiodysplasia.

Clinical features

General

Many patients do not have GI symptoms, although any symptoms found may prioritize subsequent investigation.

History

In pre-menopausal women a menstrual history should be taken. Previous gastric surgery may predispose to iron deficiency through duodenal bypass (i.e. gastroenterostomy) or gastric cancer. Vegans have reduced dietary iron, and thresholds for investigations should be raised.

Examination

In elderly people, an underdiagnosed cause of iron deficiency is intestinal angiodysplasia—small angiodysplastic lesions may be seen on the lips or buccal mucosa. There is an association between angiodysplasia and aortic stenosis; as aortic stenosis can induce functional von Willebrand's disease, iron deficiency may complicate the natural history of this valve lesion. Lymphadenopathy should be sought (i.e. Virchow's node). An abdominal mass may be present and each iliac fossa should be carefully palpated. Even without altered bowel habit or rectal bleeding, a rectal examination and sigmoidoscopy are required.

Investigations
• **Blood tests**: full blood count (FBC) shows a microcytic anaemia,
• **Ferritin and transferrin saturation (serum iron divided by total iron binding capacity)** are low. Ferritin is an acute phase reactant and may be raised (or inappropriately 'normal') in the presence of any coexisting inflammation. A microcytic anaemia should always be confirmed as being caused by iron deficiency before treatment/GI investigation.
• **Faecal occult blood (FOB)**: chemical tests for haem oxygenase (Haemoccult) are very sensitive—persistently strongly positive results suggest significant GI blood loss. Up to 30% of colonic cancers are FOB negative (see p. 240).
• **Endoscopy and colonoscopy**: most patients with iron deficiency require examination of both upper and lower GI tracts. At upper endo-scopy, duodenal biopsies should be taken to exclude coeliac disease. Polyps identified at colonoscopy are snared and removed.
• **Barium enema**: barium contrast radiology is an alternative way to image the colon.
• **Small bowel imaging**: if no source is identified, consideration should be given to small bowel imaging (small bowel enema, enteroscopy).
• **Endomysial antibodies**: persistent or recurrent iron deficiency in the absence of obvious loss requires investigation for malabsorption. Endomysial antibody or tissue transglutaminase antibody must be done to exclude coeliac disease.

Management
• **Treat underlying cause**: gastrointestinal angiodysplasia usually responds to continuous oral iron replacement (for gastric and colorectal cancer, see pp. 238 and 240).
• **If no source of GI blood loss is identified**, consideration should be given to either continuous oral iron replacement or a course of replacement and repeat investigation should the problem recur.

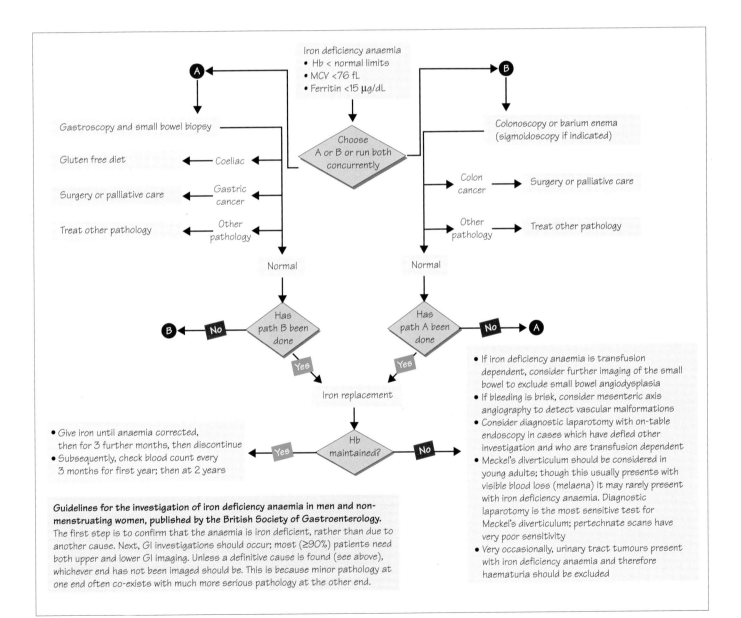

Guidelines for the investigation of iron deficiency anaemia in men and non-menstruating women, published by the British Society of Gastroenterology.
The first step is to confirm that the anaemia is iron deficient, rather than due to another cause. Next, GI investigations should occur; most (≥90%) patients need both upper and lower GI imaging. Unless a definitive cause is found (see above), whichever end has not been imaged should be. This is because minor pathology at one end often co-exists with much more serious pathology at the other end.

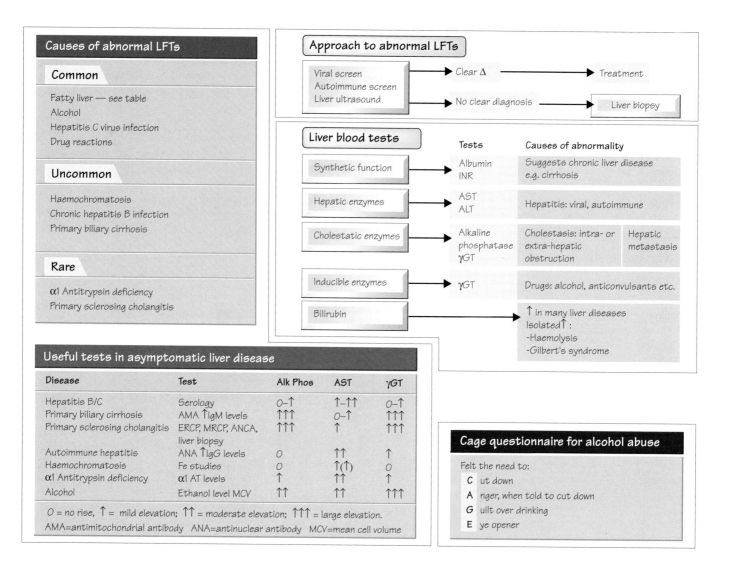

Causes of abnormal LFTs

Common

Fatty liver — see table
Alcohol
Hepatitis C virus infection
Drug reactions

Uncommon

Haemochromatosis
Chronic hepatitis B infection
Primary biliary cirrhosis

Rare

α1 Antitrypsin deficiency
Primary sclerosing cholangitis

Approach to abnormal LFTs

Viral screen
Autoimmune screen → Clear Δ → Treatment
Liver ultrasound → No clear diagnosis → Liver biopsy

Liver blood tests

	Tests	Causes of abnormality	
Synthetic function	Albumin INR	Suggests chronic liver disease e.g. cirrhosis	
Hepatic enzymes	AST ALT	Hepatitis: viral, autoimmune	
Cholestatic enzymes	Alkaline phosphatase γGT	Cholestasis: intra- or extra-hepatic obstruction	Hepatic metastasis
Inducible enzymes	γGT	Drugs: alcohol, anticonvulsants etc.	
Bilirubin		↑ in many liver diseases Isolated↑: -Haemolysis -Gilbert's syndrome	

Useful tests in asymptomatic liver disease

Disease	Test	Alk Phos	AST	γGT
Hepatitis B/C	Serology	O–↑	↑–↑↑	O–↑
Primary biliary cirrhosis	AMA ↑IgM levels	↑↑↑	O–↑	↑↑↑
Primary sclerosing cholangitis	ERCP, MRCP, ANCA, liver biopsy	↑↑↑	↑	↑↑↑
Autoimmune hepatitis	ANA ↑IgG levels	O	↑↑	↑
Haemochromatosis	Fe studies	O	↑(↑)	O
α1 Antitrypsin deficiency	α1 AT levels	↑	↑↑	↑
Alcohol	Ethanol level MCV	↑↑	↑↑	↑↑↑

O = no rise, ↑ = mild elevation; ↑↑ = moderate elevation; ↑↑↑ = large elevation.
AMA=antimitochondrial antibody ANA=antinuclear antibody MCV=mean cell volume

Cage questionnaire for alcohol abuse

Felt the need to:

C ut down
A nger, when told to cut down
G uilt over drinking
E ye opener

Overall approach

Abnormalities in liver function tests (LFTs) accompanied by symptoms are described in the relevant chapters. Abnormalities of LFTs in asymptomatic individuals are a frequent reason for outpatient hospital referral. Although these individuals are often not ill at the time of the consultation, the abnormal test may herald an underlying disease and an attempt is made to reach a diagnosis to make prognostic and therapeutic decisions. For differential diagnosis, see figure and Table 112.1.

Clinical features

General

Often there is little in the clinical history, although there are many features that should be specifically sought:

• Alcohol intake is **commonly** underestimated **by the patient**. The CAGE questionnaire **may be** useful. Two or more positive answers has a 90% correlation with alcohol dependence.

• Features suggesting hepatitis B or C, including foreign travel (Far East and Africa), sexual preferences and intravenous drug use (past or present). Previous jaundice.

• Full current and recent (< few months) medication history, including over-the-counter drugs, herbal and alternative medicines.

• Family history of liver disease or multi-organ pathology such as alcohol, diabetes (haemochromatosis) or emphysema (α_1-antitrypsin deficiency).

• Other illnesses.

Examination

For signs of chronic liver disease, although these are rarely found. Record the patient's weight and body mass index (see p. 56).

Investigations

Blood tests

LFTs usually show an isolated rise in AST or ALT—a **hepatitic** pattern, rather than a predominant rise in alkaline phosphatase that indicates a 'cholestatic' pattern. Random ethanol levels may help diagnose occult alcoholic liver disease (and this may also be suggested by increased γ-glutamyl transferase [γGT] levels, **erythrocyte mean** red cell volume [MCV]). **Other** routine tests include:

- **Viral serology**: hepatitis A does not cause persistently abnormal LFTs, though hepatitis B and C can.
- **Autoantibodies and immunoglobulins**: primary biliary cirrhosis may present with non-specific malaise and pruritus. Anti-mitochondrial antibodies (anti-M2) will be present in 95% and will often be accompanied by an elevated IgM. Autoimmune hepatitis is usually accompanied by auto-antibodies to ds-DNA, smooth muscle, soluble liver antigen, liver cytosol and liver-kidney microsomes. The IgG and IgA are usually elevated. Sclerosing cholangitis is associated with atypical ANCA.
- **Iron studies to detect haemochromatosis**: the early identification of this common inborn error of metabolism is very important (see p. 237).
- **α_1-Antitrypsin (α_1-AT) levels**: the relationship between α_1-AT deficiency and liver disease is very complex but patients **should be counselled against smoking**.
- **Fasting glucose**: diabetes can cause abnormal LFTs, as can obesity and, paradoxically, starvation.

- **Depressed albumin or prolonged prothrombin** indicates **impaired liver function**.
- **The lipid profile** is often deranged in significant chronic liver disease and should be measured.

Liver ultrasonography

This is mandatory to exclude focal liver abnormality, such as malignancy, and may occasionally identify features suggesting chronic liver disease (e.g. splenomegaly, ascites, intra-abdominal varices).

Liver biopsy

Liver biopsy remains the definitive way of determining prognosis (i.e. the presence of fibrosis), even if a formal diagnosis is not possible.

Management

Management depends on the underlying pathology. Often the need is for qualified reassurance and an opinion about prognosis.

Table 112.1 Non-alcoholic steatosis—common cause of abnormal liver function tests.

	Non-alcoholic fatty liver disease (NAFLD)	Non-alcoholic steato-hepatitis (NASH)	Cirrhosis, due to NASH
Epidemiology	• Also known as simple steatosis • Affects 10–25% of the population • Found in 70% of obese subjects • Increasing rates in older subjects	• May affect 2–3% of USA population • Found in 25% of those undergoing anti-obesity surgery • 40% overweight/obese • 20% diabetic • 20% dyslipidaemic • 50% men	• Occurs in a variable number with NASH—± 3% at 10 years with simple steatosis or non-specific inflammation on biopsy • Occurs in 25–30% at 8–10 years in those with NASH and hepatocyte necrosis on biopsy • 80% of those developing cirrhosis have fibrosis on preceding biopsy for NASH
Clinical features	• Usually asymptomatic • Small proportion 'tired', upper abdominal discomfort	50% have persistent fatigue and/or upper abdominal discomfort	Features of chronic liver disease • Tired • Other features—see figure, p. 233
Cause	Relates to 'the metabolic syndrome' (insulin resistance)	Primary NASH: • Obesity; especially central pattern Secondary NASH: • Drugs, including amiodarone, methotrexate • Sudden weight loss (e.g. jejuno-ileal bypass surgery) or weight-cycling • Wilson's disease, lipodystrophy	• Genetic factors may promote progression from NASH to cirrhosis • Cytokines, and reactive oxygen species may also promote cirrhosis
Laboratory data	Biochemistry usually normal	• ALT and AST raised. ALT/AST ratio > 1 (in EtOH-related disease ratio usually < 1) • TNFα may promote progression from simple steatosis to NASH • 20–50% have ↑ ferritin levels	• Features in common to other cirrhosis patients • Liver enzymes may be normal ↔ abnormal • ±↓ Albumin; ±↑ INR
Imaging	Ultrasound, CT and MRI can diagnose moderate-severe steatosis	Imaging cannot distinguish NAFLD from NASH	Liver often small, spleen large
Histology	Normal liver architecture + lipid accumulation in hepatocytes (lipids comprise 5–10% by weight)	• Steatosis + some inflammation ± fibrosis • BMI > 28, ALT > 2× normal, age > 50 years, triglycerides > 1.8, hypertension and diabetes predict fibrosis (confirmatory biopsy needed) • Biopsy shows liver inflammation + variable fibrosis	• Frank cirrhosis
Treatment	• Weight loss (must be gradual) • Exercise	• Control hyperglycaemia • Remove any contributor drugs • Possibly probiotics to reduce gut-derived cytokines, LPS. Possibly vitamin E, etc.	• Standard care for chronic liver disease • Accounts for 3% of liver transplants
Prognosis	Excellent—probably the same as age-matched controls	Reasonable—though some increase in mortality	• Poor. 15% of hepatoma's may relate to NASH or NASH-related cirrhosis

Diseases and Treatments at a Glance

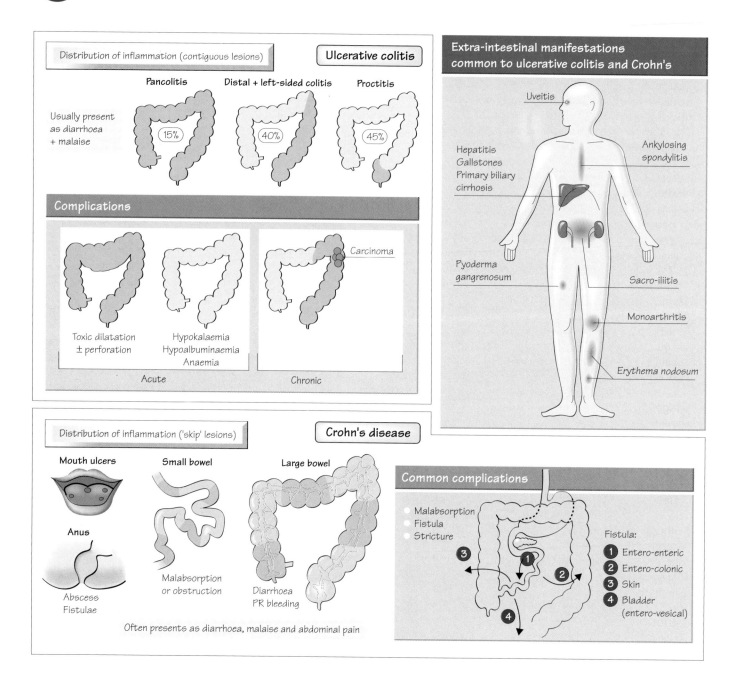

Ulcerative colitis

Distribution of inflammation (contiguous lesions)

Pancolitis Distal + left-sided colitis Proctitis

Usually present as diarrhoea + malaise

15% 40% 45%

Complications

Toxic dilatation ± perforation

Hypokalaemia Hypoalbuminaemia Anaemia

Carcinoma

Acute Chronic

Crohn's disease

Distribution of inflammation ('skip' lesions)

Mouth ulcers Small bowel Large bowel

Anus

Malabsorption or obstruction

Diarrhoea PR bleeding

Abscess Fistulae

Often presents as diarrhoea, malaise and abdominal pain

Extra-intestinal manifestations common to ulcerative colitis and Crohn's

Uveitis
Hepatitis
Gallstones
Primary biliary cirrhosis
Ankylosing spondylitis
Pyoderma gangrenosum
Sacro-iliitis
Monoarthritis
Erythema nodosum

Common complications

- Malabsorption
- Fistula
- Stricture

Fistula:
1. Entero-enteric
2. Entero-colonic
3. Skin
4. Bladder (entero-vesical)

Idiopathic inflammatory bowel disease (IBD) comprises ulcerative colitis (UC), Crohn's disease and a much rarer state of microscopic colitis. In some patients the distinction between these conditions may prove difficult and the term 'indeterminate colitis' may be used.

Ulcerative colitis

This is the most common form of IBD, affecting 80–160 per 100 000 of the population. It commonly presents in young adults. No unifying cause has been identified, although genetic factors play a major role with 15% of cases having a clear family history. Smoking appears to protect against UC for unknown reasons. Jewish people have two- to fourfold and white people have more than fourfold higher incidences.

Pathophysiology

The pathological hallmarks of ulcerative colitis are:
- Inflammation is always present in the rectum.
- This extends a variable distance proximally in the colon.
- The inflammation is continuous.
- Inflammation is limited to the mucosa of the bowel.

Clinical features

This depends largely on the extent of the inflammation.
- **Total colitis (pancolitis)** presents with chronic diarrhoea (> 6 weeks), sometimes with constitutional upset and objective biochemical markers of inflammation.

- **Distal ulcerative colitis** (**left-sided colitis, proctosigmoiditis, proctitis**) more often presents with rectal bleeding associated with urge and tenesmus. Constitutional disturbance is less frequent.

With either presentation there may be extra-intestinal manifestations of disease (arthralgia, iritis, skin lesions). Pain is an infrequent feature.

Investigations

The diagnosis is made on the basis of history, histology and imaging. It is crucial to recognize severe colitis early and treat vigorously. The Truelove–Witts criteria for severe colitis are: stool frequency > 6/day; T°C > 38°C; pulse > 90 beats/min, Hb < 10.5 g/dL; ESR > 30 mm/h.
- **Rectal biopsy** may differentiate a short-lived infective colitis (hallmarks of chronicity being distortion of colonic crypts and depletion of goblet cell stores of mucus).
- **Flexible sigmoidoscopy, colonoscopy** is used to delineate the disease extent. Longstanding total colitis is a risk for colonic carcinoma. Reassessment of extent of disease by colonoscopy is recommended 8–10 years from diagnosis. Surveillance colonoscopy with biopsies of the colon looking for dysplasia may be appropriate and should occur every 2 years initially. In some patients yearly surveillance may be necessary (those with coexistent primary sclerosing cholangitis and those with a disease history of over 20 years).
- **Abdominal X-ray**: in severe colitis a plain abdominal X-ray confirms the extent of disease (inflamed bowel being empty) and excludes 'toxic dilatation'—a life-threatening complication with a high risk of perforation, which **requires consideration of emergency surgery**.
- **Stool culture**: to exclude infective diarrhoea.

Management

- **Steroids**: severe acute colitis requires hospital admission and intravenous steroids. Less severe attacks require oral or topical steroids depending on disease extent.
- **Ciclosporin** may be of benefit for severe acute colitis that fails to respond to initial treatment.
- **5-Aminosalicylic acid (5-ASA) compounds** are effective in mild attacks and reduce the risk of subsequent episodes.
- **Azathioprine** is used in those experiencing frequent relapses.
- **Surgery**: the indications for surgery are a colon that is life threatening (i.e. perforation, cancer or severe dysplasia) or one that is incompatible with a reasonable quality of life (i.e. unacceptable symptoms despite maximal medical therapy).

Prognosis

After the first attack, 5% die < 1 year, 10% have continually active disease, 75% intermittently active disease and 10% a long-lasting (> 15 years) remission. There is a 20% risk of colon cancer after 30 years.

Crohn's disease

A chronic granulomatous inflammatory disease affecting the small and large bowel, characterized by 'skips' lesions (i.e. normal mucosa interspersed with areas of abnormal mucosa) and fistula formation, resulting in considerable ill health to sufferers. Unlike UC, Crohn's disease is characterized by deep ulceration, often resulting in strictures and fistulae.

Incidence

Uncommon. UK prevalence is 40–80 cases per 100 000 population.

Clinical features

The cardinal symptoms are: diarrhoea (80%), abdominal pain (50%),

weight loss (70%) and fever (40%). The presence of these depends on:
- **The site of disease**: small bowel disease is more likely to present with malabsorption and features of small bowel obstruction than colonic disease, which causes diarrhoea.
- **The extent and severity of inflammation** are easily underestimated in young adults—many patients present with pronounced fatigue, anorexia and poor general health.
- **Secondary complications**: such as abscess, stricture and fistulae.
- **Extra-intestinal manifestations** may be related to disease activity (e.g. aphthous ulceration, erythema nodosum, acute arthropathy, eye complications) or occur independently from disease flares (sacroiliitis, ankylosing spondylitis).

The **differential diagnosis** includes yersinia infection and intestinal tuberculosis.

Investigations

- **Systemic markers of inflammation**: the ESR and C-reactive protein are useful in making a diagnosis of Crohn's disease and in monitoring disease activity.
- **Barium contrast radiology**: small bowel Crohn's disease can be demonstrated on a small bowel enema or follow-through study. This gives important information about the extent of small bowel disease and the degree of intestinal obstruction.
- **Endoscopy**: allows for diagnostic biopsy. Colonoscopy with terminal ileoscopy is useful for delineating the extent and severity of colonic disease.
- **Capsule endoscopy**: may be of use in identifying subtle mucosal inflammation but the presence of intestinal strictures is a contra-indication (risk of capsule impaction).
- **Ultrasonography/computed tomography (CT) of abdomen**: useful for excluding abscess formation in sick patients with a palpable abdominal mass. Magnetic resonance imaging (MRI) is useful for the investigation of perianal and pelvic Crohn's disease.

Management and prognosis

Multi-disciplinary, involving physicians, surgeons and nutritionists.

Crohn's disease is an incurable illness, which follows a remitting/relapsing course, causes considerable morbidity and has a 15% mortality rate.
- **Steroids**: remain the most potent medical treatment. Other than in isolated distal colonic disease, these must be administered systemically (e.g. oral prednisolone or intravenous hydrocortisone), with the attendant long-term risks of adrenal suppression and osteopenia.
- **5-ASA compounds**, such as sulfasalazine and mesalazine, are used as maintenance treatment of colonic Crohn's disease.
- **Other immunosuppressive agents**: azathioprine and methotrexate are effective maintenance treatments and are used in those with frequent or severe relapses. Antibodies to TNFα have been licensed for treating steroid-resistant disease and perineal fistulae.
- **Surgery**: given the patchy and recurrent nature of Crohn's disease, surgery tends to be conservative and reserved for symptoms due to structural disease (i.e. strictures) not responding to medical therapy and other specific complications, e.g. abscesses and fistulae.
- **Nutrition**: nutritional support presents specific challenges, given the combination of the high metabolic demand of acute inflammation with small intestinal dysfunction. Liquid diets are very effective. An 'elemental diet' is a liquid diet in which the nitrogen source is in the form of amino acids. A 'polymeric diet' provides short peptides.

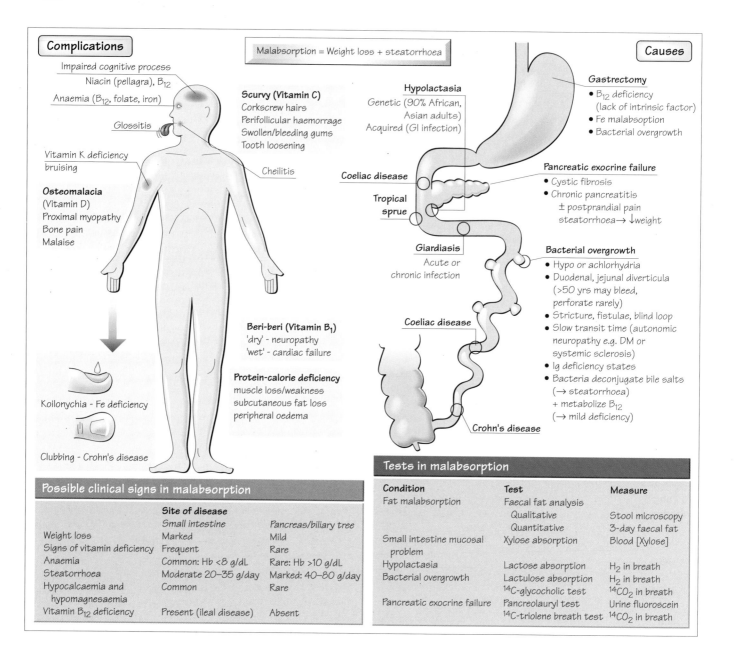

Malabsorption = Weight loss + steatorrhoea

Complications

Impaired cognitive process
Niacin (pellagra), B_{12}
Anaemia (B_{12}, folate, iron)
Glossitis
Vitamin K deficiency bruising

Osteomalacia (Vitamin D)
Proximal myopathy
Bone pain
Malaise

Koilonychia - Fe deficiency

Clubbing - Crohn's disease

Scurvy (Vitamin C)
Corkscrew hairs
Perifollicular haemorrage
Swollen/bleeding gums
Tooth loosening

Cheilitis

Beri-beri (Vitamin B_1)
'dry' - neuropathy
'wet' - cardiac failure

Protein-calorie deficiency
muscle loss/weakness
subcutaneous fat loss
peripheral oedema

Hypolactasia
Genetic (90% African, Asian adults)
Acquired (GI infection)

Coeliac disease
Tropical sprue

Giardiasis
Acute or chronic infection

Coeliac disease

Crohn's disease

Causes

Gastrectomy
• B_{12} deficiency (lack of intrinsic factor)
• Fe malabsoption
• Bacterial overgrowth

Pancreatic exocrine failure
• Cystic fibrosis
• Chronic pancreatitis ± postprandial pain steatorrhoea→ ↓weight

Bacterial overgrowth
• Hypo or achlorhydria
• Duodenal, jejunal diverticula (>50 yrs may bleed, perforate rarely)
• Stricture, fistulae, blind loop
• Slow transit time (autonomic neuropathy e.g. DM or systemic sclerosis)
• Ig deficiency states
• Bacteria deconjugate bile salts (→ steatorrhoea) + metabolize B_{12} (→ mild deficiency)

Possible clinical signs in malabsorption

	Site of disease	
	Small intestine	Pancreas/biliary tree
Weight loss	Marked	Mild
Signs of vitamin deficiency	Frequent	Rare
Anaemia	Common: Hb <8 g/dL	Rare: Hb >10 g/dL
Steatorrhoea	Moderate 20–35 g/day	Marked: 40–80 g/day
Hypocalcaemia and hypomagnesaemia	Common	Rare
Vitamin B_{12} deficiency	Present (ileal disease)	Absent

Tests in malabsorption

Condition	Test	Measure
Fat malabsorption	Faecal fat analysis	
	Qualitative	Stool microscopy
	Quantitative	3-day faecal fat
Small intestine mucosal problem	Xylose absorption	Blood [Xylose]
Hypolactasia	Lactose absorption	H_2 in breath
Bacterial overgrowth	Lactulose absorption	H_2 in breath
	^{14}C-glycocholic test	$^{14}CO_2$ in breath
Pancreatic exocrine failure	Pancreolauryl test	Urine fluoroscein
	^{14}C-triolene breath test	$^{14}CO_2$ in breath

Malabsorption is suggested by the combination of chronic diarrhoea and weight loss despite preservation of appetite (see p. 30). Thyrotoxicosis can also cause these symptoms. The **causes of malabsorption** include:
• **Common**: coeliac disease, pancreatic exocrine insufficiency and Crohn's disease
• **Uncommon**: hypolactasia, small bowel bacterial overgrowth, giardiasis and HIV
• **Rare**: tropical sprue, Whipple's disease and amyloidosis

Clinical features (see figure)

Most patients describe weight loss, general fatigue and diarrhoea, often steatorrhoea (pale offensive stools that float in the toilet pan and require two or more flushes of the toilet). In malabsorption caused by pan-creatic exocrine failure, a history of excess alcohol or **previous acute pancreatitis** may be found. In malabsorption relating to gastrointestinal (GI) infection, a travel history may be relevant.

In the physical examination look specifically for:
• Objective evidence of weight loss.
• Markers of malnutrition: leukonychia, glossitis, cheilitis, anaemia (folate, vitamin B_{12}, protein).
• Markers of specific nutritional deficiencies: scurvy (vitamin C), koilonychia (iron), osteomalacia (vitamin D and calcium), bruising (vitamin K).
• Clinical features of thyrotoxicosis: tremor, tachycardia, exophthalmos.
• Lymphadenopathy: Virchow's node—representing intra-abdominal malignancy.

Abdominal examination: a mass may be palpable in ileal Crohn's disease. The stool on rectal examination often appears pale and smells offensively. It may also be 'oily'.

Investigations

Investigations should objectively evaluate the effects of malnutrition and seek to identify the underlying disease.
- **Blood tests**:
  - Determine the severity of malnutrition (full blood count, liver function tests, albumin, international normalized ratio [INR], calcium, magnesium, zinc, vitamin B_{12}, folate).
  - Exclude certain conditions (thyroxine, thyroid-stimulating hormone, EMA for coeliac disease/TTG).
  - Raise the possibility of certain diseases (erythrocyte sedimentation rate (ESR)/C-reactive protein in Crohn's disease)
- **Endoscopy and duodenal biopsies** are used to exclude coeliac disease.
- **Small bowel imaging** is used when non-coeliac small bowel mucosal disease is suspected. The two principal tests are small bowel enema and enteroscopy.
- **Testing of stool** for the presence of undigested faecal fat is rarely performed now.
- **Tests of small bowel function**:
  - **Hydrogen breath tests**: H_2 appears in the breath when lactose (hypolactasia) or lactulose (small bowel overgrowth) are given.
  - **^{14}C-labelled triolene breath test** measures the ability of the small bowel to absorb fat. Triolene is not absorbed in pancreatic exocrine failure. This test is rarely used.
- **Pancreatic imaging**: pancreatic ultrasonography, computed tomography and endoscopic retrograde cholangiopancreatography are indicated when chronic pancreatitis is suspected to underlie pancreatic exocrine failure. There is an increasing role for magnetic resonance imaging.
- **Tests of pancreatic function**:
  - **Pancreolauryl test**: fluorescein dilaurate is ingested, and if pancreatic exocrine enzymes are present, fluorescein is split off, absorbed and passed into the urine, where it can be detected.
  - **Faecal elastase**: pancreatic elastase is not found in the stool in moderate–severe pancreatic exocrine failure.

Management

- **Treat underlying cause**: see relevant sections.
- **Dietary advice and supplementation** vitamin and nutrient replacement may be indicated (folate, vitamin B_{12}, iron).
- **Think about the bones**: osteopenia is a significant long-term problem in malabsorption (see p. 394).

Diseases causing malabsorption

Coeliac disease

Coeliac disease (gluten-sensitive enteropathy) is the most common cause of malabsorption in the West. It is common, especially in northwest Europe. The prevalence in west Ireland is 1 : 150, in England 1 : 300. The incidence is increasing, although better diagnostic tests may contribute to this. The peak incidence is 20–40 years, although it can present at any age.

Coeliac disease is the result of an allergic reaction to the gliaden fraction of wheat germ. Initially this causes an increase in the intraepithelial lymphocytes in the small intestinal epithelium. This subsequently progresses to flattening of the intestinal villi (villous atrophy). There are strong HLA (human leukocyte antigen) associations.

Clinical features
- **Iron deficiency**: the diagnosis is often made during investigation of iron deficiency.
- **Malabsorption**: coeliac disease now rarely presents with classic sprue (diarrhoea, weight loss, oedema).
- **Case finding**: although there is no mandate for screening for coeliac disease, the increasing recognition of a strong genetic component has led to a lowered threshold for making the diagnosis in first-degree relatives of affected individuals.
- **Dermatitis herpetiformis**: this rare but characteristic blistering eruption may lead to the diagnosis of coeliac disease.

Investigations
- **Endoscopy and distal duodenal biopsy**: traditionally, this is repeated after a period on a gluten-free diet.
- **Antibodies**: IgA class endomysial antibodies or tissue transglutaminase antibodies are highly sensitive and specific for coeliac disease. IgA deficiency is a risk factor for development of coeliac disease: under these circumstances the normal IgA class antibodies will be undetectable, but IgG-class antibodies may be found.
- **Bone densitometry**: even in the absence of significant weight loss, bone density may be significantly reduced at the time of presentation.

Management and prognosis
- **Gluten-free diet** completely reverses the histological and nutritional changes.
- **Vitamin and iron replacement** with iron, folate and vitamin B_{12} are needed in malabsorption.
- **Osteopenia**: with effective treatments for osteopenia now available, this important feature should be prospectively monitored and treated.
- **Small intestinal cancers** (enteropathy-associated T-cell lymphoma and adenocarcinoma): these are rare complications for which no surveillance is possible. They are important to consider in refractory disease or individuals who relapse clinically.

Other causes of malabsorption

- **Small bowel bacterial overgrowth** results from either structural or functional disorders which cause relative stasis (e.g. hypo- or achlorhydria, jejunal diverticulosis, post-surgical blind loops, intestinal strictures, autonomic neuropathy, scleroderma). Diagnosis is confirmed with a lactulose breath test or empirical treatment with antibiotics. Small bowel imaging for structural lesions is usually unnecessary. Treatment is with antibiotics (metronidazole and tetracyline), which may need to be repeated.
- **Giardiasis**: persistent infection with *Giardia lamblia* may cause diarrhoea and malabsorption.
- **Hypolactasia**: loss of lactase from the small intestinal brush border may be primary or secondary following a gastrointestinal infection. This results in milk intolerance, which causes bloating, nausea, wind and diarrhoea. The diagnosis is confirmed by a lactose breath test. Treatment is with a low-lactose diet.
- **Other diseases**: including pancreatic exocrine failure, Crohn's disease (see p. 222).

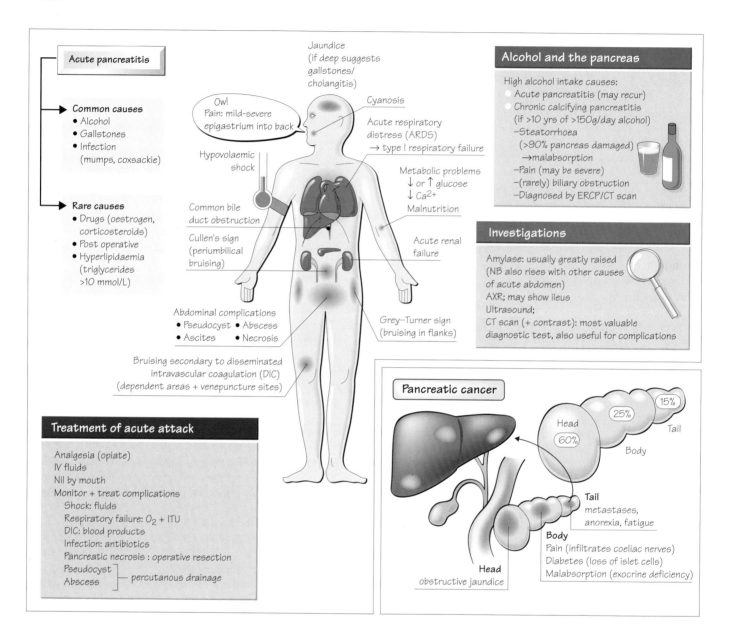

Acute pancreatitis

Common causes
- Alcohol
- Gallstones
- Infection (mumps, coxsackie)

Rare causes
- Drugs (oestrogen, corticosteroids)
- Post operative
- Hyperlipidaemia (triglycerides >10 mmol/L)

Jaundice
(if deep suggests gallstones/ cholangitis)

Cyanosis

Ow! Pain: mild–severe epigastrium into back

Acute respiratory distress (ARDS)
→ type I respiratory failure

Hypovolaemic shock

Metabolic problems
↓ or ↑ glucose
↓ Ca2+
Malnutrition

Common bile duct obstruction

Cullen's sign (periumbilical bruising)

Acute renal failure

Abdominal complications
- Pseudocyst
- Abscess
- Ascites
- Necrosis

Grey–Turner sign (bruising in flanks)

Bruising secondary to disseminated intravascular coagulation (DIC) (dependent areas + venepuncture sites)

Alcohol and the pancreas

High alcohol intake causes:
- Acute pancreatitis (may recur)
- Chronic calcifying pancreatitis (if >10 yrs of >150g/day alcohol)
  - Steatorrhoea (>90% pancreas damaged) →malabsorption
  - Pain (may be severe)
  - (rarely) biliary obstruction
  - Diagnosed by ERCP/CT scan

Investigations

Amylase: usually greatly raised (NB also rises with other causes of acute abdomen)
AXR; may show ileus
Ultrasound;
CT scan (+ contrast): most valuable diagnostic test, also useful for complications

Treatment of acute attack

Analgesia (opiate)
IV fluids
Nil by mouth
Monitor + treat complications
  Shock: fluids
  Respiratory failure: O₂ + ITU
  DIC: blood products
  Infection: antibiotics
  Pancreatic necrosis : operative resection
  Pseudocyst ⎤
  Abscess ⎦— percutanous drainage

Pancreatic cancer

15% Tail

25%

Head 60%

Body

Tail metastases, anorexia, fatigue

Body
Pain (infiltrates coeliac nerves)
Diabetes (loss of islet cells)
Malabsorption (exocrine deficiency)

Head
obstructive jaundice

Acute pancreatitis

Acute pancreatitis results from a sudden onset of pancreatic inflammation associated with varying degrees of 'auto-digestion'. The incidence in the UK is currently 20 per 100 000 population with a 43% increase in the last decade, probably as a result of increased alcohol consumption nationally.

Pathophysiology

The common causes of acute pancreatitis are: 1) Gallstones 30–50% 2) Alcohol 10–40% 3) Idiopathic 15% 4) Rarer (but important other) causes include trauma (endoscopic retrograde cholangiopancreatography [ERCP], postoperative, blunt trauma), 5% drugs (including loop diuretics), pancreas divisum, hypertrigly-ceridaemia, viral (mumps, Coxsackie virus).

Once the process has started there is a variable degree of pancreatic necrosis, in part related to proteolytic autodigestion of the gland.

Clinical features

- **Abdominal pain**: characteristically sudden onset (< 30 min) epigastric, radiating through to the back.
- **Hypovolaemia/Shock**: the degree of circulating volume depletion may be underestimated and contribute significantly to the associated renal failure.
- **Vomiting**, which contributes to hypovolaemia.
- **Jaundice**: suggests the presence of an associated cholangitis.

Various scoring systems are used to grade the severity of pancreatitis (Ranson, Glasgow, APACHE II). In general prognosis is determined more by markers of shock (acidaemia, hypoxia, etc.) than by the level

Table 115.1 Markers of severe pancreatitis (most reliable when used at 48 h after the onset of pain; > 3 = severe disease).

Assessment of severity of pancreatitis	
White cell count	$> 15 \times 10^9$/L
Urea	> 16 mmol/L
Calcium	< 2.0 mmol/L
Albumin	< 32 g/L
Glucose	> 10 mmol/L
P_{O_2}	< 8 kPa
AST	> 200 IU/L
LDH	> 600 IU/L
CRP	> 150 mg/L

of serum amylase recorded on admission. Mortality rate varies from 2% in mild attacks to > 50% in severe disease.

Investigations (see figure and Table 115.1)

Management and prognosis

The key to managing pancreatitis is restoration of euvolaemia and, once stable, determination and treatment of the underlying cause:
- **Resuscitation**: intravenous fluids, central venous pressure (CVP) monitoring and oxygen. The routine use of broad-spectrum antibiotics is unproven.
- **Treat underlying cause**: clinical features of cholangitis raise the possibility of a gallstone impacted at the ampulla and is an indication to consider early ERCP. If gallstones are confirmed to be the underlying cause of the pancreatitis, early cholecystectomy is recommended.

Complications

Mild cases of pancreatitis usually resolve without complications; the more severe the acute attack, the more likely are complications:
- **Pancreatic pseudocyst/abscess**: suggested by persistent pain and/or fever, diagnosed by CT, and often drained percutaneously.
- **Adult respiratory distress syndrome**.
- **Portal vein/mesenteric thrombosis**.

Chronic pancreatitis

Chronic pancreatitis may result as a consequence of repeated attacks of acute pancreatitis Some patients present with clinical features of pancreatic insufficiency in the absence of pain. The prevalence is 40–75 per 100 000 and the incidence 8/100 000.

Pathophysiology
- Recurrent acute pancreatitis.
- Alcohol: the most common cause in the UK.
- Idiopathic: accounts for 20% of cases.

Clinical features

The cardinal features of chronic pancreatitis are:
- **Pain**: in 85%, typical pancreatic pain is epigastric radiating through to the back, often precipitated by eating. The severity is very variable.
- **Exocrine pancreatic insufficiency**: produces steatorrhoea and weight loss.
- **Endocrine pancreatic insufficiency (i.e. diabetes)**: in 30%.

There are often no abnormal physical signs, despite dramatic symptoms.

Investigations

Pancreatic enzymes raised in attacks of acute pancreatitis are normal in chronic disease.
- **Faecal elastase (or chymotrypsin)** has now largely replaced tests quantifying faecal fat. Tests of exocrine pancreatic function (e.g. pancreolauryl test) may still be useful in difficult cases, although more often than not a clinical response to pancreatic enzyme replacement is sufficient.
- **Abdominal CT**: **may** show pancreatic calcification and small pseudocysts. It might also be used to identify pancreatic masses (i.e. tumour).
- **MRCP** (or **less commonly** ERCP): demonstrates pancreatic duct irregularity and pseudocystic change.

Management and prognosis

Pancreatic enzyme replacement with preparations such as Creon and Pancrex often improves both the pain and the malabsorption of chronic pancreatitis. The diabetes associated with chronic pancreatitis frequently requires insulin therapy. Opioid analgesia is frequently needed where pancreatic pain is dominant: a coeliac axis block may be necessary in selected cases.

Pancreatic cancer

Cancer of the pancreas remains a major source of mortality in the developed world. The incidence is increasing, and is now 11 per 100 000. The disease is more common in men (1.3 : 1) and African–Caribbean people (50% higher). Smoking and a high fat/meat diet are risk factors. Most primary malignant tumours of the pancreas are adenocarcinoma although neuroendocrine tumours are not uncommon.

Clinical features

Pancreatic cancer is notorious for producing few or non-specific signs in the early stages. Painless jaundice caused by biliary obstruction is the most common presentation as the commonest location for pancreatic tumours is in the pancreatic head. Tumours in the body or tail of the gland will present with weight loss and abdominal pain.

Investigations
- **Abdominal CT**: is presently the best first-line investigation in patients where pancreatic cancer is suspected clinically. This is useful in establishing a diagnosis and may identify tumours that are potentially resectable (i.e. no invasion into important local structures or metastases).
- **MRCP** should now become the first-line investigation for painless obstructive jaundice.
- **ERCP** should be reserved until endoscopic therapy is expected/planned.

Management and prognosis

Too often carcinoma of the pancreas is advanced at the time of presentation and there is no possibility of cure. Overall 90% of individuals presenting with carcinoma of the pancreas will have succumbed to their disease within a year. Five-year survival is only 2%.
- **Surgery**: in some patients pancreatico-duodenectomy (Whipple's procedure) offers the possibility of a surgical cure. Surgery may also be beneficial in patients with advanced disease in providing combined biliary and gastroduodenal bypass.
- **Palliative measures**: stenting of biliary obstruction by either ERCP or PTC may relieve jaundice. Pancreatic pain may require opioid analgesia. Palliative chemotherapy with gemcitabine may slow the progression of the disease. Anorexia and weight loss remain major problems.

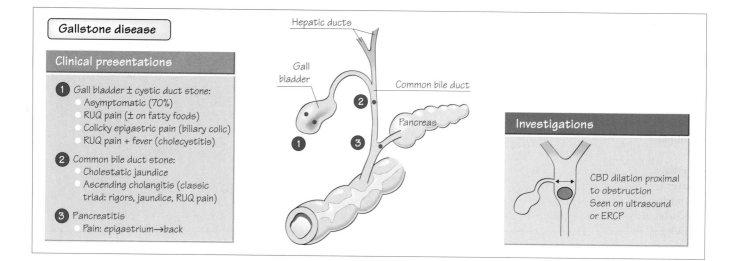

Gallstone disease

Clinical presentations

1. Gall bladder ± cystic duct stone:
   - Asymptomatic (70%)
   - RUQ pain (± on fatty foods)
   - Colicky epigastric pain (biliary colic)
   - RUQ pain + fever (cholecystitis)
2. Common bile duct stone:
   - Cholestatic jaundice
   - Ascending cholangitis (classic triad: rigors, jaundice, RUQ pain)
3. Pancreatitis
   - Pain: epigastrium→back

Hepatic ducts
Gall bladder
Common bile duct
Pancreas

Investigations
CBD dilation proximal to obstruction
Seen on ultrasound or ERCP

Gallstone disease

The prevalence of gallstones is underestimated, because around 90% remain asymptomatic. Stones occur in 7% of men and 15% of women aged 18–65 years. There is a 3 : 1 female predominance in those aged < 40 years, which disappears in elderly people.

Pathophysiology

Gallstone formation results from precipitation of cholesterol crystals in supersaturated bile. Ultimately stones form that contain a combination of calcium salts; they increase in size at a rate of 2.5 mm/year. Less commonly, pigment stones occur from chronic haemolysis (see p. 320).

Clinical features

- **Asymptomatic**: gallstones may be an incidental finding.
- **Biliary colic**: recurrent right upper quadrant (RUQ) pain, often precipitated by fatty food.
- **Cholecystitis** typically presents with acute right hypochondral pain and fever. If the neck of the gall bladder becomes obstructed, an empyema of the gall bladder (with a 20–30% mortality rate) may occur.
- **Cholestatic jaundice**: jaundice with pale stools and dark urine indicates biliary obstruction as a result of the migration of a stone into the common bile duct (choledocolithiasis). With clinical evidence of superadded infection (fever, rigors), this is known as cholangitis.
- **Pancreatitis**: gallstones are a major cause of pancreatitis in the developed world, usually caused by migration of stones down the comon bile duct and through the ampulla of Vater.
- **Carcinoma of the gall bladder** is rare and in 90% occurs in association with gallstones. Extensive gall bladder calcification ('porcelain gall bladder') is a particularly powerful risk factor.
- Rare presentations and complications include **biliary peritonitis**, resulting from perforation (30% mortality) and **small bowel obstruction** (gallstone ileus) caused by a large gallstone being held up at the ileo-caecal valve.

Investigations

Only 20% of gallstones are visible on plain X-rays.

- **Transabdominal ultrasonography** is most commonly used to identify gallstones. Bile duct dilatation (intra-hepatic or extra-hepatic) raises the possibility of common bile duct (CBD) stones although transabdominal ultrasonography can rarely prove or exclude this (30–40% of patients with stones in the CBD have 'normal' ultrasound scans). Endoscopic ultrasonography has greater sensitivity but is more invasive and less widely available.
- **Liver transaminases** should be checked in any patient considered for cholecystectomy. If these are abnormal, endoscopic retrograde cholangiopancreatography (ERCP) should be considered before surgery, because they may reflect stones in the common bile duct.
- **Magnetic resonance cholangiopancreatography (MRCP)**: with improvement in magnetic resonance imaging, this is becoming widely available as an alternative to ERCP for demonstration of stones in the biliary tree.
- **Endoscopic ultrasound** is an alternative if stones in the common bile duct are clinically suspected.
- **Endoscopic retrograde cholangiography (ERCP)** provides simultaneous imaging of the biliary tree and the opportunity to relieve biliary obstruction by endoscopic sphincterotomy and removal of CBD stones.
- **Percutaneous transhepatic cholangiography (PTC)**: this is an alternative approach to achieving direct visualization of the biliary tree. The transhepatic approach is potentially more traumatic to the patient and is reserved for when ERCP is technically impossible.

Management and prognosis

- **Watchful waiting**: the incidental finding of gallstones requires no treatment.
- **ERCP**: this is both an investigation and treatment in patients with cholestatic jaundice in the presence of gallstones. For elderly or otherwise unwell patients, ERCP sphincterotomy may be sufficient because the risk of further problems is probably low.
- **Surgery**: in patients with symptomatic gallstones or after a significant complication, the definitive treatment is cholecystectomy.

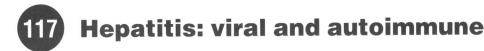

117 Hepatitis: viral and autoimmune

Viral hepatitis

Hepatitis A virus (HAV)

Common cause of transient hepatitis. Faeco-oral transmission.
- **Subclinical**: 50% of adults have IgG antibodies to HAV without previous jaundice.
- **Jaundice/acute hepatitis**: the most common presentation is an acute hepatitis, occasionally with a prolonged cholestatic phase. Fatigue, malaise, anorexia and nausea are prominent.
- **Fulminant liver failure**: very rarely.

Investigations
- **Liver blood tests** usually show an acute hepatocellular abnormality (i.e. predominant rise in aspartate transaminase (AST), with less marked rises in bilirubin and alkaline phosphatase).
- **HAV IgM serology** in high titre is diagnostic of acute infection.

Management and prognosis
Clinical hepatitis usually settles with symptomatic management and rarely requires hospital admission. Evidence of liver failure (i.e. encephalopathy, coagulopathy) requires referral to a transplant centre. No risk of chronic liver disease/cirrhosis.
- **Similar pathogens**: hepatitis E gives a similar clinical picture, although the risk of fulminant hepatic failure in pregnancy is particularly high. Cytomegalovirus (CMV) and Epstein–Barr virus (EBV) are rare causes of fulminant hepatitis.

Hepatitis B virus (HBV)

Worldwide HBV is the most common cause of chronic liver disease and hepatoma. In the UK, HBV is common among intravenous drug users and homosexuals. It is a parenterally transmitted hepatotrophic DNA virus. Genetic factors relating to the host immune response may account for the variability in clinical manifestations.

Clinical features
- **Acute hepatitis**: an acute jaundiced illness occurs in 15% of individuals exposed to HBV.
- **Fulminant liver failure** is rare with HBV but more likely in those co-infected with HCV, HIV or the δ agent.
- **Chronic liver disease**: 5% of adults exposed to HBV develop chronic infection, more so in immunocompromised individuals (50% or more) and in neonates (90%).
- **Hepatocellular carcinoma (HCC)** rates are increased tenfold in HBV carriers.

Investigations
- **Liver function tests**: show a non-specific hepatitic picture.
- **HBV serology**: see figure.
- **Other tests**: liver ultrasonography is needed if there is doubt about the biliary tree or the presence of other structural liver pathology. Liver biopsy is sometimes performed if there is a prominent cholestatic phase.

Management and prognosis
- **Prevention**: individuals at risk (e.g. health-care workers) should be immunized. Known virus carriers should know the risks to others of exposure to body fluids and should use barrier contraception.
- **General**: acute HBV infection rarely requires hospital admission. Follow-up is necessary to determine whether or not the virus has been cleared.
- **Antiviral therapy**: there is no helpful antiviral therapy during acute infection. Chronic infection may be clinically stable in many patients. Active hepatitis may require viral suppression with antiviral drugs (e.g. lamivudine, adefovir).
- **Screening for HCC**: regular surveillance with liver ultrasonography and α-fetoprotein measurement.
- **Liver transplantation**: indicated for decompensated cirrhosis and small unifocal hepatoma.

Hepatitis C virus (HCV)

Common. Accounts for 25% of the liver disease burden in the UK. One of the major causes of chronic liver disease and transplantation in the developed world. The RNA HCV virus is transmitted parenterally. It relies on a reverse transcriptase for replication, which has an inherently high error rate, resulting in high rates of viral mutation. This, among other features, means that the virus commonly escapes the immune response, and chronicity of viraemia is the consequence.

Clinical features
- **Acute hepatitis**: this occurs in only a small number of patients.
- **Asymptomatic carriage**: in the majority of cases the recipient is oblivious to the fact that they have acquired the virus, yet 85–90% of those exposed will develop chronic viraemia.
- **Chronic liver disease**: 20% of patients with chronic viraemia eventually develop liver fibrosis and clinical chronic liver disease. The rate of progression varies but the clinical course is accelerated by concurrent infection with HBV and excess of alcohol consumption.

Investigations
- **Liver blood tests**: show relatively modest elevation in transaminases. The degree of liver blood test derangement bears little relation to the degree of underlying liver fibrosis.
- **Tests for HCV** are by serological antibody tests. The virus is identified in blood by the polymerase chain reaction (PCR) and levels of viraemia can be quantified. Virus genotyping may determine the duration of antiviral therapy.
- **Liver biopsy** remains the only way to grade the disease in terms of necro-inflammatory change in the liver, and also to stage the condition by defining the degree of liver fibrosis.

Management and prognosis
- **Prevention**: public health measures and education are important. There is no vaccine available or likely.
- **Antiviral therapy** with sustained release (PEGylated) interferon-α with ribavirin is used in patients with HCV. Overall, antiviral therapy leads to a 60% sustained response (i.e. long-term viral clearance).
- **Liver transplantation**: transplantation remains an important mode of therapy for patients with end-stage chronic liver disease. Viral recurrence in the transplanted organ is common.

Autoimmune hepatitis

Rare. Acute autoimmune inflammation centred predominantly on the

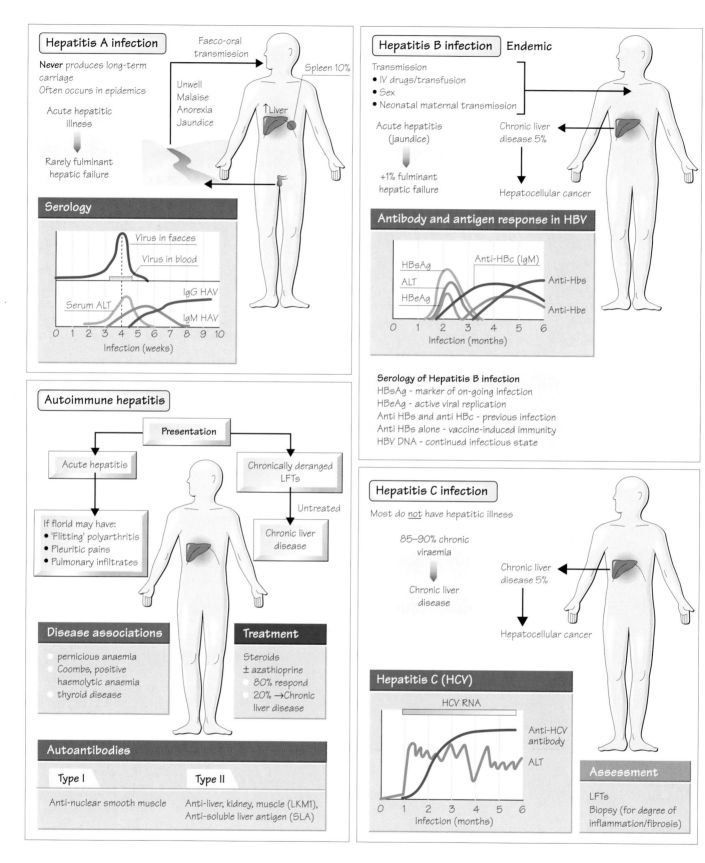

Hepatitis A infection

Never produces long-term carriage
Often occurs in epidemics

Acute hepatitic illness
↓
Rarely fulminant hepatic failure

Faeco-oral transmission

Unwell
Malaise
Anorexia
Jaundice

Spleen 10%

↑Liver

Serology

Virus in faeces
Virus in blood
IgG HAV
Serum ALT
IgM HAV

Infection (weeks)

Autoimmune hepatitis

Presentation

Acute hepatitis

Chronically deranged LFTs

Untreated

If florid may have:
• 'Flitting' polyarthritis
• Pleuritic pains
• Pulmonary infiltrates

Chronic liver disease

Disease associations

○ pernicious anaemia
○ Coombs, positive haemolytic anaemia
○ thyroid disease

Treatment

Steroids
± azathioprine
○ 80% respond
○ 20% →Chronic liver disease

Autoantibodies

Type I	Type II
Anti-nuclear smooth muscle	Anti-liver, kidney, muscle (LKM1), Anti-soluble liver antigen (SLA)

Hepatitis B infection   Endemic

Transmission
• IV drugs/transfusion
• Sex
• Neonatal maternal transmission

Acute hepatitis (jaundice)
↓
+1% fulminant hepatic failure

Chronic liver disease 5%
↓
Hepatocellular cancer

Antibody and antigen response in HBV

HBsAg
ALT
HBeAg
Anti-HBc (IgM)
Anti-Hbs
Anti-Hbe

Infection (months)

Serology of Hepatitis B infection
HBsAg - marker of on-going infection
HBeAg - active viral replication
Anti HBs and anti HBc - previous infection
Anti HBs alone - vaccine-induced immunity
HBV DNA - continued infectious state

Hepatitis C infection

Most do not have hepatitic illness

85–90% chronic viraemia
↓
Chronic liver disease

Chronic liver disease 5%
↓
Hepatocellular cancer

Hepatitis C (HCV)

HCV RNA
Anti-HCV antibody
ALT

Infection (months)

Assessment

LFTs
Biopsy (for degree of inflammation/fibrosis)

hepatic lobule, causing a range of clinical manifestations, ranging from fulminant hepatic failure to chronic liver disease and cirrhosis. Presentation is typically with:

• Jaundice
• Fatigue
• Arthralgia
• Associated autoimmune conditions.

Less commonly autoimmune hepatitis presents with a persistent abnormality of liver blood tests.

- **Liver blood tests** usually show a predominant hepatocellular derangement of transaminases. A high titre of antinuclear antibodies (ANAs) often with smooth muscle (antiactin) antibodies (SMAs) are found. In a few others, classified as having type II autoimmune hepatitis, autoantibodies may be demonstrable (e.g. liver/kidney microsomal antibody—LKM-1; soluble liver antigen—SLA). IgG is usually high.
- **Viral serology** must, given the usual acute presentation, be tested.
- **Liver biopsy** shows an acute lobular inflammation with interface hepatitis and may demonstrate features of chronicity (i.e. fibrosis).

Management and prognosis

- **Immunosuppression**: acute autoimmune hepatitis is very sensitive to high-dose steroids. Longer-term control often requires azathioprine.
- **Liver transplantation**: for fulminant liver failure and decompensated chronic liver disease.

Primary biliary cirrhosis (PBC)

Rare (prevalence 90–150 per million), disease of mid-life women (male : female ratio 1 : 9). The pathology is of a non-suppurative granulomatous inflammation centred predominantly on the small interlobular bile ducts, resulting in progressive fibrosis and ultimately cirrhosis. The cause is unknown, but PBC may be triggered by a bacteria (?E. Coli) in those genetically predisposed.

Clinical features

The typical symptomatic presentation is of **chronic progressive cholestasis** with pruritis, lethargy and fatigue, progressing to steatorrhoea, and possibly with fat soluble vitamin deficiency (A, D and K) syndromes. Some patients present with established **chronic liver disease** without prior symptomatic cholestasis. Increasingly **asymptomatic** individuals are identified by abnormal liver blood tests with a positive mitochondrial antibody. Associated autoimmune conditions: rheumatoid disease; autoimmune thyroid disease; coeliac disease.

Investigations

- **Liver blood tests** demonstrate a cholestatic picture (raised alkaline phosphatase with features of chronic liver disease in the advanced stages (i.e. low albumin). Elevated (sometimes massively) levels of alkaline phosphatase may be the only abnormality on 'simple' blood tests. The antimitochondrial antibody and the M2 antibody directed at the 2-oxoacid dehydrogenase (E2) complex of the inner mitochondrial membrane are specific **autoantibodies**, and are found in 95% of patients with PBC. Antibodies against the mitochondrial m4/m8 complex may occur in those with more aggressive disease. IgM is often raised.
- **Liver imaging** (ultrasonography, should be considered if extra-hepatic biliary disease needs to be excluded (gallstones, primary sclerosing cholangitis [PSC]).
- **Liver biopsy** shows features of PBC and fibrosis, the extent of which has prognostic value.

Management and prognosis

Primary biliary cirrhosis progresses slowly, ultimately resulting in cirrhosis. Treatment of pruritis and fatigue is disappointing, although ursodeoxycholic acid may help. Chronic cholestasis increases the risk of osteopenia (see p. 394). **Liver transplantation** is excellent for persistent jaundice and decompensated chronic liver disease.

Primary sclerosing cholangitis

Primary sclerosing cholangitis is an uncommon, complex, probably autoimmune disorder, strongly associated with inflammatory bowel disease. The pattern varies considerably. Inflammation may predominantly involve the intralobular bile ducts—**intra-hepatic (small duct) PSC**—or the extra-hepatic biliary strictures—**extra-hepatic (large duct) PSC**. Many patients have both small and large duct disease.

Clinical features

- **Abnormal liver function tests** are the most common presentation, (especially increased alkaline phosphatase). Positive ANCA occurs in 80%; antimitochondrial antibodies are not found.
- **Recurrent bacterial cholangitis** with RUQ pain, fever and jaundice may occur in those with dominant extra-hepatic disease.
- **Chronic cholestasis and chronic liver disease** are common.
- **Inflammatory bowel disease** may be diagnosed after PSC.

Investigations

- **Liver function tests** often demonstrate a mixed pattern of 'hepatitic' and 'cholestatic' abnormalities.
- **Tumour marker** CA19–9 may indicate cholangiocarcinoma.
- **Anti-neutrophil cytoplasmic antibody**
- **Liver ultrasonography** to exclude focal liver lesions (i.e. cholangiocarcinoma).
- **MRCP or ERCP** may demonstrate multiple biliary strictures. Dominant strictures should be brushed and bile aspirated for cytology.
- **Liver biopsy** demonstrates features consistent with PSC—the onion-skin lesion around an obliterated bile duct.

Management and prognosis

The clinical course varies considerably and unpredictably. Symptomatic patients are largely dead in 10–15 years, though some 75% of asymptomatic patients are alive after 15 years. Bacterial cholangitis requires antibiotics. Pruritis may improve with ursodeoxycholic acid. There is no specific therapy. **Liver transplantation** is used for those with a rapidly progressive clinical course and decompensated chronic liver disease. **Cholangiocarcinoma** risk is increased and has a very poor prognosis.

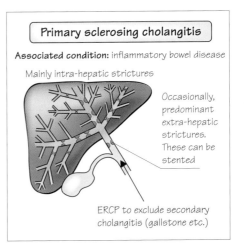

Primary sclerosing cholangitis

Associated condition: inflammatory bowel disease

Mainly intra-hepatic strictures

Occasionally, predominant extra-hepatic strictures. These can be stented

ERCP to exclude secondary cholangitis (gallstone etc.)

Pathological features of hepatitis and cirrhosis

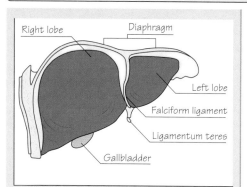

Normal liver: the normal liver is one of the largest organs in the body. It has a key role in producing vital proteins, and detoxifying externally ingested and internally produced toxins

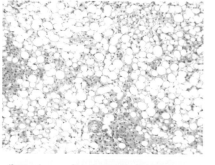

Fatty change of the liver: this slide shows extensive fatty change, now called steatosis (when there is no evidence of inflammation) and steatohepatitis (when there is evidence of inflammation)

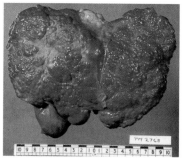

Macronodular cirrhosis; it is reputed that viral infection of the liver results in a macronodular form of cirrhosis (as does Wilson's disease, and α1-antitrypsin deficiency), whereas alcohol leads to a micronodular form

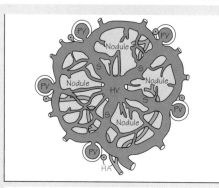

Cirrhosis of the liver showing the formation of portal venous (PV)/hepatic venous (HV) anastomoses or internal Eck fistulae at the site of pre-existing sinusoids (S). Note that the regeneration nodules are supplied by the hepatic artery (HA)

High power appearance of liver in acute alcoholic hepatitis; within this slide can be seen areas of (purplish-red) hyaline within the hepatocytes. These finding, called Mallory's hyaline, are believed to indicate the presence of alcohol abuse

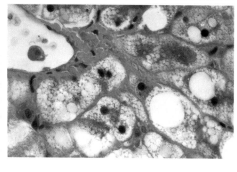

Cardiac cirrhosis: this occurs when the right side of the heart has been failing for a long time. Fibrosis, extending from central vein to central vein isolating nodules of liver cells is seen. Chronic heart failure is the commonest cause of this, and may explain some chronic ill health in heart failure

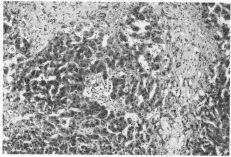

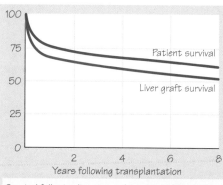

Survival following liver transplantation: this graph shows the survival of the patient, and the liver graft, following liver transplantation. Patients who survived without their graft were retransplanted. Adverse factors for survival were transplantation for cancer, donor age > 55 years, recipient age > 15 years and transplantation for acute liver failure

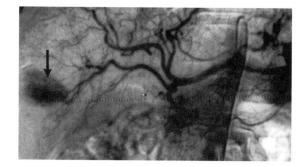

Hepatocellular carcinoma; selective hepatic arterial angiography confirms tumour in right lobe (arrow)

All pictures from *Diseases of the Liver and Biliary System*, 11th edition, by Sheila Sherlock and James Dooley, Blackwell Publishing, 2001, except graph showing survival following liver transplantation

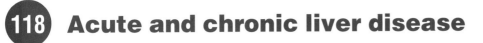

118 Acute and chronic liver disease

Acute hepatitis

This non-specific term refers to a short-term (self-limiting) liver inflammation. There are many causes (see figure). Jaundice, nausea and anorexia, right upper quadrant discomfort, fever and fatigue occur.

Investigations

• **Liver function test**: hepatitic enzymes aspartate transaminase (AST), alanine transaminase (ALT); cholestatic enzymes—alkaline phosphatase; synthetic function tests—prothrombin time, albumin.
• **Tests to determine the cause**: viral serology, immunoglobulins and autoantibody profile, copper.
• **Liver ultrasonography** to exclude structural lesions (e.g. neoplasia, biliary disease, etc.).

Management and prognosis

Stop all potentially harmful drugs. Prognosis is usually good.

Fulminant liver failure

The term fulminant liver failure traditionally describes the progression from normal liver function to liver failure, i.e. hepatic encephalopathy within 8 weeks.

Clinical features

• **Encephalopathy** is the clinical hallmark of liver failure, characterized by a progressive deterioration in cognitive function from a shortened attention span through a reversal of sleep pattern to deep coma. The characteristic clinical sign is the metabolic flap or asterixis.
• **Jaundice**: depending on the rate of deterioration, jaundice may not initially be clinically evident.
• **Haemorrhage** may be confined to the gastrointestinal (GI) tract or occur widely as a result of haemostatic failure.

Investigations

• **Prothrombin time** is the single best prognostic marker. Coagulopathy should not necessarily be corrected (with fresh frozen plasma FFP) unless bleeding is otherwise life threatening.
• **Blood glucose** should be measured frequently. Hypoglycaemia is an ominous sign.
• **Electrolytes**: renal impairment most commonly relates to a degree of acute tubular necrosis on admission, rather than reflecting a true hepatorenal syndrome.
• **Arterial blood gases**: metabolic acidosis is a poor sign.
• **Paracetamol level** should be measured in all cases and is the most common cause of fulminant liver failure in the UK; it is amenable to medical treatment (*N*-acetylcysteine).

Management and prognosis

• **Airway management**: patients can deteriorate quickly. Those with progressive coma should undergo early intubation and ventilation, especially if between-hospital transfer occurs.
• **Optimize circulatory state**: patients have a hyperdynamic circulation with lowered systemic vascular resistance. The degree of volume depletion on admission is often underestimated.
• ***N*-Acetylcysteine** is the antidote to paracetamol poisoning, although

Table 118.1 Indications for referral to a liver transplant unit in fulminant liver failure.

Paracetamol poisoning
pH < 7.3
INR > 6.5
Creatinine > 300 mmol/L

Other pathologies (viruses, drugs, etc.)
INR > 6.5

And any three of:
Aetiology being drug or non-A, non-B
Age < 10 years or > 40 years
Jaundice for 7 days before encephalopathy
Bilirubin > 300
INR > 3.5

INR, international normalized ratio.

increasing evidence suggests that it might benefit patients with fulminant liver failure from all causes.
• **Broad-spectrum antibiotics** and systemic antifungals.
• Indications for liver transplant unit referral and possible transplantation (Table 118.1).

Chronic liver disease

Much liver pathology follows an indolent course and presents with clinical features of **chronic liver disease**. Compensated chronic liver disease implies a (relatively) well patient, whereas those with decompensated chronic liver disease have substantial symptoms and/or signs.

Pathophysiology and clinical features

Long-term, low-grade liver damage results in progressive liver fibrosis, which results in a combination of reduced liver cell mass and portal hypertension. These cause the clinical features—the relative dominance of one over the other varies between patients:
• Weakness, anorexia, muscle and adipose tissue loss
• GI bleeding: from portosystemic venous anastomoses (i.e varices)
• Ascites: possibly complicated by spontaneous bacterial peritonitis
• Jaundice
• Encephalopathy.

Problems caused by reduced liver cell mass

• **Encephalopathy**: the hallmark of liver cell failure and a common albeit subtle feature of most patients with chronic liver disease, causing a reduced attention span and reversed sleep pattern (insomnia and daytime somnolence). A metabolic flap may be found. With more advanced encephalopathy patients demonstrate a constructional dyspraxia and ultimately progress to hepatic coma. Encephalopathy can be worsened by portosystemic shunting (which is sometimes used in treatment).
• **Loss of lean body mass** is usually most evident at the shoulders. The accumulation of body water (oedema and ascites) means that the extent of muscle loss is underestimated.
• **Coagulopathy**.

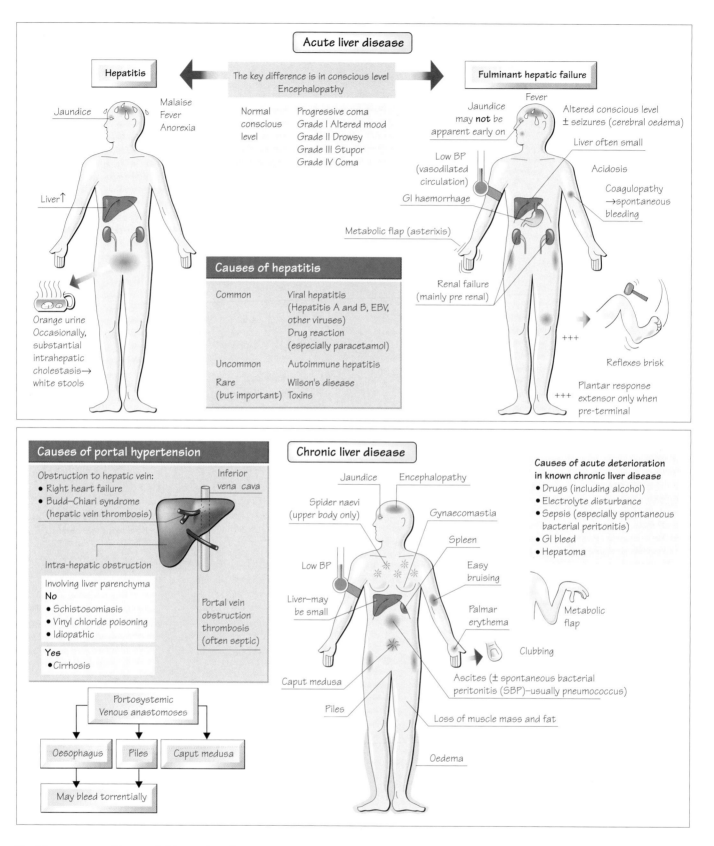

Acute liver disease

Hepatitis

Jaundice

Malaise
Fever
Anorexia

Liver↑

Orange urine
Occasionally,
substantial
intrahepatic
cholestasis→
white stools

The key difference is in conscious level
Encephalopathy

Normal conscious level	Progressive coma
	Grade I Altered mood
	Grade II Drowsy
	Grade III Stupor
	Grade IV Coma

Causes of hepatitis

Common	Viral hepatitis (Hepatitis A and B, EBV, other viruses)
	Drug reaction (especially paracetamol)
Uncommon	Autoimmune hepatitis
Rare (but important)	Wilson's disease Toxins

Fulminant hepatic failure

Fever

Jaundice may **not** be apparent early on

Altered conscious level ± seizures (cerebral oedema)

Liver often small

Acidosis

Coagulopathy →spontaneous bleeding

Low BP (vasodilated circulation)

GI haemorrhage

Metabolic flap (asterixis)

Renal failure (mainly pre renal)

+++

Reflexes brisk

Plantar response extensor only when pre-terminal

+++

Causes of portal hypertension

Obstruction to hepatic vein:
- Right heart failure
- Budd–Chiari syndrome (hepatic vein thrombosis)

Inferior vena cava

Intra-hepatic obstruction

Involving liver parenchyma
No
- Schistosomiasis
- Vinyl chloride poisoning
- Idiopathic

Yes
- Cirrhosis

Portal vein obstruction thrombosis (often septic)

Portosystemic Venous anastomoses

Oesophagus | Piles | Caput medusa

May bleed torrentially

Chronic liver disease

Jaundice | Encephalopathy

Spider naevi (upper body only)

Gynaecomastia

Spleen

Low BP

Easy bruising

Liver–may be small

Palmar erythema

Caput medusa

Piles

Ascites (± spontaneous bacterial peritonitis (SBP)–usually pneumococcus)

Loss of muscle mass and fat

Oedema

Causes of acute deterioration in known chronic liver disease
- Drugs (including alcohol)
- Electrolyte disturbance
- Sepsis (especially spontaneous bacterial peritonitis)
- GI bleed
- Hepatoma

Metabolic flap

Clubbing

Problems caused by portal hypertension

• **Varices**: form at sites of portosystemic communication, most commonly in the lower oesophagus. GI bleeding, sometimes torrential, may be the first presentation of chronic liver disease and can provoke decompensation of the chronic liver disease.

• **Ascites**: is the result of sodium retention, possibly contributed to by high portal pressure and low albumin. It is important to exclude spontaneous bacterial peritonitis (SBP), as this commonly complicates low protein ascites resulting from cirrhosis.

Investigations

These are directed to identify the cause of the underlying liver disease and to identify the triggers for decompensation (infection, bleeding, drugs, electrolyte disturbance, hepatoma):

• **Haematology**: haemoglobin may be low, as a result of bleeding and hypersplenism. The prothrombin time is prolonged, as a result of synthetic failure ± disseminated intravascular coagulation (DIC).

• **Autoimmune** profile/immunoglobulins.

• **Iron studies** (haemochromatosis) and **copper** studies (Wilson's disease).

• **Viral** serology (hepatitis B and C virus [HBV, HCV]).

Management

Identify and treat the cause of the clinical decompensation (see figure).

Treatment of acute complications

• **Variceal bleeding**: blood product support, urgent endoscopy, with band ligation of the varices. Vasoconstrictors (glypressin) are a short-term but complementary measure. In overwhelming haemorrhage balloon tamponade (Sengstaken-Blakemore tube) may be tried. Acute percutaneous portosystemic shunting (TIPSS—trans-jugular intra-hepatic portosystemic stent shunt) can also control bleeding. In the long term, injection/banding of varices and/or beta-blockers reduces the risk of haemorrhage.

Table 118.2 Pugh–Child scoring system. A = 5–6. B = 7–9. C = 10–15.

	1	2	3
Bilirubin (mmol/L)	< 35	35–51	> 51
Albumin (g/L)	> 35	30–35	< 30
Ascites	None	Controlled	Poorly controlled
Encephalopathy	None	Minimal	Advanced
Nutrition	Excellent	Good	Poor

• **Ascites**: spironolactone and salt restriction are useful.

• **Encephalopathy**: provoking factors are removed/treated. Minimize absorption of dietary nitrogenous substances using lactulose).

Long-term management and prognosis

Prognosis is unpredictable but relates to Pugh-Child class (Table 118.2).

• If a clear aetiology is identified, treatment can restore good health even if cirrhosis is present (e.g. haemochromatosis).

• **Hepatoma**: may complicate long-standing cirrhosis from some aetiologies (viral hepatitis, haemochromatosis, alcohol). Frequent liver ultrasonography and α-fetoprotein measurements are indicated for early tumour detection.

• Treatment-refractory symptoms may be relieved by liver transplantation in selected cases.

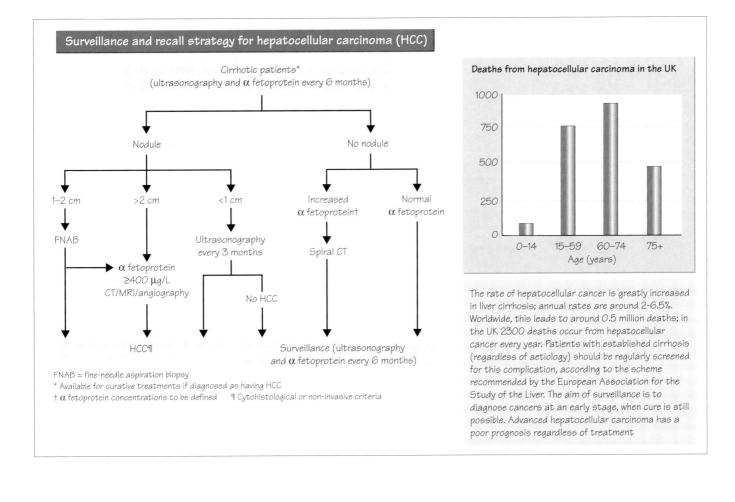

Surveillance and recall strategy for hepatocellular carcinoma (HCC)

Cirrhotic patients*
(ultrasonography and α fetoprotein every 6 months)

Nodule — No nodule

1–2 cm — >2 cm — <1 cm — Increased α fetoproteint — Normal α fetoprotein

FNAB

α fetoprotein ≥400 µg/L CT/MRI/angiography

Ultrasonography every 3 months

Spiral CT

No HCC

HCC¶

Surveillance (ultrasonography and α fetoprotein every 6 months)

FNAB = fine-needle aspiration biopsy
* Available for curative treatments if diagnosed as having HCC
† α fetoprotein concentrations to be defined   ¶ Cytohistological or non-invasive criteria

Deaths from hepatocellular carcinoma in the UK

The rate of hepatocellular cancer is greatly increased in liver cirrhosis; annual rates are around 2–6.5%. Worldwide, this leads to around 0.5 million deaths; in the UK 2300 deaths occur from hepatocellular cancer every year. Patients with established cirrhosis (regardless of aetiology) should be regularly screened for this complication, according to the scheme recommended by the European Association for the Study of the Liver. The aim of surveillance is to diagnose cancers at an early stage, when cure is still possible. Advanced hepatocellular carcinoma has a poor prognosis regardless of treatment

Diseases and Treatments at a Glance

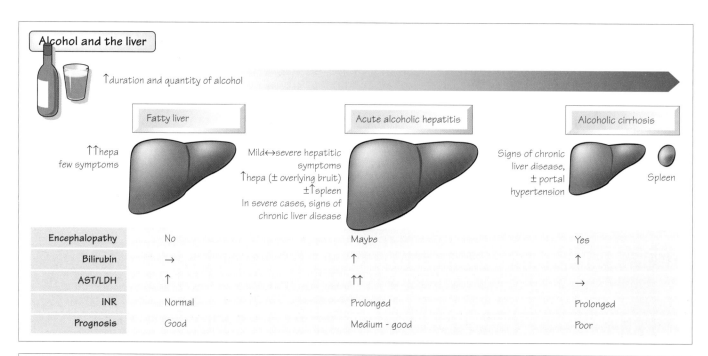

Alcohol and the liver

↑duration and quantity of alcohol

Fatty liver

↑↑hepa
few symptoms

Acute alcoholic hepatitis

Mild↔severe hepatitic symptoms
↑hepa (± overlying bruit)
±↑spleen
In severe cases, signs of chronic liver disease

Alcoholic cirrhosis

Signs of chronic liver disease, ± portal hypertension

Spleen

	Fatty liver	Acute alcoholic hepatitis	Alcoholic cirrhosis
Encephalopathy	No	Maybe	Yes
Bilirubin	→	↑	↑
AST/LDH	↑	↑↑	→
INR	Normal	Prolonged	Prolonged
Prognosis	Good	Medium - good	Poor

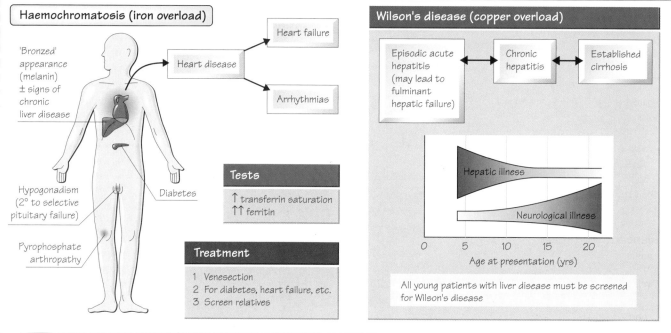

Haemochromatosis (iron overload)

'Bronzed' appearance (melanin) ± signs of chronic liver disease

Heart disease → Heart failure
Heart disease → Arrhythmias

Hypogonadism (2° to selective pituitary failure)

Diabetes

Pyrophosphate arthropathy

Tests

↑ transferrin saturation
↑↑ ferritin

Treatment

1 Venesection
2 For diabetes, heart failure, etc.
3 Screen relatives

Wilson's disease (copper overload)

Episodic acute hepatitis (may lead to fulminant hepatic failure) ↔ Chronic hepatitis ↔ Established cirrhosis

Hepatic illness

Neurological illness

| 0 | 5 | 10 | 15 | 20 |

Age at presentation (yrs)

All young patients with liver disease must be screened for Wilson's disease

Alcoholic liver disease

The relationship between alcohol and chronic liver disease is complex. Clearly, excess alcohol consumption is a risk factor for chronic liver disease. However, individual susceptibility varies considerably and typical alcohol-related pathology is increasingly seen in individuals who drink minimal amounts of alcohol (non-alcoholic steatohepatitis [NASH]—see p. 221).

Incidence

Common. Alcohol remains the most tolerated substance of abuse in the world. Despite this only a fifth of people with alcohol problems develop features of chronic liver disease.

Pathophysiology

Many theories have been proposed to explain alcohol-related liver injury. Many focus on the acetaldehyde derivatives of alcohol. There may be important genetic factors. There are three pathological forms of alcoholic liver disease:

1 Fatty liver: occurs in 50% of heavy drinkers—reversible on alcohol cessation.

2 Acute alcoholic hepatitis: occurs in 40% of heavy drinkers.

3 Cirrhosis: needs > 30 units/week. A man consuming 210 g ethanol (= 2.5 bottles wine)/day for 22 years has a 50% chance of developing cirrhosis.

Clinical features

Alcohol-related liver injury may present in many different ways:
- Chance finding of abnormal liver blood tests.
- **Decompensated chronic liver disease** (gastrointestinal bleeding, ascites).
- **Acute alcoholic hepatitis**: this presentation is particularly challenging. Often there is a long history of alcohol use and, then, the apparently sudden onset of jaundice often with anorexia, nausea, malaise, fever and neutrophil leukocytosis.

Investigations

There are no clinically useful objective markers of alcohol abuse other than a random ethanol level taken on admission. This may be of limited value in many cases because often patients will have stopped drinking before admission.

Management and prognosis

Management of patients with alcohol-related liver injury involves:
- Addressing the difficult challenge of total abstinence from alcohol. In alcoholic cirrhosis 5-year survival is 70% in abstinent patients and only 35% in drinkers.
- Objectively assessing the degree of chronic liver disease (biopsy for fibrosis).
- Hepatocellular carcinoma occurs in 15% of people with alcoholic cirrhosis: surveillance for this may be indicated.

Haemochromatosis

Haemochromatosis is the term used to describe primary iron overload (total body iron of > 5 g vs normal stores of < 3 g). In most cases iron overload is the result of increased gastrointestinal absorption of iron. The excess iron is deposited in many organs, resulting in damage.

Incidence

The mutation in the *HFE* gene responsible for haemochromatosis (*C282Y*) is very common in white people, with a prevalence of up to 1 : 150 in populations with a strong Celtic ancestry (e.g. the Irish). This makes haemochromatosis the most common single gene disorder to affect northwest European populations. Despite this, symptomatic presentation remains rare. The reason for this disparity is not clear.

Pathophysiology

The *C282Y* mutation in the *HFE* gene prevents cell surface expression of the protein. How this leads to the demonstrable increase in gastrointestinal iron absorption is still not clear. Once absorbed, excess iron is deposited in the liver and other organs (pancreas, heart, joints). This leads to liver fibrosis and ultimately a risk of hepatoma.

Clinical features

Although the original 'classic' descriptions of haemochromatosis were of bronzed diabetes, i.e.:

- Diabetes
- Skin involvement leading to a bronzed appearance
- Cardiac failure
- Joint involvement, often producing a pyrophosphate arthropathy—in many cases the most disabling symptom.

This 'full-blown' clinical presentation is rarely seen today. Increasingly the diagnosis is made in patients without distinctive clinical symptoms or physical signs.

Investigations

- **Liver blood tests**: non-specific hepatitis.
- **Iron indices**: transferrin saturation > 80%. Ferritin levels are often very high, not infrequently > 1–2000 mg/L (normal < 300 mg/L). Liver biopsy shows a characteristic distribution of iron and provides important information on staging (i.e. the degree of liver fibrosis).
- **Genetic mutation analysis**: 90% of white people with haemochromatosis are homozygous for the *C282Y* mutation in *HFE*.

Management and prognosis

- **Venesection**: 500 g of whole blood removed weekly until excess iron stores removed (which takes up to 12–18 months in heavily iron-loaded individuals). Thereafter, venesection should continue every 3 months indefinitely.
- **Surveillance for hepatoma**: in patients who have developed cirrhosis before the diagnosis has been made there remains a risk of developing hepatoma and in these cases it may be appropriate to regularly test α-fetoprotein and undertake liver ultrasonography.
- **Screening first-degree relatives**: this process has been greatly facilitated by *HFE* mutation analysis.

Wilson's disease

Rare (worldwide incidence 1–30/million), autosomal recessive disorder of copper metabolism resulting in copper overload. Arises when mutations in the gene coding for a copper transport protein (*ATP7B*, chromosome 13q14.3) lead to failure of biliary excretion of copper and thus progressive copper accumulation. This often results in hepatic and neurological damage. Usually presents in children and young adults. Equal sex incidence. Kayser-Fleischer rings may be identified in the eyes by slit-lamp examination. There are various presentations:

- **Hepatic**: acute hepatitis. Fulminant liver failure or chronic liver disease/cirrhosis.
- **Neuropsychiatric**: extrapyramidal disturbance/psychosis.
- **Haematological**: acute intravascular haemolysis.

Investigations

- **Copper studies**: serum copper (low); ceruloplasmin (low in 80%); 24-h urinary copper (increased).
- **Liver biopsy**: defines degree of fibrosis as well as quantifies copper load.
- Cerebral computed tomography/magnetic resonance imaging (CT/MRI).

Management and prognosis

- **Liver disease**: penicillamine is used to chelate copper, which is then excreted in the urine. Severe liver disease has been successfully treated with liver transplantation.
- **Neurological disease** is permanent.
- **Screening of first-degree relatives**.

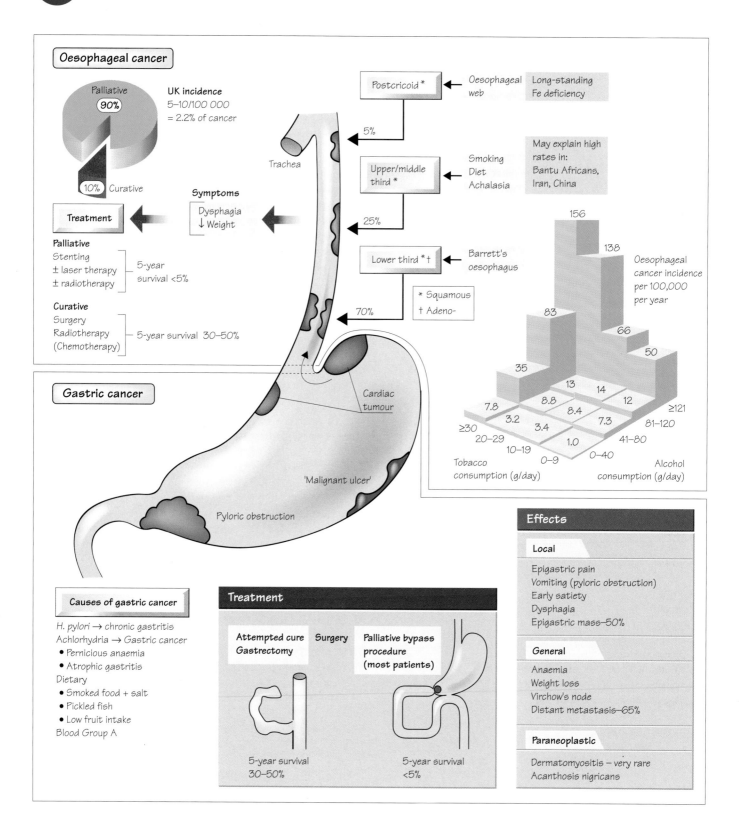

Oesophageal cancer

Palliative **90%**

10% Curative

UK incidence
5–10/100 000
= 2.2% of cancer

Symptoms
Dysphagia
↓ Weight

Treatment

Palliative
Stenting
± laser therapy
± radiotherapy
5-year survival <5%

Curative
Surgery
Radiotherapy
(Chemotherapy)
5-year survival 30–50%

Postcricoid *
Oesophageal web
Long-standing Fe deficiency

5%

Trachea

Upper/middle third *
Smoking Diet Achalasia
May explain high rates in: Bantu Africans, Iran, China

25%

Lower third *†
Barrett's oesophagus

* Squamous
† Adeno-

70%

Oesophageal cancer incidence per 100,000 per year

156
138
83
66
50
35
13
14
12
7.8
8.8
3.2
8.4
7.3
3.4
1.0
≥121
81–120
41–80
0–40
≥30
20–29
10–19
0–9

Tobacco consumption (g/day)
Alcohol consumption (g/day)

Gastric cancer

Cardiac tumour

'Malignant ulcer'

Pyloric obstruction

Causes of gastric cancer

H. pylori → chronic gastritis
Achlorhydria → Gastric cancer
• Pernicious anaemia
• Atrophic gastritis
Dietary
• Smoked food + salt
• Pickled fish
• Low fruit intake
Blood Group A

Treatment

Attempted cure
Gastrectomy

Surgery

Palliative bypass procedure (most patients)

5-year survival 30–50%

5-year survival <5%

Effects

Local
Epigastric pain
Vomiting (pyloric obstruction)
Early satiety
Dysphagia
Epigastric mass–50%

General
Anaemia
Weight loss
Virchow's node
Distant metastasis–65%

Paraneoplastic
Dermatomyositis – very rare
Acanthosis nigricans

Oesophageal carcinoma

Incidence

Although squamous carcinoma is declining in the western world in keeping with the reduction in cigarette smoking, adenocarcinoma of the distal oesophagus/gastric cardia is increasing throughout the world. The UK incidence is 12 per 100 000, with a 50% increase in incidence over the last 20 years.

Pathophysiology

Two different histological types of oesophageal cancer exist:

1 Squamous carcinoma most commonly affects the middle third of the oesophagus. There is a strong association with cigarette smoking.

2 Adenocarcinoma most commonly affects the lower third of the oesophagus and merges pathologically with carcinoma of the gastric cardia. Most theories relating the cause of the distal oesophageal adenocarcinoma involve chronic gastro-oesophageal reflux of both acid and possibly bile.

Clinical features

- **Dysphagia**: the major clinical feature relating to oesophageal malignancy is dysphagia. Rapidly progressive dysphagia (i.e. dysphagia to solids progressing to dysphagia to soft food and liquids) and weight loss at the time of presentation are particularly worrying features.

Investigations

Progressive dysphagia always requires urgent investigation (see p. 42):

- **Endoscopy**: will achieve a histological diagnosis and allows symptoms relief (oesophageal dilatation).
- **Computed tomography (CT)**: in patients suitable for consideration of surgery (bearing in mind the high prevalence of significant co-morbidity) a CT of the chest and upper abdomen will exclude gross pulmonary and/or hepatic metastases and may identify local invasion into important other structures such as the pericardium or aorta.
- **Endoscopic ultrasonography**: this is more sensitive than CT for detecting local tumour invasion.
- **Staging laparoscopy** is occasionally undertaken before attempted curative surgery, because malignant spread to lymph nodes may be missed on CT scan.

Management and prognosis

The prognosis is poor, 5-year survival 9%.

- **Surgery**: this offers the best chance of cure which justifies the efforts put into preoperative staging, although even with 'curative' resection 5-year survival rate is < 20%.
- **Radiotherapy and chemotherapy**: squamous carcinoma of the oesophagus is sensitive to radiotherapy and newer combination regimens are proving beneficial in adenocarcinoma as well.

- **Palliative procedures**: even without the possibility of cure, it is possible to alleviate the distressing symptom of dysphagia.
  - **Dilatation**: in many cases dilatation of the oesophagus will relieve dysphagia, although this may have to be repeated.
  - **Laser or argon beam ablation**: laser can be used in the oesophagus to ablate exophytic tumour.
  - **Stenting**: in tumours causing mediastinal encasement stenting with self-expanding metal stents provides reasonable palliation.

Gastric carcinoma

Incidence

The incidence of gastric carcinoma (other than that of the gastric cardia—see above) is decreasing (17 per 100 000). There is a higher incidence in males than in females.

Pathophysiology

Predisposing factors include atrophic gastritis and previous surgery for peptic ulcer disease. The role of *H. pylori* in the aetiopathogenesis of upper gastrointestinal (GI) malignancy is controversial. There is an association between *H. pylori* infection and the development of gastric lymphoma (MALToma, where MALT is mucosa-associated lymphoid tissue), but the relationship with adenocarcinoma is less clear.

Clinical features

Gastric cancer often presents late, because there are no early clinical symptoms. Although dyspepsia remains a common prompt for diagnostic endoscopy, ironically patients with gastric cancer often have reduced gastric acid output (e.g. gastric atrophy). Many gastric cancers will prove to be at an advanced stage at the time they are identified.

- **Anaemia**: occult GI bleeding and the resulting iron deficiency is probably the most common way in which gastric carcinoma presents (see p. 218).
- **Weight loss** is common and suggests advanced metastatic disease.
- **Vomiting**: indicates impending gastric outflow obstruction.

Investigations

- **Endoscopy**: including biopsies for histological confirmation of the diagnosis.
- **Abdominal CT** for staging, i.e. to detect hepatic and other metastasis.

Management and prognosis

The prognosis is poor, with 5-year survival 12%.

- **Surgery** should be considered in most cases because, even in tumours that are advanced at the time of presentation, a surgical bypass (i.e. gastrojejunostomy) can provide good palliation. Increasingly, laparoscopy is being used to stage the tumour before any attempted resection.
- **Chemotherapy and radiotherapy**: these modalities tend to be less useful in gastric carcinoma.

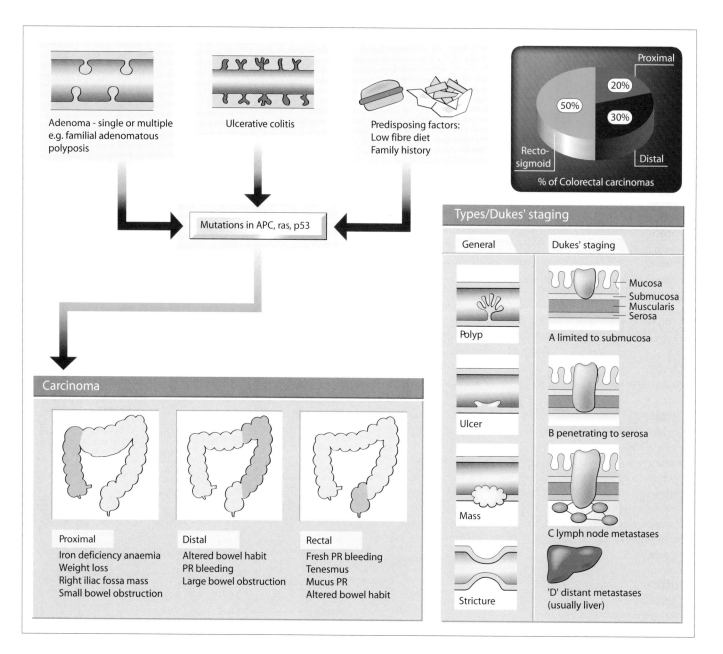

Adenoma - single or multiple e.g. familial adenomatous polyposis

Ulcerative colitis

Predisposing factors:
Low fibre diet
Family history

Proximal
20%
30%
50%
Recto-sigmoid
Distal
% of Colorectal carcinomas

Mutations in APC, ras, p53

Types/Dukes' staging

General | Dukes' staging

Polyp

Mucosa
Submucosa
Muscularis
Serosa

A limited to submucosa

Ulcer

B penetrating to serosa

Mass

C lymph node metastases

Stricture

'D' distant metastases (usually liver)

Carcinoma

Proximal	Distal	Rectal
Iron deficiency anaemia	Altered bowel habit	Fresh PR bleeding
Weight loss	PR bleeding	Tenesmus
Right iliac fossa mass	Large bowel obstruction	Mucus PR
Small bowel obstruction		Altered bowel habit

Colorectal cancer is a major public health problem in the developed world and increasingly efforts are being directed to identifying the condition early in individuals considered to be at risk.

Incidence

The incidence of colorectal cancer increases with age and overall this has increased over the last 50 years (currently 55 per 100 000 in men, 40 per 100 000 in women). Colorectal cancer now accounts for 20 000 deaths/year in the UK, with an additional 6000 successful resections. Colorectal cancer accounts for 39% of all cancer deaths in the UK with 5-year survival of 36% for men and 41% for women. Probably the single greatest determinant of prognosis is early detection, which has led to the principle of screening the population for colorectal cancer.

Pathophysiology

There are several conditions that are recognized to predispose to colorectal cancer.

Adenomatous polyps of the colon

Particularly tubulovillous adenomas. Colorectal cancer usually develops in pre-existing adenomatous polyps in the colon. The risk of finding cancer depends upon the size of the polyp (Table 121.1).

Table 121.1 Colonic polyp size and risk of cancer.

Polyp size (cm)	Cancer risk (%)
< 1	1–10
1–2	7–10
> 2	35–55

Table 121.2 Family history and lifetime risk of colorectal cancer.

Family history	Lifetime risk
None	1 : 40
One first-degree relative > 45 years	1 : 17
One first-degree and one second-degree relative	1 : 12
One first-degree relative < 45 years	1 : 10
Two first-degree relatives (any age)	1 : 8
Hereditary non-polyposis colon cancer	1 : 2

Ulcerative colitis

Longstanding total ulcerative colitis predisposes to colorectal cancer and patients with a 10-year history of total colitis should be offered 2-yearly surveillance colonoscopy with random colonic biopsies taken to detect severe dysplasia.

Family history

A greater understanding of the genetic predisposition to colorectal cancer is resulting in an increasing number of individuals referred for colonoscopic screening/surveillance. Surveillance colonoscopy is beneficial at risk ratios ≥ 1 : 12 (Table 121.2).

Familial cancer syndromes

There are some rare but important hereditary cancer syndromes. The most important of these are familial adenomatous polyposis (FAP) and hereditary non-polyposis colon cancer (HNPCC). In FAP, affected individuals have hundreds of adenomatous polyps throughout the colon evident from an early age. The risk of neoplasia is such that prophylactic colectomy is performed before the age of 20. HNPCC is inherited in an autosomal dominant fashion and is the result of mutations in DNA-mismatch repair genes. Individuals at risk are offered colonoscopic screening.

Clinical features

The clinical presentation of sporadic colorectal cancer depends to a degree on the site of the tumour. Proximal colonic cancers may present with features of subacute bowel obstruction or may be identified during the investigation of iron deficiency anaemia. Distal colon cancers will often cause a change in bowel habit (either constipation or diarrhoea) or present with overt rectal bleeding.

Investigations

• **Barium enema**: this is often the way in which the tumour is first identified. If the appearances are unequivocal and there are signs of impending bowel obstruction, a tissue diagnosis before laparotomy is unnecessary.
• **Colonoscopy**: if a tumour is identified at colonoscopy, it is worth completing the examination to exclude the presence of synchronous

Table 121.3 Five-year survival after resection of colorectal cancer.

Dukes' stage		5-year survival rate (%)
A	Limited to bowel wall	95–100
B	Penetrated bowel wall —no metastases	65–75
C	Lymph node metastases	30–40
	Distant metastases	< 1

tumours or polyps. If this has not been performed before resection, it ought to be done subsequently (see Follow-up/secondary prevention, below).
• **Full blood count**: iron deficiency anaemia.
• **Search for metastatic disease**: liver function tests, abdominal and thoracic CT. Although surgery is required in most cases it is useful to identify whether or not the patient has metastatic disease before laparotomy.
• **Carcinoembryonic antigen (CEA)**: this tumour marker is not useful for diagnosis, but is useful in monitoring the patient's response to treatment and for the identification of disease relapse.

Management and prognosis

• **Surgery**: surgery is required in most cases of colorectal cancer. The extent of bowel resection depends on the site of the tumour. Attempts are made to resect at least 5 cm of normal bowel either side of the tumour, and regional lymph nodes should also be resected. Prognosis after surgery depends on the histological grade of the tumour and the Dukes' stage (Table 121.3).
• **Chemotherapy**: chemotherapy with 5-fluorouracil (5FU) improves survival for Dukes' B and C cancers.
• **Radiotherapy**: preoperative radiotherapy to 'down-stage' rectal tumours is gaining popularity.
• **Follow-up/secondary prevention**: patients with a prior history of either colorectal cancer or tubulovillous adenoma of the colon should undergo surveillance colonoscopy.
• **Palliative approaches**: although surgery has been considered the appropriate treatment of patients with impending colonic obstruction, stenting of tumours with self-expanding metal stents offers an alternative approach for the palliative relief of obstruction.

Screening

Following a successful feasibility study a national programme for bowel cancer screening is about to be launched in England. This will take the form of screening the UK population over the age of 60 by faecal occult blood (FOB) testing. Patients identified as FOB positive will be invited to attend for colonoscopy. This process will identify patients with early stage (Dukes' A) cancer that should result in improved survival. Furthermore the process will identify colonic polyps, which if removed endoscopically will not develop into cancer (i.e. the process might actually *prevent* rather than just detect cancer). In time flexible sigmoidoscopy or even total colonoscopy might increasingly be seen as the best primary screening tool although there are issues of safety, quality assurance, staffing and patient acceptability that will need to be addressed.

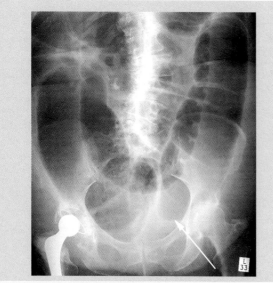

This image shows large bowel obstruction secondary to sigmoid carcinoma. There is gaseous distension of the large bowel down to the left pelvis, at the level of the obstruction (arrow). A plain (erect) abdominal film is a very useful examination in many patients acutely unwell with abdominal pain, especially in the elderly. Though the history usually gives vital clues as to whether or not bowel obstruction is present, many very elderly patients present with very non-specific symptoms, such as vague abdominal pains, without a clear history of absolute constipation. In the presence of abdominal discomfort in the elderly, always consider bowel obstruction, commonly resulting from cancer, ischaemia, or sigmoid volvulus (where the 'upside-down' bowel can often be seen)

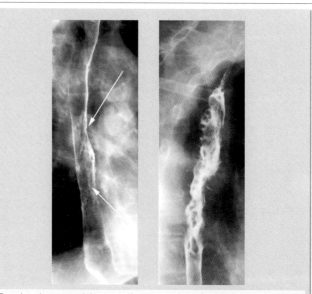

Though endoscopy with biopsy is the main modality for diagnosing most GI tract malignancies (see other chapters), there remains an important role for barium based examinations. 1) Left-hand image: this image demonstrates a superficial spreading oesophageal cancer (arrows). 2) Image right hand side. This barium swallow demonstrates a very abnormal oesophagus; there is a large polypoidal mass with structuring, mucosal irregularity and ulceration. The appearances are due to advanced oesophageal cancer

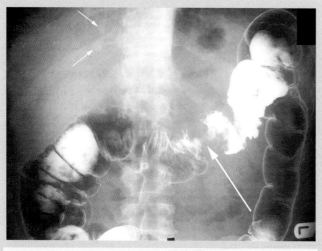

Double contrast barium enema. A cancer of the transverse colon is seen. There is irregular structuring of the bowel, resulting in an 'apple core' lesion. This appearance is highly likely to be due to cancer, and very unlikely to be due to a benign process. This film also shows (arrows) metastasis in the lungs; patients with known GI malignancy usually need a radiological search for secondaries. Plain Xrays can offer much; for example, many GI malignancies spread to the lungs – so the chest Xray can be useful. Likewise, if any bones hurt, plain Xrays may show secondaries. CT scanning is the usual means to assess occult pulmonary and hepatic metastasis. They do however carry quite a radiation dose (see right), though this is usually not relevant to patients with a known serious malignancy

Photos from *The Hands on Guide to Imaging*, by Howlett and Ayers

Typical doses from diagnostic medical exposure

Diagnostic procedure	Typical effective dose (mSv)	Equivalent no. of chest X-rays	Approx. equivalent period of natural background radiation
Radiographical examinations			
Limbs and joints (except hip)	<0.01	<0.5	<1.5 days
Chest (single PA film)	0.02	1	3 days
Skull	0.06	3	9 days
Thoracic spine	0.7	35	4 months
Lumbar spine	1	50	5 months
Hip	0.4	20	2 months
Pelvis	0.7	35	4 months
Abdomen	0.7	35	4 months
IVU	2.4	120	14 months
Barium swallow	1.5	75	8 months
Barium meal	2.6	130	15 months
Barium follow-through	3	150	16 months
Barium enema	7.2	360	3.2 years
CT head	2	100	10 months
CT chest	8	400	3.6 years
CT abdomen or pelvis	10	500	4.5 years
Radionuclide studies			
Lung ventilation (^{133}Xe)	0.3	15	7 weeks
Lung perfusion (^{99}mTc)	1	50	6 months
Bone (^{99}mTc)	4	200	1.8 years

Abbreviations: CT, computed tomography; IVU, intravenous urogram; PA, posteroanterior. UK average background radiation = 2.2mSv/year; regional averages range from 1.5 to 7.5mSv/year.

(Modified from Royal College of Radiologists handbook, *Making the Best Use of the Radiology Department*, 4th edn. 2003)

Functional gastrointestinal disorders

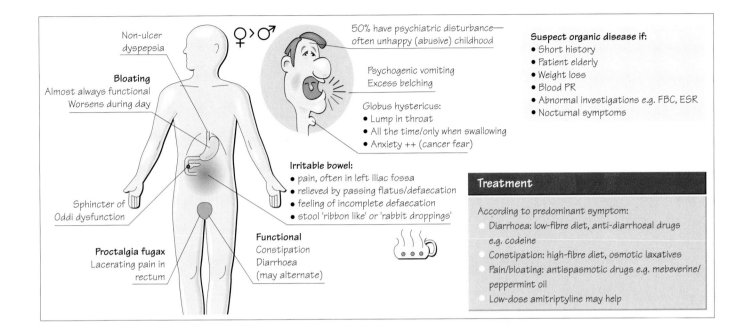

Non-ulcer dyspepsia

Bloating
Almost always functional
Worsens during day

Sphincter of
Oddi dysfunction

Proctalgia fugax
Lacerating pain in
rectum

♀ > ♂

50% have psychiatric disturbance—
often unhappy (abusive) childhood

Psychogenic vomiting
Excess belching

Globus hystericus:
• Lump in throat
• All the time/only when swallowing
• Anxiety ++ (cancer fear)

Irritable bowel:
• pain, often in left iliac fossa
• relieved by passing flatus/defaecation
• feeling of incomplete defaecation
• stool 'ribbon like' or 'rabbit droppings'

Functional
Constipation
Diarrhoea
(may alternate)

Suspect organic disease if:
• Short history
• Patient elderly
• Weight loss
• Blood PR
• Abnormal investigations e.g. FBC, ESR
• Nocturnal symptoms

Treatment

According to predominant symptom:
○ Diarrhoea: low-fibre diet, anti-diarrhoeal drugs
e.g. codeine
○ Constipation: high-fibre diet, osmotic laxatives
○ Pain/bloating: antispasmotic drugs e.g. mebeverine/
peppermint oil
○ Low-dose amitriptyline may help

Irritable bowel syndrome is a widely used term with relatively limited clinical value. It represents one of many functional syndromes of gut sensitivity and/or motility that affect any part of the gastrointestinal tract. Examples include: globus hystericus, non-ulcer dyspepsia, irritable bowel syndrome, functional diarrhoea, functional constipation, proctalgia fugax and sphincter of Oddi dysfunction.

The common link between these conditions is that they have characteristic symptom complexes without clinical or laboratory features to suggest progressive intestinal pathology.

Incidence and pathophysiology

The prevalence depends on definition. Ten per cent of the population consult doctors with functional gastrointestinal (GI) complaints; 20% who consider themselves normal admit to symptoms consistent with irritable bowel. Other overlapping symptom complexes include chronic fatigue syndrome and functional gynaecological symptoms. In some individuals, episodes of gut insult, e.g. severe gastroenteritis, may have triggered the problem (post-infective irritable bowel). Sufferers may have heightened visceral sensory awareness.

Clinical features

Although the symptoms vary enormously there are some patterns that dominate:
• **Bloating**.
• **Marked gastrocolic reflex** (the need to defecate shortly after eating).
• **Identifiable dietary precipitants**: specific foods may cause symptoms, e.g. dairy products, fatty or spicy foods and alcohol.
• **Pain relieved by defaecation**.
• **Chaotic bowel habit**: patients often describe an increased frequency of defecation with clustering in the morning—the 'cork out of the champagne bottle' effect.

Some symptoms should not be put down to a functional cause without further investigation: dysphagia; anorexia and/or weight loss; mouth ulcers; nocturnal diarrhoea; rectal bleeding.

Stress may be a dominant feature. Unfortunately it is not possible to quantify stress and, more importantly, it is difficult to avoid.

Management and prognosis

The extent of clinical investigation to exclude a progressive intestinal pathology must be individually tailored. A detailed history (including dietary) from the patient is central to the correct diagnosis and management. A full examination including rigid sigmoidoscopy should be undertaken. Thereafter investigations depend largely on the patient's particular symptom complex. As a minimum, a full blood count and erythrocyte sedimentation rate (ESR) should be performed.

A thorough history and physical examination is the most important diagnostic and therapeutic tool. The **most important** part of the management is to listen to the patient. Often the qualified reassurance of being told that there is no objective evidence of physical disease is sufficient to improve symptoms (or at least the resulting concern).
• **Antispasmodic drugs**: mebeverine or alverine are useful for colicky abdominal pain.
• **Anticholinergics**: low doses of amitriptyline help those with depressive features (low mood, anhedonia, rumination, poor sleep, etc.). Relaxation therapy may also help.
• **Dietary measures**: patients resistant to the above measures or those with clearly identifiable dietary intolerances may benefit from dietary intervention (low-lactose diet, exclusion diet). Paradoxically, many patients with an irritable bowel find that their symptoms worsen with a high-fibre diet.

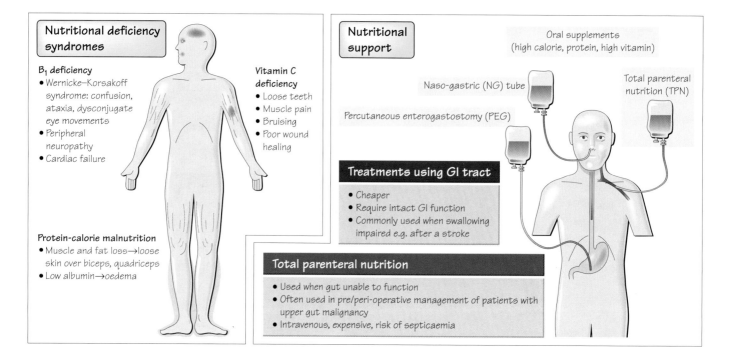

The extent of malnutrition in hospital inpatients is often under-estimated. Many diseases lead to anorexia and a reduction in calorific intake, and this is especially relevant when placed in the context of the increased nutritional requirements resulting from the catabolic state of malignant or inflammatory disease.

Identification of malnutrition in hospital patients

General (protein–calorie malnutrition)

Protein–calorie malnutrition is easy to miss in the hospitalized patient, because the primary disease often dominates the clinical picture. Starvation is, however, very common, and can be recognized by weight loss > 10% in < 3 months (when the body mass index or BMI < 19 kg/m^2), muscle wasting, peripheral oedema (with an albumin < 35 g/L). Lymphocytes < 1.5×10^9/L.

Specific (vitamin and mineral deficiencies)

Acute vitamin deficiency is much more frequent with the water-soluble vitamins (particularly vitamin B$_1$ [thiamine] and vitamin C; Table 124.1), rather than those that are fat soluble, for which there are substantial body stores.

• **Thiamine** deficiency can develop quickly (within 3 weeks), and leads to Wernicke's encephalopathy. People with alcohol problems are particularly predisposed, but so are patients with prolonged (> 3 weeks) vomiting.

• **Folate stores** are relatively small and deficiency can occur quickly, causing a macrocytic anaemia.

• **Vitamin C deficiency** (scurvy) is much commoner than realized, and impairs wound healing. If prolonged, classic scurvy may occur, with the development of unusual 'corkscrew'-shaped hair, haemorrhages around the hair follicle, swollen spongy gums, leading to loose teeth, spontaneous bruising and bleeding. Anaemia, which is usually hypochromic but can be normochromic, occurs. Vitamin C levels can be measured in the plasma, and also in the leukocyte-platelet layer of centrifuged blood—the 'buffy' layer. Treatment is with ascorbic acid.

• **Iron** (microcytic anaemia, glossitis, cheilosis, koilonychia), **calcium** (proximal myopathy, perioral paraesthesia and tetany) and **magnesium** (myopathy not responding to calcium) deficiency can all occur in hospitalized patients.

Nutritional support

Indications

In patients considered to be malnourished, consideration should always be given to nutritional support.

Forms of nutritional support (see figure)

Therapeutic diets (Table 124.2)

Many diets are useful for the treatment of specific gastrointestinal conditions and for non-specific symptoms. Low-protein diets tend not to be advised nowadays for either renal failure or hepatic encephalopathy.

Table 124.1 Feature of water-soluble vitamin deficiency (for features of vitamin C deficiency see text, folate deficiency see p. 318, for B_{12} deficiency see p. 318).

	Vitamin B_1	Vitamin B_2	Niacin	Vitamin B_6
Solubility	Water			
Common name	Thiamine	Riboflavin		Pyridoxine
Occurrence	• Cereals • Beans • Nuts • Pork, duck	• Dairy products • Offal • Leafy vegetables	• Plants • Meat • Fish	Found widely in plant and animal derived foods
Function	Essential cofactor in many enzyme systems, especially involving carbohydrate metabolism		Hydrogen acceptor in many oxidative reactions	Cofactor in metabolism of many amino acids
Cause of deficiency	• Dietary deficiency, e.g. milled rice • Alcoholism (usually due to dietary deficiency) • Prolonged vomiting, e.g. hyperemesis gravidarum, cancer especially with chemotherapy	Low dietary intake	Lost during the milling process of cereals—unless replaced deficiency occurs in those with cereal-only diet • Isoniazid therapy • Malabsorption syndromes (rare) • Carcinoid syndrome	• Dietary deficiency is very rare • Drugs can produce deficiency (e.g. isoniazid, hydralazine penicillamine
Consequence of deficiency	• 'Dry' beriberi; polyneuropathy, ± cerebral involvement with Wernicke-Korsokoff syndrome (causing dementia, ataxia, external ophthalmoplegia, nystagmus) • 'Wet' beriberi: oedema of the legs → ascites, pleural effusions (largely due to cardiac failure) • Vasodilatation (due to lactic acid) → bounding pulse	Clinical deficiency very rare: • Angular stomatitis • Red inflamed tongue • Seborrhoeic dermatitis • Conjunctivitis	Pellagra (→ the 3 Ds): • Dermatitis: in sun-exposed areas of the skin → thickening, dry, hyperpigmentation • Diarrhoea: other GI symptoms include a red raw tongue, glossitis, angular stomatitis • Dementia: in severe cases, in milder cases, depression, apathy ad thought disorders	• Polyneuropathy • Rarely, some sideroblastic anaemias respond to B_6 • Some premenstrual tension symptoms may respond to B_6 supplementation
Diagnosis	• Clinical response to thiamine • Red cell (transketolase) before and after added thiamine		Clinical features	Clinical features
General treatment	Most vitamin deficiencies are not isolated, and accordingly multiple different vitamin supplements should be given, along with protein and calories			
Treatment	Supplemental thiamine—if due to EtOH abuse, thiamine MUST be given prior to carbohydrates	Riboflavin supplementation	Niacin supplementation	Vitamin B_6
Excess	Ataxia	No data		

Table 124.2 Indications for specific diets.

Diet	Indication	Principle
Gluten free	Coeliac disease	Total gluten withdrawal
Low lactose	Hypolactasia	Low in dairy products
High-fibre	Constipation/Diverticular change	High content of insoluble fibre (e.g. bran)
Low residue	Subacute small bowel obstruction (e.g. Crohn's disease)	Low in fibre to reduce obstructive symptoms
Exclusion	Intractable irritable bowel	Bland diet for control of irritable bowel symptoms
Low salt	Cirrhosis, heart failure	Useful adjunct to diuretics in control of oedema and/or ascites
Elemental/Peptide	Crohn's disease	Liquid diet with nitrogen as either short peptides or amino acids

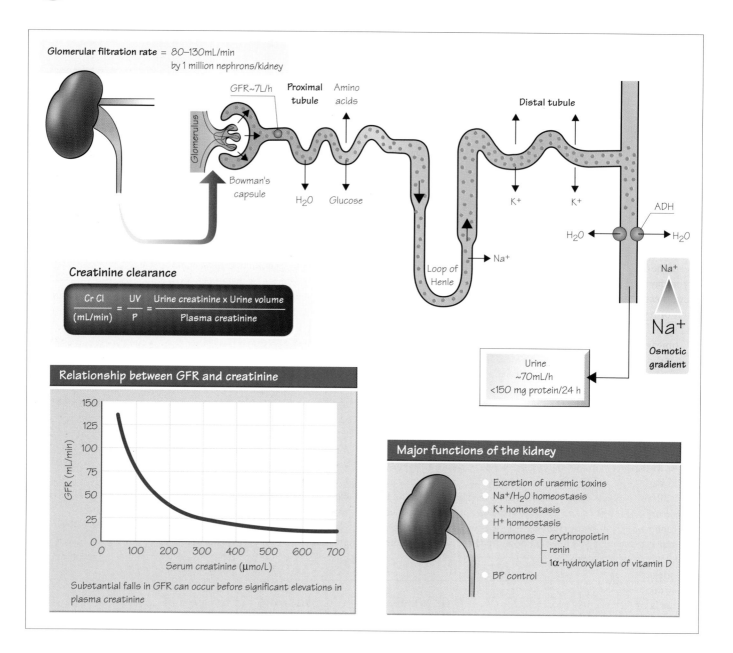

Glomerular filtration rate = 80–130mL/min
by 1 million nephrons/kidney

GFR~7L/h | Proximal tubule | Amino acids

Glomerulus

Bowman's capsule

Distal tubule

H_2O Glucose

K^+ K^+

ADH

H_2O H_2O

Loop of Henle

Na^+

Na^+

Na^+

Osmotic gradient

Creatinine clearance

$$\frac{Cr\ Cl}{(mL/min)} = \frac{UV}{P} = \frac{Urine\ creatinine \times Urine\ volume}{Plasma\ creatinine}$$

Urine
~70mL/h
<150 mg protein/24 h

Relationship between GFR and creatinine

GFR (mL/min) vs Serum creatinine (μmol/L)

Substantial falls in GFR can occur before significant elevations in plasma creatinine

Major functions of the kidney

- Excretion of uraemic toxins
- Na^+/H_2O homeostasis
- K^+ homeostasis
- H^+ homeostasis
- Hormones — erythropoietin
  — renin
  — 1α-hydroxylation of vitamin D
- BP control

Each kidney consists of approximately one million nephrons. Each nephron has a glomerulus, which is located mainly in the renal cortex and which filters into a renal tubule. The tubule consists of proximal and distal tubules, and the loop of Henle in which reabsorption of water, electrolytes and other important solutes occurs; this produces urine which drains into the collecting ducts, undergoes further water absorption and then drains into the renal pyramids. The thick ascending limb of the loop of Henle possesses a specialized plaque of cells which attaches to the extra-glomerular mesangium and afferent arteriole to form the juxtaglomerular apparatus; this secretes renin and is involved in the regulation of glomerular blood flow and filtration rate. The kidneys receive 20% of the cardiac output and filter 7 L of fluid/h to produce 50–100 mL of urine/h, showing the efficiency with which water and other solutes are reabsorbed by the renal tubules.

The key functions of the kidney are therefore to excrete/secrete the waste products of metabolism, and other substances harmful to the body, while conserving useful constituents of blood. In addition the kidney has major endocrine functions. Although often renal disease leads to failure in all three of these key functions, equally often disease can affect the first two functions independently. It is convenient to consider how the different functions of the kidney can be measured according to anatomical location:

• **Glomerular function—toxin/metabolic waste product elimination**: the key variable reflecting the efficiency of the kidney in waste products disposal is the glomerular filtration rate (GFR). The most commonly used measure of GFR is serum creatinine, an end-product of skeletal muscle metabolism (higher in those with large muscle bulk). The relationship between GFR and serum creatinine is not linear (see

Diseases and Treatments at a Glance

Table 125.1 Proteinuria in renal disease.

	Glomerulonephritis	Tubular disease	Overflow proteinuria
Amount of proteinuria	+ to ++++	+ to ++	+ to ++++
Nephrotic syndrome present	0 to ++++	No	0 to ++ (amyloid in multiple myeloma)
Dipstick positive for protein	Yes	No	No
κ or λ free chains	No	Yes	Monoclonal Ig κ or λ

figure), and it is important to emphasize that highly significant falls in GFR can occur before serum creatinine rises. If impairment of GFR is suspected, it is insufficient to rely on plasma creatinine; a more accurate measure of GFR should be used instead, such as the creatinine clearance. The principle underlying this measure is that creatinine is an inert molecule, passively filtered by the kidney, and a knowledge of urine creatinine quantity (Urine$_{Cr}$) and plasma creatinine concentration (P$_{Cr}$) (over 24 h) allows calculation of the GFR, from:

$$GFR = (Urine_{Cr} \times Urine\ volume)/P_{Cr}$$

Creatinine clearance measurements are usually sufficiently accurate for day-to-day clinical practice, although the GFR measured this way may overestimate the true GFR by up to 100% in severe renal disease, as a result of renal tubule secretion of creatinine (thus overestimating the amount of urine creatinine derived from glomerular filtration).

• **Glomerular function—conservation of normal blood constituents**: glomerular function can be disturbed such that plasma protein is no longer conserved. This leak of protein can range from the mild, significant as a marker of renal disease, to devastating, associated with profound hypoalbuminaemia and substantial oedema. In addition to defective glomerular function, mild proteinuria also results from defects in tubular function (see Table 125.1) and as an overflow phenomenon (e.g. multiple myeloma, Ig κ or λ light chains: acute leukaemia, lysozymuria). These three different kinds of mild proteinuria are distinguished on the basis of electrophoretic properties. Urine dipsticks primarily detect albumin, which is found in glomerular disease and not in tubular disease or multiple myeloma. If these conditions are suspected, urine electrophoresis should be performed.

• **Renal concentrating ability**: the loop of Henle, via the countercurrent mechanism, establishes an osmotic gradient that increases from the cortex to the inner medulla. Water excretion is adjusted in the collecting ducts, which pass through the medulla and where permeability of water is controlled by the antidiuretic hormone (ADH). The ability of the kidney to concentrate urine is disturbed in many intrinsic renal diseases, particularly tubulointerstitial ones, as well as in actual or functional deficiency of ADH (diabetes insipidus). The renal concentrating power can be measured by (1) osmolality of early morning urine, which is the easiest and safest test, and (2) concentrating ability when faced with 24-h fluid deprivation, which is uncomfortable (so compliance is an issue) and which may induce hypovolaemic renal failure. It is usual to admit patients to hospital for this.

• **Amino acid conserving function**: amino acids are filtered at the glomerulus, and reabsorbed in the proximal tubules. Diffuse proximal tubular damage results in generalized aminoaciduria, whereas specific lesions cause specific patterns of amino acid loss. The pattern of aminoaciduria is detected by two-dimensional chromatography.

• **Renal acid–base control**: a major function of the proximal and distal tubules is acid–base balance. Advanced renal failure gives rise to the retention of metabolic acids (exacerbating renal bone disease), which may provoke myocardial depression and death. Specific tubular lesions may, in the absence of filtration failure, produce retention of metabolic acid—the so-called renal tubular acidosis.

• **Electrolyte control**: the kidney is central in the control of potassium, as a result of secretion of potassium into the tubular fluid in exchange for sodium or hydrogen ions, and in the regulation of urinary pH. In advanced renal failure, the distal tubule cannot exchange plasma K$^+$/H$^+$ for tubule Na$^+$, leading to hyperkalaemia, which when profound may lead to cardiac arrest.

• **Hormonal function**: the kidney has hormonal functions, notably in the production of renin and erythropoietin, and the 1α-hydroxylation of vitamin D from an inactive to an active form. When renal function is globally disturbed, renal hormone production is usually diminished, provoking anaemia (erythropoietin deficiency) and exacerbating renal bone disease. Other hormones, especially the renin-angiotensin system, are involved in **blood pressure control**. Renal diseases such as renal ischaemia (e.g. unilateral renal artery stenosis) or glomerulonephritis are commonly associated with hypertension.

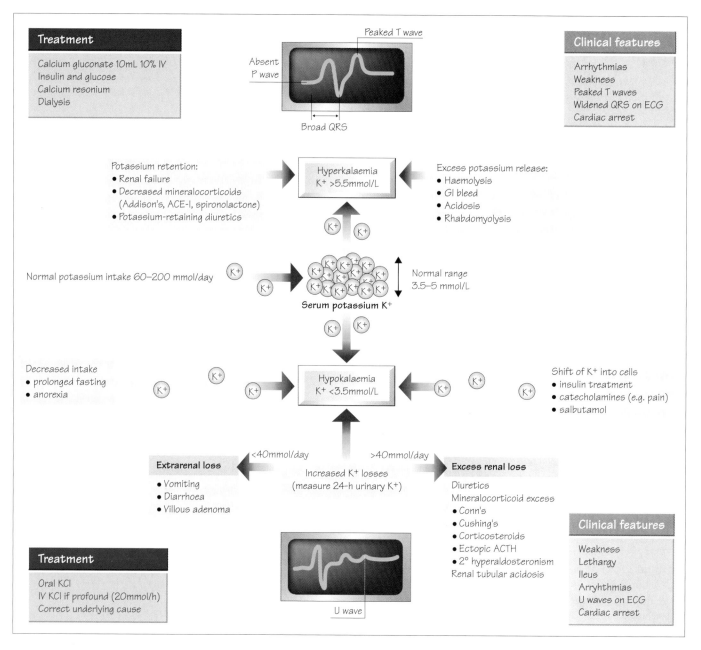

Treatment

Calcium gluconate 10mL 10% IV
Insulin and glucose
Calcium resonium
Dialysis

Clinical features

Arrhythmias
Weakness
Peaked T waves
Widened QRS on ECG
Cardiac arrest

Peaked T wave
Absent P wave
Broad QRS

Potassium retention:
• Renal failure
• Decreased mineralocorticoids (Addison's, ACE-I, spironolactone)
• Potassium-retaining diuretics

Hyperkalaemia
K+ >5.5mmol/L

Excess potassium release:
• Haemolysis
• GI bleed
• Acidosis
• Rhabdomyolysis

Normal potassium intake 60–200 mmol/day

Normal range 3.5–5 mmol/L

Serum potassium K+

Decreased intake
• prolonged fasting
• anorexia

Hypokalaemia
K+ <3.5mmol/L

Shift of K+ into cells
• insulin treatment
• catecholamines (e.g. pain)
• salbutamol

<40mmol/day   >40mmol/day

Extrarenal loss
• Vomiting
• Diarrhoea
• Villous adenoma

Increased K+ losses (measure 24-h urinary K+)

Excess renal loss
Diuretics
Mineralocorticoid excess
• Conn's
• Cushing's
• Corticosteroids
• Ectopic ACTH
• 2° hyperaldosteronism
Renal tubular acidosis

Clinical features

Weakness
Lethargy
Ileus
Arryhthmias
U waves on ECG
Cardiac arrest

Treatment

Oral KCl
IV KCl if profound (20mmol/h)
Correct underlying cause

U wave

Hypokalaemia

Hypokalaemia is a serum potassium of less than 3.5 mmol/L. It is the most common electrolyte disorder in hospitalized patients, mostly attributable to diuretic therapy. It can occur as a result of increased losses from the urinary or gastrointestinal tract, poor intake (such as in eating disorders) or a shift to the intracellular compartment (insulin treatment or familial periodic paralysis—p. 383). Gastrointestinal losses may occur as a result of diarrhoea, vomiting, laxative abuse or villous adenomas of the colon. Renal losses may occur as the result of diuretic therapy, mineralocorticoid excess (Conn's syndrome, Cushing's syndrome, ectopic adrenocorticotrophic hormone [ACTH], secondary hyperaldosteronism [renal artery stenosis, hypertension, heart failure]) or renal tubular acidosis. β-Receptor stimulation moves potassium into

cells, which explains why hypokalaemia is common in the sick and in those treated with salbutamol.

Common causes (see Table 126.1)
• Diuretic therapy
• Acute illness
• Gastrointestinal losses.

Clinical features
Often asymptomatic when mild, but hypokalaemia can produce weakness, intestinal ileus, decreased renal concentrating ability and ECG changes of T-wave flattening, the appearance of U-waves and an increased incidence of tachyarrhythmias. Long-standing hypokalaemia

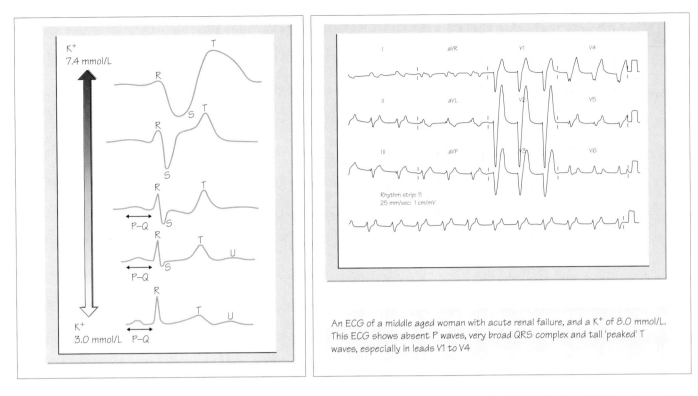

An ECG of a middle aged woman with acute renal failure, and a K$^+$ of 8.0 mmol/L. This ECG shows absent P waves, very broad QRS complex and tall 'peaked' T waves, especially in leads V1 to V4

Table 126.1 Causes of renal potassium wasting.

Blood pressure	Plasma renin activity	Cause
High BP	High PRA	Malignant hypertension, renal artery stenosis, (diuretics)
	Low PRA	Conn's, Cushing's, Liddle's, CAH
Normal BP	Low HCO$_3$	RTA 1,2
	High HCO$_3$	Diuretics, Bartter's, carbenoxolone

CAH = congenital adrenal hyperplasia; RTA = renal tubular acidosis.

can lead to (poorly reversible) damage to the distal tubule, leading to a failure of renal-concentrating properties, and polyuria, with compensatory polydipsia.

When severe (K$^+$ < 2 mmol/L) skeletal muscle weakness, which may be profound, dominates the clinical picture and flaccid paralysis may be seen. Very rarely, respiratory failure can occur in this situation.

Management

Treat the underlying cause. If potassium is < 2.5 mmol/L or < 3.0 mmol/L in a patient at risk of arrhythmias (e.g. post-myocardial infarction), give intravenous potassium chloride as an infusion not exceeding 20 mmol/h at a concentration not exceeding 40 mmol/L because concentrated potassium will damage peripheral veins. If potassium is between 2.5 and 3.5 mmol/L, give oral replacement therapy (unless the patient is nil-by-mouth or vomiting) at 80–120 mmol/day in divided doses.

Hyperkalaemia

The main cause of hyperkalaemia is renal failure (because potassium excretion is impaired). Other causes include reduced mineralo-corticoids, such as in Addison's disease, spironolactone (aldosterone antagonist), and angiotensin-converting enzyme (ACE) inhibitors or potassium-retaining diuretics such as amiloride. Cell destruction in haemolysis, cytotoxic therapy and rhabdomyolysis can liberate large amounts of potassium and cause hyperkalaemia. The hyperkalaemic effects of ACE inhibitors or potassium-retaining diuretics such as amiloride can be very marked in patients with renal impairment.

Hyperkalaemia can be artifactual as a result of the haemolysis of blood during venepuncture, so treat an unsuspected/anomalous finding of hyperkalaemia with suspicion, and repeat the measurement.

Common causes

- Renal failure
- Drugs, in those with borderline or frankly abnormal renal function, e.g. ACE inhibitors or spironolactone in elderly people.

Clinical features

Even very severe hyperkalaemia is usually asymptomatic although it can very rarely be accompanied by muscular weakness. It may be associated with ECG abnormalities of T-wave peaking, QRS widening, prolonged PR interval, loss of P waves and a sine wave appearance, leading to cardiac arrest.

Management

In mild hyperkalaemia (potassium < 6.0 mmol/L), oral or intravenous potassium should be restricted. Severe hyperkalaemia (potassium > 6.5 mmol/L or hyperkalaemic ECG changes) is a medical emergency. The patient should receive intravenous calcium gluconate (10 mL of 10% over 2 minutes), which stabilizes the myocardium. Measures to lower potassium should be instituted: the administration of intravenous glucose with insulin (50 mL of 50% glucose and 10 units of short-acting insulin), the potassium-binding resin, Calcium Resonium, and dialysis may be required.

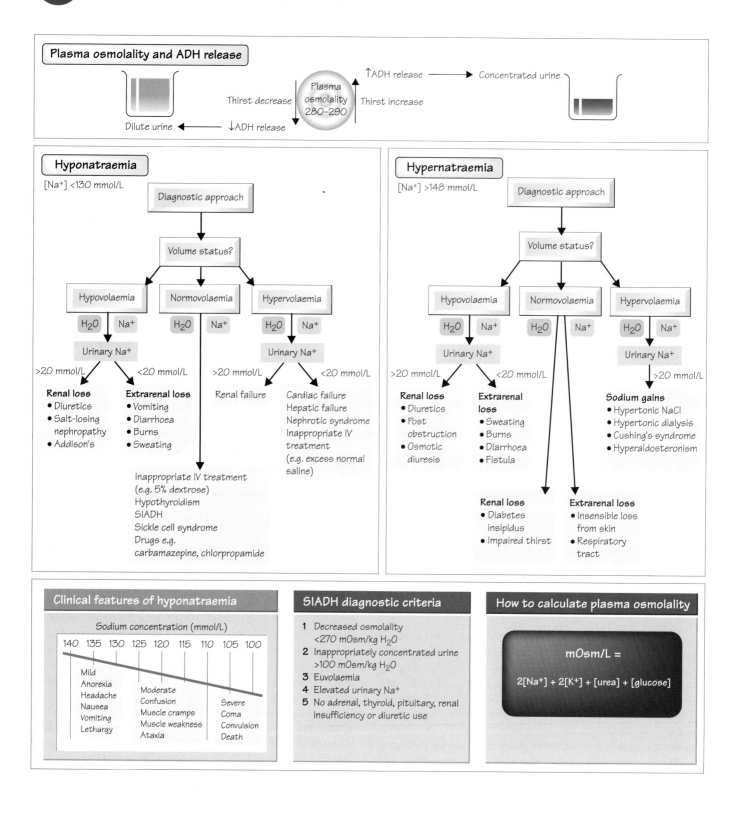

Plasma osmolality and ADH release

Thirst decrease · Plasma osmolality 280–290 · Thirst increase

↑ADH release → Concentrated urine

Dilute urine ← ↓ADH release

Hyponatraemia

[Na⁺] <130 mmol/L

Diagnostic approach

Volume status?

Hypovolaemia — H₂O Na⁺ — Urinary Na⁺
- >20 mmol/L — **Renal loss**
  - Diuretics
  - Salt-losing nephropathy
  - Addison's
- <20 mmol/L — **Extrarenal loss**
  - Vomiting
  - Diarrhoea
  - Burns
  - Sweating

Normovolaemia — H₂O Na⁺
- Inappropriate IV treatment (e.g. 5% dextrose)
- Hypothyroidism
- SIADH
- Sickle cell syndrome
- Drugs e.g. carbamazepine, chlorpropamide

Hypervolaemia — H₂O Na⁺ — Urinary Na⁺
- >20 mmol/L — Renal failure
- <20 mmol/L
  - Cardiac failure
  - Hepatic failure
  - Nephrotic syndrome
  - Inappropriate IV treatment (e.g. excess normal saline)

Hypernatraemia

[Na⁺] >148 mmol/L

Diagnostic approach

Volume status?

Hypovolaemia — H₂O Na⁺ — Urinary Na⁺
- >20 mmol/L — **Renal loss**
  - Diuretics
  - Post obstruction
  - Osmotic diuresis
- <20 mmol/L — **Extrarenal loss**
  - Sweating
  - Burns
  - Diarrhoea
  - Fistula

Normovolaemia — H₂O Na⁺
- **Renal loss**
  - Diabetes insipidus
  - Impaired thirst
- **Extrarenal loss**
  - Insensible loss from skin
  - Respiratory tract

Hypervolaemia — H₂O Na⁺ — Urinary Na⁺
- >20 mmol/L — **Sodium gains**
  - Hypertonic NaCl
  - Hypertonic dialysis
  - Cushing's syndrome
  - Hyperaldosteronism

Clinical features of hyponatraemia

Sodium concentration (mmol/L)

140 135 130 125 120 115 110 105 100

Mild
- Anorexia
- Headache
- Nausea
- Vomiting
- Lethargy

Moderate
- Confusion
- Muscle cramps
- Muscle weakness
- Ataxia

Severe
- Coma
- Convulsion
- Death

SIADH diagnostic criteria

1. Decreased osmolality <270 mOsm/kg H₂O
2. Inappropriately concentrated urine >100 mOsm/kg H₂O
3. Euvolaemia
4. Elevated urinary Na⁺
5. No adrenal, thyroid, pituitary, renal insufficiency or diuretic use

How to calculate plasma osmolality

$$mOsm/L = 2[Na^+] + 2[K^+] + [urea] + [glucose]$$

Abnormalities of serum sodium are closely linked to water balance. The most common causes of altered serum sodium are the result of excessive losses or administration of water.

Hyponatraemia

Hyponatraemia is defined as a serum sodium < 130 mmol/L and is found in 5% of hospital inpatients. Hyponatraemia may be asymptomatic, but can produce confusion, coma and convulsions.

In hyponatraemia there is an excess of extracellular water relative to the sodium content of the extracellular compartment. This can occur in three different circumstances:
1 Hypovolaemia (body Na⁺ and water deficit).
2 Normovolaemia (no change in body Na⁺ but a modest increase in water).
3 Hypervolaemia (increase in body Na⁺ and water).

Common causes
• Syndrome of inappropriate secretion of antidiuretic hormone (SIADH—see below).
• Heart failure (severity of hyponatraemia relates to severity of heart failure and prognosis).
• Inappropriate over-vigorous intravenous dextrose in post-operative patients.
• Iatrogenic Addison's disease (over-rapid corticosteroid withdrawal in elderly patients on large doses of steroids or with failure to increase corticosteroids when ill).

Management
The underlying aetiology should be sought and corrected where possible. The volume status of the patient should be determined. If signs of hypovolaemia are present (thirst, tachycardia, hypotension, postural fall in blood pressure, reduced skin turgor, etc.) then sodium chloride should be administered intravenously. In mild hyponatraemia, treatment may not be necessary, but if symptoms are present and there is no evidence of hypovolaemia the patient's fluid intake should be restricted. If there is evidence of hypervolaemia (oedema, elevated jugular venous pressure [JVP], hypertension) diuretics and water restriction may be necessary. Cautious correction of Na⁺ is essential to avoid central pontine myelinolysis, a syndrome of encephalopathy, cranial nerve palsies and quadriplegia, which occurs after rapid correction of Na⁺. In chronic hyponatraemia, the Na⁺ should be corrected at less than 0.5 mmol/L per h, although in acute hyponatraemia, if neurological symptoms are present, more rapid correction may be appropriate.

Syndrome of inappropriate antidiuretic hormone release
This is a relatively common cause of hyponatraemia in hospital patients. However, the diagnosis requires the exclusion of adrenal, thyroid, pituitary or renal insufficiency, no diuretic usage and euvolaemia. For the plasma tonicity, there is inappropriate elevation of ADH (vasopressin) levels which leads to an inappropriate urinary concentration. There are a large number of possible causes (see Table 127.1) which can be broadly grouped into carcinomas, particularly of the lung, pulmonary disorders including pneumonia, central nervous system (CNS) disorders such as meningitis and head trauma, and drugs.

Treatment of SIADH involves removing the precipitating cause wherever possible. Fluid restriction, of increasing degree with increas-

Table 127.1 Some causes of the syndrome of inappropriate antidiuretic hormone release.

Commonest causes	Idiopathic
Post-operative pain	Lung infection + COPD Drugs (see below)
CNS causes	Infection Stroke Neoplasia
Lung causes	Infection Tumour
Oncological causes	Lung cancer—commonest Prostate, GI tract, haematological malignancies
Drugs	↑ H₂O permeability of nephron, e.g. vasopressin ↑ ADH release, e.g. carbamazepine ↑ ADH action, e.g. cyclophosphamide ↓ Prostaglandin synthesis e.g. aspirin

ingly lower sodium is usually effective and tolerable. Demeclocycline (which inhibits the action of ADH on the distal tubule) may be used if these simple manoeuvres are ineffective.

Hypernatraemia

Hypernatraemia is defined as a serum sodium > 145 mmol/L caused by a relative water deficit and the major defence against it is thirst. It therefore occurs more commonly in patients who are unable to increase their water intake. As for hyponatraemia, the causes can be grouped into three categories depending on volume status.
1 Hypovolaemia (low body sodium with loss of water exceeding that of Na⁺).
2 Normovolaemia (normal body Na⁺ but water loss).
3 Hypervolaemia (increased total body Na⁺).

As with hyponatraemia, assessment of volume status and determination of urinary sodium are central to the diagnostic approach.

Common causes
• Fluid (water) deprivation, particularly in elderly people
• Hyperosmolar diabetic coma

Management
The underlying cause requires identification and correction. In patients with hypovolaemia, the volume deficit should be corrected with physiological saline until haemodynamics are normalized and then water may be required. In hypervolaemic hypernatraemia, the excess sodium requires removal, often with diuretics. In euvolaemic hypernatraemia, water is given intravenously as 5% dextrose. In all cases, careful monitoring of volume status and serum sodium concentration is necessary and correction of Na⁺ should be made at a rate of less than 0.5 mmol/L per h.

Diabetes insipidus is characterized by polyuria and polydipsia and is the result of defects in ADH action. It can produce hypernatraemia and is discussed in greater detail in Chapter 149.

Diseases and Treatments at a Glance

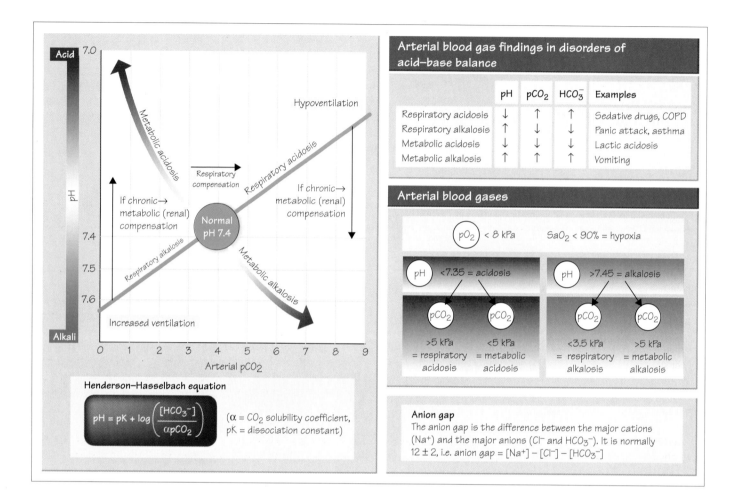

Henderson–Hasselbach equation

$$pH = pK + \log\left(\frac{[HCO_3^-]}{\alpha pCO_2}\right)$$

(α = CO_2 solubility coefficient, pK = dissociation constant)

Arterial blood gas findings in disorders of acid–base balance

	pH	pCO$_2$	HCO$_3^-$	Examples
Respiratory acidosis	↓	↑	↑	Sedative drugs, COPD
Respiratory alkalosis	↑	↓	↓	Panic attack, asthma
Metabolic acidosis	↓	↓	↓	Lactic acidosis
Metabolic alkalosis	↑	↑	↑	Vomiting

Anion gap

The anion gap is the difference between the major cations (Na$^+$) and the major anions (Cl$^-$ and HCO$_3^-$). It is normally 12 ± 2, i.e. anion gap = [Na$^+$] − [Cl$^-$] − [HCO$_3^-$]

In many ill patients important acid–base disturbances occur. They may lack specific symptoms, and in any seriously ill patient arterial blood gases should be determined. The type of acid–base disturbance can be determined from the pH and PCO$_2$ (see figure).

Metabolic acidosis

Metabolic acidosis is seen most commonly in diabetic ketoacidosis, lactic acidosis and renal failure. The presence of a significant metabolic acidosis is important and requires urgent diagnosis and treatment. It can be grouped into four major categories by aetiology:

1 Ingestion of acid, such as salicylate, methanol or ethylene glycol poisoning.

2 Accumulation of endogenous acids, such as lactic acid in tissue hypoperfusion or ketones in diabetic ketoacidosis.

3 Loss of alkali in severe diarrhoea, with biliary or enteric fistulae or renal loss in proximal renal tubular acidosis.

4 Failure of elimination of acid in renal failure and distal tubular acidosis.

Severe acidosis results in cardiac depression and death.

The anion gap can be useful in the diagnosis of metabolic acidoses. The anion gap is the difference between the major cation (sodium) and the major measured anions (chloride and bicarbonate). It is normally 12

$\pm$ 2. An elevated anion gap suggests the presence of additional anions such as lactate (in lactic acidosis) or ketones (in diabetic ketoacidosis), whereas a normal or reduced anion gap (or hyperchloraemic acidosis) suggests bicarbonate loss or renal tubular acidosis (Tables 128.1 and 128.2).

Table 128.1 Anion gap and metabolic acidosis.

Anion gap	Disease
Normal (=hyperchloraemic acidosis)	Renal tubular acidosis Extrarenal HCO$_3^-$ loss Hyperparathyroidism Hypoaldosteronism $\pm$ Diabetic ketoacidosis
Increased (> 20 mmol/L)	Renal parenchymal disease Ingestion of acid Acid metabolized from endogenous substances Lactic acidosis $\pm$ Diabetic ketoacidosis

Diabetic ketoacidosis may give rise to either normal or high anion gap acidosis

Table 128.2 Causes of lactic acidosis.

Mechanism	Disease
Increased rate of lactate production	Any cause of decreased tissue perfusion Hypoxia Increased skeletal muscle activity (e.g. status epilepticus or marathon runners) Destruction of large tumour masses (e.g. lymphoma or leukaemia) Poisoning (e.g. CO or cyanide)
Decreased lactate transport	Decreased cardiac output due to any cause
Decreased lactate metabolism	Liver failure (any cause) Intoxication (phenformin or alcohol) Diabetes mellitus Liver hypoxia
Miscellaneous	Haemofiltration with lactate buffer Pregnancy

Traditionally lactic acidosis is divided into type A (clinical evidence of poor tissue perfusion/oxygenation) and type B (no clinical evidence of poor tissue perfusion/oxygenation). B1 associated with underlying diseases. B2 due to drugs and toxins. B3 due to inborn errors of metabolism.

The body will usually respond to the acidaemia with respiratory compensation, an increase in respiratory rate causing a fall in carbon dioxide, which in turn increases the blood pH. Metabolic acidosis may be associated with the signs or symptoms of the precipitating cause, the increased rate and depth of respiration, sometimes described as Kussmaul's respiration, or if severe it may itself be associated with the signs of shock.

The treatment should be directed towards reversing the underlying cause. In exceptional circumstances sodium bicarbonate may be administered and haemodialysis or haemofiltration used.

Metabolic alkalosis

Metabolic alkalosis rarely gives rise to symptoms from the alkalosis alone. The aetiologies of metabolic alkalosis include:

- Loss of acid such as in vomiting, particularly with pyloric stenosis.
- Increased renal loss of bicarbonate which can occur with hyperaldosteronism or severe hypokalaemia.
- Excess intake of alkali (e.g. the milk–alkali syndrome, where large quantities of alkaline antacids are ingested, often with milk).

There may be respiratory compensation with a reduction in respiratory rate, a rise in carbon dioxide and a fall in pH.

Treatment involves the identification and treatment of the underlying cause.

Respiratory acidosis (see also Chapter 88)

The primary control of ventilation is achieved by monitoring of blood pH by the respiratory centre, and appropriate changes in ventilatory rate to alter the blood partial pressure of carbon dioxide, which in turn leads to changes in blood pH. The development of respiratory acidosis is a concern and may indicate the need for ventilatory support.

A reduction in ventilation leads to an accumulation of carbon dioxide and the development of acidosis. This may be the result of a wide variety of causes of ventilatory impairment and commonly include:

- Sedation, particularly with opiates.
- Respiratory muscle weakness, e.g. Guillain–Barré syndrome, poliomyelitis or myasthenia gravis.
- Severe chronic obstructive pulmonary disease.

The accumulation of carbon dioxide can sometimes be associated with clinical signs, which include a bounding pulse, papilloedema or a metabolic flap. If the carbon dioxide retention has been chronic, there may be metabolic renal compensation with an elevated blood bicarbonate concentration.

Treatment usually involves attempts to improve the underlying ventilatory defect. Rarely respiratory stimulants may be used, whereas in particular patients with acute ventilatory failure artificial ventilation may be appropriate.

Respiratory alkalosis

This arises as a consequence of increased ventilation causing the partial pressure of carbon dioxide in the blood to fall, with a resultant rise in blood pH. The causes include:

- A response to hypoxaemia or tissue hypoxia.
- Increased ventilation, e.g. in panic attacks.
- Excessive artificial ventilation.
- Stimulation of respiration by drugs, central nervous system stimulation or pulmonary disease in which there is stimulation of chest receptors.

The fall in carbon dioxide and rise in pH can be associated with a fall in ionized calcium which can produce symptoms of peripheral and circumoral paraesthesia, light-headedness and carpopedal spasm. Chvostek's sign may be present (tapping of the facial nerve elicits brief facial muscle contraction, reflecting latent hypocalcaemic tetany).

Treatment is directed towards ensuring that there is correction of any concomitant hypoxaemia and reversal of the underlying cause.

Mixed acid–base disorders

The ability of the body to compensate for pH disturbances with respiratory or metabolic compensations and the presence of more than one cause of acid–base disturbance in a particular patient can produce complex disturbances. In such cases a detailed history, complete examination, consideration of the blood gases and determination of the anion gap are critical in establishing the correct diagnosis.

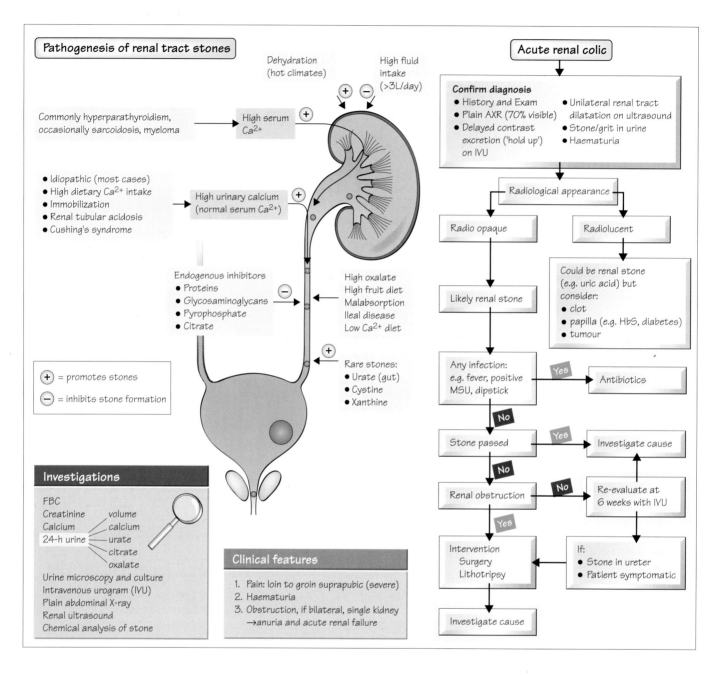

Urinary calculi are very common, with a prevalence of 2%. There is a peak prevalence at age 30–40 years and a 3 : 1 male predisposition. Most calculi contain calcium oxalate; the remainder consists of mixed calcium and ammonium phosphate (usually caused by infection), urate, cystine and xanthine stones.

Aetiology

Most calculi are idiopathic; the remainder may be associated with hypercalciuria, hypercalcaemia, recurrent urinary tract infection (UTI), hyperuricosuria or cystinuria. Urinary calculi form when urinary solutes exceed their maximum urinary solubility. Conditions producing excretion of a high solute load or reduced urine volume will promote

calculus formation (see Table 129.1). Urine is usually supersaturated for some solutes and crystallization inhibitors such as citrate tend to prevent calculus formation.

Presentation

Urinary calculi can cause haematuria (both macroscopic and microscopic), loin pain, renal colic, suprapubic pain, dysuria, UTIs, urinary tract obstruction, and acute or chronic renal failure as a result of obstruction ± infection. The pain of renal colic may be excruciating and commonly localizes to the flank, although radiation to the anterior abdomen, groin or scrotum can occur.

Table 129.1 Conditions predisposing to renal stones.

Metabolic syndromes
Hypercalciuria: present in 70% of renal stones
Hyperoxaluria: idiopathic, genetic (type I or II) or secondary to GI disease
Hypocitraturia: distal renal tubular acidosis, K^+ depletion, renal failure
   Chronic hypercalcaemia: usually hyperparathyroidism
   Rare genetic metabolic diseases (e.g. cystinuria, etc.)
Repeated infection
Concentrated urine
Chronically low fluid intake (< 2 L/day)/high insensible losses (e.g. in hot
   countries)
Structural abnormality
Renal tract obstruction (e.g. sloughed papilla, prostate, neurogenic
   bladder)
Nephrocalcinosis
   Renal tubular acidosis (distal—type 1)

Investigations

- Full blood count (FBC) to exclude the very rare association with haematological malignancies (urate stones).
- Creatinine, urea, electrolytes, plasma calcium and urate.
- 24-h urine collection for urine volume, calcium, urate, citrate and oxalate.
- Urine microscopy and culture because recurrent UTIs may be the cause or consequence of urinary calculi.
- Intravenous urogram (IVU), renal tract ultrasonography and plain abdominal X-ray to exclude obstruction and demonstrate the position of calculi.
- Chemical analysis of calculi.

Imaging of calculi

- **Ultrasonography**: 20% sensitivity, 97% specificity. Accessible, good for diagnosing hydronephrosis and renal stones, requires no ionising radiation. Poor at visualizing ureteral stones.
- **Plain radiography** is 50% sensitive, 75% specific. Accessible and inexpensive. Problems: stones in the middle section of the ureter, phleboliths, radiolucent calculi, extra-urinary calcifications and non-genitourinary conditions.
- **Intravenous pyelography** is 65% sensitive and 90% specific. Advantages: accessible. Provides information on anatomy and functioning of both kidneys. Problems: variable-quality imaging, requires bowel preparation and use of contrast media, poor visualization of non-genitourinary conditions, delayed images required in high-grade obstruction.
- **Non-contrast helical computed tomography**: 95% sensitive, 95% specific. Advantage: most sensitive and specific radiological test (i.e. facilitates fast, definitive diagnosis). Provides information on non-genitourinary conditions. Problems: indirect signs of the degree of obstruction, less accessible and relatively expensive, no direct measure of renal function.

Management

Renal colic can be particularly painful, so adequate analgesia is important, often requiring non-steroidal anti-inflammatory drugs (NSAIDs) and/or opiate analgesia. Fluid intake should be increased to > 3 L/day. Surgical treatment (required in 20%) of calculi or extra-corporeal shock wave lithotripsy, where ultrasonic energy sufficient to fragment the calculus is transmitted from a probe placed on the skin over the renal tract, may prove necessary if the calculus is causing renal obstruction, particularly if infection is present. Renal failure (anuria) can occur if ureteric obstruction to a sole remaining kidney occurs. This is a medical emergency and requires immediate diagnosis and treatment.

Prevention

General measures include increasing endogenous inhibitors of stone formation, by giving oral potassium citrate, lemon juice and avoiding low potassium diets. Specific preventive treatments include:
- **Infection** associated with stones: prophylactic antibiotics.
- **Hypercalciuria**: the amount of calcium in the urine can be lessened with thiazide diuretics, and by reducing the amount of sodium in the diet. The relationship between a high protein diet and an excess incidence of upper renal tract stones may be explained by dietary protein increasing renal calcium excretion.
- **Urate calculi**: both gouty and calcium oxalate renal stones can be prevented with allopurinol. In oxalate stones, the amount of oxalate in the diet (e.g. rhubarb or spinach) should be reduced.
- **Phosphate stones**: the urine should be acidified with ammonium chloride to decrease progression.
- **Oxalate stones**: increasing dietary vitamin B_6 intake decreases urinary oxalate.
- **Cystinuria** is treated with urinary alkalinization, or dissolution with penicillamine (although side effects limit its use).

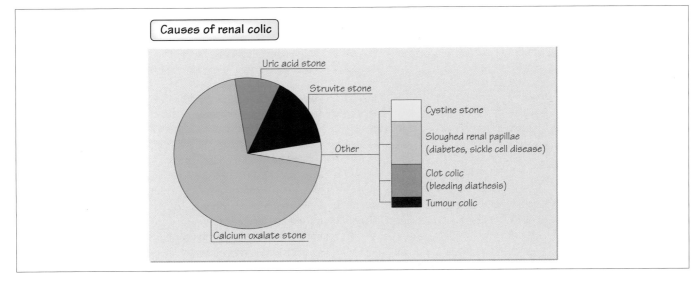

Causes of renal colic

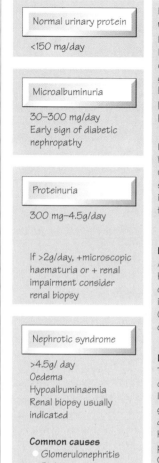

Normal urinary protein

<150 mg/day

Microalbuminuria

30–300 mg/day
Early sign of diabetic
nephropathy

Proteinuria

300 mg–4.5g/day

If >2g/day, +microscopic
haematuria or + renal
impairment consider
renal biopsy

Nephrotic syndrome

>4.5g/ day
Oedema
Hypoalbuminaemia
Renal biopsy usually
indicated

Common causes
● Glomerulonephritis
● Diabetes
● Amyloid

Histology in glomerulonephritis associated with the nephrotic syndrome

Normal kidney
Normal electron micrograph of the foot processes of the glomerular endothelial cells; beautiful discrete foot processes are seen on the podocytes

Minimal change disease
Whereas in minimal changes GN, the light microscope shows no change, the EM image shows fusion of the foot processes

Lupus nephritis
A large number of different histological appearances occur in lupus nephritis – this image shows staining for the C1q component of complement.

Diabetic glomerular damage
This image shows the characteristic sclerotic lesions found in diabetic glomerular damage. Early on, diabetes leads to glomerular hyperfiltration; later proteinuria and decreases in GFR occur, often culminating in renal failure with the nephrotic syndrome

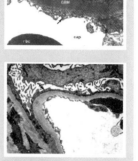

Cause of proteinuria as related to quantity	
Daily protein excretion	Cause
0.15 to 2.0 g	Mild glomerulopathies
	Tubular proteinuria
	Overflow proteinuria
2.0 to 4.0 g	Usually glomerular
>4.0 g	Always glomerular

From McConnell KR, Bia MJ. Evaluation of proteinuria: an approach for the internist. *Resident Staff Phys* 1994; 40:41-8

Features of the nephrotic syndrome

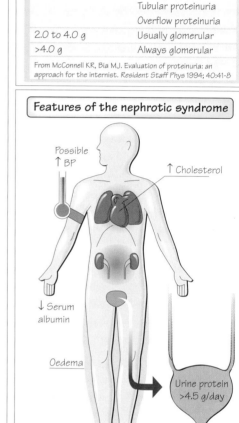

Possible ↑ BP

↑ Cholesterol

↓ Serum albumin

Oedema

Urine protein >4.5 g/day

Proteinuria and nephrotic syndrome

The normal amount of protein in urine is < 150 mg/day. Most of this is the result of a physiological, rather viscous glycoprotein that is secreted by tubular cells, termed 'Tamm-Horsfall protein'. The presence of higher amounts of protein may indicate significant renal disease, often glomerulonephritis. Dipsticks detect mainly albumin and will not detect pathological proteins, such as immunoglobulin light chains (Bence-Jones protein) in myeloma. Microalbuminuria (urinary albumin excretion 30–300 mg/day) is an early sign of diabetic nephropathy.

In patients with proteinuria, a careful **history and examination** should be performed, looking for causes of renal disease. Hypertension, evidence of renal failure and oedema may be found on examination. Renal function should be assessed with serum creatinine and electrolytes, and a 24-h urine collection performed to determine creatinine clearance and 24-h protein excretion. A 'spot' urine protein : creatinine ratio correlates well with 24-h protein excretion, and can be used as a simple estimate of renal protein loss.

If these results confirm significant proteinuria (see Table 130.1) or renal dysfunction, further investigations should include ultrasonography of the renal tract, and blood glucose (to exclude diabetes, a common cause of the nephrotic syndrome) and immunological investigations to exclude myeloma and autoimmune conditions such as systemic lupus erythematosus (SLE) or systemic vasculitis (anti-nuclear factor [ANF] and anti-neutrophil cytoplasmic antibody [ANCA]). If significant proteinuria is present (> 2 g/day) a renal biopsy may be appropriate to define the cause of the proteinuria.

Levels of proteinuria > 4.5 g in 24 h may produce the **nephrotic syndrome** which is characterized by:
• Proteinuria (usually 3 – 4 + on dipstick testing; 24-h urine excretion of protein is often > 4 g/24 h).
• Hypoalbuminaemia (usually albumin < 30 g/dL).
• Peripheral oedema.
• Unlike the nephritic syndrome (see below), haematuria (either macroscopic or on dipstick testing) is rare and blood pressure is normal or only mildly elevated.

The nephrotic syndrome is usually a consequence of:
• Glomerular disease, commonly glomerulonephritis. The types of glomerulonephritis most commonly found to be responsible for nephrotic

Diseases and Treatments at a Glance

Table 130.1 Classification of proteinuria.

Type	Pathophysiological features	Cause
Glomerular	Increased glomerular capillary permeability to protein	Primary or secondary glomerulopathy
Tubular	Decreased tubular reabsorption of proteins in glomerular filtrate	Tubular or interstitial disease
Overflow	Increased production of low-molecular-weight proteins	Monoclonal gammopathy, leukaemia

Source: Abuelo JG. Proteinuria: diagnostic principles and procedures. *Ann Intern Med* 1983; 98: 186–91.

syndrome on renal biopsy are minimal change disease (overwhelmingly the most likely cause for nephrotic syndrome in childhood), membranous nephropathy and focal segmental glomerulo-sclerosis (FSGS).
• Diabetes.
• Renal amyloid, which may relate to primary or secondary amyloidosis, or multiple myeloma
• Drugs (particularly those used in rheumatology, such as non-steroidal anti-inflammatory agents, penicillamine and gold) are occasionally the cause.
• Other causes include SLE.

Complications of nephrotic syndrome relate in part to the low albumin, and partly to more complex pathophysiological changes induced by the nephrotic condition:
• Oedema is found in dependent sites (i.e. the lower limbs in ambulant and the sacral area in bed-bound patients), but can also be found in the face (e.g. periorbitally) and hands.
• Hypercoagulability may lead to renal vein thrombosis and a dramatic worsening of renal function, or may produce deep venous thrombosis. There is no evidence that prophylactic routine anticoagulation in nephrotic syndrome is indicated.
• Hypercholesterolaemia: may play a large role in the accelerated atheroma that may be found in longstanding nephrotic syndrome. The reason why hypercholesterolaemia occurs is not clear; it may relate to hypersynthesis of apolipoproteins, resulting from the general increase in protein synthesis found in many nephrotic patients.
• Infection: nephrotic syndrome is associated with hypogamma-globulinaemia and impairment of the immune system. Infection, which may be overwhelming, can occur, particularly with pneumococci. Immunization against the pneumococcus should be given.

Treatment of nephrotic syndrome

Any underlying cause should be fully diagnosed and treated with specific therapy. General management includes the use of diuretics to reduce oedema (although their use must be balanced against the possibility of diuretic-induced hypovolaemia, which itself will worsen renal function) and angiotensin-converting enzyme (ACE) inhibitors

may be used to reduce proteinuria and treat hypertension aggressively to slow the progression of renal impairment, particularly in diabetes. If thrombotic episodes occur, anticoagulation may be instituted, whereas hyperlipidaemia commonly requires treatment. Specific treatment exists for certain types of glomerulonephritis, e.g. minimal change disease commonly responds well to corticosteroids. Unfortunately, some diseases are very resistant to treatment, such as the nephrotic syndrome related to renal amyloid.

The nephritic syndrome

Previously this was a widely used term describing an acute renal illness with the following features:
• Haematuria (occasionally macroscopic) and mild proteinuria, i.e. usually only 1–2+ on dipstick testing, which is insufficient to cause a depression in serum albumin, unlike the nephrotic syndrome.
• Inability of the kidney to excrete fluids, leading to fluid retention (oedema), hypertension and occasionally oliguria.
• Decreased glomerular filtration rate, producing varying degrees of uraemia.

This term was used when streptococcal infection was common, because nephritic syndrome not infrequently followed 2–3 weeks after a throat infection with group A β-haemolytic streptococci. The prognosis of post-streptococcal glomerulonephritis is excellent, the need for dialysis in the acute stage is low, and the likelihood of spontaneous and full recovery of renal function is very high. The differential diagnosis of the nephritic syndrome is wide and includes most of the diseases capable of producing glomerulonephritis (see Chapter 131). Immunological tests and a renal biopsy are usually indicated.

Treatment of nephritic syndrome

It is important to treat any underlying cause with specific therapies. Oedema, hypertension and renal impairment should be treated as for the nephrotic syndrome, although as hypertension is more common and more severe, it should be looked for assiduously and treated aggressively with hypotensive drugs (often ACE inhibitors). Dialysis is more likely to be needed for uraemia than in the nephrotic syndrome.

131 Glomerulonephritis

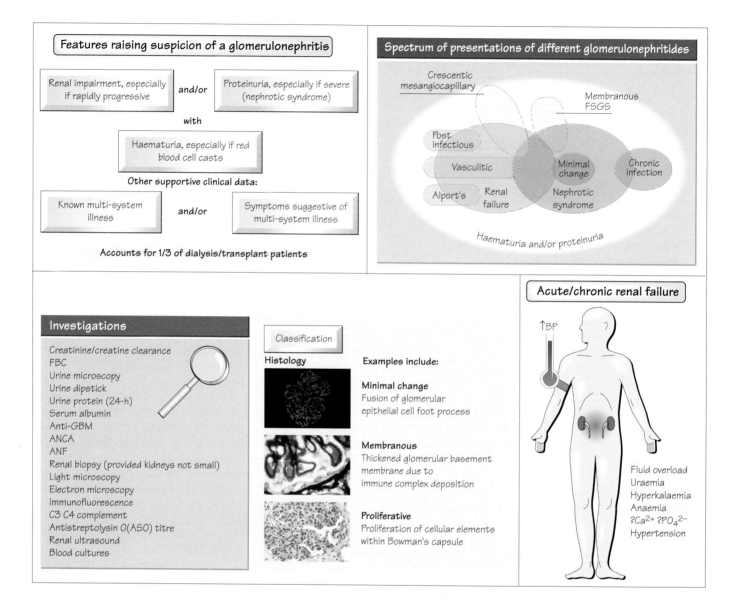

Features raising suspicion of a glomerulonephritis

Renal impairment, especially if rapidly progressive

and/or

Proteinuria, especially if severe (nephrotic syndrome)

with

Haematuria, especially if red blood cell casts

Other supportive clinical data:

Known multi-system illness

and/or

Symptoms suggestive of multi-system illness

Accounts for 1/3 of dialysis/transplant patients

Spectrum of presentations of different glomerulonephritides

Crescentic
mesangiocapillary

Membranous
FSGS

Post infectious

Vasculitic

Minimal change

Chronic infection

Alport's

Renal failure

Nephrotic syndrome

Haematuria and/or proteinuria

Investigations

Creatinine/creatine clearance
FBC
Urine microscopy
Urine dipstick
Urine protein (24-h)
Serum albumin
Anti-GBM
ANCA
ANF
Renal biopsy (provided kidneys not small)
Light microscopy
Electron microscopy
Immunofluorescence
C3 C4 complement
Antistreptolysin O(ASO) titre
Renal ultrasound
Blood cultures

Classification

Histology

Examples include:

Minimal change
Fusion of glomerular epithelial cell foot process

Membranous
Thickened glomerular basement membrane due to immune complex deposition

Proliferative
Proliferation of cellular elements within Bowman's capsule

Acute/chronic renal failure

↑BP

Fluid overload
Uraemia
Hyperkalaemia
Anaemia
?Ca^{2+} ?PO$_4$$^{2-}$
Hypertension

Glomerulonephritis (GN) can present in a variety of ways: 1) acute or chronic renal failure; 2) the nephrotic syndrome (oedema, proteinuria and hypoalbuminaemia); 3) haematuria; 4) proteinuria and hypertension.

It accounts for the cause of renal failure in up to one-third of patients requiring dialysis or transplantation. The cardinal features of glomerular abnormalities are:
1) proteinuria 2) haematuria 3) urinary casts.

Glomerulonephritis affects both kidneys symmetrically. The disease may affect primarily the kidneys (primary GN) or be associated with systemic illnesses such as Wegener's granulomatosis, systemic lupus erythematosus (SLE) and other vasculitides (secondary GN). The type of glomerulonephritis is usually established by renal biopsy (light microscopy, immunofluorescence and electron microscopy). The different histological types of glomerulonephritis (see figure) each have a different spectrum of presentation, and vary in their prognosis and response to treatment.

Acute glomerulonephritis

A confusing aspect of glomerular disease is that many different histological subtypes can produce the same clinical syndrome and, conversely, that each histological form can produce different clinical patterns. It is therefore usual to classify glomerulonephritis in terms of both the clinical syndrome and the pathological diagnosis. The different pathological forms underlying the different clinical syndromes are:
• **Acute renal failure**: glomerulonephritis can underlie acute renal failure, when it is termed 'rapidly progressive glomerulonephritis' (RPGN). This is usually characterized by the presence of crescents (a crescentic-shaped proliferation of cells in Bowman's capsule) and is most commonly seen with the glomerulonephritis associated with the vasculitic conditions such as Wegener's granulomatosis, Goodpasture's syndrome (acute renal failure and pulmonary haemorrhage caused by a circulating anti-glomerular basement membrane antibody) and post-infectious glomerulonephritis after a streptococcal infection.

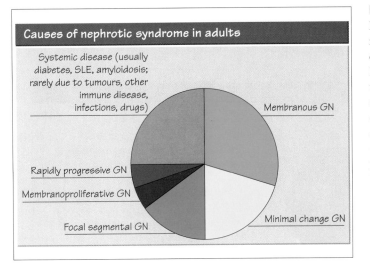
Time is of the essence, because many patients progress from normal renal function to dialysis-dependent renal failure within days, and RPGN is therefore a medical emergency. Early aggressive treatment often stabilizes or improves renal function, whereas late (i.e. occurring by the time renal support is needed, or when the patient is oliguric) treatment is usually much less effective.

• **Nephrotic syndrome**: the most common causes of nephrotic syndrome in adults are shown in the figure.

Renal histology

• **In membranous GN** the light microscopic appearances are of a thickened basement membrane, which on electron microscopy is the result of numerous subepithelial immune complex deposits of IgG and complement C3. Although usually idiopathic, it can be secondary to underlying malignancy in 10% of cases, and can relate to SLE, drugs or infections.

• **In minimal change glomerulonephritis**, light microscope and immunological studies are normal, but podocyte foot processes are fused on electron microscopy. Focal segmental glomerulosclerosis (FSGS) is similar, except some glomeruli have segmental sclerotic lesions.

• The renal histology in **incidental haematuria and/or proteinuria** varies. The most common finding at renal biopsy is of IgA nephropathy (Berger's disease). Clinically, patients often have marked haematuria after upper respiratory tract infections. Histologically, the condition is characterized by mesangial deposition of IgA with variable segmental mesangial proliferation. Although most patients have a benign prognosis, 20–40% of patients progress to renal failure. IgA nephropathy also occurs in people with longstanding alcohol problems who have liver disease, although rarely is it of clinical importance.

Chronic glomerulonephritis

Patients presenting with chronic renal failure may have small, shrunken kidneys on ultrasonography and chronic fibrotic changes with glomerulosclerosis on biopsy. The disease underlying the renal failure is then presumed to be a glomerulonephritis, particularly if there is a history of previous proteinuria or haematuria. The process is usually burnt out and does not respond to any treatment. Renal biopsy does not usually alter treatment and is contraindicated when small kidneys are found in view of the risks posed by renal biopsy.

Management

Important **investigations** in a patient with suspected glomerulonephritis include assessment of renal function with serum creatinine and creatinine clearance, urine dipstick and microscopy examining particularly for red cells and casts, 24-h urinary protein excretion and renal ultrasonography for renal size. Significant proteinuria (> 1 g/day) is strongly suggestive of a glomerulonephritis. Immunological tests are essential in establishing whether the glomerulonephritis is secondary and should include antineutrophil cytoplasmic antibodies (ANCA) (Wegener's granulomatosis—p. 262), antinuclear factor (ANF), complement C3 and C4 (SLE—p. 263), anti-glomerular basement membrane (anti-GBM) antibodies (Goodpasture's syndrome—p. 262) and anti-streptolysin O (ASO) titre (poststreptococcal GN). Renal biopsy is necessary to establish an accurate diagnosis; however, this will not usually be undertaken if the kidneys are small (see above).

The **treatment** of glomerulonephritis depends on the precise type:

• In minimal change glomerulonephritis, corticosteroid treatment can often produce remission. Half of adult patients relapse once after initial remission: a second course of steroids is then indicated. Further relapses or failure to induce remission are indications for more aggressive immunosuppression.

• The prognosis in membranous GN is variable. At 10 years, 25% have remitted spontaneously, 25% have persistent non-nephrotic proteinuria, 25% have nephrotic proteinuria and 25% have renal failure. In those with deteriorating renal function, regimens including steroids and chlorambucil (Ponticelli regimen) are beneficial. Drug-induced membranous GN may remit after drug cessation.

• In rapidly progressive glomerulonephritis, more aggressive immunosuppressive regimens are commonly advocated and include corticosteroids, cyclophosphamide and plasmapheresis.

In GN, aggressive blood pressure treatment can reduce the speed of disease progression, control of lipids is important and nephrotoxic drugs should be avoided.

Renal consequences of immune complex deposition

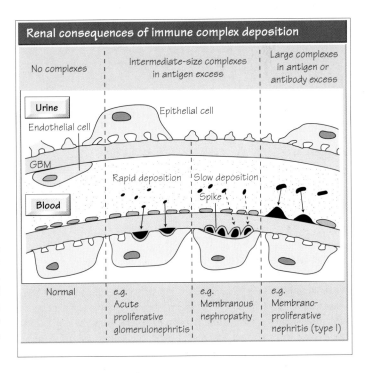

Diseases and Treatments at a Glance

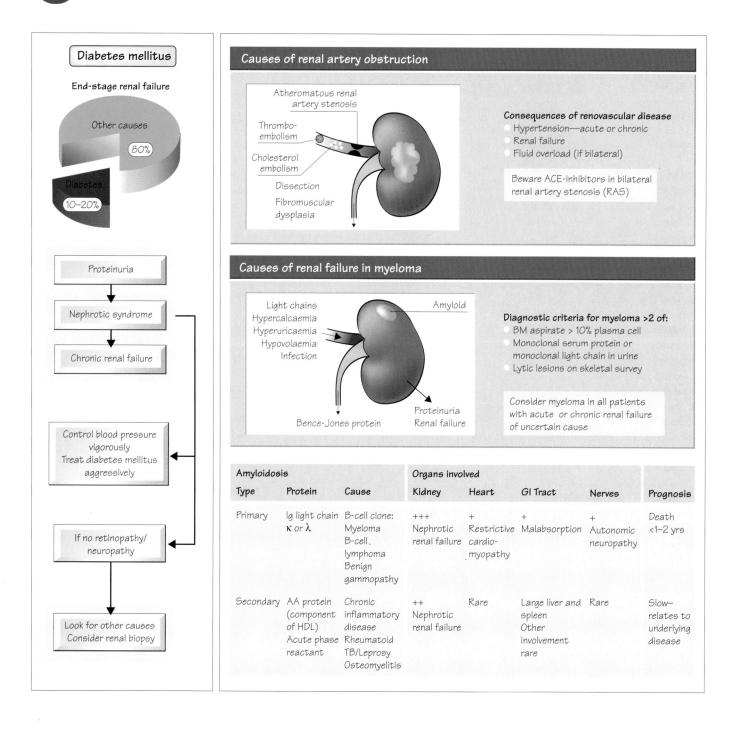

Diabetes mellitus

Diabetes mellitus causes renal disease; the incidence increases with longer duration of disease, with 30% having nephropathy 20 years after diagnosis. It accounts for 10% of patients on renal replacement therapy. The initial diabetic renal lesion is manifest as microalbuminuria, which progresses to increasing levels of proteinuria or even nephrotic syndrome. There may be a gradual loss of excretory function manifest as rising creatinine and urea. Patients with diabetic nephropathy commonly suffer from diabetic retinopathy or neuropathy. If absent, this should prompt a search for alternative causes of renal impairment or nephrotic syndrome. If doubt remains about whether the renal dysfunction is attributable to diabetes, a renal biopsy should be performed.

In diabetes, very aggressive blood pressure lowering, often with angiotensin-converting enzyme (ACE) inhibitors and/or angiotensin II receptor blockers (ARBs), can slow the progression of the renal disease. Similarly, excellent glycaemic control may reduce the development and progression of renal disease.

Myeloma

Myeloma commonly produces renal impairment. In patients with acute or chronic renal impairment of unknown cause, myeloma should be considered in the differential diagnosis and protein electrophoresis (for paraproteinaemia), urine electrophoresis (for Bence-Jones proteins) and immunoglobulin estimations undertaken. Renal impairment in myeloma has several causes, including the direct toxicity of Ig light chains to the tubular cells, hypercalcaemia, dehydration, hyperuricaemia, renal amyloid, hyperviscosity and infection. Treatment involves that of the underlying myeloma and rapid correction of hypovolaemia and hypercalcaemia. Plasma exchange has a role in rapidly removing myeloma protein in some patients with renal failure.

Amyloidosis

Amyloidosis is characterized by the deposition of protein fibrils in many organs including the kidney. It may be primary in association with myeloma (amyloid AL) or secondary to chronic infections or inflammation (amyloid AA). The most common renal presentation is with proteinuria, often sufficient to produce the nephrotic syndrome. Renal biopsy demonstrates an eosinophilic tissue infiltration which stains positive with Congo red and exhibits green birefringence under polarized light. The prognosis for renal function is poor.

Haemolytic/uraemic syndrome

This syndrome is characterized by haemolysis and acute renal failure. It may be associated with diarrhoea, particularly in children, when *Escherichia coli* serotype O157 produces verocytotoxin which causes endothelial damage. Investigations reveal haemolysis, thrombocytopenia and renal failure. Renal biopsy shows fibrin thrombi occluding glomerular tufts. In the diarrhoea-associated disease, spontaneous remission is common but in severe forms plasmapheresis is often advocated.

Renovascular disease

There are two pathologies causing renovascular disease:
1 Atherosclerotic renal artery stenosis: this presents with hypertension, renal impairment or, if bilateral, fluid overload manifesting as pulmonary oedema. A renal bruit may rarely be audible and renal ultrasonography may show small or asymmetrical kidneys. Renal angiography or magnetic resonance angiography can demonstrate the stenosis. Cardiovascular risk factors should be treated. Angioplasty and/or stenting has a variable effect on subsequent renal function and hypertension; they are reserved for patients with resistant hypertension or deteriorating renal function. Obstruction of renal blood flow can also occur with embolism of the renal arteries or renal artery dissection, and classically presents with loin pain and impairment of renal function. Atherosclerosis of intrarenal vessels may occur with or without real artery stenosis and contribute to renal impairment and hypertension.
2 Fibromuscular dysplasia: produces a beaded appearance of the renal artery on angiography, occurs more commonly in younger females and is an important cause of hypertension.

Renal vasculitis

The UK prevalence of systemic vasculitis affecting the kidney is 10 000.

Wegener's granulomatosis

This rare condition (600 new cases/year) is characterized by granulomatous disease of the upper airway (including nose, sinuses, trachea), the lung and renal impairment resulting from a focal necrotizing glomerulonephritis. It is part of the differential diagnosis in patients with upper airway disease, lung masses or rapidly progressive glomerulonephritis. If suspected, an antineutrophil cytoplasmic antibody (ANCA) test should be performed, where the pattern of staining of the cytoplasmic components of neutrophils after applying serum IgG antibodies is studied. Two patterns of staining are found: one where staining is principally cytoplasmic (cANCA—the antigen is principally a proteinase) and the other where staining is principally perinuclear (pANCA—the antigen is predominantly myeloperoxidase). Although both forms of ANCA are occasionally found in normal individuals, especially elderly people, both are also associated with disease: pANCA is found in microscopic polyangiitis (see below) and cANCA is positive in over 90% of cases of Wegener's granulomatosis, in which its titre can reflect disease activity. A renal biopsy shows a focal necrotizing glomerulonephritis, sometimes with crescent formation and granuloma. Treatment should be prompt because patients can deteriorate rapidly and is aggressive immunosuppression; corticosteroids, cyclophosphamide, plasmapheresis.

Microscopic polyangiitis

This rare vasculitis (400 cases/year UK) produces inflammation of small blood vessels and can present with multi-system or single-organ involvement. The kidneys, skin, brain and nerves are the most common organs affected. Rapidly progressive renal impairment can result. Testing for ANCA usually reveals a positive staining with a perinuclear pattern (pANCA). Treatment is as for Wegener's granulomatosis.

Table 132.1 Renal vasculitis.

	Incidence	F : M	Organ involvement						Diagnostic test	Treatment
			Kidney	Lung	Heart	Skin	URT/ Sinus	GI tract		
Goodpasture's syndrome	±	1 : 1	+++	+++	0	0	0	0	GBM antibody	St, CyP, PE
Microscopic polyarteritis	+	1 : 1	+++	+	0	+	0	+	pANCA	St, CyP, PE
Churg–Strauss syndrome	±	1 : 1	++	+++	++	++	++	0	Eosinophils/CXR	St
Henoch–Schönlein purpura	+++	1 : 2	+	0	0	+++	0	++	None	None
Wegener's granulomatosis	+(+)	1 : 2	+++	++	0	0	+++	0	cANCA	St, CyP, PE
SLE	++	9 : 1	++	+	+	++	+	+	Anti-dsDNA	St, AM, CyP
Scleroderma	++	4 : 1	+	++	+	+++	0	+++	ANA, Scl-70	ACE inhibitors, None
Cryoglobulinaemia	+	1 : 1	++	0	0	+++	0	0	See text	St, PE

AM, antimalarials (chloroquine); ANA, antinuclear antibodies; ANCA, antineutrophil cytoplasmic antibodies; CyP, cyclophosphamide; CXR, chest X-ray; GI, gastrointestinal; GBM, glomerular basement membrane; PE, plasma exchange; SLE, systemic lupus erythematosus; St, corticosteroids.

Diseases and Treatments at a Glance

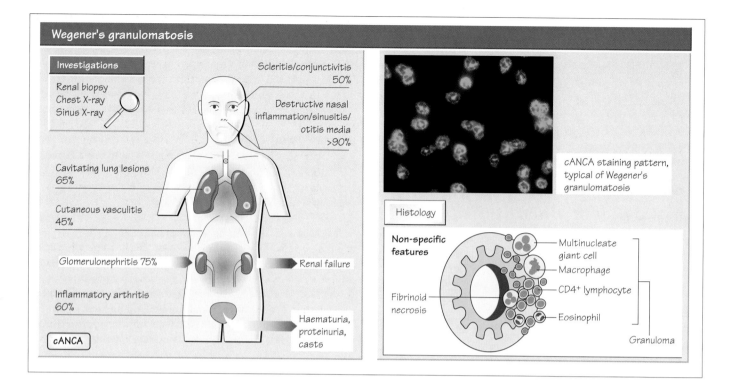

Wegener's granulomatosis

Investigations

Renal biopsy
Chest X-ray
Sinus X-ray

Scleritis/conjunctivitis 50%

Destructive nasal inflammation/sinusitis/otitis media >90%

Cavitating lung lesions 65%

Cutaneous vasculitis 45%

Glomerulonephritis 75% → Renal failure

Inflammatory arthritis 60%

Haematuria, proteinuria, casts

cANCA

cANCA staining pattern, typical of Wegener's granulomatosis

Histology

Non-specific features

Multinucleate giant cell
Macrophage
CD4+ lymphocyte
Eosinophil

Fibrinoid necrosis

Granuloma

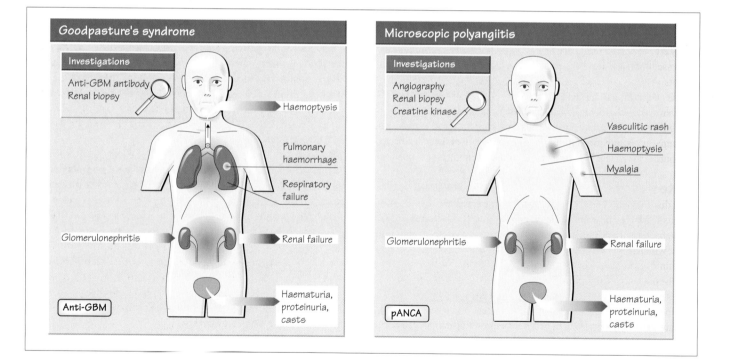

Goodpasture's syndrome

Investigations

Anti-GBM antibody
Renal biopsy

Haemoptysis

Pulmonary haemorrhage

Respiratory failure

Glomerulonephritis → Renal failure

Haematuria, proteinuria, casts

Anti-GBM

Microscopic polyangiitis

Investigations

Angiography
Renal biopsy
Creatine kinase

Vasculitic rash

Haemoptysis

Myalgia

Glomerulonephritis → Renal failure

Haematuria, proteinuria, casts

pANCA

Goodpasture's syndrome

Very rare (50/year). This syndrome is characterized by pulmonary haemorrhage (which is more common in people who smoke), haematuria and rapidly progressive renal failure. It is caused by an autoantibody directed against a collagen found only in basement membrane—the anti-glomerular basement membrane (anti-GBM) antibody. The antibody can be detected in blood. Renal biopsies demonstrate a crescentic glomerulonephritis with linear antibody staining along the GBM on immunofluorescence. Lung function tests may reveal an elevated carbon monoxide transfer factor (K_{CO}), consistent with pulmonary haemorrhage because haemoglobin binds CO very avidly. Treatment; plasmapheresis to remove the antibody, immunosuppression with corticosteroids ± cyclophosphamide to reduce its production.

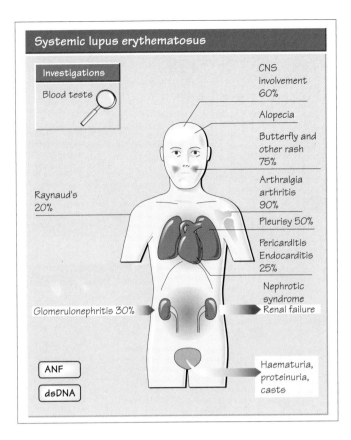

Systemic lupus erythematosus

Investigations

Blood tests

Raynaud's 20%

Glomerulonephritis 30%

ANF

dsDNA

CNS involvement 60%

Alopecia

Butterfly and other rash 75%

Arthralgia arthritis 90%

Pleurisy 50%

Pericarditis Endocarditis 25%

Nephrotic syndrome Renal failure

Haematuria, proteinuria, casts

Polyarteritis nodosa

This vasculitis (incidence 150/year) affects larger blood vessels and presents with non-specific symptoms such as weight loss, fever, malaise and abdominal pain. Arteriography demonstrates micro-aneurysms and arterial narrowing, and biopsies of affected tissue may be diagnostic. ANCA tests are usually negative. There is an association with hepatitis B infection. Renal involvement causes haematuria and proteinuria or with renal impairment. Treatment is immunosuppression.

Systemic lupus erythematosus

Renal disease occurs in half the patients with systemic lupus erythematosus (SLE), with an annual incidence of 3000 patients in the UK. Involvement ranges from mild, with proteinuria and haematuria, to severe, with nephrotic syndrome or rapidly progressive renal failure. In determining the nature of renal involvement urine microscopy is important. The presence of significant haematuria, proteinuria or red cell casts implies a significant glomerular lesion. Renal biopsy is then undertaken to define the glomerular pathology. Several patterns of renal involvement are seen including a focal and segmental proliferative glomeru-

lonephritis (GN), a membranous GN or a diffuse proliferative GN with crescents. The immunology varies: 90% of patients have a positive antinuclear antibody test (i.e. IgG staining of the nucleus, often of discrete nuclear or nucleolar elements). Although antibodies to double-stranded DNA (anti-dsDNA antibodies) are highly specific for SLE, in renal disease their titre may paradoxically be de-pressed. Some 40% have antibodies to extractable nuclear antigens (ENAs, such as Smith Sm or Ro–SS-A). Antibodies to platelets, red cells and phospholipid are also common. There is often complement consumption with lowered levels of C3 and C4. The erythrocyte sedimentation rate (ESR) (but not the C-reactive protein) is elevated. Treatment depends on histology but often involves corticosteroids and immunosuppressive agents such as cyclophosphamide and azathioprine.

Henoch–Schönlein purpura

Although common in children, Henoch-Schönlein purpura is rare in adults (< 300/year). The aetiology is not known, but it may reflect an autoimmune response to an infective agent, which in part explains the seasonal variation and that one-third have a preceding upper respiratory tract infection. Malaise, arthralgia, abdominal pain and, most typically, a purpuric rash on the extensor surfaces (elbows, buttocks, knees) characterize the illness. Renal involvement consists of a usually self-limiting focal GN. Occasionally progressive renal failure occurs.

Scleroderma

Renal involvement complicates 25% of scleroderma, occurs early or late on in the course of the disease, and accounts for 40% of deaths. Incidence is about 200/year. It may present as an active sediment (i.e. haematuria, sometimes severe enough to produce 'red cell casts'), or ominously as a 'scleroderma renal crisis', with treatment-resistant hypertension, rapidly progressive uraemia and characteristic 'onion skin' appearance of blood vessels on renal histology. Immunological tests show antibodies to Scl-70 (the enzyme topoisomerase I) and often to RNA polymerases 1–3. Anti-centromere antibodies are associated with mild cutaneous disease. ACE inhibitor therapy may help.

Cryoglobulinaemia

Cryoglobulins are abnormal immunoglobulins that precipitate when cooled. If this occurs in superficial blood vessels, then obstruction of the vessel and tissue necrosis may occur. Type I cryoglobulins are monoclonal proteins, and found in association with myeloma, Waldenstrom's macroglobulinaemia and lymphoma. Type II cryoglobulins comprise a monoclonal component which has rheumatoid factor activity and binds to normal immunoglobulins. These are found in chronic infections such as hepatitis C, bacterial endocarditis, as well as connective tissue disease and myeloma or lymphoma. Type III cryoglobulins are polyclonal with rheumatoid factor activity and are usually associated with SLE and rheumatoid arthritis.

133 Hereditary renal disorders

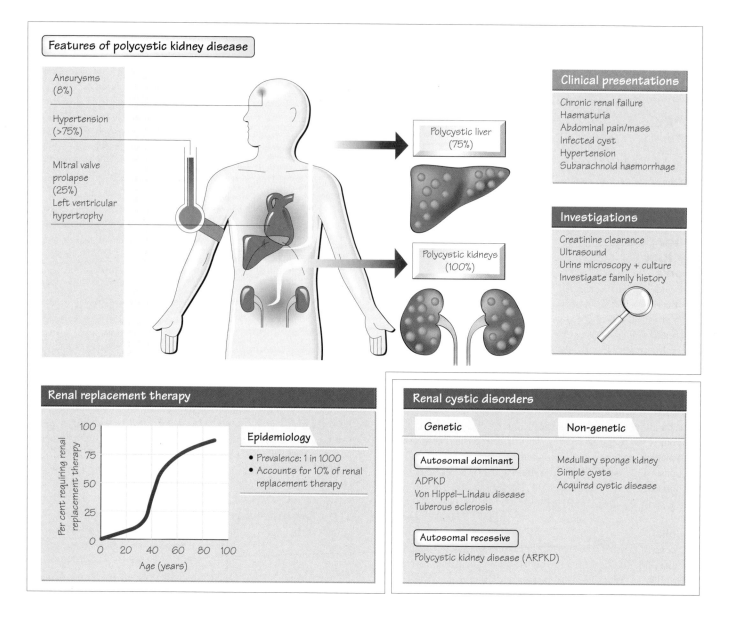

Autosomal dominant polycystic kidney disease

A variety of inherited conditions affect the kidney, but adult polycystic kidney disease (APKD) is by far the most common, affecting 1 in 1000 individuals and accounting for 8–10% of patients with end-stage renal disease. It usually presents in adult life (the rarer autosomal recessive form presents in infancy). Inheritance is autosomal dominant. Children of an affected parent have a 50% chance of inheriting the condition. About 25% of cases are the result of spontaneous mutation. The genetic defect is on chromosome 16 (*PKD1*, which accounts for 95% of cases) or more rarely on chromosome 4 (*PKD2*).

The condition is characterized by a progressive appearance and enlargement of renal cysts. These may bleed, producing haematuria and loin pain, or may become infected. As the cysts gradually enlarge, there is a slowly progressive and inexorable decline in renal function.

Patients may also present with abdominal masses, hypertension and chronic renal failure, and subarachnoid haemorrhages occur in some 10% as a result of the associated berry aneurysms that affect intracranial arteries. Polycystic kidneys may be found incidentally on ultrasonography during investigations for other indications. Cysts also occur in the liver, pancreas, spleen and ovaries, although these rarely cause clinical problems.

Investigations

The condition is usually suspected from the clinical features and family history and confirmed with ultrasonography or computed tomography (CT). Renal function should be determined with serum creatinine, and creatinine clearance and urinary infection excluded.

There are no specific treatments to slow the disease progression—as usual it is important to control any hypertension. Infections require appropriate antibiotic treatment and pain caused by haemorrhage may require analgesia. As renal failure progresses, renal replacement therapy with dialysis or transplantation is required, at a mean age in *PKD1* of 55–60 years. Sometimes nephrectomy is required to permit space so that peritoneal dialysis or transplantation can be undertaken. Genetic counselling is important and screening of children of affected individuals should be delayed until cysts are identifiable on ultrasonography—usually > 18 years unless there is renal impairment or hypertension.

Simple cysts

These become increasingly common with age and can be detected in > 12% of individuals aged over 50 years. They are usually asymptomatic and are detected incidentally. It is important to distinguish them from the multiple cysts of APKD, other cystic diseases and renal cell carcinoma. On ultrasonography simple cysts have smooth walls and no intracystic debris. If doubt exists then CT scanning is necessary.

Other inherited disorders affecting the kidney

Alport's syndrome

This syndrome is characterized by haematuria, sensorineural deafness (overt in 40%), and progressive renal impairment with proteinuria and ocular abnormalities in 15%. It is caused by mutations in the basement membrane type IV collagen gene (most commonly) *COL4A5*; 20% are the result of new mutations. It is X-linked in 80% of patients, producing a more severe phenotype in males. The diagnosis is confirmed on renal biopsy, where thickening and splitting of the glomerular basement membrane on electron microscopy is found. End-stage renal failure (ESRF), i.e. disease requiring dialysis, develops usually between 16 and 35 years of age in virtually all affected males with X-linked Alport's syndrome, and males and females with the autosomally inherited form. Transplantation, although not contraindicated, can rarely result in a Goodpasture's disease-like syndrome caused by the immunological reaction to the previously 'unseen' type IV collagen in the transplanted kidney.

Medullary sponge kidney

This condition, which is often inherited, is characterized by dilated medullary collecting ducts and can affect both, one or part of one kidney. It is often asymptomatic, but small calculi can form which may produce haematuria and predispose to urinary tract infection, or larger calculi may produce obstruction. Renal failure is rare. The diagnosis is established by intravenous urogram (IVU) which shows a typical blush-like opacity in the medulla corresponding to accumulation of contrast in the dilated collecting ducts.

Tuberous sclerosis

In this rare (1–2/100 000) autosomal dominant condition, tumour-like malformations called hamartomas develop in the CNS (often causing learning disorders and epilepsy) and produce skin lesions including facial angiofibromas and hypomelanotic macules, and the kidneys can develop angiomyolipomas, cysts and renal malignancies.

von Hippel–Lindau syndrome

This is a very rare autosomal dominantly inherited condition characterized by tumours affecting the kidney (renal cell carcinoma), the brain (haemangioblastomas) and the adrenals (phaeochromocytoma). Occasionally bilateral nephrectomy for tumours leads to the patient requiring dialysis. Mutations in the von Hippel–Lindau (VHL) gene are also commonly found in cells from patients with sporadic renal cell carcinomas.

Anderson–Fabry disease

This X-linked recessive disorder is the result of mutations in the gene encoding α-galactosidase A. Anderson–Fabry disease results in the intracellular accumulation of glycosphingolipids, which leads to progressive renal failure, autonomic dysfunction and skin lesions called angiokeratomas (dark-red macules or papules). Diagnosis is confirmed by the demonstration of reduced urinary α-galactosidase A. It occurs in two forms, typical Anderson–Fabry disease, where there is no α-galactosidase A activity, and atypical Anderson–Fabry disease, where there is some, albeit greatly reduced α-galactosidase A activity. Patients with typical Anderson–Fabry disease develop symptoms when very young, in many organs, whereas patients with atypical Anderson–Fabry disease develop symptoms later, typically only affecting the heart.

Typical Anderson–Fabry disease

Affects about 1200 patients in the UK. The first symptoms usually occur around the age of 10 years; unfortunately, they are often ignored or misdiagnosed, and in the typical patient the actual diagnosis of Anderson–Fabry disease is not made until 18 years later. Patients can however present at any age: **symptoms in children** include pain (especially of the hands and feet) and painful crises (often starting in the hands and feet, spreading to other parts of the body, lasting minutes to days), angiokeratomas, peripheral vasospasm, and ophthalmological abnormalities. **Later on (ages 10–30 years)** the following can occur: renal dysfunction, fever, reduced sweating, heat sensitivity, exercise intolerance, diarrhoea and abdominal pain, an increase in angiokeratomas. **In later adulthood (age > 30)** the following can occur:

- Heart disease
- Impaired renal function
- Stroke or transient ischaemic episodes
- Epilepsy.

Atypical Anderson–Fabry disease

Affects many 1000s in the UK (maybe 6000–10 000). Atypical Anderson–Fabry disease usually presents in adulthood (20–70 years). It is increasingly recognized; by far the commonest manifestation is left ventricular hypertrophy. Typically, the heart is the only organ affected. **Atypical Anderson–Fabry disease should be considered in all with unexplained LV hypertrophy, especially if LV outflow tract gradient is present.** Indeed, atypical Anderson–Fabry disease may account for some 3% of all cases of LV hypertrophy (and a higher percentage in those suspected of having hypertrophic cardiomyopathy). ECG evidence of LV hypertrophy (sometimes with pre-excitation) is usually present which is confirmed by cardiac ultrasound. Some (1–30%) α-galactosidase A activity is found.

Treatment

To treat, consider α-galactosidase A enzyme replacement therapy.

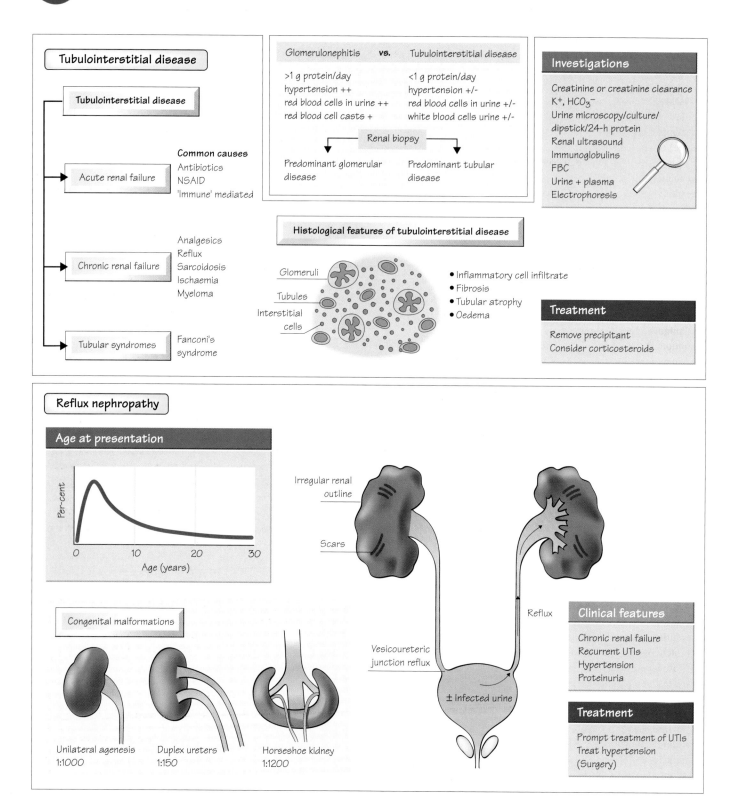

Tubulointerstitial disease

Tubulointerstitial disease

Acute renal failure

Common causes
Antibiotics
NSAID
'Immune' mediated

Chronic renal failure

Analgesics
Reflux
Sarcoidosis
Ischaemia
Myeloma

Tubular syndromes

Fanconi's syndrome

Glomerulonephitis	vs.	Tubulointerstitial disease
>1 g protein/day		<1 g protein/day
hypertension ++		hypertension +/–
red blood cells in urine ++		red blood cells in urine +/–
red blood cell casts +		white blood cells urine +/–

Renal biopsy

Predominant glomerular disease

Predominant tubular disease

Histological features of tubulointerstitial disease

Glomeruli
Tubules
Interstitial cells

• Inflammatory cell infiltrate
• Fibrosis
• Tubular atrophy
• Oedema

Investigations

Creatinine or creatinine clearance
K^+, HCO_3^-
Urine microscopy/culture/dipstick/24-h protein
Renal ultrasound
Immunoglobulins
FBC
Urine + plasma
Electrophoresis

Treatment

Remove precipitant
Consider corticosteroids

Reflux nephropathy

Age at presentation

Per-cent
Age (years)

Irregular renal outline

Scars

Reflux

Vesicoureteric junction reflux

± Infected urine

Congenital malformations

Unilateral agenesis
1:1000

Duplex ureters
1:150

Horseshoe kidney
1:1200

Clinical features

Chronic renal failure
Recurrent UTIs
Hypertension
Proteinuria

Treatment

Prompt treatment of UTIs
Treat hypertension
(Surgery)

Diseases affecting the renal interstitium and tubules can present with renal impairment, proteinuria, haematuria or tubular syndromes and, in some, prominent abnormalities in electrolyte balance. The most common of these conditions is interstitial nephritis which, in its chronic form, accounts for 20% of end-stage renal failure (ESRF) and in its acute form is a common cause of acute renal failure.

Acute interstitial nephritis

Acute inflammation of the renal interstitium is a common consequence of drug hypersensitivity, particularly to antibiotics and non-steroidal anti-inflammatory drugs (NSAIDs). Some 30% of those with drug-induced acute interstitial nephritis (AIN) have fever, rash and eosinophilia. AIN may also relate to infection (leptospirosis, cytomegalovirus, hantavirus).

Cholesterol emboli

Cholesterol emboli can produce renal failure and result when an atheromatous plaque in the aorta ruptures, either spontaneously (in elderly people) or after angiography, with systemic emboli resulting in fever, myalgia, skin rash, retinal emboli (amaurosis fugax), high white blood cell count (WCC) and C-reactive protein (CRP), and a variable decline in renal function.

Chronic interstitial nephritis and chronic pyelonephritis

Chronic interstitial nephritis may present more insidiously with a progressive decline in renal function, small kidneys on ultrasonography, severe electrolyte disturbance, including, in 10–15% of cases, a salt-losing nephropathy leading to sodium depletion and hypotension. Causes include:

- **Analgesics**: analgesic nephropathy requires > 700 g analgesic consumption (often denied), and is four times more common in women than in men. Features include polyuria, mild proteinuria, insidious progressive renal failure, and hypertension in 60%, often complicated by renal papillary necrosis, and renal colic.
- **Reflux nephropathy** (see below), **obstructive uropathy**, either of which may be complicated by infection; when chronic interstitial nephritis results primarily from chronic infection, it is termed 'chronic pyelonephritis'.
- **Primary glomerular disease**.
- **Other causes** (in 15%), include sarcoidosis, ischaemia, hyperuricaemia, myeloma, chronic hypokalaemia. Longstanding hypercalcaemia produces chronic interstitial inflammation, possibly related to calcium salt deposition. Medullary sponge kidney and hyperoxaluria (genetic, high ascorbic acid consumption, longstanding gastrointestinal disease).
- **Chronic poisoning with heavy metals** (lead, cadmium, mercury): common in industrial workers, and especially in certain developing countries, and Chinese herbs (aristolochic acid), which are often found in over-the-counter herbal preparations.

Features that can help distinguish glomerulonephritis from tubulo-interstitial disease are that, in glomerulonephritis, there is usually > 1 g of proteinuria/day, hypertension is more common, casts and red blood cells are found in the urine and, in the renal biopsy (which is the diagnostic test), the glomeruli are primarily affected.

Isolated/specific tubular defects

Other rare disorders exist in which there are specific tubular defects, including distal tubular syndromes such as nephrogenic diabetes insipidus and proximal tubular syndromes (Fanconi's defects) which are often congenital, such as renal tubular acidoses. There may be other tubular defects associated with Fanconi's syndrome resulting in aminoaciduria, glycosuria, phosphaturia and bicarbonaturia.

Investigations and treatment

In investigating the patient in whom interstitial nephritis is suspected, important investigations include examining for peripheral blood eosinophilia (which when present may suggest a drug allergy), immunoglobulins, urine and plasma electrophoresis to exclude myeloma, urine microscopy and culture, renal ultrasonography and renal biopsy.

Treatment consists of removing the precipitating cause. There is no effective treatment for many forms of interstitial nephritis but in others corticosteroids can produce important responses. Spontaneous improvement of interstitial nephritis does occur.

Reflux nephropathy

The vesicoureteric junction normally prevents reflux of urine up the ureter—congenital incompetence at this junction can lead to renal damage. 'Reflux nephropathy' is the term given to the scarred and shrunken kidney with chronic tubulointerstitial nephritis that results. This usually presents during childhood with urinary tract infection, hypertension, proteinuria or renal failure. For unknown reasons, it is more common in females. Urinary tract infection may be important in the genesis of damage by the refluxing urine.

Investigations

Renal function should be assessed, proteinuria quantified and urine culture performed to exclude active infection. Intravenous urograms (IVUs) characteristically show an irregular renal outline with clubbed calyces and kidney size is often reduced. A micturating cystogram can demonstrate vesicoureteric reflux whereas DMSA ($[^{99m}Tc]$mercapto-succinic acid) scanning can reveal scars. A renal biopsy is not usually appropriate but would show chronic tubulointerstitial nephritis.

Treatment

Any acute urinary tract infection should be treated promptly, although in some individuals there may be a role for prophylactic antibiotics. Any associated hypertension should be treated aggressively, asymptomatic infection should be looked for and renal function carefully monitored. The role of surgical ureteric reimplantation to prevent reflux is controversial. There is a strong familial predisposition to reflux and it may be sought in family members.

If there has been substantial scarring, progressive renal failure may develop. However, if renal function is normal during adolescence, the development of renal failure in adulthood is unusual.

Other congenital malformations of the urinary tract

Congenital malformations may affect the kidney, ureter or bladder.
- **Kidney**: unilateral renal agenesis occurs in 1 : 1000 of the population and is not normally associated with renal impairment. Horseshoe kidneys are fused at their lower pole and are found in 1 : 1200 individuals and sometimes present with reflux or obstruction.
- **Ureters**: duplex ureters are the most common congenital malformation of the renal tract occurring in 1 : 150 individuals, but they rarely cause clinical problems. Pelviureteric junction obstruction is a common cause of urinary tract obstruction in children and young adults. There may be hyperplasia of the smooth muscle of the renal pelvis. It may present with loin pain after high fluid intake or even with hydronephrosis. An IVU may suggest the diagnosis and surgical treatment may be necessary.
- **Bladder**: congenital disorders of the bladder include a neuropathic bladder, prune-belly syndrome (abdominal muscle agenesis, undescended testes and urinary tract malformations, including renal dysplasia and bladder dilatation) and posterior urethral valves.

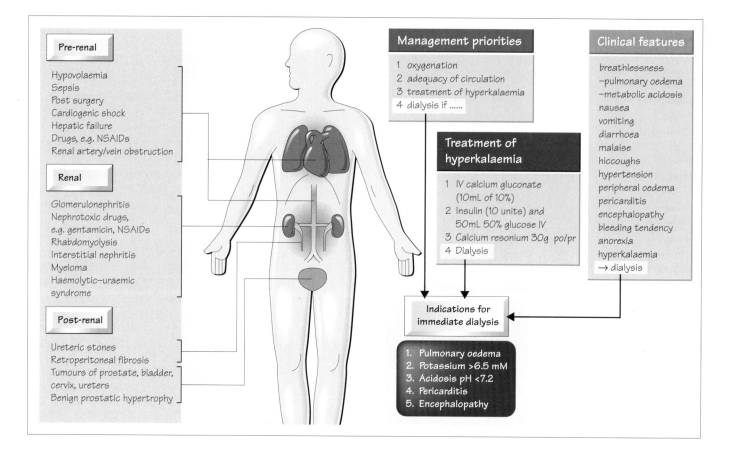

Acute renal failure is a syndrome characterized by a rapid decline in glomerular filtration rate over days to weeks with the accumulation of nitrogenous waste. It is often recognized by a rapidly rising serum urea and creatinine (see Table 135.1). It may be accompanied by reduced urine output. The symptoms of acute renal failure include those of the precipitating aetiology (e.g. shock or sepsis) and those resulting from renal failure itself, including fluid overload, nausea, malaise and encephalopathy. The annual incidence of acute renal failure in developed countries is 180 cases/million. The causes of renal failure are conventionally divided into pre-renal, renal and post-renal.

Pre-renal

The kidneys need an adequate perfusion pressure for normal function. This depends on the systemic blood pressure being high enough, and the post-glomerular arteriole being able to constrict. If either the systemic blood pressure falls too low (the most common cause) or the post-glomerular arteriole dilates inappropriately, glomerular perfusion falls and the kidneys fail. Pre-renal renal failure usually occurs in the context of a seriously ill patient. There are often several systemic insults which produce renal hypoperfusion sufficient to lead to renal failure, including:

- Hypovolaemia from haemorrhage, severe diarrhoea or vomiting.
- Cardiogenic shock.
- Sepsis.

- Drugs such as angiotensin-converting enzyme (ACE) inhibitors and non-steroidal anti-inflammatory drugs (NSAIDs).
- Severe liver disease leading to renal failure, termed the 'hepatorenal syndrome'.

The common histological pattern seen in the kidney in response to severe injury of this nature is acute tubular necrosis (ATN), which usually recovers over several weeks. In very severe and prolonged hypotensive insults, acute cortical necrosis can also occur, from which recovery is less certain. In established renal failure caused by ATN, the concentrating ability of the kidney is lost and urinary sodium is > 40 mmol/L. This contrasts with early pre-renal failure which may be reversible, with attention to haemodynamics and fluid balance when the urine is concentrated (urinary sodium usually < 40 mmol/L).

Renal

There are many causes of renal failure as a result of disease affecting the kidney itself. These include glomerulonephritis, vasculitis, nephrotoxic drugs, rhabdomyolysis, interstitial nephritis, haemolytic/uraemic syndrome and myeloma.

Post-renal

Urinary tract obstruction can occur at any site in the urinary tract and produce renal failure. Common causes include prostatic hypertrophy, carcinoma of the prostate, ureteric stones, tumours of the renal pelvis, ureters or bladder, external compression of ureters by tumour or retroperitoneal fibrosis. Advanced renal failure will only occur with the obstruction of both kidneys.

Diagnostic approach

The rapid diagnosis of the cause of acute renal failure is important because a reversible cause may be present that will respond to specific treatment. A careful history and examination often point towards the likely cause of acute renal failure. Examination should include palpation and percussion of the bladder, the prostate gland in men and the pelvis for a mass in women. In pre-renal failure, the insults are often apparent, such as significant surgical operation, shock, sepsis or perhaps all three! In any patient with pre-renal failure examination for hypovolaemia is vital, and is suggested by:

- **Decreased skin turgor** (an unreliable sign).
- **Tachycardia**, often > 100 beats/min.
- **Hypotension**, with systolic blood pressures (BPs) < 90 mmHg, and a postural systolic BP fall between lying and sitting/standing of > 20 mmHg.
- **Low venous pressure**—if the jugular venous pressure (JVP) is not reliably seen, the central pressure should be measured invasively. The response (urine output) to a small intravenous bolus of fluid (e.g. 250 mL physiological saline) may clarify if the venous pressure is right for that individual patient.

Any pre-renal precipitants should be rapidly corrected. Renal ultrasonography is important to examine for urinary tract obstruction which will be manifest as urinary tract dilatation, particularly hydronephrosis. It will also provide information about renal size and symmetry (small kidneys indicating chronic renal disease).

If the renal size is normal, the kidneys are not obstructed and the history and examination do not suggest a pre-renal cause, further blood tests including immunology should be undertaken and the urine examined for the presence of red cells, protein and casts, which may suggest a renal cause such as glomerulonephritis. A renal biopsy may be necessary for accurate definition of the cause of the acute renal failure.

Management

As in any seriously ill patient, the priorities in acute renal failure are in ensuring adequate oxygenation and circulation. In acute renal failure, the most dangerous threat to oxygenation is fluid overload resulting in pulmonary oedema. The accurate assessment of the fluid status of the patient is thus crucial. In patients with fluid overload who are in established renal failure, oxygen should be administered and fluid removed. Diuretics will not work, vasodilators such as intravenous nitrates may provide temporary benefit, but definitive treatment with haemodialysis, haemofiltration or peritoneal dialysis should be performed. Evidence of hypovolaemia should result in treatment with intravenous fluids.

The other major life-threatening complication of acute renal failure is the presence of hyperkalaemia, which can result in cardiac dysrhythmias (especially ventricular fibrillation and cardiac asystole). The potassium should be measured urgently, ECG changes of hyperkalaemia sought (peaked T waves, widened QRS, absent P waves, sine wave appearance) and, if the potassium is > 6 mmol/L or if ECG abnormalities are present, treatment with intravenous calcium, insulin and glucose, and oral or rectal Calcium Resonium, and urgent dialysis treatment arranged.

The other serious complications of acute renal failure that may require urgent treatment with dialysis include metabolic acidosis, encephalopathy and pericarditis.

Once these priorities have been addressed, specific treatments for the cause of the renal failure may be necessary. These might include the relief of obstruction, the treatment of sepsis or the administration of immunosuppression for a rapidly progressive glomerulonephritis.

136 Chronic renal failure and the dialysis patient

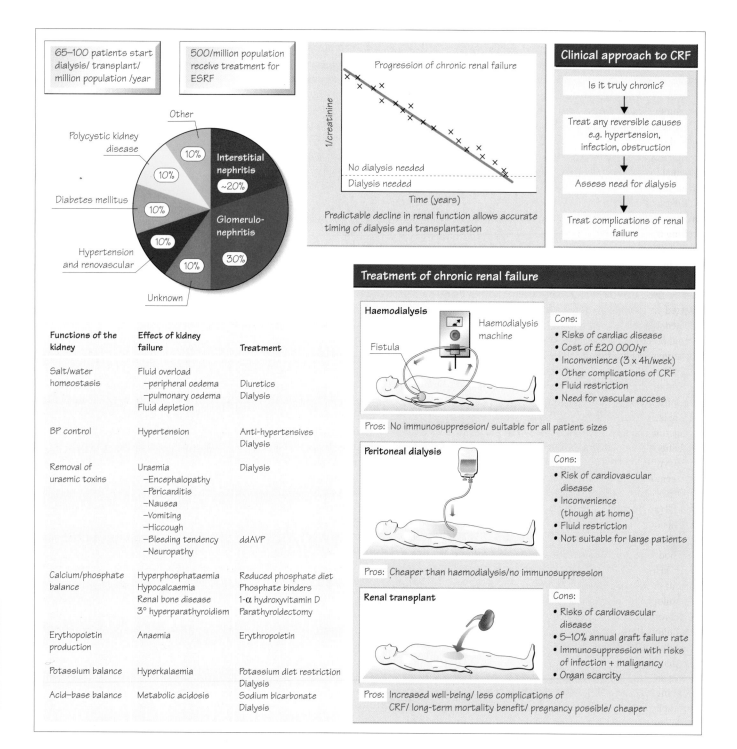

65–100 patients start dialysis/ transplant/ million population /year

500/million population receive treatment for ESRF

Progression of chronic renal failure

1/creatinine

No dialysis needed

Dialysis needed

Time (years)

Predictable decline in renal function allows accurate timing of dialysis and transplantation

Clinical approach to CRF

Is it truly chronic?

↓

Treat any reversible causes e.g. hypertension, infection, obstruction

↓

Assess need for dialysis

↓

Treat complications of renal failure

Other

Polycystic kidney disease — 10%

Diabetes mellitus — 10%

Hypertension and renovascular — 10%

Unknown — 10%

10%

Interstitial nephritis ~20%

Glomerulo-nephritis 30%

Functions of the kidney	Effect of kidney failure	Treatment
Salt/water homeostasis	Fluid overload	
	—peripheral oedema	Diuretics
	—pulmonary oedema	Dialysis
	Fluid depletion	
BP control	Hypertension	Anti-hypertensives Dialysis
Removal of uraemic toxins	Uraemia	Dialysis
	—Encephalopathy	
	—Pericarditis	
	—Nausea	
	—Vomiting	
	—Hiccough	
	—Bleeding tendency	ddAVP
	—Neuropathy	
Calcium/phosphate balance	Hyperphosphataemia	Reduced phosphate diet
	Hypocalcaemia	Phosphate binders
	Renal bone disease	1-α hydroxyvitamin D
	3° hyperparathyroidism	Parathyroidectomy
Erythopoietin production	Anaemia	Erythropoietin
Potassium balance	Hyperkalaemia	Potassium diet restriction Dialysis
Acid–base balance	Metabolic acidosis	Sodium bicarbonate Dialysis

Treatment of chronic renal failure

Haemodialysis

Haemodialysis machine

Fistula

Cons:
- Risks of cardiac disease
- Cost of £20 000/yr
- Inconvenience (3 x 4h/week)
- Other complications of CRF
- Fluid restriction
- Need for vascular access

Pros: No immunosuppression/ suitable for all patient sizes

Peritoneal dialysis

Cons:
- Risk of cardiovascular disease
- Inconvenience (though at home)
- Fluid restriction
- Not suitable for large patients

Pros: Cheaper than haemodialysis/no immunosuppression

Renal transplant

Cons:
- Risks of cardiovascular disease
- 5–10% annual graft failure rate
- Immunosuppression with risks of infection + malignancy
- Organ scarcity

Pros: Increased well-being/ less complications of CRF/ long-term mortality benefit/ pregnancy possible/ cheaper

Chronic renal failure (CRF) is defined as an abnormally low glomerular filtration rate (GFR) for > 3 months. Numerous disorders produce CRF, including glomerulonephritis (30%), interstitial nephritis and reflux nephropathy (20%), polycystic kidney disease (10%), diabetes mellitus (10%), renovascular disease/hypertension (10%), obstructive uropathy and unknown causes (20%). The incidence of chronic renal failure suitable for renal replacement therapy is 65–100/million population/year, with 500/million patients receiving end-stage renal failure (ESRF) treatment.

The normal functions of the kidney include the maintenance of sodium and water balance, control of blood pressure, excretion of nitrogenous waste products, potassium and acid excretion, and hormonal functions in erythropoietin production and vitamin D metabolism. In CRF, perturbations may occur to any or all of these and produce symptoms:

Diseases and Treatments at a Glance

- Failure of regulation of salt and water excretion can produce oedema (peripheral and pulmonary) or more rarely fluid depletion. Failure of concentrating power leads to nocturia.
- Hypertension is common and occasionally severe enough to cause encephalopathy. Premature cardiovascular disease (particularly coronary artery disease) accounts for much of the excess mortality of CRF; this may relate to dyslipidaemia (commonly found in CRF), hypertension, chronic anaemia, abnormalities of calcium metabolism and renin-angiotensin system activation.
- Accumulation of nitrogenous waste products in the blood (and of metabolic products with molecular weight of 500–2000—the 'middle molecules') produces symptoms that include encephalopathy, hiccough, pericarditis, nausea, vomiting, pruritus, malaise, impotence, menstrual irregularities and (mixed motor/sensory) neuropathy. Uraemia causes anorexia and complex disturbances in protein metabolism, resulting in malnutrition, such that maintenance of lean body mass becomes difficult. Muscle wasting causes weakness and inactivity, resulting in further muscle loss.
- Metabolic acidosis and hyperkalaemia.
- Anaemia, principally resulting from erythropoietin deficiency, with contributions from a reduced red cell lifespan, occasionally iron deficiency from gastrointestinal bleeding, etc. Anaemia is milder than expected in polycystic kidney disease and can be more severe than expected in diabetics.
- Renal bone disease: this can be profound and disabling. This relates to osteomalacia (failure of renal hydroxylation of vitamin D), secondary hyperparathyroidism driven by chronic hypocalcaemia (caused by high phosphate and low vitamin D) and nutritional osteoporosis. Aluminium bone toxicity may complicate haemodialysis.
- There is an increased bleeding tendency, largely as a result of platelet dysfunction and depressed activity of von Willebrand's factor.
- Infection is common, because immunity is impaired.

The symptoms of CRF may have an insidious onset, or may present as a uraemic emergency with life-threatening complications.

Management (see Table 136.1)

A full history and examination may provide important clues to the aetiology of the renal failure. A history of frequent urinary tract infections in childhood may suggest a diagnosis of reflux nephropathy, whereas a family history may suggest polycystic kidney disease. Haematuria found at previous medical examinations might point towards chronic glomerulonephritis. It is important to establish that the renal failure is truly chronic to ensure that there is no acute and reversible cause of renal failure. Previous estimations of renal function are of greatest help in determining this; furthermore, the absence of anaemia usually suggests that the renal failure is acute rather than chronic, although small kidneys are usually found in chronic (irreversible) disease.

The investigation of patients with CRF includes renal tract ultrasonography to exclude obstruction and document size. If the cause is unclear and the kidneys are of normal size, a renal biopsy is undertaken. Tests to exclude myeloma and autoimmune disease (systemic lupus erythematosus [SLE], vasculitis) and urinalysis for proteinuria, haematuria and urinary infection are indicated. The severity of the renal failure is determined from creatinine, urea and creatinine clearance.

Once significant renal dysfunction develops, there is an inexorable deterioration in renal function over several years (possibly caused by hyperfiltration in the remaining glomeruli). Apart from treatments directed against the specific cause of the renal failure, the main therapy reducing the speed of deterioration is aggressive blood pressure control.

Table 136.1 Management of chronic renal failure.

GFR	Management
< 15 mL/min	Severe renal failure: if new → urgent specialist referral
> 15 & < 30mL/min	Significant impairment of renal function → prompt assessment and referral
> 30 & 60 mL/min	May reflect age, biological variation or renal disease (suggested by proteinuria, haematuria ± ↑ BP). Evaluate, repeat after 1 week in unwell patients & 1 month in the well. Refer all those with renal damage, any with a GFR < 3rd centile for age

The Glomerular Filtration Rate can be estimated from the serum creatinine using the following formulas:

MDRD $\quad$ GFR (mL/min/1.73m^2) = $186 \times$ (PCR)$^{-1.154} \times$ (Age)$^{-0.203}$ $\times$ (0.742 if female) $\times$ (1.210 if African American)

Cockcroft-Gault $\quad \dfrac{(140\text{-age}) \times \text{weight} \times 1.23 \times (0.85 \text{ if female})}{\text{Creat[micromol/L]}}$

Normal Glomerular Filtration Rate in Male/Female (mL/min)

Centile	40 years	50 years	60 years	70 years
50th	95/85	85/75	70/65	65/55
10th	75/65	65/60	55/50	45/40
3rd	65/55	60/50	45/40	35/35

'End-stage renal failure' (ESRF) is a term used when patients would not survive without renal replacement therapy (haemodialysis, peritoneal dialysis or renal transplantation). Patients are prepared for renal replacement therapy by creating dialysis access before the renal failure progresses to cause uraemic symptoms. Before dialysis, calcium and phosphate balance are corrected, using 1α-hydroxycholecalciferol and phosphate binders, anaemia is improved by erythropoietin, acidosis is ameliorated with sodium bicarbonate, hypertension is treated and sodium and water retention are controlled with diuretics.

Indications for dialysis are:
- Uraemic symptoms—the usual indication, often when creatinine is > 500 μmol/L.
- Life-threatening complications (hyperkalaemia, acidosis, fluid overload, uraemic pericarditis or encephalopathy).

In **haemodialysis** vascular access is achieved forming an arteriovenous fistula (which needs 8 weeks to 'mature' before use) or by using double-lumen jugular, subclavian or femoral lines. The diffusion of solutes and water occurs across a semipermeable membrane, which separates blood and dialysate flow in opposite directions. The major difficulties with haemodialysis are cardiovascular instability (from concurrent cardiovascular disease and drugs used for its treatment, as well as the major fluid shifts that occur during dialysis) and difficulties with vascular access. Dialysis membranes activate the clotting cascade, so heparin is used to prevent this. Most membranes do not allow the removal of β_2-microglobulin, which accumulates causing carpal tunnel syndrome and arthropathy. Over-rapid removal of toxic metabolites causes a profound illness—dialysis 'disequilibrium'—particularly during the first dialysis treatments, prevented by frequent 'small' dialysis schedules.

In **continuous ambulatory peritoneal dialysis** (CAPD) patients instill several litres of isotonic or hypertonic glucose solution four times a day into the peritoneal cavity via a permanent catheter. The peritoneal lining acts as the dialysis membrane. After several hours, the fluid containing solutes and waste products is drained out. Excess body fluid is removed by using hypertonic solutions.

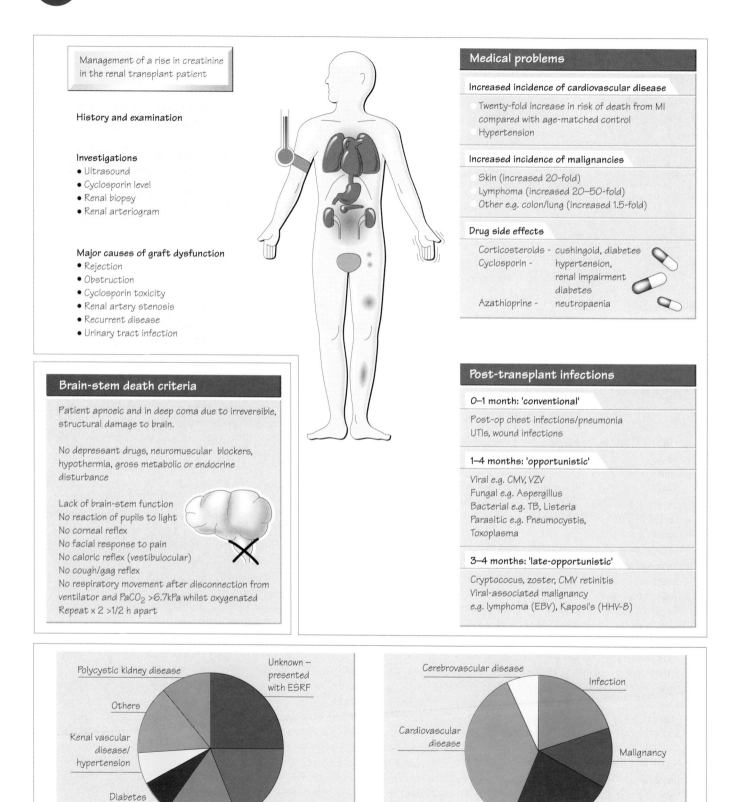

Management of a rise in creatinine in the renal transplant patient

History and examination

Investigations
- Ultrasound
- Cyclosporin level
- Renal biopsy
- Renal arteriogram

Major causes of graft dysfunction
- Rejection
- Obstruction
- Cyclosporin toxicity
- Renal artery stenosis
- Recurrent disease
- Urinary tract infection

Medical problems

Increased incidence of cardiovascular disease
- Twenty-fold increase in risk of death from MI compared with age-matched control
- Hypertension

Increased incidence of malignancies
- Skin (increased 20-fold)
- Lymphoma (increased 20–50-fold)
- Other e.g. colon/lung (increased 1.5-fold)

Drug side effects

Corticosteroids - cushingoid, diabetes
Cyclosporin - hypertension, renal impairment diabetes
Azathioprine - neutropaenia

Brain-stem death criteria

Patient apnoeic and in deep coma due to irreversible, structural damage to brain.

No depressant drugs, neuromuscular blockers, hypothermia, gross metabolic or endocrine disturbance

Lack of brain-stem function
No reaction of pupils to light
No corneal reflex
No facial response to pain
No caloric reflex (vestibulocular)
No cough/gag reflex
No respiratory movement after disconnection from ventilator and $PaCO_2$ >6.7kPa whilst oxygenated
Repeat x 2 >1/2 h apart

Post-transplant infections

0–1 month: 'conventional'

Post-op chest infections/pneumonia
UTIs, wound infections

1–4 months: 'opportunistic'

Viral e.g. CMV, VZV
Fungal e.g. Aspergillus
Bacterial e.g. TB, Listeria
Parasitic e.g. Pneumocystis, Toxoplasma

3–4 months: 'late-opportunistic'

Cryptococus, zoster, CMV retinitis
Viral-associated malignancy
e.g. lymphoma (EBV), Kaposi's (HHV-8)

Polycystic kidney disease
Others
Renal vascular disease/hypertension
Diabetes
Pyelonephritis
Glomerulonephritis
Unknown – presented with ESRF

Indications for renal transplantation

Cerebrovascular disease
Infection
Cardiovascular disease
Malignancy
Other

Causes of mortality following renal transplantation

Stages of renal dysfunction (adapted from National Kidney Foundation—K/DOQI)

Stage	Description	Creatinine clearance (~GFR) (mL/min/1.73 m²)	Metabolic consequences
1	Normal or increased GFR—people at increased risk or with early renal damage	>90	
2	Early renal insufficiency	60–89*	Concentration of parathyroid hormone starts to rise (GFR ~ 60–80)
3	Moderate renal failure (chronic renal failure)	30–59*	Decrease in calcium absorption (GFR <50) Lipoprotein activity falls Malnutrition Onset of left ventricular hypertrophy Onset of anaemia (erythropoietin deficiency)
4	Severe renal failure (pre-end-stage renal disease)	15–29	Triglyceride concentrations start to rise Hyperphosphataemia Metabolic acidosis Tendency to hyperkalaemia
5	End-stage renal disease (uraemia)	<15	Azotaemia develops

GFR = Glomerular filtration rate   * May be normal for age (see Chapter 136)

Table 137.1 Relative contraindications to transplantation.

Age > 70 years
HIV positive
Bacterial infection
Recent/current malignancy
Severe cardiac disease
Renal disease with high risk of recurrence

In the UK, 2000 patients receive renal transplants every year, compared with the 3500 who are taken on for renal replacement treatment. Not all patients with end-stage renal failure are suitable for renal transplantation (Table 137.1). Transplantation is limited by the availability of donor organs. Organs are most commonly obtained from donors in whom brain-stem death has been diagnosed. Increasingly, kidneys are being transplanted from living related (or spouse) donors. In diabetic patients dual kidney-pancreas transplants may be undertaken.

In the immediate post-operative period, the patient faces the risks of the operation and of infection resulting from heavy immunosuppression. In the longer term, the renal transplant recipient faces a variety of medical problems, including those related to immunosuppression, the increased incidence of cardiovascular and cerebrovascular disease, hypertension, increased incidence of a variety of malignancies, notably of the skin and lymphoma, the consequences of previous chronic renal failure, the underlying renal disorder and the problems of graft failure.

Recipients of renal transplants are commonly immunosuppressed with a combination of drugs, including prednisolone, azathioprine, mycophenolate, cyclosporin, tacrolimus and specific therapeutic antibodies (e.g. anti-IL2 receptor). These agents share the general side effects of an increased incidence of infections resulting from immunosuppression, but each has important unique side effects. Examples of these include the cushingoid features that occur with corticosteroid administration, the hypertension, tremor and renal impairment that can occur with cyclosporin, and the neutropenia that can occur with azathioprine and mycophenolate.

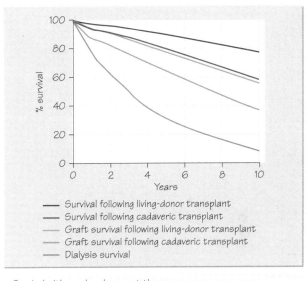

— Survival following living-donor transplant
— Survival following cadaveric transplant
— Graft survival following living-donor transplant
— Graft survival following cadaveric transplant
— Dialysis survival

Survival with renal replacement therapy

The survival of renal transplants at 1, 5 and 10 years is 90, 70 and 55%, respectively. Graft survival is enhanced by careful HLA antigen matching of donor and recipient.

The success of renal transplantation is largely the result of the ability to follow renal function precisely and frequently with measurements of serum creatinine. Any significant rise in creatinine should prompt investigation for rejection, cyclosporin toxicity, problems with the renal vasculature or the obstruction of urine flow. Rejection is usually diagnosed with renal biopsy and is treated with high-dose methylprednisolone or anti-T-cell antibodies. Obstruction can usually be diagnosed with ultrasonography; cyclosporin levels determined to exclude toxicity and angiography may be required to demonstrate normal renal blood supply.

The following categories contain examples only and are not exhaustive

Drugs usually excreted by the kidney which can accumulate in renal failure

- Digoxin
- Lithium
- Morphine (+ metabolites), pethidine (+ metabolites)
- Penicillins, gentamicin, vancomycin, erythromycin, acyclovir

Drugs which require higher dosage in renal failure

- Frusemide

Drugs which can exacerbate metabolic effects in pre-existing renal failure

- K^+ sparing diuretics → hyperkalaemia
- Corticosteroids → ↑uraemia
- NaCl, $NaHCO_3$ → Na^+/ H_2O retention

Drugs which can produce idiosyncratic renal toxicity

- NSAIDs
- Penicillins
- Gold, penicillamine

Drugs which can reduce renal function and should be used with caution in renal failure

- NSAIDs
- Angiotensin-converting enzyme inhibitors
- Cyclosporin, acyclovir
- Contrast media

Drugs which can produce renal failure in overdose

- Gentamicin
- Paracetamol
- Ethylene glycol

Drugs often prescribed for patients with chronic renal failure

	Intended effect
Erythropoietin	↓anaemia
1α vitamin D	↑Ca^{2+}
Phosphate binders	↓PO_4^-
Antihypertensives	↓BP
Diuretics (loop)	↓Na^+ / H_2O
Iron	↓anaemia

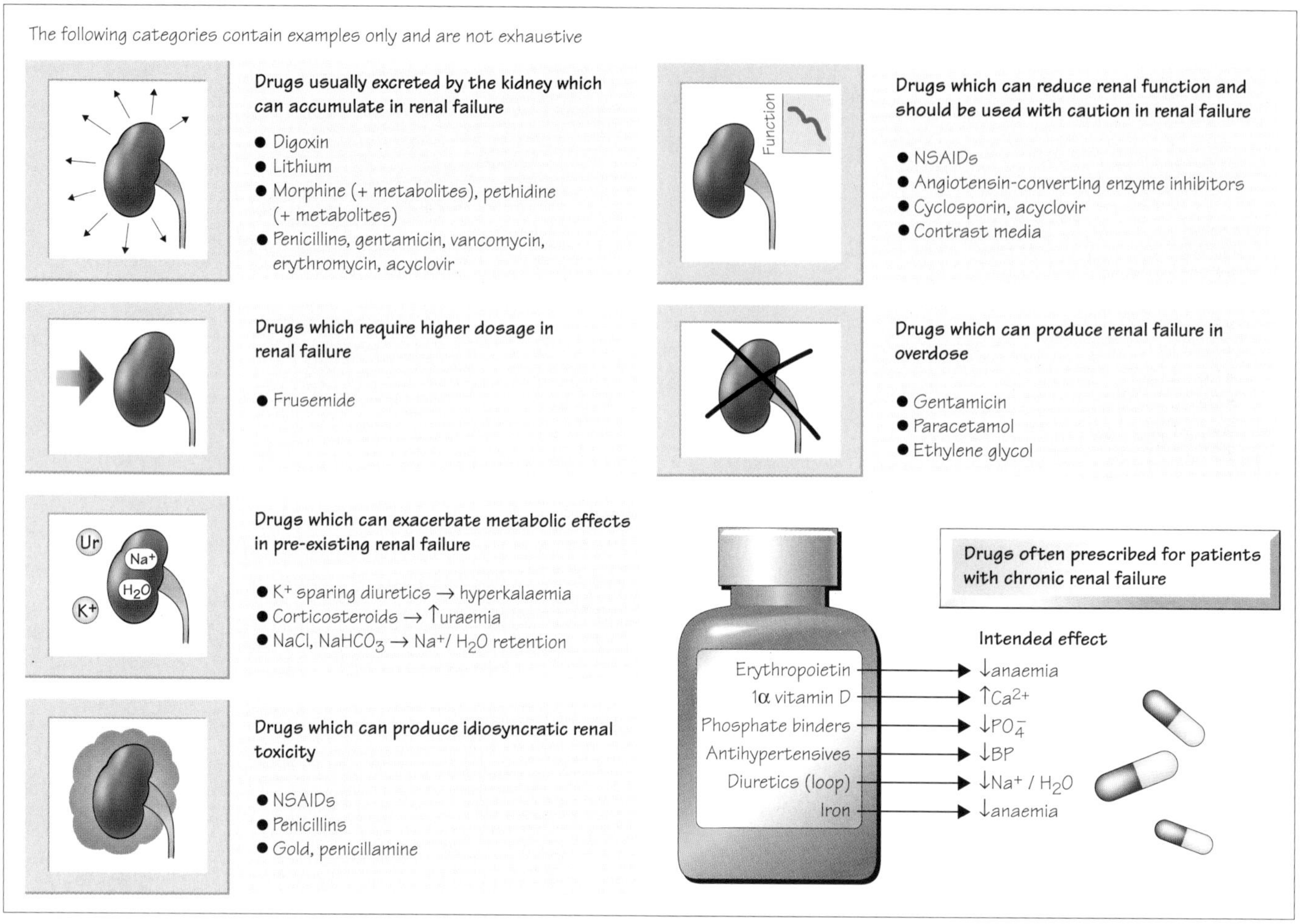

When prescribing a drug for a patient with renal failure several issues need to be addressed:

- What is the effect of the renal impairment on renal excretion of the drug?
- What is the effect of the renal impairment on drug action?
- What is the effect of the drug on the kidneys?
- How should the prescription be altered in view of the renal impairment?

The golden rule when prescribing in all patients with renal failure is to 'use drugs very sparingly', and 'always check the dose in a pharmacopoeia such as the *BNF*'.

Effect of renal impairment on excretion

Nearly all drugs are excreted to some extent by the kidneys. Furthermore, in patients with renal impairment there may be differing bioavailability, and alterations in volume of distribution and in plasma protein binding. If there is significant renal impairment, appropriate dosing should be prescribed based on recommended guidelines. For some drugs, such as morphine and pethidine, active drug metabolites may be excreted by the kidney and produce toxicity in renal impairment. The

monitoring of blood levels (for drugs such as digoxin or gentamicin) may be essential to achieve appropriate dosing.

Effect of the renal impairment on drug action

Uraemia may produce increased or decreased end-organ sensitivity, e.g. loop diuretics such as furosemide must be prescribed in much larger doses in renal impairment to achieve the same therapeutic effect.

Effect of the drug on the kidneys

Drugs may produce an idiosyncratic renal toxicity such as the interstitial nephritis produced by antibiotics and non-steroidal anti-inflammatory drugs (NSAIDs) or have a predictable adverse effect such as the exacerbation of renal hypoperfusion by angiotensin-converting enzyme (ACE) inhibitors and NSAIDs.

In patients undergoing dialysis treatment, it is also necessary to know whether the drug is removed by dialysis. In transplant recipients, there are many important and potentially dangerous interactions with the immunosuppressive agents.

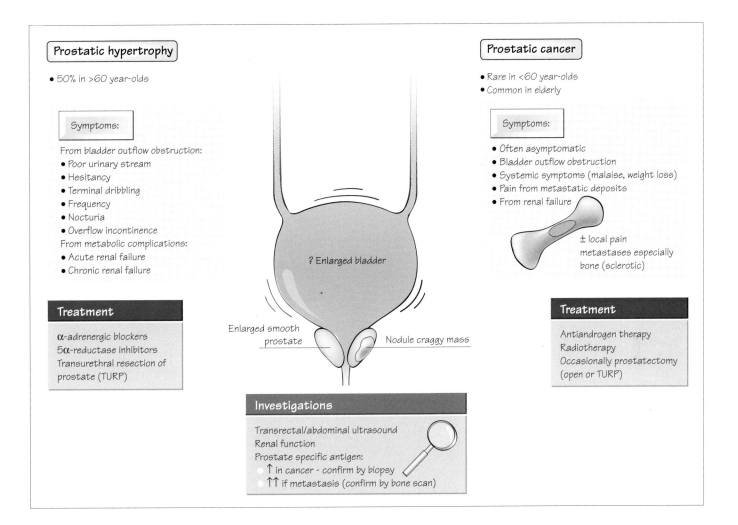

Prostatic hypertrophy

- 50% in >60 year-olds

Symptoms:

From bladder outflow obstruction:
- Poor urinary stream
- Hesitancy
- Terminal dribbling
- Frequency
- Nocturia
- Overflow incontinence

From metabolic complications:
- Acute renal failure
- Chronic renal failure

Treatment

α-adrenergic blockers
5α-reductase inhibitors
Transurethral resection of prostate (TURP)

Prostatic cancer

- Rare in <60 year-olds
- Common in elderly

Symptoms:

- Often asymptomatic
- Bladder outflow obstruction
- Systemic symptoms (malaise, weight loss)
- Pain from metastatic deposits
- From renal failure

± local pain
metastases especially
bone (sclerotic)

Treatment

Antiandrogen therapy
Radiotherapy
Occasionally prostatectomy
(open or TURP)

? Enlarged bladder

Enlarged smooth prostate

Nodule craggy mass

Investigations

Transrectal/abdominal ultrasound
Renal function
Prostate specific antigen:
- ↑ in cancer - confirm by biopsy
- ↑↑ if metastasis (confirm by bone scan)

Benign prostatic hypertrophy (BPH) is characterized by enlargement of the prostate gland and is very common, being present in over 50% of men aged over 60 years, and 80% over the age of 80. It most commonly presents with features of bladder outflow obstruction—poor urinary stream, hesitancy, terminal dribbling, and frequency. Other symptoms can include dysuria and overflow incontinence. Alternatively, patients may present with symptoms of chronic renal failure or acute urinary retention.

Examination

On examination a bladder may be palpable or detected by percussion. An enlarged smooth prostate is found on digital rectal examination.

Investigations

These may include measurement of serum creatinine, ultrasonography of the renal tract, urodynamics and determination of prostate-specific antigen (PSA) levels because these are raised in prostate malignancy (see Chapter 180).

Management

The medical management includes the use of α-adrenergic blockers such as prazosin (which relax the smooth muscle of the prostate and bladder neck) or finasteride (a 5α-reductase inhibitor that inhibits the conversion of testosterone to its active metabolite dihydrotestosterone, thus reducing prostatic hypertrophy). **Surgery** is often necessary to improve urine flow and transurethral resection of the prostate (TURP) is undertaken endoscopically.

Diseases and Treatments at a Glance

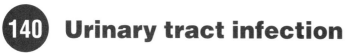

140 Urinary tract infection

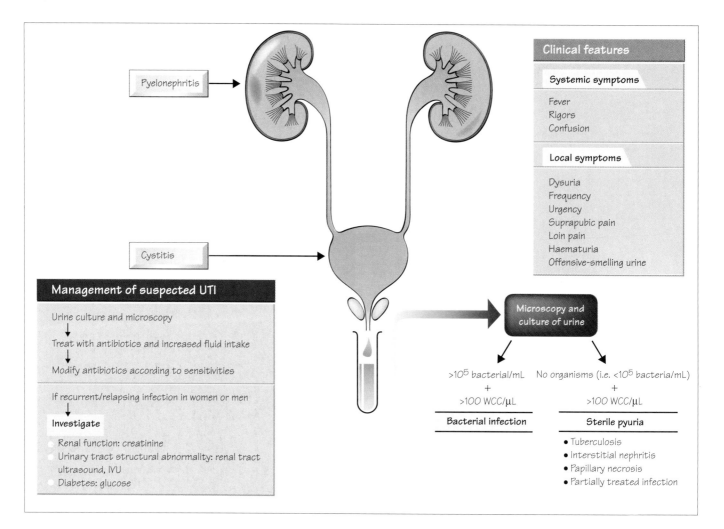

Clinical features

Systemic symptoms

Fever
Rigors
Confusion

Local symptoms

Dysuria
Frequency
Urgency
Suprapubic pain
Loin pain
Haematuria
Offensive-smelling urine

Pyelonephritis

Cystitis

Management of suspected UTI

Urine culture and microscopy

Treat with antibiotics and increased fluid intake

Modify antibiotics according to sensitivities

If recurrent/relapsing infection in women or men

Investigate

○ Renal function: creatinine
○ Urinary tract structural abnormality: renal tract ultrasound, IVU
○ Diabetes: glucose

Microscopy and culture of urine

>10⁵ bacterial/mL
+
>100 WCC/μL

Bacterial infection

No organisms (i.e. <10⁵ bacteria/mL)
+
>100 WCC/μL

Sterile pyuria

• Tuberculosis
• Interstitial nephritis
• Papillary necrosis
• Partially treated infection

Urinary tract infection (UTI) is very common, accounting for 1–2% of general practice consultations. They occur much more commonly in females and in young, sexually active women, in whom the annual incidence may be as high as 0.5/woman per year. Most infections arise from the introduction of bowel flora via the urethra into the bladder. The increased frequency of UTIs in women is attributed to short urethral length; a UTI can commonly follow sexual intercourse. Other host factors associated with an increased risk of UTI include: 1) Pregnancy. 2) Incomplete bladder emptying (e.g. neurogenic bladder in multiple sclerosis, spinal cord injury). 3) Urinary calculi. 4) Diabetes mellitus (all suspected UTIs should have urine dipstick tested for glucose). 5) Structural abnormality of the urinary tract (e.g. reflux). 6) Instrumentation of the urinary tract (e.g. urethral catheterization).

The causative organisms are usually coliforms (70%) but other bacterial pathogens include *Proteus mirabilis*, *Staphylococcus epidermidis* and *Streptococcus faecalis*. Certain cell surface antigens may enhance pathogenicity by aiding the adhesion of bacteria to uroepithelial surfaces. The typical symptoms of urinary tract infection are dysuria, urinary frequency and urgency, suprapubic discomfort, loin pain, fever, haematuria and offensive smelling urine. Sometimes, particularly in the elderly, local symptoms may be absent but the patient may present with

confusion or general deterioration. If the infection primarily causes symptoms in the bladder it can be termed 'cystitis' whereas infection affecting the kidney is termed 'pyelonephritis'.

Investigations

A number of investigations are helpful:

• **Urine dipsticks**: Gram-negative bacteria, the most common organisms implicated in UTIs, convert nitrate, a normal constituent of urine, to nitrite, which is detected by dipstick. The presence of nitrite is therefore a useful guide to the presence of pathogenic Gram-negative organisms. Finding leukocytes in the urine suggests an inflammatory process in the renal/urinary tract. The most common cause of this is infection by conventional bacteria; if these cannot be found (so-called sterile pyuria), other causes should be considered, such as tuberculosis of the renal tract, cancer and renal or bladder stones.

• **Microscopy and culture of a midstream specimen of urine (MC&S of MSU)**: if a UTI is suspected, a sample of urine (preferably obtained as a 'clean catch' from mid-stream urine) should be microscoped and cultured. A finding of more than 10⁵ organisms/mL urine is significant. Culture enables the causative organism to be identified and its antibiotic susceptibilities defined. Organisms may be cultured from

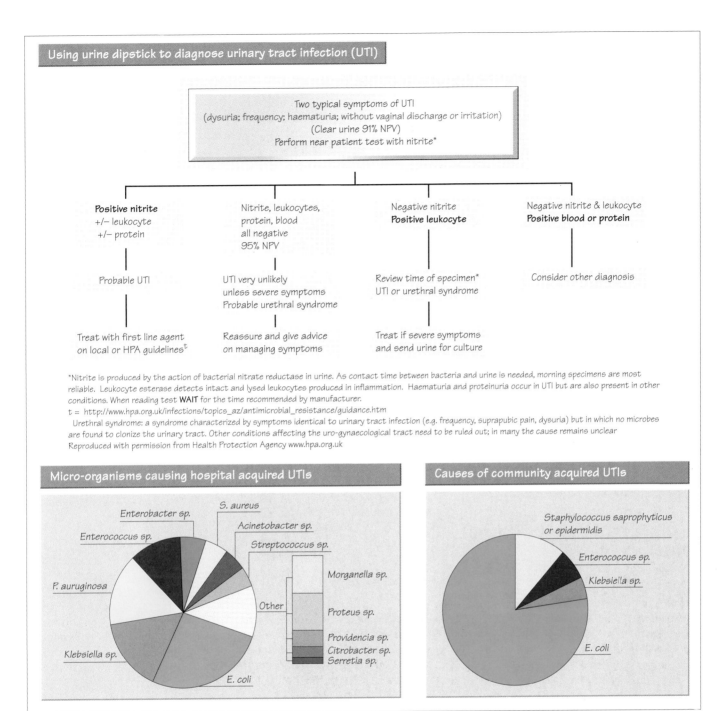

Using urine dipstick to diagnose urinary tract infection (UTI)

Two typical symptoms of UTI
(dysuria; frequency; haematuria; without vaginal discharge or irritation)
(Clear urine 91% NPV)
Perform near patient test with nitrite*

Positive nitrite
+/− leukocyte
+/− protein

Nitrite, leukocytes,
protein, blood
all negative
95% NPV

Negative nitrite
Positive leukocyte

Negative nitrite & leukocyte
Positive blood or protein

Probable UTI

UTI very unlikely
unless severe symptoms
Probable urethral syndrome

Review time of specimen*
UTI or urethral syndrome

Consider other diagnosis

Treat with first line agent
on local or HPA guidelines^t

Reassure and give advice
on managing symptoms

Treat if severe symptoms
and send urine for culture

*Nitrite is produced by the action of bacterial nitrate reductase in urine. As contact time between bacteria and urine is needed, morning specimens are most reliable. Leukocyte esterase detects intact and lysed leukocytes produced in inflammation. Haematuria and proteinuria occur in UTI but are also present in other conditions. When reading test **WAIT** for the time recommended by manufacturer.

t = http://www.hpa.org.uk/infections/topics_az/antimicrobial_resistance/guidance.htm

Urethral syndrome: a syndrome characterized by symptoms identical to urinary tract infection (e.g. frequency, suprapubic pain, dysuria) but in which no microbes are found to clonize the urinary tract. Other conditions affecting the uro-gynaecological tract need to be ruled out; in many the cause remains unclear
Reproduced with permission from Health Protection Agency www.hpa.org.uk

Micro-organisms causing hospital acquired UTIs

Enterobacter sp.
S. aureus
Enterococcus sp.
Acinetobacter sp.
Streptococcus sp.
P. auruginosa
Morganella sp.
Other
Klebsiella sp.
Proteus sp.
Providencia sp.
Citrobacter sp.
Serretia sp.
E. coli

Causes of community acquired UTIs

Staphylococcus saprophyticus
or epidermidis
Enterococcus sp.
Klebsiella sp.
E. coli

---

urine without being of pathogenic significance, e.g. because of perineal contamination; but the presence of > 100 leukocytes/mm³ urine usually characterizes significant bacterial infections.

• **Renal tract imaging**: if there are multiple infections in a woman, or a first UTI in a child or man, investigations for a predisposing cause should be undertaken and these include tests of renal function (any structural abnormality of the kidneys or renal tract can predispose to infection), glucose, intravenous urogram (IVU) or ultrasonography (to detect renal calculi, abnormalities of the urinary tract and incomplete bladder emptying) and micturating cystogram (particularly in children to exclude reflux).

Management

Urine should be sent for microscopy and culture before starting antibiotic treatment. In uncomplicated UTIs short (5-day or even single-dose) duration antibiotic therapy is usually adequate. Trimethoprim, nitrofurantoin or amoxicillin is commonly prescribed, but the prescription may need to be altered in the light of the antibiotic sensitivities of the causative organism. Acute pyelonephritis or prominent systemic symptoms of infection may require intravenous antibiotics. A high fluid intake (> 3 L/day) is recommended to prevent urinary stasis in the bladder and decrease bacterial replication.

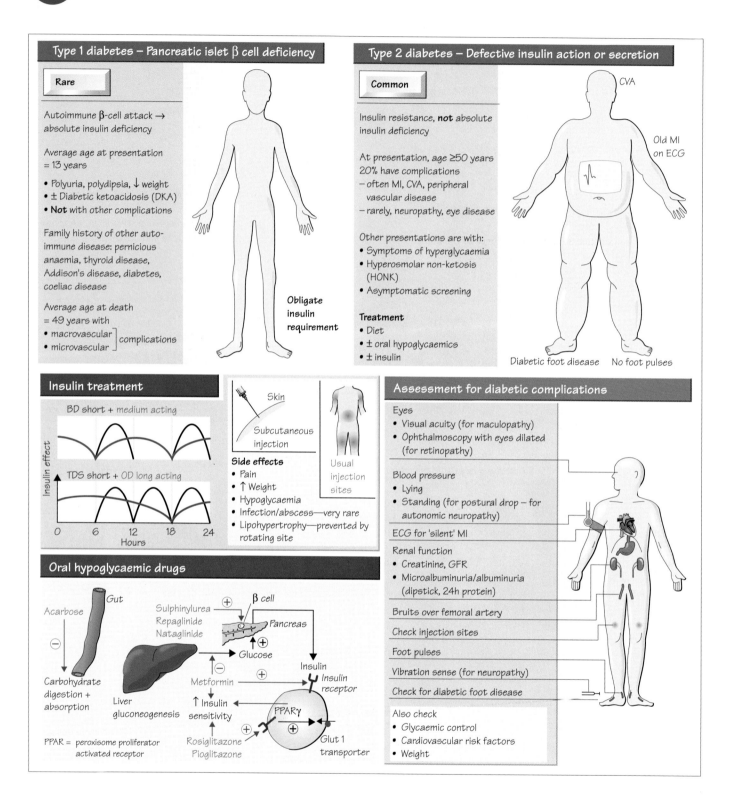

Type 1 diabetes – Pancreatic islet β cell deficiency

Rare

Autoimmune β-cell attack → absolute insulin deficiency

Average age at presentation = 13 years

- Polyuria, polydipsia, ↓ weight
- ± Diabetic ketoacidosis (DKA)
- **Not** with other complications

Family history of other auto-immune disease: pernicious anaemia, thyroid disease, Addison's disease, diabetes, coeliac disease

Average age at death = 49 years with
- macrovascular ⎤ complications
- microvascular ⎦

Obligate insulin requirement

Type 2 diabetes – Defective insulin action or secretion

Common

Insulin resistance, **not** absolute insulin deficiency

At presentation, age ≥50 years 20% have complications
– often MI, CVA, peripheral vascular disease
– rarely, neuropathy, eye disease

Other presentations are with:
- Symptoms of hyperglycaemia
- Hyperosmolar non-ketosis (HONK)
- Asymptomatic screening

Treatment
- Diet
- ± oral hypoglycaemics
- ± insulin

CVA

Old MI on ECG

Diabetic foot disease   No foot pulses

Insulin treatment

BD short + medium acting

TDS short + OD long acting

Insulin effect

0   6   12   18   24
Hours

Skin

Subcutaneous injection

Side effects
- Pain
- ↑ Weight
- Hypoglycaemia
- Infection/abscess—very rare
- Lipohypertrophy—prevented by rotating site

Usual injection sites

Oral hypoglycaemic drugs

Gut

Acarbose

⊖

Carbohydrate digestion + absorption

Liver gluconeogenesis

Sulphinylurea
Repaglinide
Nataglinide

⊕

β cell

Pancreas

⊕

Glucose

Metformin

⊖

⊕

↑ Insulin sensitivity

Rosiglitazone
Pioglitazone

⊕

PPARγ

⊕

Insulin

Insulin receptor

Glut 1 transporter

PPAR = peroxisome proliferator activated receptor

Assessment for diabetic complications

Eyes
- Visual acuity (for maculopathy)
- Ophthalmoscopy with eyes dilated (for retinopathy)

Blood pressure
- Lying
- Standing (for postural drop – for autonomic neuropathy)

ECG for 'silent' MI

Renal function
- Creatinine, GFR
- Microalbuminuria/albuminuria (dipstick, 24h protein)

Bruits over femoral artery

Check injection sites

Foot pulses

Vibration sense (for neuropathy)

Check for diabetic foot disease

Also check
- Glycaemic control
- Cardiovascular risk factors
- Weight

Definition

Diabetes mellitus is characterized by chronically elevated glucose. Fasting plasma glucose levels are (mmol/L): diabetes ≥ 7.0, impaired glucose tolerance 6–7, normal < 6; 2-h post 75 g glucose plasma glucose levels are: diabetes ≥ 11.1, impaired glucose tolerance 7.8–11.1; normal < 7.8.

Classification and pathophysiology

Type 1 diabetes mellitus (pancreatic islet beta cell deficiency)

This is a rare disease, essentially of white northern Europeans (25/10 000 population), presenting when aged < 30 years, where absolute insulin deficiency occurs after autoimmune β-cell destruction in the genetically predisposed. Various antibodies are found up to 10 years before clinical disease and disappear several years later. Associated autoimmune conditions may be found in the family (see figure).

Clinical features: at presentation patients are often thin and have symptoms of polyuria, polydipsia, weight loss, fatigue and infections (abscesses, fungal infections, e.g. candidiasis). Ketoacidosis may occur, with nausea, vomiting, drowsiness and tachypnoea. Patients have an obligate need for insulin.

Type 2 diabetes mellitus (defective insulin action or secretion)

This is a very common illness (current prevalence of 2% in the UK and 6.6% in USA, increasing rapidly as a result of dietary/lifestyle factors) of middle-aged and elderly people, caused principally by resistance to the peripheral action of insulin. Although inadequate secretion of insulin may occur late on, absolute insulin deficiency is not found. There is a substantial genetic contribution. The identical twins concordance rate is 90%, but there is no strong human leukocyte antigen (HLA) association.

Clinical features: 80% overweight; 20% present with complications (ischaemic heart disease, cerebrovascular disease, renal failure, foot ulcers, visual impairment). May present with insidious polyuria and polydipsia. Many patients can be managed with diet and hypoglycaemic drugs, though some require insulin.

Other forms of diabetes include:
- **Exocrine pancreas failure**: pancreatitis, pancreatectomy, destruction (carcinoma, cystic fibrosis, haemochromatosis).
- **Endocrine disease**: Cushing's syndrome, acromegaly, glucagonoma and phaeochromocytoma.
- **Gestational diabetes**, which usually occurs in the last trimester of pregnancy, has a similar pathophysiology to type 2 diabetes. Not surprisingly, some 30–50% of patients develop overt type 2 diabetes within 10 years.
- **Malnutrition-related diabetes mellitus**: found in developing countries.
- **Genetic causes**: are all very rare. Maturity-onset diabetes in the young (MODY) relates to defects of β-cell function, e.g. MODY 1—abnormal hepatocyte nuclear factor HNF-4α; MODY 2—glucokinase defect; MODY 3—abnormal HNF-1α, MODY 4—IRF-1 defect, mitochondrial DNA mutations. Other genetic defects are of insulin action (e.g. leprechaunism type A insulin resistance).

Management of diabetes mellitus

- **Patient education**: use of nurse practitioners, self-education, etc. is vital.
- **Clinical assessment**: after diagnosing diabetes mellitus, treating any acute metabolic complications (see later) and initiating life-long hypoglycaemic therapy, assessment of end-organ damage should occur every 6–12 months—eyesight (retinopathy and cataracts), cardiovascular system (peripheral pulses, signs of cardiac failure, hypertension), nervous system (peripheral sensory and/or autonomic neuropathy) and feet (ulceration, gangrene and infections). Renal function (creatinine and albuminuria) must be measured.
- **Treatment** should minimize symptoms and avoid complications, while allowing a normal life—this requires patient education and support. Maximizing prognosis depends on optimal blood glucose control and eliminating coexisting cardiovascular risk factors such as smoking, hypertension (aim for a BP of < 130/80 mmHg) and hyperlipidaemia. Optimal glycaemic control by itself improves cholesterol levels but, if the cholesterol remains high despite this, aggressive lipid-lowering therapy with statins may be justified. Indeed nearly all people with diabetes who have vascular disease should be on statins.

Specific treatment of diabetes mellitus

- **Dietary advice**: aim for ideal body weight (obesity increases insulin resistance, and weight reduction lessens it in type 2 diabetes). Restrict refined carbohydrate and increase complex carbohydrate intake. Reduce saturated fat. Avoid excessive alcohol.
- **Oral hypoglycaemic agents** are indicated in type 2 diabetes if there is inadequate metabolic control by diet alone.
- **Sulphonylureas**: gliclazide, glibenclamide, glimepride, tolbutamide. Increases insulin release from β cells (closes K^+ channels → cell depolarization). May cause weight gain or hypoglycaemia.
- **Biguanides**: metformin. Mechanism of action is unclear. Mild anorectic action and thus indicated in obese individuals. Reduces insulin resistance and hepatic gluconeogenesis. Side effects: gastrointestinal upset and rarely lactic acidosis.
- **α-Glucosidase inhibitors**: acarbose inhibits carbohydrate digestion, reducing intestinal glucose absorption. Side effects: bloating and diarrhoea.
- **Post-prandial glucose regulators** (PPGRs): repaglinide and nateglinide—stimulate insulin release from β cells. Short duration of action makes hypoglycaemia less common than with sulphonylureas. Side effect: hepatic dysfunction.
- **Thiazolidinediones**: troglitazone (withdrawn), rosiglitazone, pioglitazone. Insulin-sensitizing agents, which activate the peroxisome proliferator-activated receptor (PPAR-γ), stimulating transcription of the glucose transporter molecules glut-1 and glut-4. Side effect: hepatotoxicity.
- **Insulin** is given subcutaneously and is used for all those with type 1 diabetes and some people with type 2 diabetes. There are several kinds; recombinant human insulin is most commonly used, although some patients prefer porcine or bovine insulin. Different preparations have different onset and duration of actions (short, medium and long). Preparations with different combinations of short and medium/long-acting duration are often used. Insulin analogues: are chemically modified forms of insulin, e.g. lispro and Aspart, which have a rapid onset of action and shorter duration of action, allowing administration immediately before eating. Glargine is an analogue with a 22–24 h duration. Oral hypoglycaemic agents (e.g. metformin) may be added to insulin in type 2 diabetes to improve insulin sensitivity. Adverse effects of insulin are hypoglycaemia, weight gain and lipohypertrophy at injection sites.

Monitoring glycaemic control in diabetes

Tight glycaemic control improves outcome and is monitored from blood glucose levels. Those on oral agents should monitor fasting blood glucose, whereas those on insulin should check glucose more frequently, e.g. before meals. Monitoring should be more frequent if the patient is unwell. Some patients find blood monitoring difficult, and urine glucose levels are used instead, although this is less reliable than blood because the renal threshold for glucose appearing in the urine varies between 7 and 12 mmol/L. Glycated haemoglobin (HbA1c) is a good measure of glycaemic control over several weeks.

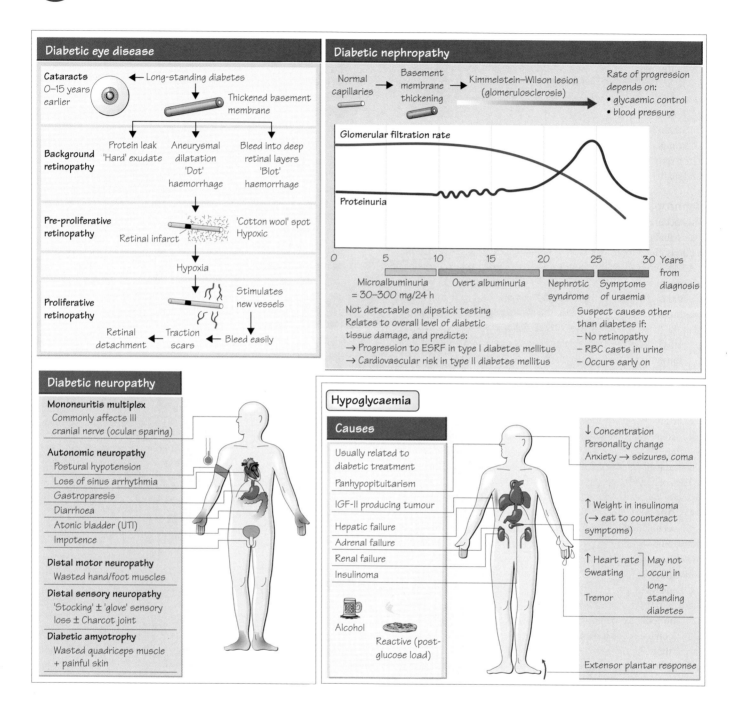

Diabetic eye disease

Cataracts 0–15 years earlier ← Long-standing diabetes

Thickened basement membrane

Background retinopathy
- Protein leak 'Hard' exudate
- Aneurysmal dilatation 'Dot' haemorrhage
- Bleed into deep retinal layers 'Blot' haemorrhage

Pre-proliferative retinopathy
Retinal infarct — 'Cotton wool' spot Hypoxic

Hypoxia

Proliferative retinopathy — Stimulates new vessels

Retinal detachment ← Traction scars ← Bleed easily

Diabetic nephropathy

Normal capillaries → Basement membrane thickening → Kimmelstein–Wilson lesion (glomerulosclerosis)

Rate of progression depends on:
- glycaemic control
- blood pressure

Glomerular filtration rate

Proteinuria

0   5   10   15   20   25   30   Years from diagnosis

Microalbuminuria = 30–300 mg/24 h | Overt albuminuria | Nephrotic syndrome | Symptoms of uraemia

Not detectable on dipstick testing
Relates to overall level of diabetic tissue damage, and predicts:
→ Progression to ESRF in type I diabetes mellitus
→ Cardiovascular risk in type II diabetes mellitus

Suspect causes other than diabetes if:
– No retinopathy
– RBC casts in urine
– Occurs early on

Diabetic neuropathy

Mononeuritis multiplex
Commonly affects III cranial nerve (ocular sparing)

Autonomic neuropathy
Postural hypotension
Loss of sinus arrhythmia
Gastroparesis
Diarrhoea
Atonic bladder (UTI)
Impotence

Distal motor neuropathy
Wasted hand/foot muscles

Distal sensory neuropathy
'Stocking' ± 'glove' sensory loss ± Charcot joint

Diabetic amyotrophy
Wasted quadriceps muscle + painful skin

Hypoglycaemia

Causes

Usually related to diabetic treatment
Panhypopituitarism
IGF-II producing tumour
Hepatic failure
Adrenal failure
Renal failure
Insulinoma

Alcohol

Reactive (post-glucose load)

↓ Concentration
Personality change
Anxiety → seizures, coma

↑ Weight in insulinoma (→ eat to counteract symptoms)

↑ Heart rate
Sweating — May not occur in long-standing diabetes
Tremor

Extensor plantar response

Diabetic complications arise from acute metabolic derangement (hypo- or hyperglycaemia) or, late on, from micro- or macrovascular damage, the risk of which relates to the tightness of glycaemic and conventional vascular risk factor control.

Microvascular complications of diabetes

Small vessel disease is the hallmark of diabetes and takes 10 years or more to develop.

Eye disease (retinopathy)

One in three people with diabetes develop eye disease and 5% are blind at 30 years. Retinopathy results from capillary basement membrane thickening, leading to leaky vessels (haemorrhage and hard exudates) occluded vessels (retinal ischaemia and new vessels) and macular oedema.

- **Background retinopathy**: blot haemorrhage, 'dot' microaneurysms, hard exudates not involving the macula. No effect on sight.
- **Maculopathy**: macular oedema, haemorrhages, hard exudates—very difficult to diagnose ophthalmoscopically and suspected from a de-

crease in visual acuity, which should therefore be checked routinely in all people with diabetes.

- **Pre-proliferative retinopathy**: cotton-wool spots (retinal ischaemia interrupts axoplasmic transport). Venous beading and IRMAs (intra-retinal microvascular abnormalities) caused by dilated capillaries. Not sight threatening.
- **Proliferative retinopathy**: retinal ischaemia induces new vessels, which are fragile and bleed easily. Retinal detachment from traction scars occurs, leading to further bleeding. The closer to the disc, the greater the risk to sight.
- **Cataract**: occurs 10–15 years earlier in people with diabetes.
- **Management**: annual eye checks, good glycaemic and BP control. Laser retinal photocoagulation in pre-proliferative and proliferative retinopathy as well as in maculopathy.

Nephropathy

This occurs 15–25 years after diagnosis in 35–45% of patients with type 1 diabetes and < 20% of patients with type 2 diabetes. The initial lesion is glomerular hyperfiltration (increased glomerular filtration rate [GFR]), which leads on to diffuse thickening of the glomerular basement membrane (GBM), manifest as microalbuminuria (urinary albumin 30–300 mg/day), a highly accurate marker of overall vascular damage and thus a predictor of impending cardiovascular death. Persistent albuminuria (urinary albumin > 300 mg/day) is initially associated with normal GFR but, as overt proteinuria (urinary protein > 0.5 g/24 h) develops, GFR progressively falls and overt renal failure develops.

- **Clinical features**: asymptomatic early on, later hypertension, oedema and uraemia occur.
- **Management**: antihypertensive treatment with angiotensin-converting enzyme (ACE) inhibitor as first-line therapy. ACE inhibitors are also beneficial if there is any proteinuria, regardless of blood pressure. Good glycaemic control. Lipid lowering agents and aspirin. Chronic renal failure requires renal replacement therapy with dialysis or transplantation.

Neuropathy

This occurs through multiple mechanisms including damage to the small blood vessels nourishing the peripheral nerves, and abnormal sugar metabolism. There are several manifestations:

- **Peripheral sensory neuropathy** which progresses from a 'loss of vibration sense' early on to a 'glove and stocking' sensory loss 'as if walking on cotton wool'.
- **Mononeuropathies** can affect any nerve, but have a predilection for those controlling eye movements, especially the oculomotor nerve, where the pupillary reactions are spared.
- **Amyotrophy**: painful wasting of thigh muscles.
- **Autonomic neuropathy**: postural hypotension, absent cardiac vagal tone (no sinus arrhythmia), gustatory sweating, gastroparesis, nocturnal diarrhoea, bladder dysfunction (increased infections, incontinence), and erectile impotence.

    Management: treatment is unsatisfactory and mainly supportive.

Macrovascular complications of diabetes mellitus

Diabetes is a major risk factor for development of atherosclerosis. Cerebrovascular risk is increased twofold, coronary artery disease three- to fivefold and peripheral vascular disease 40-fold. Diabetes synergizes strongly with other macrovascular risk factors. People with asymptomatic type 2 diabetes have the same cardiovascular mortality as those who do not have diabetes but have symptomatic vascular disease. These facts justify highly aggressive antiatherogenic treatments in all people with diabetes.

Foot disease

This occurs as a result of peripheral vascular disease (cold painful foot), peripheral neuropathy (warm foot, often without much pain) and increased susceptibility to infection, and results in ulceration, infection (cellulitis and osteomyelitis), gangrene and Charcot's foot (warm/hot foot with destruction of joint).

    Management: prevention is by patient education, good footwear and podiatry, with antibiotic treatment of infection, debridement of ulcers and reconstructive arterial surgery for peripheral vascular disease. Amputation is occasionally required for gangrene and ischaemia. Immobilization of Charcot's foot ± bisphosphonates are also used.

Prevention of complications

Good glycaemic control delays the onset of progression of all microvascular disease. Macrovascular disease is less likely in patients with good blood pressure control (< 130/80 mmHg), and when all other risk factors are under optimal control. This means that highly aggressive cholesterol and blood pressure-lowering therapy is indicated. Smoking in diabetes leads to a very premature death.

Hypoglycaemia

This is a common complication in people with diabetes who are treated with insulin and occasionally occurs in those on sulphonylureas. Symptoms occur when the blood glucose is ≤ 2.2 mmol/L, although many people with diabetes, who are used to higher blood glucose, have symptoms at higher blood glucose levels. Causes other than diabetic treatment are rare:

- Alcohol.
- Renal or hepatic failure.
- Very rare causes include: reactive hypoglycaemia—rebound hypoglycaemia after a glucose load, insulinoma (pancreatic tumour producing insulin inappropriately), endocrine disease (adrenocortical failure, hypopituitarism) and insulin-like growth factor II (IGF-II)-producing tumours (pleural fibroma, sarcoma).

Clinical features and treatment

The cardinal features of hypoglycaemia are initially anxiety, poor concentration with impaired cognition, proceeding to a decrease in conscious level, which may progress to coma and seizures. The signs are of sweating, tremor and tachycardia, and there may be an extensor plantar response. Immediate treatment with glucose should be given—oral if possible, otherwise intravenously (50 mL of 50% glucose into a large vein). If veins cannot be cannulated, intramuscular glucagon is helpful. The underlying cause also clearly needs to be addressed.

Investigation

The cause is readily apparent in people with diabetes who are treated with insulin and those on sulphonylureas, and extensive investigations are not needed. In those who are not on such treatment, glucose, insulin and C-peptide levels are taken before giving glucose. A raised insulin and C-peptide suggests an insulinoma, whereas raised insulin and low C-peptide suggests exogenous insulin administration. If there is no obvious precipitant it is also important to exclude Addison's disease, and if this is negative to search for IGF-II-producing tumours, including using pancreatic magnetic resonance imaging and chest computed tomography. Urine assay for sulphonylureas may be diagnostic.

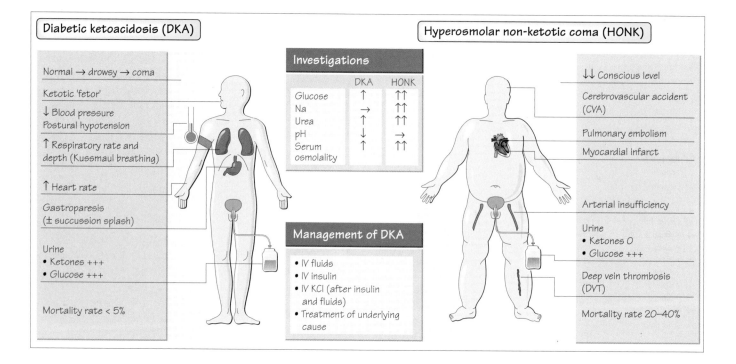

Diabetic ketoacidosis (DKA)

Normal → drowsy → coma

Ketotic 'fetor'

↓ Blood pressure
Postural hypotension

↑ Respiratory rate and
depth (Kussmaul breathing)

↑ Heart rate

Gastroparesis
(± succussion splash)

Urine
• Ketones +++
• Glucose +++

Mortality rate < 5%

Hyperosmolar non-ketotic coma (HONK)

↓↓ Conscious level

Cerebrovascular accident
(CVA)

Pulmonary embolism

Myocardial infarct

Arterial insufficiency

Urine
• Ketones 0
• Glucose +++

Deep vein thrombosis
(DVT)

Mortality rate 20–40%

Investigations

	DKA	HONK
Glucose	↑	↑↑
Na	→	↑↑
Urea	↑	↑↑
pH	↓	→
Serum osmolality	↑	↑↑

Management of DKA

• IV fluids
• IV insulin
• IV KCl (after insulin
  and fluids)
• Treatment of underlying
  cause

Diabetic ketoacidosis

Diabetic ketoacidosis (DKA) relates to absolute insulin deficiency and therefore occurs in type 1 but not in type 2 diabetes. Lack of insulin causes hyperglycaemia (osmotic diuresis and dehydration) and raises ketone bodies levels, so inducing a metabolic acidosis.

• **Precipitants** are common and should always be sought—infections, omitting insulin (sometimes for psychological reasons), myocardial infarction (MI), surgery/trauma; undiagnosed type 1 diabetes.

• **Features**: thirst, polyuria and dehydration (even hypovolaemic shock), vomiting and abdominal pain, tachypnoea (from acidosis—Kussmaul's respiration); decreased consciousness.

• **Investigations**: blood glucose typically > 20 mmol/L; urine—large amount of ketones, high potassium as a result of acidosis, although total body potassium is depleted. Arterial acidosis (pH usually 7.0–7.2), decrease in bicarbonate as a result of metabolic acidosis and decrease in $P\text{CO}_2$ (carbon dioxide tension) as a result of hyperventilation.

• Investigation of precipitant: microbiology, chest X-ray, ECG. Full blood count (FBC)—neutrophilia is common and does not necessarily indicate infection.

• **Management**: fluid replacement, often 3–5 L in < 6 h. Insulin intravenously, e.g. 6 units soluble insulin, followed by infusion. Potassium replacement (10–20 mmol/h) after initial insulin and fluid replacement (danger of hypokalaemia because insulin drives potassium into cells). Close monitoring of electrolytes. Occasionally need bicarbonate. Nasogastric tube for gastroparesis. Treatment of the underlying cause.

• **Prognosis**: always need insulin long term. Overall mortality during DKA is low (< 5%).

Hyperosmolar non-ketotic coma (HONK)

Found in type 2 but not in type 1 diabetes because insulin levels are insufficient to prevent hyperglycaemia, but sufficient to prevent ketosis.

• **Precipitant**: infection, MI, excessive sugary drinks.

• **Features**: thirst and polyuria; impaired concentration level; hyperviscosity leads to thrombotic complications (deep vein thrombosis [DVT], pulmonary embolism, stroke).

• **Investigations**: glucose is often very high (> 50 mmol/L), sodium often > 160 mmol/L; plasma osmolality is increased; acidosis is absent or mild.

• Investigation of precipitant: ECG, cardiac enzymes, and microbiology.

• **Management**: often need central venous monitoring if patients are elderly or have cardiac disease. Intravenous fluids ± K^+ replacement. Intravenous insulin 3 units/h; anticoagulation.

• **Prognosis**: mortality from HONK is very high at 20–40%. After the acute episode has resolved, the diabetes can often be managed with diet or oral hypoglycaemic agents.

Lactic acidosis

This is a very rare complication of metformin treatment. Patients present with symptoms of acidaemia (malaise, anorexia, vomiting) and signs of hyperventilation (Kussmaul's breathing). Glucose levels are usually normal; there are no ketones in the urine and blood gases show a (profound) acidosis, with high base excess. The anion gap is increased (see p. 252). Treatment is supportive and by the withdrawal of metformin.

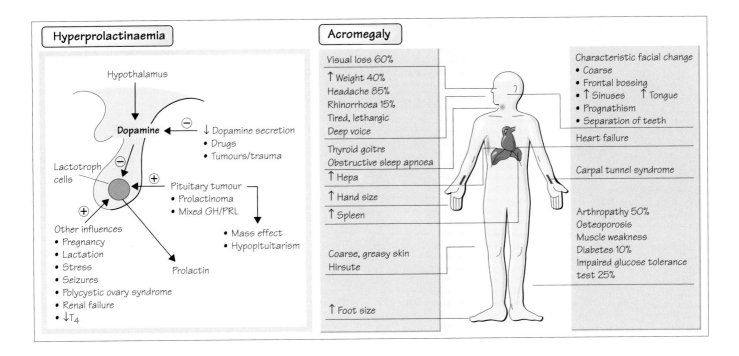

Hyperprolactinaemia

This is more obvious in women, because of presentation with menstrual disturbance or infertility.

• Females: milk production (galactorrhoea) in 30–80%, menstrual irregularity (oligo-/amenorrhoea), infertility.

• Males: galactorrhoea (< 30%), erectile impotence, infertility ± features of a macroadenoma (mass effect—see Chapter 149).

Investigations in hyperprolactinaemia: prolactin levels can be very high. If the pathology is a macroadenoma, a full assessment of anterior pituitary function is needed. Women, probably because of the earlier presentation, are more likely to have a microprolactinoma. Stress, renal failure, hypothyroidism and polycystic ovary syndrome are all potent causes of hyperprolactinaemia and should be excluded. Other tests: magnetic resonance imaging (MRI) of the pituitary and visual field measurement.

Management of prolactinomas

• **Drug treatment**: dopamine agonists (bromocriptine or cabergoline) inhibit prolactin secretion and cause tumour shrinkage. Side effects include nausea, vomiting and postural hypotension.

• **Surgery**: trans-sphenoidal removal if there is drug intolerance or if tumour fails to shrink on dopamine agonist therapy.

• **Radiotherapy**: to prevent tumour regrowth after drug treatment or surgery for macroadenoma.

Acromegaly

This is the clinical condition resulting from prolonged excessive growth hormone (GH) secretion in adults (excessive GH in children results in gigantism). Extremely rare: $5/10^6$ population; males = females. Usually diagnosed at age 40–60 years. The underlying pathology is: (i) benign pituitary tumour (macroadenomas more common than microadenomas);

(ii) pituitary carcinoma (very rare); and (iii) GH-releasing hormone (GHRH)-secreting carcinoid tumours (very rare).

The clinical syndrome results from insulin-like growth factor I (IGF-I) which mediates the effects of GH: increased sweating, headache (independent of tumour size), tiredness and lethargy; joint pains; and effects of a mass in the pituitary fossa (visual field defects, hypopituitarism).

• **Examination**: characteristic facial appearance (see figure), deep voice, carpal tunnel syndrome, hand and foot enlargement and organomegaly (goitre, hepatosplenomegaly).

• **Complications**: acromegaly increases cardiovascular morbidity and mortality, from hypertension, impaired glucose tolerance and diabetes mellitus. Cardiac failure (heart muscle disease), ischaemic heart and cerebrovascular disease are all increased. Obstructive sleep apnoea occurs. There may be an increased risk of colonic polyps and carcinoma.

Investigations and management

• **Laboratory tests**: IGF-I is high and GH levels are not suppressed by oral glucose.

• **Other investigations**: MRI scan of pituitary and visual field assessment.

The aim of treatment is to normalize GH and reduce the associated high mortality:

• **Surgery**: trans-sphenoidal adenomectomy or craniotomy for very large tumours.

• **Pituitary radiotherapy**: useful if tumour not fully removed and reduces GH progressively over years.

• **Drugs**: somatostatin analogues (octreotide, lanreotide) suppress GH in 60%. Dopamine agonists (bromocriptine, cabergoline) lower but rarely normalize GH. GH receptor antagonist (pegvisomant) normalizes IGF-I in > 90% of patients.

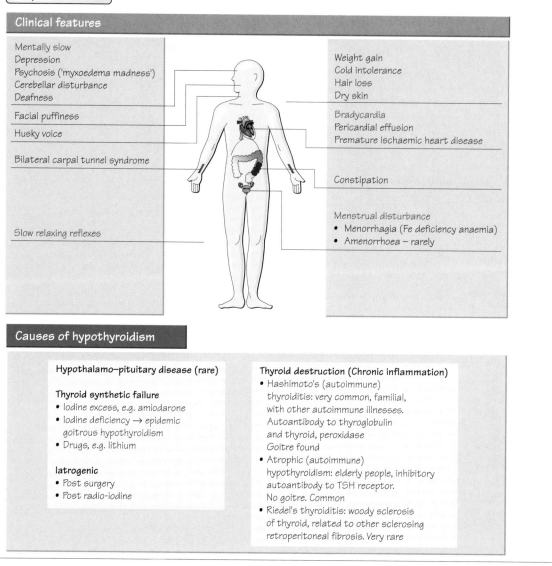

Hypothyroidism

Clinical features

Mentally slow
Depression
Psychosis ('myxoedema madness')
Cerebellar disturbance
Deafness

Facial puffiness

Husky voice

Bilateral carpal tunnel syndrome

Slow relaxing reflexes

Weight gain
Cold intolerance
Hair loss
Dry skin

Bradycardia
Pericardial effusion
Premature ischaemic heart disease

Constipation

Menstrual disturbance
• Menorrhagia (Fe deficiency anaemia)
• Amenorrhoea – rarely

Causes of hypothyroidism

Hypothalamo–pituitary disease (rare)

Thyroid synthetic failure
• Iodine excess, e.g. amiodarone
• Iodine deficiency → epidemic
  goitrous hypothyroidism
• Drugs, e.g. lithium

Iatrogenic
• Post surgery
• Post radio-iodine

Thyroid destruction (Chronic inflammation)
• Hashimoto's (autoimmune)
  thyroiditis: very common, familial,
  with other autoimmune illnesses.
  Autoantibody to thyroglobulin
  and thyroid, peroxidase
  Goitre found
• Atrophic (autoimmune)
  hypothyroidism: elderly people, inhibitory
  autoantibody to TSH receptor.
  No goitre. Common
• Riedel's thyroiditis: woody sclerosis
  of thyroid, related to other sclerosing
  retroperitoneal fibrosis. Very rare

Hypothyroidism is the clinical state arising from decreased production of and/or the effect of thyroid hormones.

Epidemiology
The female/male ratio is 6 : 1 in primary hypothyroidism. The prevalence is 1–5%, and the incidence 2/1000. It is most common from middle age onwards and often associated with a family history of autoimmune disease.

Causes
Thyroid failure can be caused by disease of the thyroid (primary hypothyroidism), the pituitary gland (secondary) or the hypothalamus (tertiary). Primary hypothyroidism is common and in Europe/North America is usually the result of autoimmune disease or previous radio-iodine treatment for hyperthyroidism (50% hypothyroid at 10 years). Worldwide, the most common cause is iodine deficiency.

Although hypothyroidism can be congenital, the important causes in adult life are:
• **Autoimmune**: there are two forms of autoimmune thyroiditis, which are easily distinguished by the presence (Hashimoto's thyroiditis/lymphocytic) or absence (atrophic) of a goitre. In both, autoantibodies are found (see below). Family members may have Addison's disease, pernicious anaemia or diabetes. Occasionally Hashimoto's thyroiditis gives rise to pain during the acute phase and, rarely, to transient hyperthyroidism.

- **Post-thyrotoxicosis treatment**: radio-iodine, surgery, anti-thyroid drugs.
- **Iodine deficiency**: endemic goitre (e.g. Derbyshire neck) is the most common worldwide cause of hypothyroidism.
- **Iodine excess**: chronic excess (e.g. amiodarone) may cause hypothyroidism.

Clinical features
See figure.

Investigations
- **Haematology**: full blood count (FBC) shows a mild macrocytic (mean cell volume [MCV] = 95–110 fL) anaemia. If Hb < 10 g/dL, suspect an additional cause—if MCV > 115 fL, this may be pernicious anaemia (see p. 318), and if MCV < 85 fL iron deficiency anaemia (menorrhagia).
- **Thyroid function tests**: low thyroxine (T4) and elevated thyroid stimulating hormone or TSH (primary hypothyroidism)—low or normal TSH (secondary/tertiary hypothyroidism).
- **Cortisol**: to exclude coexistent hypoadrenalism (Addison's disease or reduced ACTH reserve in secondary hypothyroidism).
- **Thyroid antibodies**: positive peroxidase and thyroglobulin antibodies in Hashimoto's thyroiditis, and blocking thyroid hormone-stimulating hormone (TSH) in atrophic thyroiditis.
- **Other biochemistry**: cholesterol levels are raised, as may muscle enzymes (e.g. aspartate transaminase [AST] and creatine kinase [CK]).
- **ECG**: bradycardia, low-voltage complexes.

Management
This is with thyroxine, starting at 50 µg/day and increasing to 125–150 µg/day, with the dose titrated against clinical and biochemical (normal TSH) response. Lower starting doses, or triiodothyronine (T3), which has a short half-life, may be used in elderly patients and patients with ischaemic heart disease because higher doses may provoke angina or myocardial infarction.

Myxoedema coma
This is a rare complication with a mortality rate > 50%. It should be suspected in any patient with hypothermia and coma. It is difficult to distinguish from other causes of hypothermia, because the same risk factors (sedatives, age, etc.) are present. It is vital to start treatment immediately (before diagnostic biochemistry is available) with intravenous T3 (20 µg bolus, repeated 6-hourly). As thyroid failure may relate to pituitary disease (suspect when the Na^+ is low), hydrocortisone should also be given (100 mg bolus, repeated 6-hourly) until an accurate diagnosis is made. Supportive therapy, including space blankets, antibiotics, fluids and correction of acidosis, may also be needed.

Congenital hypothyroidism
Though essentially beyond this textbook, it is none-the-less important to mention congenital hypothyroidism. The incidence varies from 1 per 1300 (Middle East) to 1 per 4000 births. Worldwide, this results most commonly from low environmental iodine levels ('endemic cretinism'). In the developed world, where iodine supplementation of the drinking water is common, endemic cretinism does not occur; sporadic cretinism does, however, and is commonly due to thyroid gland agenesis (50%), ectopia (25%), errors of metabolism (10%), and rarely (15%) from disorders in the hypothalamic-pituitary axis.

While 'in utero', the fetus receives thyroid hormone through the placenta from the mother, and so develops normally. However, after birth, this exogenous supply disappears—the infant is then deprived of thyroid hormone. This results in failure of the brain to develop, leading to profound developmental retardation, and a syndrome previously called 'cretinism'. Treatment must be given early, or permanent damage occurs. Many (though not all) of the deleterious effects of thyroid hormone deficiency can be prevented by early diagnosis and treatment (i.e. diagnosis by day 13, normalization of thyroid hormone status by week 3)—since the clinical features can be far from obvious in infants, the best means of diagnosis is by biochemical assay. All children in the UK and developed countries are screened at birth for congenital hypothyroidism, by assaying TSH levels.

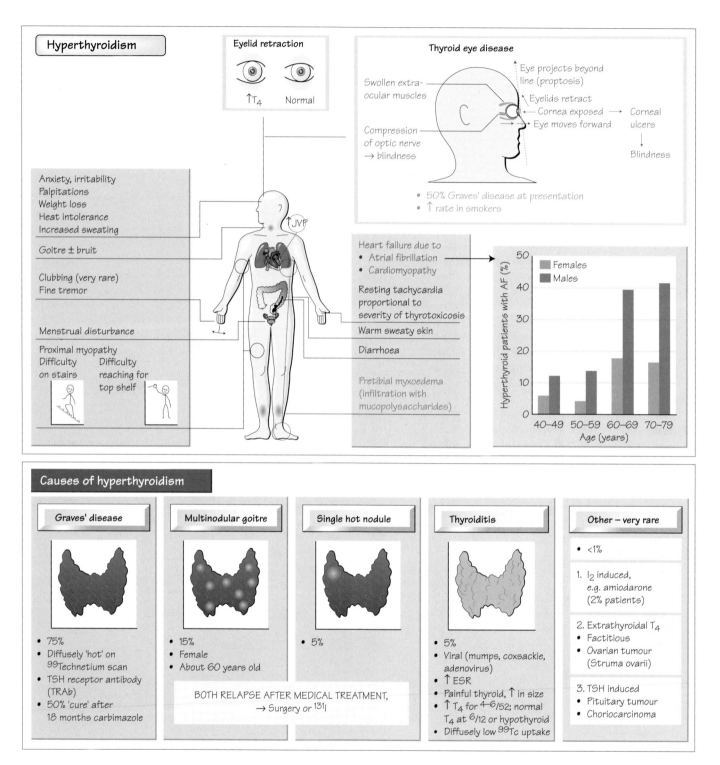

Hyperthyroidism

Eyelid retraction

↑T₄ Normal

Thyroid eye disease

Swollen extra-ocular muscles

Eye projects beyond line (proptosis)

Eyelids retract

Compression of optic nerve → blindness

Cornea exposed — Corneal ulcers

Eye moves forward

Blindness

- 50% Graves' disease at presentation
- ↑ rate in smokers

Anxiety, irritability
Palpitations
Weight loss
Heat intolerance
Increased sweating

Goitre ± bruit

Clubbing (very rare)
Fine tremor

Menstrual disturbance

Proximal myopathy
Difficulty on stairs   Difficulty reaching for top shelf

↑JVP

Heart failure due to
- Atrial fibrillation
- Cardiomyopathy

Resting tachycardia proportional to severity of thyrotoxicosis

Warm sweaty skin

Diarrhoea

Pretibial myxoedema (infiltration with mucopolysaccharides)

Females
Males

Hyperthyroid patients with AF (%)

50
40
30
20
10
0

40–49 50–59 60–69 70–79
Age (years)

Causes of hyperthyroidism

Graves' disease

- 75%
- Diffusely 'hot' on ⁹⁹Technetium scan
- TSH receptor antibody (TRAb)
- 50% 'cure' after 18 months carbimazole

Multinodular goitre

- 15%
- Female
- About 60 years old

BOTH RELAPSE AFTER MEDICAL TREATMENT,
→ Surgery or ¹³¹I

Single hot nodule

- 5%

Thyroiditis

- 5%
- Viral (mumps, coxsackie, adenovirus)
- ↑ ESR
- Painful thyroid, ↑ in size
- ↑ T₄ for ⁴⁻⁶/52; normal T₄ at ⁶/12 or hypothyroid
- Diffusely low ⁹⁹Tc uptake

Other – very rare

- <1%

1. I₂ induced, e.g. amiodarone (2% patients)

2. Extrathyroidal T₄
- Factitious
- Ovarian tumour (Struma ovarii)

3. TSH induced
- Pituitary tumour
- Choriocarcinoma

Diseases and Treatments at a Glance

Definition and epidemiology

The clinical condition is caused by increased circulating free levels of thyroid hormones. The prevalence is 2%. The male/female ratio is 1 : 5. It is most common in middle age.

Causes

The most common causes of hyperthyroidism are autoimmune thyroid disease (usually Graves' disease), a toxic nodular goitre and a toxic adenoma

- **Graves' disease**: 75% of cases. An autoimmune disorder resulting from the interaction of antibodies to immunoglobulin IgG TSH (thyroid-stimulating hormone) receptors with the thyroid gland TSH receptor, leading to thyroid gland stimulation, increased thyroxine (T4) secretion and thyroid growth. Associated with Graves' disease is eye disease (ophthalmopathy) and organ-specific autoimmune disease.
- **Toxic multinodular goitre**: 15% of cases. Hyperthyroidism may develop in a long-standing goitre. Relapses after anti-thyroid drug therapy, so definitive surgery/radiotherapy required.
- **Toxic adenoma** (single nodular goitre): 5% of cases. An autonomous hyperfunctioning nodule that produces excess thyroid hormones and suppresses TSH secretion.
- **Hashimoto's thyroiditis**: autoimmune (thyroid peroxidase antibody related), smooth thyroid enlargement, may produce hyper- and then hypothyroidism.
- **Postpartum thyroiditis**: usually self-limiting.
- Rare causes include: viral (de Quervain's) thyroiditis, drugs such as amiodarone, excessive T4 replacement, iodine excess (Jod–Basedow effect), hypothalamic-pituitary disease (TSH-secreting tumour or pituitary resistance to thyroid hormones), or hyperemesis gravidarum (human chorionic gonadotrophin [hCG]-mediated stimulation of the thyroid).

Clinical features (see figure)

Investigations
- **Thyroid function tests**: increased T4 and triiodothyronine (T3), decreased TSH (primary hyperthyroidism).
- **Thyroid autoantibodies**: thyroid peroxidase and anti-thyroglobulin antibodies suggest an autoimmune aetiology.
- **Imaging**: thyroid uptake scan differentiates Graves' disease (diffusely increased uptake) from toxic adenoma (single hot spot) and multinodular goitre (multiple hot spots).

Management
- **Drug treatment**: first-line therapy in all patients regardless of diagnosis. Carbimazole decreases thyroid hormone synthesis. Initial dose 40–60 mg/day, later reduced to a maintenance dose. The dose is titrated according to thyroid function and continued for 18 months, after which 50% patients with Graves' disease are cured. An alternative approach is to give a large dose of carbimazole with T4 to avoid hypothyroidism ('block and replace' technique). Carbimazole causes agranulocytosis in 0.1%: it should be immediately stopped if sore throat or fever occurs. Propylthiouracil is an alternative anti-thyroid drug that is often preferred in pregnancy.

- **Surgery**: thyroidectomy for multinodular goitre, toxic adenoma or relapses of Graves' disease after anti-thyroid drug therapy. The risks are small but include vocal cord palsy (recurrent laryngeal nerve damage), hypothyroidism and hypoparathyroidism.
- **Radio-iodine** is concentrated in the thyroid gland, so destroying thyroid tissue. Anti-thyroid drugs are stopped 7–10 days before administration to allow uptake of radio-iodine. Occasionally repeated doses are required. Side effects: worsening of thyroid eye disease—may be the result of the aggravating effect of hypothyroidism; transient/permanent hypothyroidism (50% at 10 years); thyrotoxic crisis (if hyperthyroidism poorly controlled before administration); pain.

Treatment of thyroid-associated ophthalmopathy
- Supportive: elevation of head of bed, artificial tears, prismatic glasses for diplopia.
- Definitive: medical with high-dose steroids ± other immunosuppressants (to decompress orbit), surgical orbital decompression or orbital radiotherapy.

Thyroid storm
This is a rare life-threatening emergency (mortality rate of 10%). Fever, anxiety, agitation, confusion and tachycardia, and occasionally heart failure, can also occur.

Management of thyroid storm
- Affects < 2% of patients with hyperthyroidism.
- Treatment MUST be started before biochemical diagnosis (which takes too long).
- Mortality 10–20%.
- 50% of patients have lost > 15 kg.
- Storm often provoked by minor physical stress.
- Severe symptoms of hyperthyroidism in most, though not always in the elderly (apathetic hyperthyroidism).
- Examination shows tachycardia, often very marked, sweating, and sometimes confusion.
- ITU admission may be required, and should be anticipated.
- β-blockers, often in high dose, are the main stay of therapy.
- Give carbimazole or propylthiouracil immediately, by NG tube if necessary.
- 1 hour later give iodide.
- IV glucocorticoids; given in large doses to inhibit the synthesis of new circulating thyroid hormone.
- Fluid and electrolyte replacement, as appropriate.

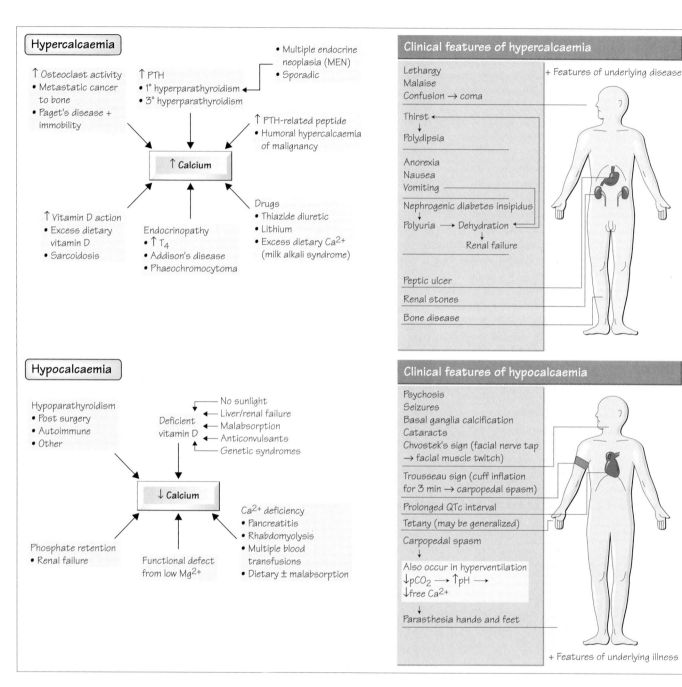

Hypercalcaemia

↑ Osteoclast activity
• Metastatic cancer to bone
• Paget's disease + immobility

↑ PTH
• 1° hyperparathyroidism
• 3° hyperparathyroidism

• Multiple endocrine neoplasia (MEN)
• Sporadic

↑ PTH-related peptide
• Humoral hypercalcaemia of malignancy

↑ Calcium

↑ Vitamin D action
• Excess dietary vitamin D
• Sarcoidosis

Endocrinopathy
• ↑ T₄
• Addison's disease
• Phaeochromocytoma

Drugs
• Thiazide diuretic
• Lithium
• Excess dietary Ca²⁺ (milk alkali syndrome)

Clinical features of hypercalcaemia

+ Features of underlying disease

Lethargy
Malaise
Confusion → coma

Thirst ←
↓
Polydipsia

Anorexia
Nausea
Vomiting

Nephrogenic diabetes insipidus
↓
Polyuria → Dehydration ←
↓
Renal failure

Peptic ulcer

Renal stones

Bone disease

Hypocalcaemia

Hypoparathyroidism
• Post surgery
• Autoimmune
• Other

Deficient vitamin D
— No sunlight
← Liver/renal failure
← Malabsorption
← Anticonvulsants
— Genetic syndromes

↓ Calcium

Phosphate retention
• Renal failure

Functional defect from low Mg²⁺

Ca²⁺ deficiency
• Pancreatitis
• Rhabdomyolysis
• Multiple blood transfusions
• Dietary ± malabsorption

Clinical features of hypocalcaemia

Psychosis
Seizures
Basal ganglia calcification
Cataracts
Chvostek's sign (facial nerve tap → facial muscle twitch)

Trousseau sign (cuff inflation for 3 min → carpopedal spasm)

Prolonged QTc interval

Tetany (may be generalized)

Carpopedal spasm
↓

Also occur in hyperventilation
↓pCO₂ → ↑pH →
↓free Ca²⁺
↓
Parasthesia hands and feet

+ Features of underlying illness

Acute hypercalcaemia

The more rapid the rise and the higher the calcium level, the more likely are patients to present with an acute brain syndrome, comprising confusion, drowsiness and coma (rarely muscle weakness or psychosis). In less marked hypercalcaemia, there can be thirst and polyuria, from calcium-induced nephrogenic diabetes insipidus, and abdominal symptoms such as anorexia, nausea and vomiting, abdominal pain and constipation. Chronic hypercalcaemia also produces renal stones and bone disease.

Aetiology

Hypercalcaemia occurs in 5–50/10 000. The diagnosis is achieved from the clinical situation and from biochemical tests. Key points are:
• Is malignancy present or likely clinically or on routine investigations?
• Is the parathyroid hormone (PTH) level high or suppressed? Normal (inappropriate in normally functioning parathyroid) or elevated PTH levels suggest primary hyperparathyroidism (far and away the most common cause), tertiary hyperparathyroidism (autonomous parathyroid glands in longstanding chronic renal failure), rarely familial

hypocalciuric or lithium-induced hypercalcaemia. Low PTH levels mean that the parathyroid gland is not responsible; causes include malignancy, sarcoidosis, thyrotoxicosis and thiazide diuretic induced.

• Presence of associated biochemical and investigative abnormalities. Elevated alkaline phosphatase, with deranged liver function tests, suggests malignancy. Paget's disease (mild hypercalcaemia on bed rest) usually has an isolated but large rise in alkaline phosphatase. Immunoglobulin electrophoresis may show a paraprotein band in myeloma. The chest X-ray may show sarcoidosis (bilateral hilar adenopathy) or cancer.

• A full dietary and drug history for excess vitamin D or calcium containing antacids (milk–alkali syndrome), thiazides and lithium.

Primary hyperparathyroidism

This is the most common cause of hypercalcaemia: female/male ratio = 2 : 1; 90% of patients are > 50 years (then female incidence is 3/1000). Symptoms of hypercalcaemia may occur, although 50% are asymptomatic patients undergoing biochemical assessment for other reasons. In 80%, the pathology is a single parathyroid adenoma; occasionally diffuse hyperplasia of all four glands occurs. Very rarely multiple endocrine neoplasia (MEN) I or II is present (see p. 293). In asymptomatic elderly patients with mild hypercalcaemia, an expectant course may be followed. In all others, definitive treatment is surgical resection, with the parathyroid adenoma being located by the surgeon at the time of operation. Imaging studies (nuclear or ultrasound scans) are required if the adenoma is not found at initial operation. Postoperative hypocalcaemia is usually transient and is treated with calcium supplements and 1α-hydroxy-vitamin D.

Hypercalcaemia of malignancy

This is the second most common cause of hypercalcaemia. There are two underlying mechanisms:

1 Tumour deposits in bone: most (> 95%) hypercalcaemia in malignancy relates to widespread metastatic disease. The most common neoplasms are lung, breast and myeloma. Patients are usually highly symptomatic both from the cancer and, as calcium levels are high and have risen quickly, from hypercalcaemia.

2 Humoral hypercalcaemia of malignancy (HHM) relates to PTH-related peptide (PTHrP), a peptide made up of 144 amino acids, which bears a structural relationship to PTH and mimics its action. The responsible neoplasm is most likely to be squamous carcinoma of the lung, although this can be a genitourinary or gynaecological malignancy. Although HHM is rare, its clinical importance is that **not all patients with malignancy and hypercalcaemia necessarily have metastatic disease**. This point is vital in deciding whether or not the primary should be resected.

Sarcoidosis and other granulomatous diseases

These are associated with hypercalcaemia, which responds readily to steroids.

Other causes of hypercalcaemia

Thyrotoxicosis and thiazide diuretics can induce hypercalcaemia. Familial hypocalciuric hypercalcaemia is an autosomal dominant inherited condition in which hypercalcaemia is associated with low renal excretion of calcium; Paget's disease.

Management

Acute/symptomatic hypercalcaemia is a medical emergency and requires urgent treatment, principally aggressive rehydration with physiological or 0.9% **saline**, which alone readily lowers calcium. **Loop diuretic** can be added to fluid therapy once adequate hydration has occurred. **Bisphosphonates** are also effective regardless of the underlying pathology. **Steroids** may be added in hypercalcaemia of malignancy and vitamin D-related hypercalcaemia. **Calcitonin** helps in Paget's disease. Definitive therapy varies according to the underlying disease.

Hypocalcaemia

Acute hypocalcaemia results in circumoral tingling, tetany, especially in the muscles supplied by long nerves, and seizures. Chvostek's sign (a tap to the facial nerve just anterior to the ear causing brief facial muscle contraction) and Trousseau's sign (inflation of a blood pressure cuff resulting in carpopedal spasm) occur. Chronic hypocalcaemia in addition results in basal ganglia calcification and cataracts.

Aetiology

Hypocalcaemia is rare, and usually relates to one of four diseases:

• **Secondary hyperparathyroidism**: the most common cause of hypocalcaemia, occurring in acute or chronic renal failure. Failure of renal vitamin D hydroxylation, together with phosphate retention (through the calcium phosphate double product), depress serum Ca^{2+}, stimulating PTH release in an attempt to normalize serum Ca^{2+}. This leads to osteoclast activation, cyst formation and bone marrow fibrosis (osteitis fibrosa cystica), which together with aluminium toxicity contribute to renal bone disease. Characteristic X-ray findings are found in the hand, skull ('pepper pot') and spine ('rugger jersey'). The diagnosis is usually obvious from creatinine and phosphate levels, and the characteristic radiology. Treatment is with vitamin D and phosphate binders. If secondary hyperparathyroidism is left untreated, parathyroid gland hyperplasia leads to autonomous production of PTH—tertiary hyperparathyroidism with frank hypercalcaemia.

• **Post-thyroid/parathyroid surgery**: transient hypocalcaemia may occur.

• **Idiopathic autoimmune parathyroid failure**: very rare. Parathyroid autoantibodies are found. Other autoimmune conditions (vitiligo, etc.) may occur.

• **Osteomalacia**: resulting from inadequate active vitamin D; associated with low calcium levels, although these are usually not so low as to cause symptoms. Osteomalacia may be compounded by dietary calcium deficiency or relate to malabsorption.

Treatment

• Acute symptoms (Ca^{2+} < 1.9 mmol/L): intravenous bolus of 10% calcium gluconate 10–20 mL with ECG monitoring followed by intravenous infusion if necessary. Oral calcium and vitamin D as soon as possible. Intravenous magnesium sulphate may be required.

• Chronic disease: vitamin D metabolites (calcitriol or alphacalcidol) and oral calcium.

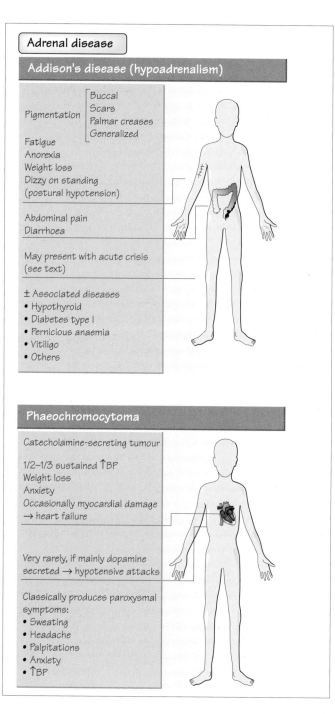

Adrenal disease

Addison's disease (hypoadrenalism)

Pigmentation
- Buccal
- Scars
- Palmar creases
- Generalized

Fatigue
Anorexia
Weight loss
Dizzy on standing
(postural hypotension)

Abdominal pain
Diarrhoea

May present with acute crisis
(see text)

± Associated diseases
- Hypothyroid
- Diabetes type I
- Pernicious anaemia
- Vitiligo
- Others

Phaeochromocytoma

Catecholamine-secreting tumour

1/2–1/3 sustained ↑BP
Weight loss
Anxiety
Occasionally myocardial damage
→ heart failure

Very rarely, if mainly dopamine
secreted → hypotensive attacks

Classically produces paroxysmal
symptoms:
- Sweating
- Headache
- Palpitations
- Anxiety
- ↑BP

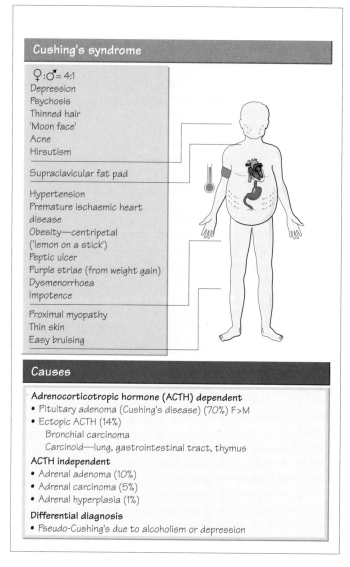

Cushing's syndrome

♀:♂ = 4:1
Depression
Psychosis
Thinned hair
'Moon face'
Acne
Hirsutism

Supraclavicular fat pad

Hypertension
Premature ischaemic heart
disease
Obesity—centripetal
('lemon on a stick')
Peptic ulcer
Purple striae (from weight gain)
Dysmenorrhoea
Impotence

Proximal myopathy
Thin skin
Easy bruising

Causes

Adrenocorticotropic hormone (ACTH) dependent
- Pituitary adenoma (Cushing's disease) (70%) F>M
- Ectopic ACTH (14%)
    Bronchial carcinoma
    Carcinoid—lung, gastrointestinal tract, thymus

ACTH independent
- Adrenal adenoma (10%)
- Adrenal carcinoma (5%)
- Adrenal hyperplasia (1%)

Differential diagnosis
- Pseudo-Cushing's due to alcoholism or depression

Adrenal failure

Failure of adrenal steroid hormone production:
- Atrophy/destruction of the adrenal gland (primary adrenal failure).
- Inadequate adrenocorticotrophin hormone (ACTH) production (secondary adrenal failure)—the most common cause, resulting from acute steroid withdrawal.

Cortisol is needed for the stress response to infection, surgery and trauma. In primary adrenal failure, cortisol deficiency increases ACTH and melanocyte-stimulating hormone (MSH) production, causing hyperpigmentation, seen in the buccal mucosa, on the palms of hands and in scars. Hyperpigmentation does not occur in secondary adrenal failure (depressed ACTH).

- **Primary adrenal failure**: rare: $50/10^6$. Autoimmune (Addison's) adrenal destruction, associated with vitiligo, premature ovarian failure and hypothyroidism. Females > males; gradual onset of symptoms; worldwide tuberculosis (TB) destruction of the adrenal glands is more common. Other causes are very rare:
  - Infection (HIV, fungi)
  - Invasion with cancer cells (lymphoma, breast, lung)
  - Haemorrhage: anticoagulants, Waterhouse-Friedrichsen syndrome from meningococcal septicaemia-induced disseminated intravascular coagulation (DIC)—adrenal failure occurs days/weeks after the initial haemorrhage-induced cortisol release
  - Infiltration (amyloid, sarcoid, haemochromatosis)
  - Congenital adrenal hyperplasia and drugs (ketoconazole).

- **Secondary adrenal failure**: common; chronic steroid therapy suppresses ACTH levels, producing adrenal cortex atrophy—physical stress or over-quick steroid withdrawal can then provoke acute adrenal failure. Pituitary failure (rare).

Clinical features of Addison's disease
- Chronic adrenal failure presents with a myriad of vague symptoms, including fatigue, weight loss, anorexia, abdominal pain, diarrhoea and postural hypotension.
- Acute adrenal failure presents with hypovolaemic shock precipitated by intercurrent stress. Untreated, this leads to refractory shock, profound hypoglycaemia and death.

Investigations
Acute adrenal failure should always be suspected in shock with hyponatraemia (± hyperkalaemia and hypoglycaemia). Hyponatraemia occurs late in the disease, but only in primary adrenal failure (mineralocorticoid deficiency) not in secondary adrenal failure where the renin-angiotensin system remains intact. Cortisol is low or normal. ACTH is high in primary failure, low in secondary failure.
- **Short synacthen test**: adrenal stimulation using synthetic ACTH fails to produce cortisol when given only once in adrenal failure from any cause.
- **Long synacthen test**: if ACTH is given repetitively over 3 days, if it has not been destroyed, the adrenal will produce cortisol.

Adrenal autoantibodies are found in autoimmune Addison's disease. Imaging (computed tomography or CT) or biopsy is used when rare diseases are suspected.

Management
- Chronic adrenal failure: glucocorticoid replacement with hydrocortisone 20 mg/day in divided doses, doubled with treatment of infection or intercurrent illness, or surgery. Mineralocorticoid replacement (fludrocortisone) only in primary adrenal failure.
- Acute adrenal failure: a medical emergency. Large volumes of intravenous fluid (physiological saline) and hydrocortisone are given at high doses. The precipitant (infection, etc.) may also need treating. Monitor electrolytes and glucose.

Hyperaldosteronism
This causes treatment-resistant hypertension (2% of hypertension) with hypokalaemia. Occasionally K^+ is normal if salt intake is low. The causes are:
- Benign adenoma (Conn's syndrome) (66%).
- Bilateral adrenal hyperplasia (30%).
- Rarely glucocorticoid remedial aldosteronism or adrenal carcinoma.

Laboratory tests demonstrate hypokalaemia, increased urinary K^+ excretion, suppressed renin and elevated aldosterone. CT scan of the adrenal glands helps define the pathology. Radiolabelled cholesterol scan and adrenal vein sampling are occasionally useful. Treatment is with surgery (adrenalectomy) for Conn's adenoma and aldosterone antagonists (spironolactone or amiloride) for other causes.

Phaeochromocytoma
This is a catecholamine-producing tumour of the adrenal medulla. It accounts for < 0.5% of hypertension and has an equal sex incidence. It is most common at age 30–50 years. The 10% rule applies: 10% malignant, 10% multiple, 10% bilateral, 10% extra-adrenal and 10% familial (von Hippel–Lindau syndrome, neurofibromatosis, multiple endocrine

neoplasia [MEN] II). Characteristically, it produces paroxysmal symptoms: labile hypertension (crises precipitated by exercise, abdominal examination, surgery, general anaesthesia, β-blockade), palpitations, sweating, headache, pallor or flushing, anxiety and glucose intolerance.

Investigations, management and prognosis
Catecholamine metabolites are detected in the urine. Adrenal imaging with magnetic resonance imaging (MRI) or MIBG scan (meta-iodobenzylguanidine, avidly taken up by chromaffin cells) may demonstrate multiple tumours or metastases.
- **Initial management**: at diagnosis α-adrenoreceptor blockade (phenoxybenzamine) before β-blockade (propranolol).
- **Definitive management**: adrenalectomy for tumour removal. Pre-operative α- and β-blockade are vital because tumour handling may precipitate a crisis. Surgery is curative in > 90% in benign disease, recurrence occurs in < 10%. The 5-year survival rate is ≥ 95% for treated benign tumours but < 50% for malignant tumours.

Cushing's syndrome
The clinical condition resulting from prolonged exposure to excessive glucocorticoids from:
- Exogenous glucocorticoid administration.
- Endogenous hypersecretion of glucocorticoids: very rare ($1–4/10^6$).

Investigations
- **Confirm Cushing's syndrome**: diagnosed when the 24-h urinary free cortisol is increased, midnight cortisol is detectable and 9 a.m. cortisol is detectable after 48 h of low-dose dexamethasone.
- **Determine the cause**: ACTH levels are normal/increased in ACTH-dependent or low in ACTH-independent cases. Serum $K^+ < 3.2$ mmol/L suggests ectopic ACTH secretion. In pituitary-dependent cases (termed Cushing's disease), there is a 50% suppression of serum cortisol with high-dose dexamethasone and no suppression in ectopic disease. Adrenal imaging can be helpful.
- **Corticotrophin (CRH)-releasing test**: administer CRH and measure cortisol. Pituitary disease—excessive rise; ectopic disease—flat response.
- **Venous sampling**: inferior petrosal sinus sampling to confirm pituitary-dependent disease. Body sampling to locate ectopic source of ACTH.
- **Imaging**: Cushing's disease is usually the result of a microadenoma, which may not be visible on MRI. CT of chest/elsewhere to locate ectopic sources of ACTH.

Management and prognosis
- Drug treatment: metyrapone (blocks cortisol synthesis) or ketoconazole (inhibits cytochrome P450 enzyme) lowers cortisol levels short-term before surgery or long-term when surgery inappropriate.
- Pituitary adenoma: trans-sphenoidal adenomectomy produces remission in > 70% cases—radiotherapy used for uncured relapse. Bilateral adrenalectomy produces aggressive pituitary tumour enlargement and hyperpigmentation as a result of excessive ACTH secretion (Nelson's syndrome) unless pituitary radiotherapy also given.
- Adrenal adenoma: adrenalectomy is curative.
- Adrenal carcinoma: surgery is not curative. Drug treatment with mitotane, an adrenolytic agent, can be helpful.
- Ectopic secretion: surgical removal of tumour if possible—otherwise medical treatment or adrenalectomy.

Untreated, Cushing's syndrome has a survival of < 5 years as a result of cardiovascular disease or infection.

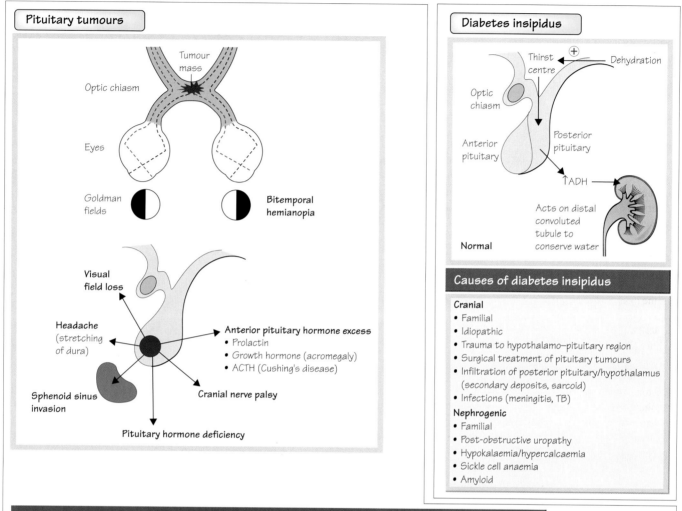

Pituitary tumours

Tumour mass

Optic chiasm

Eyes

Goldman fields — Bitemporal hemianopia

Visual field loss

Headache (stretching of dura)

Anterior pituitary hormone excess
- Prolactin
- Growth hormone (acromegaly)
- ACTH (Cushing's disease)

Sphenoid sinus invasion

Cranial nerve palsy

Pituitary hormone deficiency

Diabetes insipidus

Thirst centre ← Dehydration

Optic chiasm

Anterior pituitary

Posterior pituitary

↑ADH

Acts on distal convoluted tubule to conserve water

Normal

Causes of diabetes insipidus

Cranial
- Familial
- Idiopathic
- Trauma to hypothalamo–pituitary region
- Surgical treatment of pituitary tumours
- Infiltration of posterior pituitary/hypothalamus (secondary deposits, sarcoid)
- Infections (meningitis, TB)

Nephrogenic
- Familial
- Post-obstructive uropathy
- Hypokalaemia/hypercalcaemia
- Sickle cell anaemia
- Amyloid

Pituitary hormone deficiency

Characteristic sequence of loss in pituitary macroadenomas

Earliest ————————————————————————→ Latest

Hormone	GH	FSH/LH	ACTH	TSH	Prolactin	ADH
Clinical features	Loss of well-being	• No 2° sexual hair • Infertile • Impotent	• Pale • Hypoadrenal	• Hypothyroid	• Lactatory failure	• Diabetes insipidus
Deficiency diagnosed by	• GH after stimulation (insulin, arginine, glucagon) • Insulin-like growth factor-I (IGF-I)	♂ • [Testosterone] ♀ • Pre-menopause: periods • Post-menopause: [LH] [FSH]	• Short synacthen test • Insulin tolerance test	• TSH • T₄	Prolactin	• Serum Na⁺ • Osmolality • Water deprivation test

Table 149.1 Pathophysiology of diabetes insipidus (DI).

	[Na⁺]	Osmolality Plasma	Urine	Urine osmolality on water deprivation	Response to synthetic ADH
Cranial DI	↑	↑	↓	Fails to concentrate	Normal
Nephrogenic DI	↑	↑	↓	Fails to concentrate	Fails to concentrate
Primary polydipsia	↓	↓	↓	Concentrates	Normal

Diseases of the pituitary gland

Pituitary gland diseases are rare, and may be characterized by selective or total (panhypopituitary) pituitary failure, visual failure, selective excess in pituitary-dependent hormones (tumours) and hyperprolactinaemia (from mass lesions). Pituitary diseases include:

• Intrinsic neoplastic processes: may result in pituitary failure, mass effects (headaches and visual failure), and a selective increase in a pituitary-dependent hormone or hyperprolactinaemia.

• Inflammation (tuberculosis, sarcoidosis) and invasion by extrinsic tumours result in pituitary failure and, occasionally, in hyperprolactinaemia, by disruption of the tonic dopamine-mediated inhibition to prolactin release.

• Pituitary apoplexy: infarction not related to hypotension.

• Pituitary atrophy: infarction related to hypotension, often post partum (Sheehan's syndrome). Pituitary failure occurs early or up to 2 years after the hypotensive event.

Pituitary tumours

Pituitary tumours are the most common pituitary disorder and account for 10% of intracranial neoplasms. Tumours are classified according to size:

• Microadenoma < 1 cm in diameter—do not cause mass effects or hypopituitarism.

• Macroadenoma > 1 cm—can produce mass effects and hypopituitarism. Usually non-functioning, but can cause excessive hormonal secretion. Non-functioning macroadenomas are the most common form.

The clinical features of pituitary tumours are predictable based on which hormones have been lost or gained. **Investigations** aim to determine:

• Pituitary function: hormones (and their targets) are measured—growth hormone (insulin-like growth factor I [IGF-I]), follicle-stimulating hormone (FSH) and luteinizing hormone (LH), (testosterone/oestradiol), ACTH (cortisol ± dynamic tests), thyroid-stimulating hormone (TSH—thyroxine) and prolactin. Antidiuretic hormone (ADH) is assessed from serum Na⁺ and dynamic tests.

• Underlying disease process: assessed by magnetic resonance imaging (MRI) ± biopsy.

• Mass effect of the tumour: visual field loss (bitemporal hemianopia from compression of the optic chiasma), headache (dural stretching), cranial nerve palsies (lateral extension) or cerebrospinal fluid (CSF) rhinorrhoea/secondary meningitis (downward erosion into sphenoid sinus).

Management

• Replacement of anterior pituitary hormones: hydrocortisone and thyroxine to replace ACTH and TSH deficiency; sex hormone and growth hormone therapy.

• Treatment of underlying cause: non-functioning tumours are treated surgically (trans-sphenoidally or by craniotomy) and may need post-operative radiotherapy. Functioning tumours are treated by a combination of drugs, surgery and radiotherapy.

• Functioning tumours: prolactin (hyperprolactinaemia—see p. 283), growth hormone (acromegaly, see p. 283), ACTH (Cushing's disease —see p. 291).

Diabetes insipidus

This is the passage of large volumes of inappropriately dilute urine in the presence of concentrated plasma. It is uncommon, and has to be differentiated from other causes of polyuria (urine volume > 2.5 L/day) and polydipsia, which include:

• Diabetes mellitus.

• Renal failure.

• Primary polydipsia, usually psychogenic in origin.

• Diabetes insipidus (DI): cranial DI (relative/absolute vasopressin ADH deficiency) or nephrogenic DI (renal resistance to vasopressin, e.g. as a result of lithium toxicity).

Pathophysiology and causes are shown in the figure and investigations are shown in Table 149.1.

Treatment

This is by unrestricted access to fluid and desmopressin (long-acting ADH analogue).

Syndrome of inappropriate ADH secretion

Syndrome of inappropriate ADH secretion (SIADH) is a common cause of hyponatraemia. For a full discussion see p. 250 (Chapter 127).

Multiple endocrine neoplasia

Multiple endocrine neoplasia (MEN) syndromes are very rare conditions in which a single gene defect causes multiple endocrine tumours within a patient. MEN syndromes most commonly present with disorders of calcium metabolism (see p. 288). Probands and their families need to be regularly screened for new malignancies.

• MEN 1: parathyroid hyperplasia 95%, pituitary adenoma 70%, pancreatic islet tumour 40%; adrenal and thyroid adenomas; mutation in a recessive oncogene on chromosome 11q13—encoding menin.

• MEN 2a: medullary thyroid cancer; parathyroid hyperplasia; phaeochromocytoma 70% bilateral.

• MEN 2b also has marfanoid habitus and mucosal neuromas. Dominant oncogene on chromosome 10 (ret proto-oncogene).

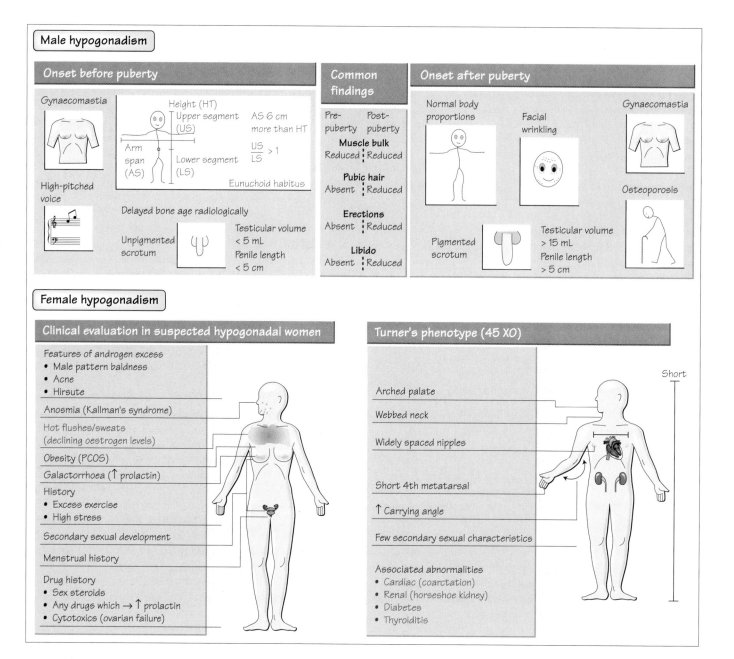

Definition

Hypogonadism is the failure of the ovaries or testis to produce sex steroids (oestrogen or testosterone) from either gonadal failure (primary hypogonadism) or hypothalamic–pituitary failure (secondary hypogonadism). The key difference between primary and secondary hypogonadism is whether luteinizing hormone (LH)/follicle-stimulating hormone (FSH) levels are high (intact hypothalamic–pituitary axis) or low (damaged hypothalamic–pituitary axis) (see Table 150.1).

Table 150.1 Differences between primary and secondary hypogonadism.

	LH/ FSH	Testosterone or oestrogen	Other tests
Primary hypogonadism	↑	↓	Karyotype
Secondary hypogonadism	↓	↓	Prolactin, MRI of pituitary fossa/ hypothalamus

Male hypogonadism

The clinical features of pre- and postpubescent male hypogonadism are shown in the figure. Acquired hypogonadism affects 20% of all men.

Primary male hypogonadism

Primary hypogonadism (testicular failure) arises from systemic disease, and renal failure and cirrhosis (especially alcohol abuse) are important causes. Of adult men with mumps, 25% develop orchitis and half of these progress to late gonadal failure (primary hypogonadism). Other viral causes of orchitis are also important. Cryptorchidism is a not uncommon cause, as are testicular trauma or torsion. Gonadal radiotherapy or systemic anticancer cytotoxic drugs are more rare but still very powerful stimuli for gonadal failure. Rare diseases causing testicular failure include Klinefelter's syndrome (XXY karyotype, 1 in 1000 births, causing small testis, gynaecomastia, eunuch-like appearance from testosterone deficiency; azoospermia contributes to infertility).

Secondary male hypogonadism

Secondary hypogonadism (hypothalamic–pituitary failure) may be caused by severe illness or malnutrition. Pituitary disease, hyperprolactinaemia. Kallman's syndrome (a genetic X-linked syndrome, autosomal dominant or autosomal recessive, with a male/female ratio of 4 : 1, a male prevalence of 1 in 10 000, and causing isolated failure of hypothalamic gonadotrophin-releasing hormone (GnRH) release with anosmia; MRI may show absent olfactory bulbs).

Management

Androgen replacement therapy: will relieve symptoms and prevent osteoporosis, but will not improve fertility, which is irreversible in primary hypogonadism. Gonadotrophins or GnRH are used to induce fertility in secondary hypogonadism.

Female hypogonadism

The symptoms of female hypogonadism are of fatigue and amenorrhoea with infertility. In primary hypogonadism, oestrogen withdrawal symptoms also occur: hot flushes and sweats, mood changes, vaginal dryness and pain on intercourse. The signs of established female hypogonadism include fine facial wrinkling, breast involution and a general reduction in body hair.

Primary female hypogonadism

Primary hypogonadism (ovarian failure): ovarian failure may relate to genetic or acquired diseases, and occurs in 1% of women aged < 40 years and accounts for 10% of secondary amenorrhoea.
• **Genetic** causes of ovarian failure: chromosomal abnormalities underlie 60% of cases of ovarian failure. Turner's syndrome (45X), affects 1 in 2000 women, causes gonadal dysgenesis and is the most common chromosomal abnormality associated with primary hypogonadism; the usual course is delayed puberty leading to premature gonadal failure. Short stature and a characteristic phenotype are found, and there may be associated cardiac (aortic coarctation), endocrine (hypothyroidism), skeletal and renal abnormalities.
• **Acquired** premature ovarian failure: results from autoimmune disease (the most common cause of premature menopause); may be idiopathic or relate to cytotoxic chemotherapy.

Secondary female hypogonadism

Secondary hypogonadism (hypothalamic–pituitary failure): hypo-gonadotrophic hypogonadism results from hypothalamic or pituitary disease, including tumours (see p. 292), hyperprolactinaemia (see p. 283), or extreme physical or psychological stress, including anorexia nervosa.

Management of female hypogonadism

In ovarian failure, treatment is with oestrogens, which alleviate deficiency symptoms and prevent long-term complications, such as osteoporosis. Progestogens are added for women with an intact uterus to avoid endometrial hyperplasia and subsequent endometrial carcinoma. Oocyte donation is needed for fertility. In secondary hypogonadism, it is vital to have a full assessment of the hypothalamic–pituitary axis functionally and structurally, to diagnose and treat any underlying disease. Gonadotrophins (FSH/hMG + human chorionic gonadotrophin (hCG), or pulsatile GnRH therapy) are used to induce fertility in hypo-gonadotrophic hypogonadism.

Menstrual failure (amenorrhoea)

Menstrual failure is associated with infertility, oestrogen deficiency (increased osteoporosis and cardiovascular disease risk) and increased risk of endometrial carcinoma (in polycystic ovary syndrome [PCOS]). The definitions of menstrual failure are: primary amenorrhoea—failure of menarche by 16 years; secondary amenorrhoea—failure of menstruation for > 6 months in women who have previously menstruated, affecting 3–9% of women of reproductive age; oligomenorrhoea—fewer than nine menstrual periods/year. Important causes of amenorrhoea are:
• **Pregnancy**: which should always be excluded by measuring hCG in the urine.
• **Illness, malnutrition and over-exercise**, all of which are usually readily apparent.
• Endocrine disease such as hyperthyroidism, or excess of androgens (see Hirsutism, p. 58).
• Primary or secondary hypogonadism, investigated as outlined above.
• **PCOS**: symptoms may be mild or severe (Stein-Leventhal syndrome). In PCOS excess androgen production occurs, mainly from the ovary (where multiple small cysts are found), but also from the adrenal glands, resulting in disruption of the menstrual cycle (mild to profound) and mild androgenization, mainly hirsutism (see p. 58) or acne. More profound virilization suggests pathology other than PCOS (particularly virilizing tumours). Insulin resistance and dyslipidaemia are also common features. Examination often shows marked obesity, with hirsutism and acne. Cushing's disease and late-onset congenital adrenal hyperplasia may need to be excluded. Investigations show mildly elevated androgen levels, normal oestrogen and normal/elevated LH. Ovarian ultrasonography may demonstrate multiple small (3–5 mm) cysts. Androgen levels are mildly elevated, oestrogen levels usually normal and LH levels may or may not be raised. There is no completely satisfactory treatment. Weight reduction, metformin (insulin sensitizer), antiandrogens (cyproterone) with contraception, ovarian suppression with the combined oral contraceptive pill, and ovarian diathermy all have a role.
• **Hyperprolactinaemia**, which although it may relate to pituitary disease, drugs, hypothyroidism or PCOS, in practice commonly relates to substantial physical or psychological stress.
• Rarely, structural disease such as an imperforate hymen or absent uterus underlies primary amenorrhoea.

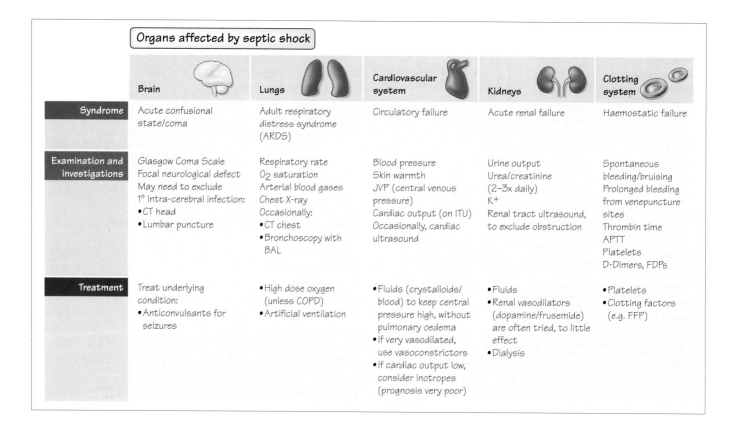

Organs affected by septic shock

	Brain	Lungs	Cardiovascular system	Kidneys	Clotting system
Syndrome	Acute confusional state/coma	Adult respiratory distress syndrome (ARDS)	Circulatory failure	Acute renal failure	Haemostatic failure
Examination and investigations	Glasgow Coma Scale Focal neurological defect May need to exclude 1° intra-cerebral infection: • CT head • Lumbar puncture	Respiratory rate O₂ saturation Arterial blood gases Chest X-ray Occasionally: • CT chest • Bronchoscopy with BAL	Blood pressure Skin warmth JVP (central venous pressure) Cardiac output (on ITU) Occasionally, cardiac ultrasound	Urine output Urea/creatinine (2–3x daily) K+ Renal tract ultrasound, to exclude obstruction	Spontaneous bleeding/bruising Prolonged bleeding from venepuncture sites Thrombin time APTT Platelets D-Dimers, FDPs
Treatment	Treat underlying condition: • Anticonvulsants for seizures	• High dose oxygen (unless COPD) • Artificial ventilation	• Fluids (crystalloids/blood) to keep central pressure high, without pulmonary oedema • If very vasodilated, use vasoconstrictors • If cardiac output low, consider inotropes (prognosis very poor)	• Fluids • Renal vasodilators (dopamine/frusemide) are often tried, to little effect • Dialysis	• Platelets • Clotting factors (e.g. FFP)

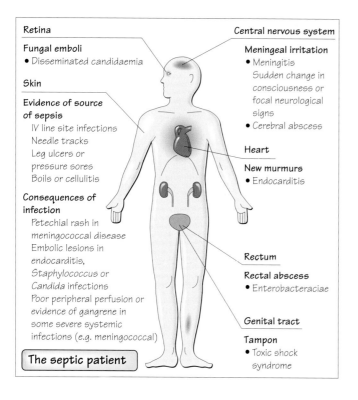

Retina

Fungal emboli
• Disseminated candidaemia

Skin

Evidence of source of sepsis
 IV line site infections
 Needle tracks
 Leg ulcers or pressure sores
 Boils or cellulitis

Consequences of infection
 Petechial rash in meningococcal disease
 Embolic lesions in endocarditis, Staphylococcus or Candida infections
 Poor peripheral perfusion or evidence of gangrene in some severe systemic infections (e.g. meningococcal)

The septic patient

Central nervous system

Meningeal irritation
• Meningitis
 Sudden change in consciousness or focal neurological signs
• Cerebral abscess

Heart

New murmurs
• Endocarditis

Rectum

Rectal abscess
• Enterobacteraciae

Genital tract

Tampon
• Toxic shock syndrome

Definitions

Bacteraemia: presence of bacteria in the blood, normally diagnosed by blood culture.

Sepsis: evidence of infection with a systemic response, including two of the following:

- temperature > 38°C or < 36°C
- respiratory rate > 20/min or P_{CO_2} < 4.3 kPa
- tachycardia > 90 beats/min
- white blood cell count (WB) > 12 000/mm³ or < 4000/mm³.

Septic shock: sepsis with organ dysfunction (from hypotension and/or 'leaky' capillaries, damaged by endotoxins and cytokines) and hypotension despite adequate fluid resuscitation. Bacteraemia and septic shock are not interchangeable:

- bacteraemia can occur with little or no clinical effect, e.g. transient bacteraemia is common after teeth brushing, etc.
- only 50% of patients with septic shock have bacteria in their blood stream.

The systemic inflammatory response syndrome (SIRS) is an identical syndrome to sepsis, but it can be triggered by a wide variety of causes, including non-infectious conditions such as pancreatitis or cardiopulmonary bypass.

Epidemiology

The most common organisms are:
• Gram positive: 55–65% (*Staphylococcus* sp., enterococci and pneumococci)

- Gram negative: 35–45% (*Escherichia coli*, *Pseudomonas* sp., *Klebsiella* sp.)
- Fungi: 3–5% (*Candida* sp. in particular).

Sepsis is the most common cause of death in intensive care units (ICUs). Mortality rates in sepsis are 20–30%, and may be much higher if there is shock or multiorgan failure. Rates are increasing as there are:
- More sick patients with diminished resistance to infections. Septic shock most often occurs in patients with underlying conditions, making them susceptible to infection.
- More aggressive surgery.
- More invasive procedures, intravascular lines, etc.

Clinical manifestations of sepsis

Fever and chills are common, non-specific signs. Patients with severe sepsis can be apyrexial, particularly if elderly—a poor prognostic sign. Symptoms/signs may relate to the source of sepsis. **Clinical assessment** should evaluate vital organ function, including:
- The heart and cardiovascular system: skin and core temperature, arterial and venous pressures.
- Peripheral perfusion: patients may be warm and vasodilated in initial stages, cold and poorly perfused in severe refractory septic shock.
- Mental state: confusion is common, especially in elderly people.
- The kidneys: urinary catheterization should be performed to measure hourly urine output as the best minute-to-minute indication of renal function.
- Lung function, as measured by respiratory rate, oxygenation and alveolar–arterial (A–a) O_2 difference (from arterial blood gases—see p. 176). These should be measured frequently, and if deterioration occurs the patient should receive mechanical ventilation.
- Vital organ perfusion, as reflected by tissue hypoxia and arterial blood gas acidaemia and lactate levels.
- Haemostatic function: assessed clinically through the presence of bruising. Spontaneous bleeding, such as from venepuncture sites, suggests haemostatic failure, which requires blood product support.

Meningococcal septicaemia

Meningococcaemia is a common cause of community-acquired sepsis and results in a characteristic illness. Fever, malaise and myalgia are associated with the development of a non-blanching rash, proceeding to hypotension and disseminated intravascular coagulation (DIC—see p. 343). Symptoms and signs of meningitis may or may not be present.

Toxic shock syndrome

Toxic shock syndrome is a specific syndrome produced by exotoxins of *Staphylococcus* or *Streptococcus* spp.: the syndrome is characterized by fever, vomiting and diarrhoea, desquamation of skin, hypotension and multisystem involvement, leading to a high mortality. Treatment is supportive (fluids and antibiotics to prevent recurrence).

Diagnosis and laboratory findings

Repeated blood, urine and sputum cultures are crucial investigations. Common laboratory findings are:
- Elevated white cell count (neutropenia also occurs with a poor prognosis).
- In DIC, low platelets (thrombocytopenia), low fibrinogen and raised D-dimers occur.

- Abnormal renal function.
- Rapid falls in albumin may occur.
- Hypoglycaemia.
- Increased lactate.

Management

High-quality nursing care is crucial, and should be obtained in specialist units rather than in general wards. Antibiotics should be started immediately, while awaiting full microbiological diagnosis. Other vital measures include:
- Localization of site/origin of sepsis, using clinical pointers, chest X-ray and 'blind' computed tomography (CT) (i.e. in the absence of localizing symptoms) of the abdomen. Infected intravascular lines are a common source of hospital-acquired sepsis and should be removed/exchanged.
- Any abscess present should be diagnosed urgently, using appropriate imaging (ultrasonography/CT), then drained.
- Optimal filling of vascular compartments: patients with septic shock are functionally hypovolaemic, with substantial ongoing invisible fluid losses (related to fever, etc.). Careful fluid replacement therapy, possibly guided by invasive central pressure monitoring, is important.
- Haemodynamic support: low blood pressure, despite an increased cardiac output, is commonly found. Provided that vital organs continue to function, this blood pressure should not be supported. However, if renal failure occurs, peripheral vasoconstrictors may be used and inotropes if there is cardiac failure.
- Ventilatory support, if respiratory failure develops or is imminent.
- Renal support for acute renal failure.
- Blood product support for anaemia, thrombocytopenia and coagulopathy.

Antimicrobial therapy

High-dose antibiotics should be started immediately. The choice should be guided by cultures (blood, urine and other appropriate fluid/tissue culture) or on the basis of the most likely organism if an obvious source exists. Antibiotic therapy should be reviewed regularly, taking clinical response into account. Empirical therapy is often necessary. Suitable choices in the absence of an obvious focus include:
- Community-acquired sepsis: second- or third-generation cephalosporin, e.g. ceftriaxone or cefotaxime, or penicillin with a β-lactamase inhibitor.
- Hospital-acquired sepsis: carbenopenem (meropenem, imipenem) or antipseudomonal penicillin and a β-lactamase inhibitor or ceftazidime and an antistaphylococcal drug.

Aminoglycosides may be added for critically ill patients or if resistant organisms are suspected. Vancomycin should be used for suspected staphylococcal sepsis in a patient at risk of methicillin-resistant *Staphylococcus aureus* (MRSA) (e.g. recent hospitalization).

Prognosis

Gram-negative sepsis has mortality rates of 25–40%; Gram-positive sepsis has slightly lower death rates of 10–20%. Mortality rates are highly dependent on factors such as age and pre-existing medical conditions.

Common viral infections in adults

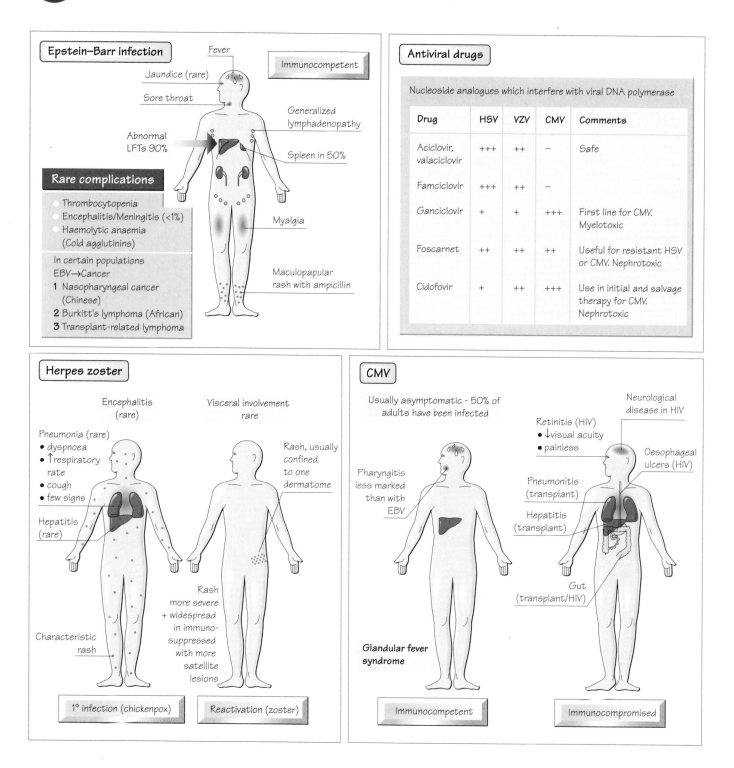

Epstein–Barr virus

Epstein–Barr virus (EBV) is common—90% of people are infected by adulthood. Half of infections occur asymptomatically in childhood. Infection in adolescent life is more commonly associated with clinical disease. EBV occurs in oropharyngeal secretions; and many cases result from intimate contact (hence the name 'kissing disease').

Symptoms are of fever, sore throat, headache, myalgia, anorexia and chills, and signs are of lymphadenopathy, prominent pharyngitis and splenomegaly in 50%—the glandular fever syndrome. A maculopapular rash often occurs if the patient has been given ampicillin. Symptoms usually resolve spontaneously over 2–3 weeks. Complications are: (i) abnormal liver function tests (common), occasional jaundice; (ii) haemolytic anaemia; (iii) rare neurological: encephalitis, aseptic meningitis; and (iv) lymphoproliferative disorder: EBV-related lymphoproliferative syndromes are common in transplant patients and late-stage HIV.

Diagnosis and treatment

• Full blood count (FBC): mononucleosis, > 10% atypical lymphocytes. Thrombocytopenia common. Serology: IgM antibodies to EBV or detection of heterophile antibodies (serum antibodies against red blood cells [RBCs] of other species) (Monospot or Paul Bunnell test).

• Differential diagnosis is from other agents causing a 'glandular fever'-type syndrome, principally cytomegalovirus (CMV) or toxoplasmosis. Streptococcal pharyngitis may give similar symptoms.

No specific antiviral treatment available. Steroids are useful in severe pharyngitis, thrombocytopenia and haemolytic anaemia.

Herpes simplex virus

Herpes simplex virus (HSV) infection is common. It has a predilection for mucocutaneous sites, affecting both normal and immunocompromised hosts, and is transmitted by direct oral or genital contact. Two types—HSV1 and HSV2—have differing epidemiology and clinical patterns, although there is considerable overlap. Most people encounter HSV1 infection in childhood, whereas acquisition of HSV2 depends on sexual contact. Recurrent infections are common, as a result of latency of the virus in sensory nerve ganglia. Identified triggers of recurrence include stress, sunlight and local trauma.

• **Oral mucocutaneous HSV**: most primary infections are asymptomatic; fever and pharyngitis or gingivostomatitis may occur. The usual manifestation is of recurrent herpes labialis (cold sores). There is a prodrome of tingling or burning, followed by painful vesicles at the edge of lip. Oral lesions may occur. Vesicles heal with crusting within 10 days.

• **Genital HSV**: the type is HSV2 in 80% of cases. Many infections are asymptomatic. Painful vesicles occur on the glans, penis shaft or vulva, perineum and vagina, 2–7 days after contact. There is dysuria. It is more common in women. Fever, malaise and tender inguinal lymphadenopathy may occur. Vesicles often ulcerate and may persist for several weeks; recurrence is common. Asymptomatic viral shedding can occur and cause transmission to sexual partners.

• **Other clinical syndromes**: (i) Primary eye infection (dendritic ulcers); (ii) Herpetic whitlow (infection of the finger); (iii) Eczema herpeticum: skin infection in atopic dermatitis; can cause severe illness; (iv) Herpes simplex encephalitis (see p. 377).

• **Treatment**: aciclovir (or alternative) is useful for severe systemic illness, e.g. encephalitis, or for primary/frequently recurrent genital herpes. In oral HSV, starting aciclovir early leads to fewer lesions and quicker healing.

Immunocompromised host

Severe mucocutaneous lesions are common in HIV-infected patients or transplant recipients. Severe proctitis and recurrent perianal disease occur in some HIV-infected gay men. HSV may affect other parts of the gut and, rarely, disseminates to involve organs such as the liver.

Varicella-zoster virus

Varicella-zoster virus (VZV) causes both varicella (chickenpox) and herpes zoster (shingles)—varicella reflects the primary infection and zoster the recurrent infection. Spread of the virus is through respiration, and 90% of primary cases occur in childhood. VZV becomes latent in the dorsal root ganglia after primary infection.

Varicella is usually a disease of children: chickenpox in adults is much more severe, with a 15-fold higher mortality. Fever and malaise precede the development of maculopapular lesions on the face and trunk, which become vesicular and crust over. In adults, particularly pregnant women, complications include: (i) varicella pneumonitis: occurs in 1 in 400 adults. Tachypnoea, cough and dyspnoea. Chest signs may not be prominent; (ii) varicella encephalitis: depressed consciousness, progressive headaches, fatal in up to 20%; (iii) varicella hepatitis.

Herpes zoster classically affects elderly people, as a result of reactivation of latent virus. A prodrome of pain is followed by a unilateral rash in a dermatomal distribution. Vesicles develop over 2–3 days, crust over and then heal.

• Lumbar or thoracic dermatomes most commonly involved.

• Trigeminal nerve involvement may lead to ocular involvement. Eye assessment is necessary.

• Ramsay Hunt syndrome. Seventh cranial nerve involved; vesicles may be hidden in auditory canal. Hearing loss and facial paralysis may occur.

Rare neurological complications include motor weakness and transverse myelitis. Post-herpetic neuralgia is distressing and occurs in up to a half of elderly patients.

VZV in immunocompromised individuals

Chickenpox causes significant morbidity and mortality; 30% of bone marrow transplant recipients without prophylaxis have infections in the first year. Dissemination occurs in 50%: lung, CNS and liver.

Zoster rash is more severe and lesions may occur outside the dermatome or be disseminated over the skin. Visceral involvement is rare.

Diagnosis and management

Diagnosis usually clinical. Vesicle fluid can be cultured or examined by electron microscopy or fluorescent antibody staining. Differential diagnosis includes impetigo, disseminated herpes simplex (rare) and disseminated Coxsackie viruses. Intravenous aciclovir is used to treat immunocompromised individuals (including those on high-dose steroids) with varicella or zoster. Treatment of chickenpox in adults may reduce complications. Early treatment reduces the number of lesions and subsequent pain in zoster.

Cytomegalovirus

Infection with CMV is common but rarely causes clinical disease: 50–95% of adults have been infected. It is, however, a major pathogen in immunocompromised individuals. Disease occurs because of: (1) reactivation or (2) transplantation of a CMV-positive organ into a CMV-negative recipient. The clinical features of infection are:

• Disease rare in healthy people. Glandular fever-like syndrome, with increased monocytes, and abnormal liver function tests may occur.

• Transplant recipients: CMV pneumonitis, hepatitis and gastrointestinal disease, such as diarrhoea.

• HIV infected: CMV retinitis, neurological infection and gut disease.

Prophylaxis is often indicated in advanced HIV and some groups of transplant recipients. Treatment is with CMV antivirals. Immunoglobulin also used for treating pneumonitis in bone marrow transplant recipients.

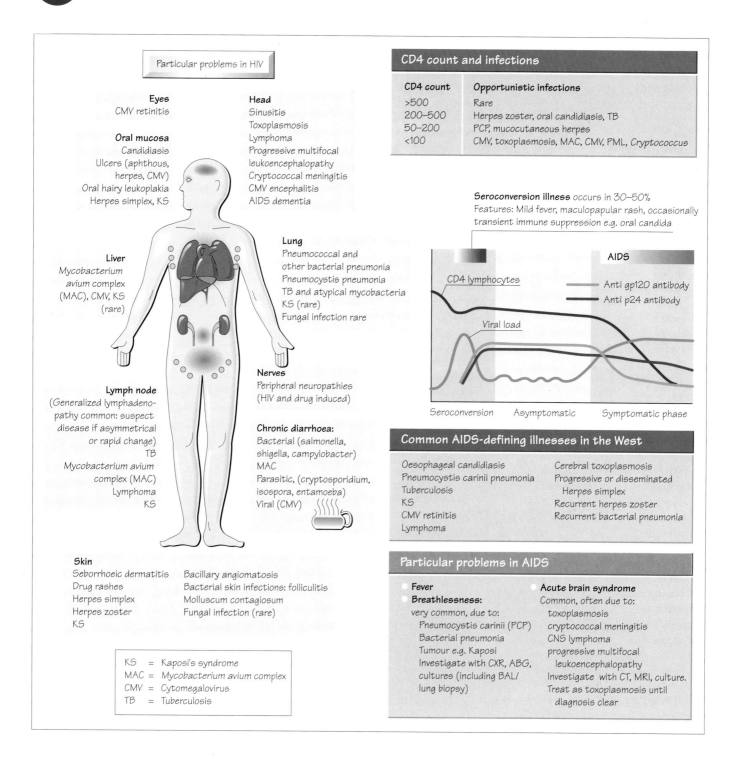

Particular problems in HIV

Eyes
CMV retinitis

Head
Sinusitis
Toxoplasmosis
Lymphoma
Progressive multifocal
leukoencephalopathy
Cryptococcal meningitis
CMV encephalitis
AIDS dementia

Oral mucosa
Candidiasis
Ulcers (aphthous,
herpes, CMV)
Oral hairy leukoplakia
Herpes simplex, KS

Liver
Mycobacterium
avium complex
(MAC), CMV, KS
(rare)

Lung
Pneumococcal and
other bacterial pneumonia
Pneumocystis pneumonia
TB and atypical mycobacteria
KS (rare)
Fungal infection rare

Lymph node
(Generalized lymphadeno-
pathy common: suspect
disease if asymmetrical
or rapid change)
TB
Mycobacterium avium
complex (MAC)
Lymphoma
KS

Nerves
Peripheral neuropathies
(HIV and drug induced)

Chronic diarrhoea:
Bacterial (salmonella,
shigella, campylobacter)
MAC
Parasitic, (cryptosporidium,
isospora, entamoeba)
Viral (CMV)

Skin
Seborrhoeic dermatitis
Drug rashes
Herpes simplex
Herpes zoster
KS

Bacillary angiomatosis
Bacterial skin infections: folliculitis
Molluscum contagiosum
Fungal infection (rare)

KS = Kaposi's syndrome
MAC = Mycobacterium avium complex
CMV = Cytomegalovirus
TB = Tuberculosis

CD4 count and infections

CD4 count	Opportunistic infections
>500	Rare
200–500	Herpes zoster, oral candidiasis, TB
50–200	PCP, mucocutaneous herpes
<100	CMV, toxoplasmosis, MAC, CMV, PML, Cryptococcus

Seroconversion illness occurs in 30–50%
Features: Mild fever, maculopapular rash, occasionally
transient immune suppression e.g. oral candida

AIDS

CD4 lymphocytes

Anti gp120 antibody
Anti p24 antibody

Viral load

Seroconversion   Asymptomatic   Symptomatic phase

Common AIDS-defining illnesses in the West

Oesophageal candidiasis
Pneumocystis carinii pneumonia
Tuberculosis
KS
CMV retinitis
Lymphoma

Cerebral toxoplasmosis
Progressive or disseminated
Herpes simplex
Recurrent herpes zoster
Recurrent bacterial pneumonia

Particular problems in AIDS

- **Fever**
- **Breathlessness:**
  very common, due to:
  Pneumocystis carinii (PCP)
  Bacterial pneumonia
  Tumour e.g. Kaposi
  Investigate with CXR, ABG,
  cultures (including BAL/
  lung biopsy)

- **Acute brain syndrome**
  Common, often due to:
  toxoplasmosis
  cryptococcal meningitis
  CNS lymphoma
  progressive multifocal
  leukoencephalopathy
  Investigate with CT, MRI, culture.
  Treat as toxoplasmosis until
  diagnosis clear

Human immunodeficiency virus (HIV) infection causes a clinical syndrome characterized by the development of progressive immuno-deficiency following a long asymptomatic period. Cellular immuno-deficiency eventually leads to severe opportunistic infection and, more rarely, malignancy.

Epidemiology
HIV infection has now reached pandemic proportions, with over 40 million people infected worldwide. Transmission of the blood-borne RNA retrovirus occurs predominantly by four mechanisms:
1 Homosexual or heterosexual intercourse
2 Intravenous drug abuse

3 Transfusion of blood products

4 Maternal–child transmission

Pathogenesis

After transmission, HIV enters lymphoid tissue where it infects CD4-bearing T lymphocytes and monocyte/macrophages. The virus enters the cell by binding to the CD4 molecule and chemokine receptors, and then replicates and integrates itself into host DNA. Latent infection or virus production follows. A total of 10^{10}–10^{11} virions are produced each day with considerable turnover of HIV-infected cells. Ultimately, progressive loss of CD4 cells and a number of other mechanisms lead to impairment of immune function.

Clinical patterns

• Primary HIV infection: 30–80% patients experience an acute clinical syndrome when viral replication occurs after HIV infection. Symptoms typically occur 2–4 weeks after infection and include fever, malaise and a maculopapular rash. A small proportion have transient immunosuppression with clinical features such as oral candida infection.

• Asymptomatic HIV: after seroconversion, most patients have a prolonged asymptomatic period (median 10 years without treatment) before the development of clinical features.

• Symptomatic HIV and acquired immune deficiency syndrome (AIDS): as HIV infection progresses, patients become symptomatic. Some symptoms are non-specific, but certain opportunistic diseases are regarded as AIDS defining (see figure), along with systemic features such as significant weight loss, persistent fever or persistent diarrhoea.

• Stage of disease can be described by (1) whether the patient is symptomatic, (2) whether an AIDS-defining illness has occurred and (3) the CD4 count. The last reflects the degree of immunosuppression and the likelihood of particular opportunistic infections.

Diagnosis of HIV infection

HIV is diagnosed by the detection of anti-HIV antibodies by ELISA (enzyme-linked immunosorbent assay). Positive samples are confirmed by Western blot. Seroconversion (i.e. acquisition of anti-HIV antibodies) occurs between 1 and 3 months after primary infection. Plasma HIV RNA can be quantified: a high viral load has a poor prognosis.

Treatment of HIV infection

The recent use of a number of drugs in combination (highly active antiretroviral therapy—HAART) has led to a significant decrease in mortality and delay in progression to AIDS. Three main classes of drugs exist:

1 Nucleoside reverse transcriptase inhibitors

2 Protease inhibitors

3 Non-nucleoside reverse transcriptase inhibitors.

A combination of three or four drugs is used to reduce the viral load (ideally below the detection limit of the assay). The viral load and CD4 response reflect the efficacy of treatment. Common problems with HAART include:

• Resistance to antiretroviral drugs, particularly common in patients who have experienced a number of different drugs.

• Side effects (e.g. neuropathy or lipodystrophy) and drug intolerance.

• Compliance problems arising from the complex multidrug regimens used.

• Antiretrovirals commonly interact with other drugs.

Common opportunistic infections

Although HAART and routine primary prophylaxis has reduced the incidence of many opportunistic infections, they still present considerable problems. The major clinical syndromes are shown in the figure.

Pneumocystis carinii pneumonia

Pneumocystis carinii pneumonia (PCP) is a major AIDS-defining illness in the West. Risk increases once the CD4 count drops below 200; primary prophylaxis with co-trimoxazole (Septrin) is effective. PCP usually presents with a non-productive cough, fever and dyspnoea. Often runs a subacute course, with mean duration of symptoms of 3–4 weeks. Physical examination is often unremarkable, fever and tachypnoea are common. Blood gases often show a moderate hypoxaemia. The chest X-ray is abnormal in 95%, classically showing fine interstitial perihilar shadowing, although the spectrum of abnormalities is wide. The demonstration of cysts in induced sputum or bronchoalveolar lavage (BAL fluid) establishes the diagnosis. Treatment is with high-dose co-trimoxazole. Addition of steroids improves the prognosis in severe disease.

Cytomegalovirus infection

Cytomegalovirus (CMV) is a late-stage infection disease (CD4 < 50). Major problem is progressive retinitis (85%); gut, nervous system and lung infection also occur. It is asymptomatic in early stages; regular ophthalmological screening is useful in advanced HIV. It is diagnosed clinically; there are white fluffy retinal lesions with perivascular haemorrhages and exudates. Treatment is with specific antiviral agents and treatment of HIV; long-term maintenance therapy is necessary and relapse is common.

Toxoplasmosis

This is a protozoa infection, which most commonly causes encephalitis (80%) in late HIV (CD4 < 100). Patients present with fever, headache, confusion, fits and focal neurological signs. MRI is more sensitive than CT in demonstrating the multiple ring-enhancing lesions, classically in the basal ganglia or corticomedullary junction, which suggest the diagnosis. Toxoplasmosis is rare in patients with no serological evidence of previous exposure. Treatment is with pyrimethamine and sulphadiazine; a clinical response confirms diagnosis.

Kaposi's sarcoma

Kaposi's sarcoma (KS) is caused by herpes virus (HHV-8) and occurs in 20% of gay men with HIV. Skin lesions are initially macular and progress to reddish-purplish indurated plaques. There is a wide spectrum from isolated skin or oral lesions to dissemination with lymph node, gastrointestinal tract or lung involvement. It is diagnosed clinically or by skin biopsy. Treatment is by localized radiotherapy, injection of lesions or systemic chemotherapy. HAART improves immunological function with improvement in KS.

Non-Hodgkin's lymphoma

Occurs in up to 10% in late stage disease—20% in the CNS. It presents with fever, sweats and organ-related symptoms; extra-nodal involvement is common. Treatment is with chemotherapy. There is a generally poor prognosis.

Progressive multifocal leukoencephalopathy

This uncommon demyelinating disease is caused by polyoma JC virus (late-stage HIV). Diagnosis is by imaging (white matter lesion) and polymerase chain reaction of the cerebrospinal fluid for JC virus. The only effective treatment is improving immune function with HAART.

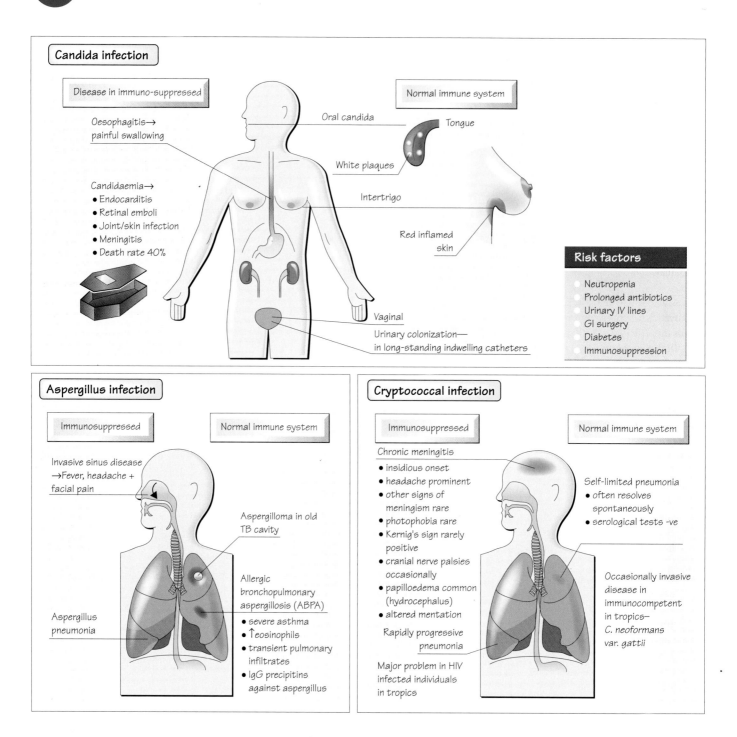

Candida infection

Disease in immuno-suppressed

Oesophagitis→
painful swallowing

Candidaemia→
- Endocarditis
- Retinal emboli
- Joint/skin infection
- Meningitis
- Death rate 40%

Normal immune system

Oral candida — Tongue

White plaques

Intertrigo

Red inflamed skin

Vaginal

Urinary colonization—
in long-standing indwelling catheters

Risk factors
- Neutropenia
- Prolonged antibiotics
- Urinary IV lines
- GI surgery
- Diabetes
- Immunosuppression

Aspergillus infection

Immunosuppressed

Normal immune system

Invasive sinus disease
→Fever, headache +
facial pain

Aspergilloma in old
TB cavity

Aspergillus
pneumonia

Allergic
bronchopulmonary
aspergillosis (ABPA)
- severe asthma
- ↑eosinophils
- transient pulmonary
  infiltrates
- IgG precipitins
  against aspergillus

Cryptococcal infection

Immunosuppressed

Normal immune system

Chronic meningitis
- insidious onset
- headache prominent
- other signs of
  meningism rare
- photophobia rare
- Kernig's sign rarely
  positive
- cranial nerve palsies
  occasionally
- papilloedema common
  (hydrocephalus)
- altered mentation

Rapidly progressive
pneumonia

Major problem in HIV
infected individuals
in tropics

Self-limited pneumonia
- often resolves
  spontaneously
- serological tests -ve

Occasionally invasive
disease in
immunocompetent
in tropics—
C. neoformans
var. gattii

In the UK and in the immunologically competent host, fungi often cause only mild disease, whereas in the immunocompromised individual, severe or life-threatening disease can result. Thus, fungal infections have assumed increasing importance as the number of immunocompromised patients increases. Many different species cause significant disease; only the main endemic fungi in the UK are discussed here.

Candida species

These are the most common invasive fungal species in the UK. The organisms are found readily in the environment and are commensals on mucous membranes in the gastrointestinal, respiratory and genitourinary tract. *Candida albicans* is the most important species, although non-albicans species are becoming more common. *Candida* spp. can cause both mucocutaneous and invasive disease.

Mucocutaneous candidiasis

May occur in immunocompetent and immunocompromised individuals: particularly common in diabetics or those with altered cellular immunity such as HIV.

- **Oral candida infection**: most common clinical manifestation is creamy white 'curd-like' patches on the mucosa and tongue. The underlying surface is raw if the exudate is scraped off. The diagnosis is usually made clinically, although hyphae can be demonstrated in lesions. Routine culture is unhelpful because *Candida* sp. is a normal mouth commensal.
- **Candidal oesophagitis**: usually in AIDS or haematological malignancy. May occur without oral lesions, and produces symptoms of dysphagia, odynophagia and retrosternal pain. Diagnosed by appearance on endoscopy and biopsies.
- **Vaginal candidiasis**: see Vaginal discharge, p. 78.
- **Intertrigo**: infection in warm damp environments between skinfolds —red macerated skin with satellite lesions.
- **Chronic mucocutaneous candidiasis**: syndrome associated with specific T-cell deficiency. Infection of skin, mucous membrane and scalp; may be disfiguring.

Invasive candidiasis

Invasive infections usually arise from endogenous colonization. Entry occurs through damaged skin or mucosa or direct access to the circulation. Both neutrophils and cell-mediated immunity are important in defences against *Candida* spp. The following are risk factors for invasive disease:

- Neutropenia increases the risk of candidaemia
- Prolonged use of antibiotics
- Indwelling urinary or intravenous catheters
- Gastrointestinal surgery
- Intravenous drug abuse

Candidaemia

Candida spp. are commonly isolated from blood cultures. Although this sometimes reflects colonization of indwelling lines rather than disseminated candidal disease, candidaemia also occurs in disseminated candidiasis, especially in immunosuppressed patients. All patients should be carefully evaluated for metastatic infection, including examination of the fundi, the heart for endocarditis, joints and skin. Candidaemia has a 40% mortality rate.

Disseminated candidiasis

Blood-borne spread can lead to infection in most organs, including the central nervous system (CNS), respiratory tract, joints, kidneys and peritoneum. Only 50% of patients with disseminated candidiasis have demonstrated candidaemia. The presence of skin or eye lesions (present in 10%) confirms the diagnosis. *Candida* sp. in the urine occurs in both invasive and disseminated candidiasis.

Treatment

- Oral or vaginal candidiasis: topical therapy or short-term systemic therapy.
- Serious mucocutaneous disease requires systemic therapy.
- Candidaemia should always be treated with azoles or amphotericin. Intravenous catheters should be removed.
- Disseminated candidiasis requires aggressive antifungal therapy.
- Surgery is usually required for endocarditis.

Antifungal prophylaxis

This is used in HIV patients with recurrent disease, and in high-risk bone marrow and most solid organ transplantations.

Aspergillus species

These mould species are found readily in the environment. Infection is acquired by inhalation of spores. Disease may be caused in three ways:
1 Allergic reactions: allergic bronchopulmonary aspergillosis (see p. 207).
2 Colonization of cavities (aspergillomas) (see p. 207).
3 Invasive aspergillosis.

Invasive aspergillosis is a disease of immunocompromised patients. Important risk factors include prolonged neutropenia, high-dose steroids or prolonged antibiotic therapy.

Clinical patterns of invasive disease

- Sinus disease: in neutropenic patients, colonizing organisms may become invasive in the nose and sinuses. Patients present with fever, headache and sinus symptoms. Soft tissue and bony invasion may lead to vascular invasion and brain involvement. Diagnosis is suspected when computed tomography shows loss of the normal bony sinus margins, confirmed by tissue biopsy.
- Aspergillus pneumonia: acute pneumonia in neutropenic patients:
  - fever, followed by pulmonary consolidation
  - rapidly progressing pneumonia, sometimes with cavitation.

Definitive diagnosis is by culture and by lung biopsy, which shows histological evidence of invasion. Aspergillus is rarely found in blood cultures in pneumonia.

Treatment

Amphotericin is the traditional drug of choice, but itraconazole and voriconazole are also effective. Caspofungin, a new class antifungal drug, may be used in refractory disease. Response rates in invasive aspergillosis are very poor and the mortality rate is about 40%.

Cryptococcal disease

Cryptococcus neoformans is a yeast-like fungus that affects both normal and immunocompromised hosts. The organism is acquired through inhalation; there are two main clinical syndromes:
- Pulmonary disease: occurs in both normal and immunocompromised hosts.
- Meningitis: usually in immunosuppressed individuals, particularly in HIV. Long non-specific history: the most common symptoms are headache and a change in mentation. There may be surprisingly few signs; neck stiffness may not be present. Papilloedema and cranial nerve palsies may occur. Skin lesions occur in 10%. Diagnosis is achieved from:
- cerebrospinal fluid (CSF): predominant lymphocytes, low glucose, high protein and high pressure; the CSF is stained using an Indian ink stain, which demonstrates yeast and capsule; this finding is then confirmed by culture;
- cryptococcal antigen titres raised in serum and CSF.

Treatment

- Normal immune system: pulmonary disease may not need treatment and can be observed. Treat meningitis as below.
- Immunocompromised: amphotericin initially, followed by azoles. Prolonged therapy is required and long-term secondary prophylaxis required. Mortality rate in meningitis in HIV is around 25%.

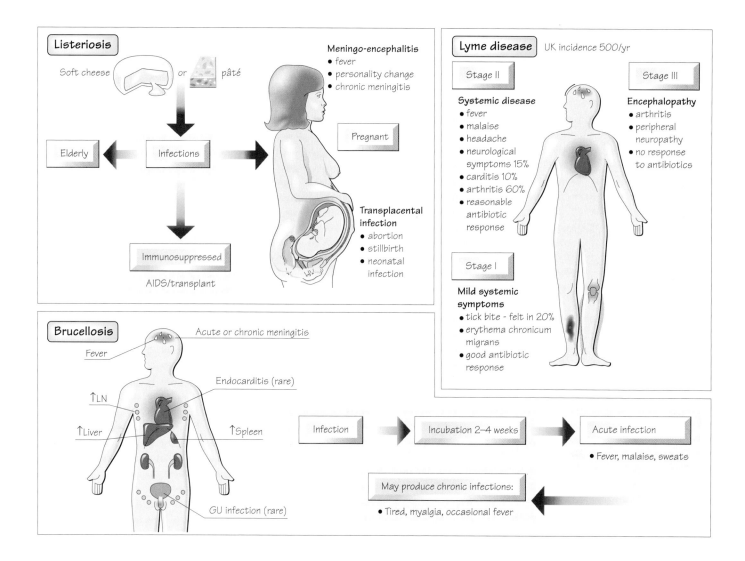

Listeriosis

Listeria monocytogenes is a Gram-positive bacillus causing disease in pregnant women, immunocompromised individuals and neonates. Infection is usually acquired through food, particularly soft cheeses and pâté. Clinical manifestations include:
• Pregnancy associated: bacteraemia producing a flu-like illness, and sometimes transplacental infection or ascending infection leading to abortion, stillbirth or neonatal sepsis. Very rarely maternal meningitis.
• Neonatal infection: high mortality.
• Meningoencephalitis is the most common manifestation, occurring in the late neonatal period, and in immunocompromised and elderly people. Wide clinical spectrum from fever with personality change to chronic meningitis.

Diagnosis and treatment

In meningitic syndromes, few organisms are present in the cerebrospinal fluid (CSF), so Gram staining may be difficult. CSF cultures are positive. In systemic disease, blood cultures may be positive. Treatment is with ampicillin and an aminoglycoside.

Brucellosis

This is caused by four species of a Gram-negative coccobacillus: *Brucella abortus*, *B. melitensis*, *B. suis* and *B. canis*. It is acquired from contact with infected animals or milk products or by inhalation of infected aerosols. Most UK infections are imported, but infection can also occur in those with occupational risks (farmers and vets). Systemic spread leads to granuloma formation in different organs. The incubation period is 2–4 weeks; fever, malaise, sweats and other non-specific symptoms occur; nausea, vomiting, gastrointestinal complaints are frequent; hepato-splenomegaly is common, lymphadenopathy occurs in 20%. May cause:
• Bone and joint infection; particularly sacroiliitis and spondylitis.
• Respiratory infection: bronchitis, abscesses.
• Acute or chronic meningitis.
• Rarely endocarditis, genitourinary infection.

Diagnosis requires a very high clinical suspicion because brucellosis can mimic many other diseases. One should attempt to culture the organism from blood or bone marrow: prolonged culture is necessary. Serology may be diagnostic.

Treatment: doxycycline is the drug of choice in combination with rifampicin, an aminoglycoside or both to prevent relapse. Treatment is for 6 weeks or longer in serious infection.

Tetanus

Tetanus is caused by infection with the anaerobic Gram-positive bacillus, *Clostridium tetani*. Spores from soil infect a wound and germinate under anaerobic conditions, producing the toxin tetanospasmin, which is transported via neurons to the CNS, where it inhibits presynaptic transmitter release from inhibitory neurons, leading to muscular rigidity.

Clinical features

The incubation period is usually 1–21 days.
• Neonatal tetanus: common in the developing world, results from infection of the umbilical stump. Initially poor feeding, trismus and spasms; high mortality.
• Generalized tetanus: initially spasm of the masseter muscles causing trismus and 'risus sardonicus', gradually spreading to spasms involving the whole of the trunk and body. Spasms may be precipitated by noise or tactile stimuli. Autonomic instability—arrhythmias or blood pressure changes may occur.

Diagnosis and management

Tetanus is diagnosed clinically. Human tetanus immunoglobulin is administered intramuscularly to neutralize circulating toxin. The wound should be debrided thoroughly and metronidazole or penicillin given to eradicate the organism. Supportive care consists of benzodiazepines to reduce rigidity and spasms; ventilation may be required. Autonomic disturbances are difficult to treat and may require inotropic support or α- and β-blockade. Mortality in 20% occurs from respiratory problems or autonomic instability. Tetanus can be prevented by primary immunization and boosting with tetanus toxoid. Dirty wounds should be debrided and a booster dose given if five or more doses of toxoid have not been given previously.

Lyme disease

Infection with the spirochaete *Borrelia burgdorferi*, transmitted by the tick *Ixodes* sp. found on infected deer or mice. Only 20% of patients recall the tick bite. Foci of disease occur in the USA, Europe and areas of Russia, China and Japan. The clinical features are:
• Localized early disease (stage 1): an annular lesion (erythema chronicum migrans) with central clearing develops at the site of the bite. Mild systemic symptoms.
• Disseminated disease (stage 2): blood spread leads to fluctuating symptoms of fever, malaise and headache. Secondary skin lesion may occur. Subsequent development of arthritis in 60% (monoarticular, affecting large joints), neurological symptoms in 15% (meningitis, peripheral or cranial neuropathy, myelitis), carditis in 10% (atrioventricular block, myopericarditis). Symptoms and signs are often self-limiting.

• Late persistent infection (stage 3): if untreated, there are chronic manifestations of recurrent arthritis (autoimmune, relates to HLA-DR2), skin changes and neurological changes (peripheral neuropathy, encephalopathy).

Diagnosis and treatment

A clinical diagnosis should be confirmed by serology and a positive immunoblot. The organism is rarely isolated. Early disease may be treated with doxycycline, amoxicillin or ceftriaxone: cephalosporins are indicated for arthritis or neurological involvement. Late disease does not respond to antibiotics.

Syphilis

Syphilis is a sexually transmitted disease caused by the spirochaete *Treponema pallidum*. Most disease occurs in developing countries, but there have been recent increases in incidence in the UK. Organisms enter the body of a sexual partner through breaches in the skin or epithelium. *Treponema pallidum* is disseminated via the blood. The clinical features are:
• Primary syphilis: median incubation period 3 weeks. An ulcerated, typically painless papule—the primary chancre—develops at the site of inoculation on the penis or cervix and labia. Inguinal lymphadenopathy occurs. The lesion heals spontaneously after several weeks.
• Secondary syphilis 6–8 weeks later, with a generalized maculopapular rash (involving palms and soles), generalized lymphadenopathy (50%) and condylomata lata (moist, broad, highly infectious plaques in warm intertriginous areas). Systemic symptoms include fever, headache and sore throat.
• Latent syphilis: symptoms and signs disappear. The only manifestation of infection is positive serology. Asymptomatic CNS infection is common.
• Tertiary syphilis: gummata (hard granulomatous lesions) occur after 3–10 years in many sites, including the skin, in which ulceration with damage to underlying cartilage or connective tissue occurs. Aortitis develops after 10–30 years and causes ascending aortic aneurysms. Neurosyphilis produces a wide spectrum of disease including:
  • meningovascular—4–7 years
  • general paresis of the insane (GPI)—10–20 years
  • tabes dorsalis—15–25 years.

Diagnosis

Identification of *Treponema pallidum*, on dark-ground microscopy of primary or secondary syphilis lesions. Serology: CSF examination in suspected neurosyphilis.

Management

Penicillin is the drug of choice. Regimen and dose depend upon stage. Alternative drugs include tetracycline and ceftriaxone. Steroids are needed to prevent the Jarisch–Herxheimer reaction (anaphylaxis to dead/dying spirochaetes) after treatment in late syphilis. Contacts should be traced and treated.

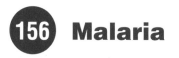

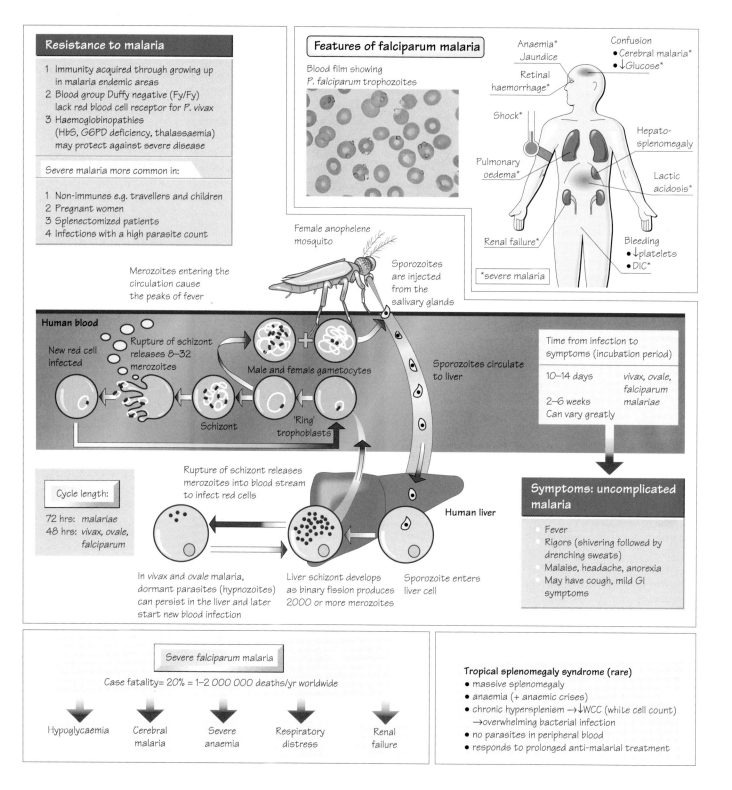

Resistance to malaria

1 Immunity acquired through growing up in malaria endemic areas
2 Blood group Duffy negative (Fy/Fy) lack red blood cell receptor for *P. vivax*
3 Haemoglobinopathies (HbS, G6PD deficiency, thalassaemia) may protect against severe disease

Severe malaria more common in:

1 Non-immunes e.g. travellers and children
2 Pregnant women
3 Splenectomized patients
4 Infections with a high parasite count

Features of falciparum malaria

Blood film showing *P. falciparum* trophozoites

Anaemia*
Jaundice
Retinal haemorrhage*
Shock*
Pulmonary oedema*
Renal failure*

Confusion
• Cerebral malaria*
• ↓Glucose*

Hepato-splenomegaly
Lactic acidosis*

Bleeding
• ↓platelets
• DIC*

*severe malaria

Female anophelene mosquito

Sporozoites are injected from the salivary glands

Merozoites entering the circulation cause the peaks of fever

Human blood

New red cell infected
Rupture of schizont releases 8–32 merozoites
Male and female gametocytes
Schizont
'Ring' trophoblasts

Sporozoites circulate to liver

Time from infection to symptoms (incubation period)

10–14 days	*vivax, ovale, falciparum*
2–6 weeks	*malariae*

Can vary greatly

Cycle length:

72 hrs: *malariae*
48 hrs: *vivax, ovale, falciparum*

Rupture of schizont releases merozoites into blood stream to infect red cells

In *vivax* and *ovale* malaria, dormant parasites (hypnozoites) can persist in the liver and later start new blood infection

Liver schizont develops as binary fission produces 2000 or more merozoites

Sporozoite enters liver cell

Human liver

Symptoms: uncomplicated malaria

• Fever
• Rigors (shivering followed by drenching sweats)
• Malaise, headache, anorexia
• May have cough, mild GI symptoms

Severe falciparum malaria

Case fatality = 20% = 1–2 000 000 deaths/yr worldwide

Hypoglycaemia | Cerebral malaria | Severe anaemia | Respiratory distress | Renal failure

Tropical splenomegaly syndrome (rare)
• massive splenomegaly
• anaemia (+ anaemic crises)
• chronic hypersplenism →↓WCC (white cell count) →overwhelming bacterial infection
• no parasites in peripheral blood
• responds to prolonged anti-malarial treatment

Epidemiology

Malaria is primarily a disease of the tropics and subtropics, but is also the most common imported infection in the UK. It causes over a million deaths per year worldwide, particularly in children in sub-Saharan Africa.

In highly endemic areas, malaria mainly causes morbidity and mortality in children, but where transmission is less intense it is a disease of both adults and children. The severity of clinical illness is highly modified by the degree of immunity of an individual. Malaria in an expatriate traveller is far more likely to be life threatening than in someone who has grown up in an endemic malarial area.

Pathogenesis

Malaria is a protozoal infection transmitted by the bite of the mosquito *Anopheles* spp. Injected sporozoites initially multiply in the liver and then invade red blood cells. Four species of *Plasmodium* infect humans: *P. falciparum, P. vivax, P. ovale* and *P. malariae. P. ovale* and *P. vivax* have forms that remain dormant in the liver for a number of years ('hypnozoites') and cause subsequent relapsing infection. Only *P. falciparum* causes severe disease as a result of its ability to infect red blood cells of all ages, and to adhere to vascular endothelium and sequester in vital organs such as the brain, liver, kidneys and muscles.

Clinical features

Incubation period is usually 10–14 days, rarely longer than 6 weeks, but may be several years (unusual in *P. falciparum*). Prophylaxis may delay onset of symptoms. The predominant symptoms are:
• Malaise, headache, fever and rigors.
• Occasionally gastrointestinal or respiratory symptoms dominate, making the clinical diagnosis difficult.

Irregular fever occurs in the acute stages of malaria: classic periodic fever occurs only if untreated. Examination is often unremarkable apart from mild hepatosplenomegaly. Malaria does not cause rashes; other diagnoses should be considered in this situation (although patients with rashes from other causes, e.g. drugs, may have malaria).

Severe malaria

Only *P. falciparum* causes severe malaria which is a medical emergency; case fatality rates may be 20% or higher:
• Cerebral malaria: coma, often with seizures. Low (< 5%) risk of long-term damage in adults, greater risk in children (hemiplegia, cortical blindness, mental handicap).
• Severe anaemia: due to haemolysis and a depressed marrow response.
• Respiratory distress: particularly prominent in children, associated with acidosis and sometimes with severe anaemia.
• Hypoglycaemia: as a result of increased glucose consumption, impaired gluconeogenesis and quinine-induced hyperinsulinaemia.
• Acute renal failure: multi-factorial in origin. Rare in children. Rarely, 'blackwater' fever occurs: intravascular haemolysis, producing haemoglobinuria and deep jaundice. Dialysis is needed in 10% of cases of severe malaria.
• Jaundice: caused by haemolysis and hepatic dysfunction, particularly in adults.
• Disseminated intravascular coagulation (see p. 343).
• Non-cardiogenic pulmonary oedema, which can be life threatening.
• Shock ('algid malaria'). May be caused by concomitant bacteraemia.

Diagnosis

Consider malaria in every febrile patient who has been in an endemic area. The gold standard of diagnosis is the demonstration of malaria trophozoites on a blood film using stains such as Giemsa or Field's stain.
• Thick blood films are used to screen for the presence of parasites.

• Thin films demonstrate detail of parasites, allowing determination of the species.

Patients may have a low parasite burden, especially if malaria prophylaxis has been used. Repeated thick blood films may be needed to make the diagnosis. Commercial 'stick' tests detect parasite proteins or metabolites—these require less expertise to perform but are less sensitive than a well-performed blood slide.

Differential diagnosis: uncomplicated malaria needs to be distinguished from the long list of tropical and non-tropical diseases that can cause a fever. The differential diagnosis of cerebral malaria includes bacterial, viral and fungal meningitis, arbovirus and other viral causes of encephalitis, and non-infectious causes of coma.

Treatment and management

Treatment of malaria depends on the malaria species. Antimalarial drug resistance is a significant problem in the treatment of *falciparum* malaria, particularly in south-east Asia.
• *P. ovale, P. vivax* and *P. malariae*: treat with chloroquine on 3 successive days to eliminate red blood cell infection. Primaquine is required in *P. vivax* and *P. ovale* malaria to eliminate hepatic forms. Glucose-6-phosphate dehydrogenase (G6PD) status should be checked to avoid primaquine-induced haemolysis.
• Uncomplicated *P. falciparum*: chloroquine resistance is present in most areas of the world. Oral quinine should be given for 7 days; usually combined with doxycycline. Other agents include mefloquine, artemisin derivatives and atovaquone-proguanil.
• Severe *P. falciparum* infection: intravenous quinine should be used. A loading dose enables therapeutic concentrations to be reached more rapidly. Parenteral artemisin derivatives are effective but are not currently licensed in the UK.

Supportive care is crucial, including careful fluid balance to prevent renal impairment or pulmonary oedema. Hypoglycaemia is common and should be anticipated. The role of exchange transfusion in severe malaria is unproven and fiercely disputed. Many advocate its use for patients with manifestations of severe malaria and high parasite counts (> 10% red cells infected).

Course and prognosis

Most patients become afebrile and aparasitaemic within 2–3 days. There is a significant case fatality rate from severe malaria, especially in non-immune patients. Antimalarials must be continued for their full course; if inadequate treatment courses are given, or if parasites are partially resistant to the drug, then recrudescence of infection can occur.

Preventing infection

Avoid mosquito bites by physical measures; long-sleeved shirts and trousers, mosquito nets, insect repellents, etc.

The choice of a chemoprophylactic regimen depends on local resistance patterns. Chloroquine and proguanil are used in the limited areas where chloroquine resistance is not a problem. Mefloquine, doxycycline and atovaquone–proguanil can all be used for most areas where chloroquine resistance occurs. In parts of south-east Asia, there is extensive resistance to antimalarial drugs; specialist advice is necessary.

157 Tuberculosis

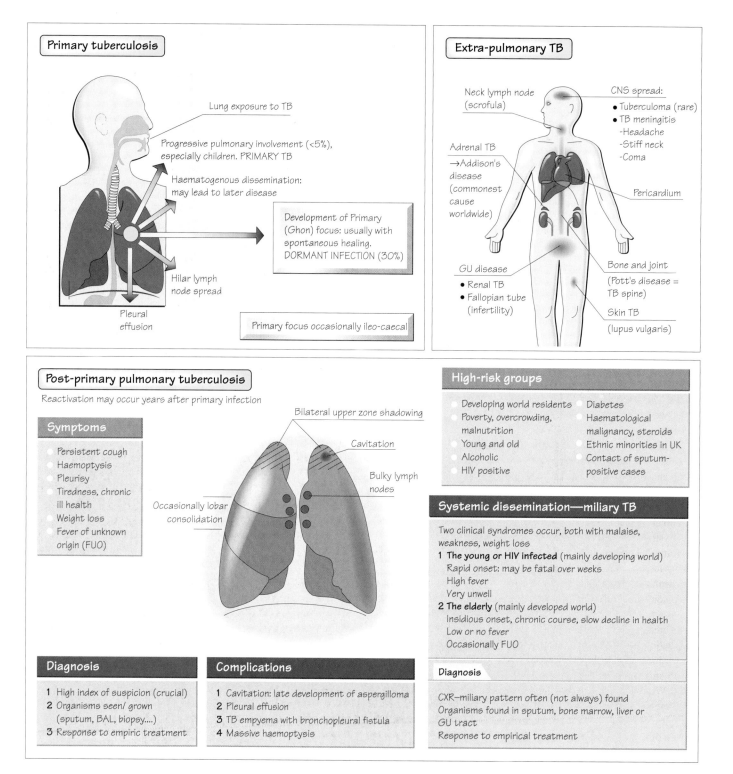

Primary tuberculosis

Lung exposure to TB

Progressive pulmonary involvement (<5%), especially children. PRIMARY TB

Haematogenous dissemination: may lead to later disease

Development of Primary (Ghon) focus: usually with spontaneous healing. DORMANT INFECTION (30%)

Hilar lymph node spread

Pleural effusion

Primary focus occasionally ileo-caecal

Extra-pulmonary TB

Neck lymph node (scrofula)

CNS spread:
- Tuberculoma (rare)
- TB meningitis
  -Headache
  -Stiff neck
  -Coma

Adrenal TB →Addison's disease (commonest cause worldwide)

Pericardium

GU disease
- Renal TB
- Fallopian tube (infertility)

Bone and joint (Pott's disease = TB spine)

Skin TB (lupus vulgaris)

Post-primary pulmonary tuberculosis

Reactivation may occur years after primary infection

Symptoms
- Persistent cough
- Haemoptysis
- Pleurisy
- Tiredness, chronic ill health
- Weight loss
- Fever of unknown origin (FUO)

Bilateral upper zone shadowing

Cavitation

Bulky lymph nodes

Occasionally lobar consolidation

High-risk groups
- Developing world residents
- Poverty, overcrowding, malnutrition
- Young and old
- Alcoholic
- HIV positive
- Diabetes
- Haematological malignancy, steroids
- Ethnic minorities in UK
- Contact of sputum-positive cases

Systemic dissemination—miliary TB

Two clinical syndromes occur, both with malaise, weakness, weight loss
1 **The young or HIV infected** (mainly developing world)
  Rapid onset: may be fatal over weeks
  High fever
  Very unwell
2 **The elderly** (mainly developed world)
  Insidious onset, chronic course, slow decline in health
  Low or no fever
  Occasionally FUO

Diagnosis

CXR—miliary pattern often (not always) found
Organisms found in sputum, bone marrow, liver or GU tract
Response to empirical treatment

Diagnosis
1 High index of suspicion (crucial)
2 Organisms seen/ grown (sputum, BAL, biopsy....)
3 Response to empiric treatment

Complications
1 Cavitation: late development of aspergilloma
2 Pleural effusion
3 TB empyema with bronchopleural fistula
4 Massive haemoptysis

TB causes more deaths worldwide than any other infection. Most infection occurs in tropical regions but numbers of patients are rising in Europe and the USA, as a result of cases in poorer, often homeless populations and in HIV-infected patients. The HIV pandemic has caused a huge global increase in cases, particularly in sub-Saharan Africa.

Diseases and Treatments at a Glance

Epidemiology

Mycobacterium tuberculosis is spread by respiratory droplets; transmission occurs from close proximity to an infected individual. Household contacts of patients with *Mycobacterium tuberculosis* in their sputum have a one in four chance of becoming infected. Clinical disease develops in 5–15% of those infected; this risk is higher in HIV.

Pathogenesis

Following inhalation of organisms, multiplication occurs in subpleural and mid-zone terminal air spaces. Bacteria ingested by alveolar macrophages survive and spread to local lymph nodes. Bloodstream spread occurs to the lung apices and other organs, where latent infection may persist for many years. The slow development of a cellular immune response leads to tuberculous granulomata in tissues and cutaneous hypersensitivity to mycobacterial antigens.

Primary infection

Exposure occurs in childhood in endemic areas, but in later life in most Western regions. The immune response limits damage to a localized area of the lung in the mid-zone with hilar node involvement, termed the primary or Ghon focus; calcification may subsequently be visible on a chest X-ray. Clinical disease is rare at the time of primary infection in adolescents and adults, although primary pulmonary TB does occur.

Pulmonary TB

Eighty per cent of TB used to be pulmonary, but the proportion of extra-pulmonary disease is increasing and is over 50% in HIV patients. The majority of cases are the result of reactivation; re-infection also occurs. The major symptoms are cough, weight loss, malaise, fever and night sweats. Haemoptysis occurs in a third. Examination findings are often unremarkable. The chest X-ray is usually abnormal—classically, apical disease with infiltration and cavitation that heals with fibrotic changes. Complications include severe haemoptysis, bronchopleural fistula and aspergilloma within cavities.

Extra-pulmonary disease

- **Pleural tuberculosis**: occurs most commonly after primary infection. Systemic symptoms, cough and pleuritic pain. Unilateral effusions are common. Often self-limiting, sometimes with resolution of symptoms. Most develop active disease within 3 years.
- **Lymph node TB**: occurs after primary infection, reactivation and contiguous spread. Cervical in 70%. Systemic symptoms in 30–60%. Painless discrete nodes enlarge in size and become matted. Nodes eventually break down with discharging sinuses and chronic skin lesions.
- **Bone/joint TB**: affects any bone or joint. Most common form is spinal (Pott's disease). Vertebral destruction leads to collapse and, sometimes, severe angulation of the spine (gibbus). Paravertebral abscesses may occur. Watch for cord compression; most can be treated medically.
- **TB meningitis**: important; risk of permanent neurological damage or death if not treated promptly. Initial blood-borne spread, followed by rupture of focus into CSF. Non-specific symptoms for 2–8 weeks, with onset that is often insidious. Fever and headache prominent. Mild neck stiffness, cranial nerve palsies, papilloedema, long tract signs. Seizures common in children. Differential diagnosis: fungal or partially treated bacterial meningitis, cerebral abscess.
- **Pericardial TB**: usually caused by spread from lungs or mediastinal lymph nodes. Three clinical syndromes: acute pericarditis ± effusion, chronic pericardial effusion and chronic constrictive pericarditis.

Systemic symptoms, shortness of breath (SOB), signs of effusion or constriction. Pericardial calcification (late) on chest X-ray in constrictive pericarditis. Echocardiography helpful.
- **Miliary TB**: disseminated disease from blood spread in those with underlying chronic disease or immunosuppression. Insidious symptoms: weight loss, fever, malaise. Pulmonary, CNS and liver involvement most frequent. Choroidal tubercles (15%) are pathognomonic. Classic chest X-ray; multiple 1–2 mm nodules in lung fields.

Diagnosis

Definitive diagnosis depends upon demonstrating or culturing the organism.

Pulmonary TB is normally diagnosed by:
- Ziehl-Neelsen staining of acid-fast bacilli (AFB) in sputum.
- Culture of samples on selective media (takes up to 8 weeks).
  Open TB describes the presence of AFB in sputum.

Extra-pulmonary TB: sputum culture occasionally positive, but the diagnosis is usually made from culture of appropriate samples (needle aspiration of lymph node or marrow and liver biopsy in miliary TB) or by histology (pleural or pericardial biopsy) showing granulomata or AFB. Classic X-ray changes (in Pott's disease) may be diagnostic. CSF in TB meningitis (lymphocytes, high protein, low sugar) likewise may be highly suggestive. The role of the polymerase chain reaction (PCR) is still being evaluated.

Mantoux test: measures delayed hypersensitivity reaction to intradermal purified protein derivative (PPD). Positive tests indicate previous exposure. Diagnostic role is debated. In UK, patients may react because of previous BCG (Bacille Calmette–Guérin) immunization. Anergy occurs in systemic illness such as miliary TB. A strongly positive reaction may be helpful clinically.

Treatment

Short-course chemotherapy (6 months) is given for most forms of TB (Table 157.1); longer courses may be needed for TB meningitis and bone/joint TB. Combinations of three or four drugs are used to prevent development of resistance. The clinical response to therapy may be important in confirming the diagnosis; reductions in fever and weight gain are helpful. Steroids are of proven benefit in pericardial disease and are commonly used in TB meningitis and genitourinary TB.

Resistance to individual TB drugs is a major clinical problem in some countries. Some isolates are resistant to multiple drugs. Prolonged treatment with second- and third-line agents is necessary with a poor response in many patients.

Surgery is useful for: chronic constrictive pericarditis, Pott's disease if there is severe cord compression or spinal instability, and intractable haemoptysis or bronchopleural fistula.

Table 157.1 Standard short-course therapy for TB.

Drug	Duration	Important side effects or problems
Isoniazid	6 months	Hepatotoxicity, neuropathy (vitamin B$_6$ prevents)
Rifampicin	6 months	Hepatotoxicity, drug interactions
Pyrazinamide	1st 2 months	Hepatotoxicity
Ethambutol or streptomycin	1st 2 months	Retrobulbar neuritis (check colour vision) (if resistance a concern)

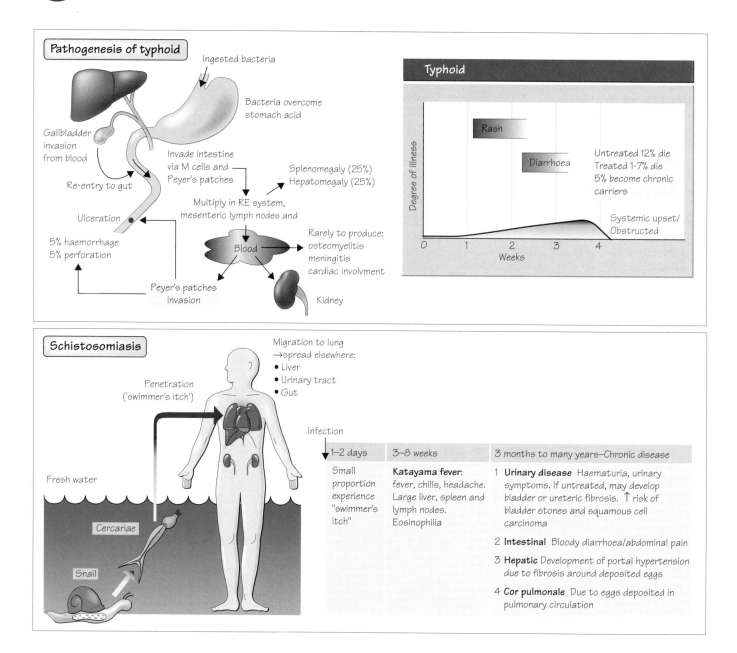

Pathogenesis of typhoid

Ingested bacteria
Bacteria overcome stomach acid
Gallbladder invasion from blood
Invade intestine via M cells and Peyer's patches
Splenomegaly (25%)
Hepatomegaly (25%)
Re-entry to gut
Multiply in RE system, mesenteric lymph nodes and
Ulceration
5% haemorrhage
5% perforation
Blood
Rarely to produce: osteomyelitis meningitis cardiac involvment
Peyer's patches invasion
Kidney

Typhoid

Degree of illness
Rash
Diarrhoea
Untreated 12% die
Treated 1–7% die
5% become chronic carriers
Systemic upset/ Obstructed
0 1 2 3 4
Weeks

Schistosomiasis

Migration to lung →spread elsewhere:
• Liver
• Urinary tract
• Gut
Penetration ('swimmer's itch')
Infection
Fresh water
Cercariae
Snail

1–2 days	3–8 weeks	3 months to many years–Chronic disease
Small proportion experience "swimmer's itch"	**Katayama fever:** fever, chills, headache. Large liver, spleen and lymph nodes. Eosinophilia	1 **Urinary disease** Haematuria, urinary symptoms. If untreated, may develop bladder or ureteric fibrosis. ↑ risk of bladder stones and squamous cell carcinoma 2 **Intestinal** Bloody diarrhoea/abdominal pain 3 **Hepatic** Development of portal hypertension due to fibrosis around deposited eggs 4 **Cor pulmonale** Due to eggs deposited in pulmonary circulation

Typhoid

Infection with the Gram-negative bacteria *Salmonella typhi* or *S. paratyphi* through ingestion of contaminated food or water. *Salmonella* sp. enters through the gut, multiplies within mesenteric lymph nodes and macrophages and enters the blood stream to be disseminated to many sites where further replication occurs.

Clinical features

The incubation period is 10–14 days. Gradually rising fever, headache, malaise and occasionally cough. Abdominal symptoms (pain, diarrhoea or constipation) are prominent during the first week, whereas diarrhoea, mild hepatosplenomegaly and rose spots (in 60%) occur during the second week. Shock, renal impairment and altered mental state, including coma, occur in severe cases. Complications include: (i) perforation or bleeding from the ileum; (ii) osteomyelitis, more common in sickle-cell disease; (iii) cholecystitis; (iv) myocarditis.

Diagnosis

Leukopenia is common and elevated transaminases may occur. Culture of the organism from stool, blood, urine or bone marrow is diagnostic. Serology (Widal test) may occasionally be helpful in non-immunized cases.

Treatment

Optimum treatment depends on the knowledge of geographical origin of isolate; drug resistance to the traditional chloramphenicol,

Diseases and Treatments at a Glance

co-trimoxazole or ampicillin is common. Sensitivity testing is useful. Fluoroquinolones are now drugs of choice and are effective in short (< 7-day) courses, although resistance is becoming problematic. Steroids are used in severe disease. Fever may take several days to respond to treatment. Relapse occurs in 10%. Long-term asymptomatic carriage may occur from persistence of organism in the gall bladder.

Dengue

Dengue is caused by an arbovirus transmitted by the mosquito *Aedes* sp. —increasingly common as its geographical distribution expands. Two main clinical syndromes occur:

1 Dengue fever, seen in most travellers.
2 Dengue haemorrhagic fever/dengue shock syndrome (DHF/DSS), usually seen in children in endemic areas as a result of an immunological response to a second infection.

Clinical features (3- to 8-day incubation)

These are sudden fever, severe headache, backache, muscle pains and rigors. Fever may be biphasic—it disappears then reappears. Maculopapular rash occurs late on in the illness. In DHS/DSS (rare in the UK) increased vascular permeability results in shock, petechiae and bleeding.

Diagnosis and treatment

Leukopenia and thrombocytopenia are common. In DHF/DSS, severe thrombocytopenia, raised haematocrit and abnormal liver enzymes are found. Diagnosis is clinical because virus isolation is not routinely available. Serology is useful for retrospective diagnosis.

No specific treatment is available. DSS/DHF requires supportive therapy and fluids and has a high case fatality.

Schistosomiasis

Two hundred million people are infected worldwide and it is common in returned travellers, although patients are rarely unwell. Schistosomal cerceriae penetrate the skin after fresh water exposure and migrate to the vessels of the bladder or gut (depending on the species), where eggs are produced. Eggs migrate back into gut lumen or urinary tract, but may cause local inflammation. Worm burdens are low in expatriates; severe disease is rare. The clinical features of disease are:
• Swimmer's itch: transient rash 1–2 days after exposure, often unrecognized.
• Katayama fever: 4–10 weeks after exposure in a small proportion of patients. Acute fever, sweats, malaise—sometimes lymphadenopathy and hepatosplenomegaly; self-limiting.
• Urinary schistosomiasis (*Schistosoma haematobium*): often asymptomatic, diagnosed because of eosinophilia. May have haematuria, urinary symptoms or altered ejaculate. Long-term complications unusual in travellers.
• Intestinal/hepatic schistosomiasis: vague abdominal symptoms/ bloody diarrhoea or asymptomatic. Significant liver disease rare in travellers, but very common worldwide.

Diagnosis and treatment

• Eosinophilia common.
• Demonstration of eggs in urine, ejaculate, stool or rectal biopsies.
• Schistosomal serology is useful, but may not be positive until several months after exposure.
• Praziquantel is effective for all species.

Tick typhus

Tick typhus is the major rickettsial disease seen in the UK, particularly in travellers from southern Africa. Tick typhus is caused by the bite of a tick which may be infected by a number of different rickettsial species with a wide geographical distribution. The clinical features are:
• Fever, headache and myalgia.
• Maculopapular rash.
• An eschar (necrotic skin lesion at the site of a tick bite) helps to confirm the diagnosis.
• Lymphadenopathy may occur.
• Rarely, severe systemic illness occurs.

Diagnosis and treatment

Diagnosis is usually clinical, with serological confirmation retrospectively. Tetracycline is extremely effective as treatment.

Leptospirosis

This occurs after contact with water infected by animal urine containing leptospires. May be contracted in the UK (sewer workers, water sports) but common in many parts of the tropics. Leptospires penetrate skin and mucosa, multiply in the blood and then localize in the liver, central nervous system (CNS), muscle and renal cortex.

Clinical features

Wide spectrum of illness from fever, headache and muscle pains to severe sepsis with conjunctivitis, pneumonitis, jaundice, renal failure and extensive haemorrhages.

Diagnosis and treatment

Leukocytosis and thrombocytopenia are common. Creatine kinase elevated in moderate or severe cases. There is abnormal liver function and renal function. Clinical suspicion may be confirmed by identification of leptospires on dark-ground microscopy of the blood. Serology gives retrospective diagnosis. Treatment is with doxycycline or parenteral penicillin in severe cases.

Haemorrhagic fevers

Although uncommon, high mortality and potential for transmission to others mean that such fevers should be considered in sick patients returning from the tropics. They are caused by a number of different RNA viruses, are predominately zoonoses and occur on every continent apart from Australia. Diseases include Lassa fever, yellow fever and Hanta viruses. Suspect on geographical grounds and history of contact with tick or animal blood, or in ill patients, often in remote areas. Clinically:
• Fevers, severe myalgia and increasing prostration.
• Pharyngitis prominent in Lassa fever. Petechiae and bleeding gums may progress to shock and frank haemorrhage.
• Severe malaria is the major differential diagnosis and must be excluded.

Diagnosis and management

Diagnosis is by virus isolation or serology in most cases, with appropriate precautions. Patients are isolated until diagnosis has been excluded —take care to avoid nosocomial transmission. Supportive care is crucial; ribavirin is useful in Lassa fever and some other viruses.

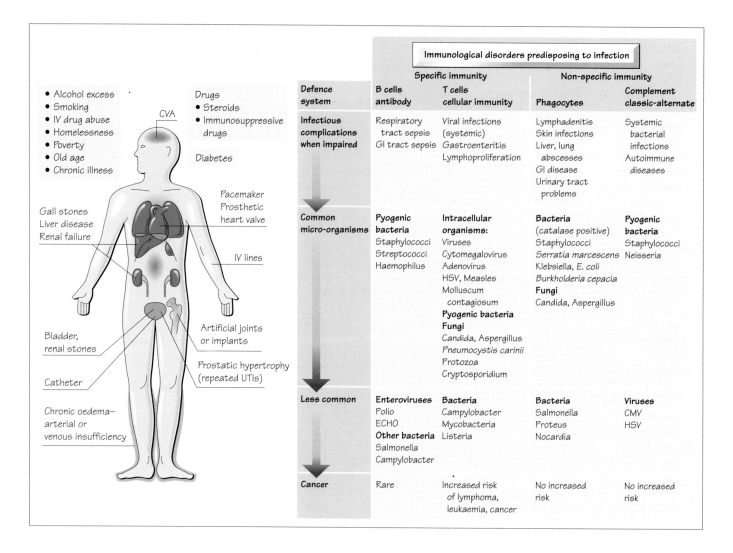

Abnormalities of host immunity predispose to:
- Unusually severe infection
- Infection in unusual sites
- Recurrent infection
- Infection with unusual pathogens, or organisms not usually regarded as pathogenic.

In a patient with any of the above, a search for diseases that alter immunity is crucial. The type of pathogen, site and extent of infection sometimes helps to identify the underlying disease.

Diseases predisposing to infections with common bacterial pathogens
Metabolic and toxic diseases
- Diabetes mellitus predisposes to infection, which may be recurrent or more severe in most tissues, especially the lung, urinary tract and skin (boils, etc.).
- Smoking has a clear role in repeated respiratory tract infections.
- Alcohol excess, even in the absence of chronic liver disease, predisposes to many infections, particularly those involving the respirat-

ory tract, e.g. pneumococcal pneumonia, Legionnaires' disease, and tuberculosis.
- Renal failure is a potent factor predisposing to infection. Not only does uraemia impair immunity, but those with renal failure also have recurrent instrumentation (e.g. intravenous cannulae, dialysis lines) which introduces infection. Infective endocarditis, often caused by *Staphyloccoccus aureus*, occurs annually in 1% of the dialysis population. The nephrotic syndrome predisposes even more powerfully to infection, possibly as the renal protein losses includes IgG, although not IgM.
- Chronic liver disease impairs immunity (e.g. bacterial uptake by the reticuloendothelial system), and contributes to infection in those with chronic abuse of alcohol, as well as in those with other forms of chronic hepatitis.
- Steroid therapy, especially high dose, impairs immunity and, although it may lead to unusual infections (see below), more frequently infection is with common pathogens (e.g. pneumococci, herpes zoster, etc.). The same is true for many other drugs that impair immunity, such as azathioprine, ciclosporin A, etc.

- Chronic inflammatory illness also impairs immunity, e.g. active rheumatoid arthritis, Crohn's disease, disseminated malignancy, etc. impair nutritional status, producing hypoalbuminaemia and hypogammaglobulinaemia.

Structural factors predisposing to infection with common bacterial pathogens

- Intravenous lines: central and peripheral venous lines are a potent source of bacteraemia, commonly with *Staphylococcus aureus*. This infection may lead to infective endocarditis, even in the absence of underlying valvular disease, or to osteomyelitis. Intravenous drug abuse (IVDA) also predisposes to infective endocarditis, particularly involving the right-sided heart valves and lung abscesses. Intravenous drug abusers may have HIV infection, hepatitis B or C, which can impair immunity and predispose to infection themselves.
- Structural abnormalities should be considered in repeated infections of the same structure, e.g. bladder and renal stones or prostatic hypertrophy may cause recurrent urinary tract infections. An obstructing bronchial carcinoma may underlie recurrent/severe pneumonia.
- Prosthetic material: niduses of bacterial infection on prosthetic material, e.g. pacemakers, heart valves, and less commonly hip replacements, can cause persistent/recurrent bacteraemia or septicaemia. Once colonized, prosthetic material can rarely be sterilized and usually needs to be removed. Usually common bacterial pathogens are involved, although occasionally infection is with fairly indolent bacteria, e.g. *Staph. epidermidis*.
- Immobility predisposes to urinary tract infection, because a low fluid intake (deliberate, to avoid unnecessary visits to the toilet) fails to 'flush' the urinary tract free of pathogens.
- Hemiparesis, especially during the acute phase, predisposes to chest infection.
- Gastroenterological pathology such as dysphagia (especially if the result of neurological disease) or gastro-oesophageal reflux can underlie recurrent pneumonia.

Miscellaneous conditions

- Homelessness is an obvious precipitant for repeated respiratory tract and skin infections.
- Cachexia impairs the ability of the body to fight infection and underlies infections in terminal illness. Milder degrees of malnutrition, such as those relating to undiagnosed inflammatory or neoplastic illness, social deprivation or psychiatric illness, are relatively easy to miss and can underlie some repeated infections.
- Failure of the immune system predisposes to infection with opportunistic pathogens (see below), as well as with common pathogens—illness in this situation is likely to be more severe and progress more rapidly. Many viral infections depress immunity transiently, predisposing to subsequent bacterial infection, e.g. influenza in elderly people, predisposing to bacterial pneumonia, and measles in malnourished individuals leading on to infective diarrhoea. Splenectomy predisposes to pneumococcal infection, often presenting as overwhelming septic shock. Previous haematological cancer or autologous bone marrow transplantation predisposes, even many years later, to infection with many common pathogens.

Diseases predisposing to infection with unusual pathogens

Defects in immune function should be considered when infection involves unusual organisms (e.g. normally non-pathogenic organisms), or if common pathogens infect patients at unexpected ages (e.g. *Neisseria meningitidis* in adults, tuberculosis in well-nourished white adults aged 16–65 years), in unusual sites (e.g. fungal pneumonia) or are particularly severe or recurrent (e.g. extensive pyogenic abscesses). Underlying conditions include diabetes, immunosuppressive drugs, and the conditions listed below.

Complement defect *predisposes to infection with staphylococci and, strikingly,* N. meningitidis *at an unusual age.*
- Acquired defects, e.g. as a result of systemic lupus erythematosus (SLE).
- Inherited deficiency is very rare. C5, C6, C7 or C8 deficiency predisposes to *N. meningitidis*.

Neutrophil defects *predispose to overwhelming sepsis with* S. aureus, *Gram-negative bacteria and fungi:*
- Neutropenia: inadequate neutrophil numbers (see p. 85). The most common causes are drugs and haematological cancer and its treatment.
- Defects in neutrophil function: myelodysplasia and haematological cancer depress neutrophil counts and the function of any remaining cells. Other functional defects include the rare inherited ones (see p. 314).

Antibody deficiency *predisposes to bacterial infection, especially with staphylococci, streptococci and haemophilus. Infections, particularly those caused by pneumococci, may be overwhelming:*
- multiple myeloma is a relatively common cause of acquired hypogammaglobulinaemia
- chronic lymphocytic leukaemia and other haematological malignancy and its treatment depress B-cell counts, both during and after treatment
- primary antibody deficiencies are all extraordinarily rare (see p. 315).

Defects in cell-mediated immunity:
- HIV infection (see p. 300)
- haematological cancer and its treatment
- primary defects (see p. 316).

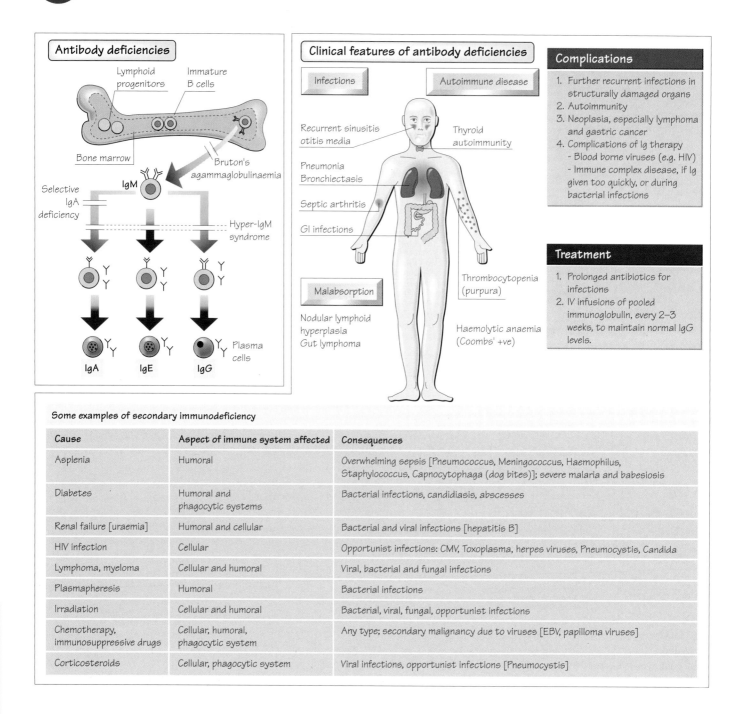

Antibody deficiencies

Lymphoid progenitors
Immature B cells
Bone marrow
Bruton's agammaglobulinaemia
IgM
Selective IgA deficiency
Hyper-IgM syndrome
IgA   IgE   IgG   Plasma cells

Clinical features of antibody deficiencies

Infections   Autoimmune disease

Recurrent sinusitis otitis media
Pneumonia Bronchiectasis
Septic arthritis
GI infections
Thyroid autoimmunity

Malabsorption

Nodular lymphoid hyperplasia
Gut lymphoma
Thrombocytopenia (purpura)
Haemolytic anaemia (Coombs' +ve)

Complications

1. Further recurrent infections in structurally damaged organs
2. Autoimmunity
3. Neoplasia, especially lymphoma and gastric cancer
4. Complications of Ig therapy
   - Blood borne viruses (e.g. HIV)
   - Immune complex disease, if Ig given too quickly, or during bacterial infections

Treatment

1. Prolonged antibiotics for infections
2. IV infusions of pooled immunoglobulin, every 2–3 weeks, to maintain normal IgG levels.

Some examples of secondary immunodeficiency

Cause	Aspect of immune system affected	Consequences
Asplenia	Humoral	Overwhelming sepsis [Pneumococcus, Meningococcus, Haemophilus, Staphylococcus, Capnocytophaga (dog bites)]; severe malaria and babesiosis
Diabetes	Humoral and phagocytic systems	Bacterial infections, candidiasis, abscesses
Renal failure [uraemia]	Humoral and cellular	Bacterial and viral infections [hepatitis B]
HIV infection	Cellular	Opportunist infections: CMV, Toxoplasma, herpes viruses, Pneumocystis, Candida
Lymphoma, myeloma	Cellular and humoral	Viral, bacterial and fungal infections
Plasmapheresis	Humoral	Bacterial infections
Irradiation	Cellular and humoral	Bacterial, viral, fungal, opportunist infections
Chemotherapy, immunosuppressive drugs	Cellular, humoral, phagocytic system	Any type; secondary malignancy due to viruses [EBV, papilloma viruses]
Corticosteroids	Cellular, phagocytic system	Viral infections, opportunist infections [Pneumocystis]

Immunodeficiency should be suspected whenever there is evidence of increased susceptibility to infection. The commonest causes of immunodeficiency are secondary to other medical or surgical problems or their therapy. Symptomatic primary immunodeficiency is rare. There are no hard and fast rules indicating that immunodeficiency is likely to be present, but two or more serious (requiring intravenous antibiotics) infections in a year are highly suspicious. Infections in unusual sites, for example liver or brain abscesses, osteomyelitis, septic arthritis, where there is no obvious structural reason, and infection with unusual or normally non-pathogenic organisms are highly suspicious of immuno-

deficiency. Primary immunodeficiency may also be accompanied by evidence of immune dysfunction such as autoimmune disease. The immune system is very adaptable and often the severity of the clinical problem is less severe than one might predict because of compensatory mechanisms. The nature of the infection gives a clue to the underlying defect (see Table 160.1). Cases of suspected primary or secondary immunodeficiency should be referred to an immunologist for formal investigation; suspected HIV infection should be referred to a consultant in infectious diseases or genitourinary medicine (GUM) experienced in the management of the condition.

Table 160.1 Classification of immunological deficiency syndromes.

Type of defect	Typical infections
B cell defect (reduced antibody)	Bacterial infections: • *Streptococcus pneumoniae* • *Haemophilus influenzae* • *Neisseria meningitidis* • *Staphylococcus aureus* • *Campylobacter* species • *Salmonella* species and other enteric pathogens • *Mycoplasma* species • *Ureaplasma* species Viral infections: • Enteroviruses (polio, echoviruses, Coxsackie viruses) Protozoal infections: • *Giardia lamblia*
T cell defect	Bacterial infections: • May be some increase in bacterial infections due to poor T cell help for B cell responses Viral infections: • All types, often persistent • Enteric viruses (Rotavirus) • Respiratory viruses (respiratory syncytial virus, parainfluenza viruses, adenoviruses) • Herpes viruses (EBV, CMV, HHV6) • Papillomaviruses (warts) • JC and BK viruses (progressive multifocal leukoencephalopathy) Fungal infections: • *Candida* • *Aspergillus* • *Pneumocystis carinii* Protozoal infections: • *Toxoplasma gondii* • Cryptosporidium • Microsporidium
Combined T and B cell defect	As for B and T cell defects Pattern may be variable
Neutrophil defects	Bacterial infections: • Catalase-positive organisms (*Staphylococcus aureus*) Fungal infections: • Any fungus (typically *Aspergillus*)
Complement deficiency	• Bacterial infections • *Neisseria* species • As for antibody deficiency (C3 deficiency only)

Antibody deficiency syndromes

In antibody deficiencies recurrent bacterial infections occur, usually with common organisms, e.g. *Haemophilus influenzae*, *Streptococcus pneumoniae*, although less usual organisms (e.g. *Mycoplasma*) are also important. Infections most frequently involve the upper and lower respiratory tract, but may involve the gastrointestinal tract (e.g. *Giardia*) and other sites. Malabsorption may be due to infection, to nodular lymphoid hyperplasia or malignancy. If the underlying disorder is untreated, the frequency and severity of the infections results in structural end-organ damage including bronchiectasis and growth retardation in children. Deficiencies are classified into primary and secondary antibody deficiencies.

Primary antibody deficiency

Primary antibody deficiency is a reduction or absence of one or more immunoglobulin isotypes when no other contributory disorder is present. There are four major forms. All are rare—prevalence 12 per million. In primary antibody deficiencies both infections and antibody-mediated autoimmune disease occur:

• **X-linked agammaglobulinaemia** (XLA, Bruton's agammaglobulinaemia): mutation in the X chromosome (*Btk* gene) prevents normal B-cell maturation. Presents aged 3–12 months: milder forms present later.
• **Hyper IgM syndrome** presents in childhood with recurrent bacterial infections and autoimmune disease (neutropenia and thrombocytopenia). The X-linked form (70% of cases) is a deficiency of CD40 ligand on T cells (a lymphocyte communication molecule). The IgM antibody response is intact. B cells cannot produce mature IgG or IgA antibody. Very high IgM, and low/undetectable IgG and IgA. Increased risk of IgM lymphomas.
• **Common variable immunodeficiency** (CVID): unknown aetiology but is partly genetic (50% have a family history of IgA deficiency). Heterogeneous laboratory findings. Serum IgG levels may be only

marginally reduced, but specific antibody production is invariably poor or absent. IgM levels may be normal. Patients present at any age, particularly adolescence and early adulthood. Autoimmune disease is common. There is a 40-fold increased risk of lymphoma, and also an increased risk of gastric cancer.

• **Selective IgA deficiency** affects 1 : 400–800. Most are asymptomatic, but an increased incidence of allergic disease and connective tissue disease. Recurrent infections are rarely a problem unless additional immune defects present. The diagnosis is made based upon *absent* serum IgA (not just low levels).

• **Specific antibody deficiency**: this is linked to CVID and selective IgA deficiency and represents failure of immune responsiveness to a single class of antigens such as bacterial polysaccharides. Serum immunoglobulins and IgG subclasses are normal.

Secondary antibody deficiency

Secondary antibody deficiency syndromes are the commonest cause of antibody deficiency and relate to conditions such as nephrotic syndrome (protein leak), protein-losing enteropathies/malabsorption (protein leak), immunosuppressive drug therapy, multiple myeloma (negative feedback), lymphoproliferative disease (especially chronic lymphocytic leukaemia) and (probably) malignancy.

Investigations

The initial investigation in suspected primary antibody deficiency is serum immunoglobulins and protein electrophoresis. These measure the ability to produce antibodies, although not their 'usefulness'. Absence of immunoglobulins is always significant, but antibody deficiency can occur with normal serum immunoglobulins and functional tests of antibody production may be required. The diagnosis in CVID is complicated, as while serum IgG may be absent or very low, this is not invariable. In such cases it is important to measure specific antibodies to antigens to which the patient has been exposed, e.g. tetanus/diphtheria vaccinations. If specific antibodies are undetectable or very low, the patient may be test-immunized with a (killed) vaccine and serology repeated 4–6 weeks later. Failure to mount a response may indicate an antibody deficiency. Secondary antibody deficiencies (see above) should be excluded.

Management and prognosis

The mainstay of treatment is long-term replacement therapy with pooled immunoglobulin, which provides passive protection from bacterial infections. Once diagnosed and treated, patients usually lead normal active lives, although recurrent infections can occur despite adequate replacement therapy if there is pre-existing structural damage. If an infection becomes established, early treatment with antibiotics is essential, usually for 10 days. Autoimmune diseases usually require corticosteroids. There is an increased incidence of malignancies, particularly lymphoma.

T cell deficiencies

These are usually secondary to another disease process (haematological malignancy, its treatment or HIV infection) but can be primary. Most are evident in childhood but may present in early adult life.

• **22q11 deletion syndrome (DiGeorge syndrome)**: complex genetic disorder (chromosome 22) with major cardiac, facial and parathyroid gland defects. Intellectual impairment is common. High risk of blood-borne infection from transfusions during cardiac surgery. The degree of immunodeficiency is very variable: severe cases have a small, atrophic thymus and no T cells and can mimic severe combined immuno-deficiency. Survival into adult life is common. Bone marrow and thymic transplants have been used.

• **Chronic mucocutaneous candidiasis**: a common, mainly T cell defect, leading to chronic candidiasis, typically of mouth and nails. Fifty per cent have an autoimmune endocrinopathy (associated with defects in autoimmune regulator gene, AIRE). Bacterial, viral and mycobacterial infections may also occur.

• **Other syndromes**: other predominantly T cell syndromes include **Wiskott-Aldrich syndrome** (eczema, thrombocytopenia with small platelets and immune deficiency), due to mutations in the WASP gene on the X-chromosome and **ataxia telangiectasia** (progressive cerebellar degeneration and immune deficiency) due to mutations in the ATM gene.

Severe combined immunodeficiency (SCID)

This only rarely presents in adult life. Features are those of bacterial, viral, fungal and opportunist infections. Genetic defects include mutations affecting the cytokine common gamma chain, Jak-3, adenosine deaminase genes. The bare lymphocyte syndrome often presents slightly later and may be due to defects in genes controlling MHC antigen expression.

Investigations

Measurement of T cell subpopulations (CD4, CD8) and MHC antigens (MHC Class I and Class II) and functional assays of T cells are required. This can only be undertaken in specialist laboratories and early referral to an immunologist is required.

Management of severe combined and T cell disorders

Prevention of infection is critical in all T cell deficiencies:

• Live vaccines (e.g. BCG) should not be given

• Concomitant humoral deficiency can be treated with immunoglobulin replacement therapy

• Blood transfused should be CMV negative and irradiated to avoid graft vs. host disease (mediated by donor lymphocytes)

• Prophylaxis against *Pneumocystis carinii* infection should be given.

• Bone marrow transplantation is indicated in severe primary disease, including all SCID patients and Wiskott-Aldrich syndrome.

Neutrophil disorders

The commonest neutrophil disorders in adults are secondary, but primary neutrophil disorders may also present in adults for the first time. Typically present with recurrent abscesses (liver), unusual granulomatous disease (mimicking sarcoidosis) and atypical Crohn's disease.

• **Chronic granulomatous disease (CGD)**: occurs due to defects in neutrophil oxidative metabolism, caused by mutations in genes for the components of the multi-protein NADPH-oxidase enzyme. X-linked and autosomal recessive forms may occur. Involvement of the bowel with consequent malabsorption and hepatosplenomegaly are common.

• **Other inherited neutrophil defects**: other genetic diseases interfere with chemotaxis (hyper IgE syndrome and Chediak-Higashi syndromes), phagocytosis (leukocyte adhesion deficiency) or numbers (cyclic neutropenia).

• **Acquired defects**: neutrophil abnormalities include deficient numbers (neutropenia, p. 85, often drug or leukaemia related), or quality (e.g. in myelodysplasia, p. 337).

Investigations

Diagnosis of CGD is made using the nitroblue tetrazolium test or a flow cytometric assay of neutrophil oxidative metabolism.

Management

Prevention of infection is critical.
- Prophylactic co-trimoxazole (active in neutrophil phagocytic granules).
- Prophylactic itraconazole to prevent fungal infections.
- Investigate for bowel involvement.
- Bone marrow transplantation (any age), as long-term outlook without is poor.

Complement deficiency

Complement deficiency is strongly associated with recurrent neisserial infection and atypical connective tissue disease (SLE) and glomerulonephritis. Any component may be deficient. Investigate every patient with more than one episode of bacterial meningitis.

Investigations

Complement deficiency can be proved by demonstration absence of haemolytic complement activity in fresh serum (CH100 and alternate pathway CH100).

Management

- Prophylactic penicillin V 500 mg bd for adults.
- Immunize against *Meningococcus* (tetravalent vaccine), *Pneumococcus*.

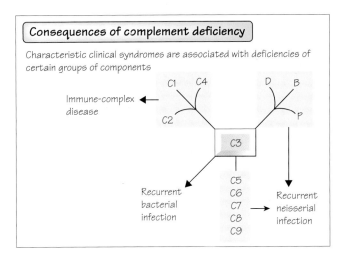

Consequences of complement deficiency

Characteristic clinical syndromes are associated with deficiencies of certain groups of components

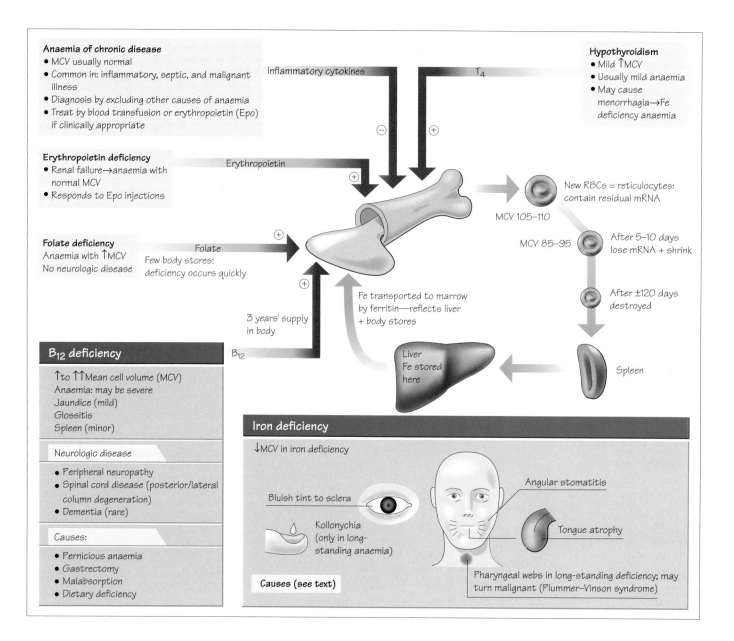

Anaemia of chronic disease
- MCV usually normal
- Common in: inflammatory, septic, and malignant illness
- Diagnosis by excluding other causes of anaemia
- Treat by blood transfusion or erythropoietin (Epo) if clinically appropriate

Inflammatory cytokines

T_4

Hypothyroidism
- Mild ↑MCV
- Usually mild anaemia
- May cause menorrhagia→Fe deficiency anaemia

Erythropoietin deficiency
- Renal failure→anaemia with normal MCV
- Responds to Epo injections

Erythropoietin

New RBCs = reticulocytes: contain residual mRNA

MCV 105–110

Folate deficiency
Anaemia with ↑MCV
No neurologic disease

Folate
Few body stores: deficiency occurs quickly

MCV 85–95

After 5–10 days lose mRNA + shrink

After ±120 days destroyed

Fe transported to marrow by ferritin—reflects liver + body stores

3 years' supply in body

B_{12}

Spleen

Liver Fe stored here

B_{12} deficiency

↑to ↑↑Mean cell volume (MCV)
Anaemia: may be severe
Jaundice (mild)
Glossitis
Spleen (minor)

Neurologic disease

- Peripheral neuropathy
- Spinal cord disease (posterior/lateral column degeneration)
- Dementia (rare)

Causes:

- Pernicious anaemia
- Gastrectomy
- Malabsorption
- Dietary deficiency

Iron deficiency

↓MCV in iron deficiency

Bluish tint to sclera

Angular stomatitis

Koilonychia (only in long-standing anaemia)

Tongue atrophy

Causes (see text)

Pharyngeal webs in long-standing deficiency; may turn malignant (Plummer–Vinson syndrome)

Iron deficiency

Iron deficiency underlies 500 million cases of anaemia worldwide. Premenopausal women are more commonly affected than men because of menstrual blood loss. Iron is absorbed from the upper small intestine from food. A normal Western diet provides 15 mg/day. Adult men have a daily iron requirement of 1 mg, menstruating females 1.5 mg and an extra 5–6 mg/day are needed in pregnancy. Iron is transported in the blood by transferrin and stored bound to ferritin.

Causes of iron deficiency

Blood loss from the gastrointestinal or genitourinary tracts is the most common cause of iron deficiency. The increased demands of pregnancy also lead to maternal iron deficiency. Malabsorption caused by coeliac disease is an uncommon, but important, cause. Iron deficiency solely caused by an inadequate diet is uncommon in the West.

Clinical features

The important clinical features relate to anaemia (fatigue, breathlessness, swollen feet and ankles, pale mucous membranes) and, more rarely, as the result of tissue iron deficiency (angular stomatitis, glossitis and, very rarely, koilonychia—spoon-shaped nails).

Diagnosis

Iron deficiency is suspected by finding microcytic (small red cells) and hypochromic (red cells with reduced haemoglobin) anaemia. Serum iron and ferritin are low and the total iron-binding capacity (transferrin) high. Ferritin is an acute phase protein and is normal or elevated in patients with inflammatory, malignant or liver disease even in the presence of iron deficiency.

Management

• Diagnose the underlying cause: it is vital to diagnose and manage appropriately the underlying illness. Blood loss is identified from the history, examination and investigation. Occult gastrointestinal malignancy may be found.

• Replace iron: oral iron, to replace and replenish body iron stores, should be given until the haemoglobin and mean cell volume (MCV) are normal, then continued for a further 3 months to build up adequate body iron stores. Side effects include nausea, diarrhoea or constipation. Intravenous iron is rarely needed.

• Blood transfusion is seldom appropriate unless the patient is severely symptomatic with angina or breathlessness. Preoperative blood transfusion may worsen the outlook in colonic cancer, through an immunomodulatory action.

Vitamin B12 deficiency

The most common cause of vitamin B12 deficiency in the UK is pernicious anaemia. Other causes include malabsorption of vitamin B12 in the terminal ileum (e.g. Crohn's disease), after a total gastrectomy, pancreatic disease, bacterial overgrowth as a result of blind loop syndrome, gut infection with the fish tapeworm and, very occasionally, dietary deficiency, usually in strict vegans.

Pernicious anaemia

There are 25 new cases of pernicious anaemia (PA) per 100 000 people every year. It is more common in elderly people. Mean age of onset is 60 years.

Pathophysiology

Vitamin B12 is synthesized by micro-organisms and humans obtain it from food of animal origin, particularly liver and kidney. Vitamin B12 absorption requires intrinsic factor (made by stomach parietal cells) and does not occur in its absence. Vitamin B12 binds to intrinsic factor and is absorbed in the terminal ileum. In pernicious anaemia there is an autoimmune gastritis and antibodies occur against:

• Gastric parietal cells, diminishing intrinsic factor secretion.

• Intrinsic factor, preventing vitamin B12 binding.

In addition to vitamin B12, methyl tetrahydrofolate (methyl-THF) is needed as a coenzyme in the methylation of homocysteine to methionine—the first step in intracellular folate production. Thus, vitamin B12 deficiency results in intracellular folate deficiency. Given this biochemical background, it is not surprising that the haematological disorder is the same in both vitamin B12 and folate deficiency.

Clinical features

Common clinical features are symptoms of anaemia, mild jaundice, glossitis and weight loss. PA is an autoimmune disease and other autoimmune diseases such as vitiligo may occur. Neurological disturbances (peripheral neuropathy or subacute combined degeneration of the cord) are rare now, as a result of earlier diagnosis. Infertility is a rare presenting symptom. Dementia may occasionally be caused by vitamin B12 deficiency in the absence of a macrocytic anaemia.

Diagnosis

Most patients have a macrocytic anaemia with a megaloblastic bone marrow (delay in nuclear maturation of red cell precursors). Mild/moderate thrombocytopenia and leukopenia are common. A small increase in the plasma bilirubin is found. The diagnosis is confirmed by finding:

• Low serum vitamin B12.

• Antibodies against gastric parietal cells and intrinsic factor: found in 50% of patients with pernicious anaemia. Also check thyroid antibodies and thyroid function in view of close association between PA and thyroid disease.

• The Schilling test: the absorption of orally administered radiolabelled vitamin B12 in the absence (part 1 of the test) or presence (part 2) of intrinsic factor (IF) is determined. In PA only vitamin B12 with intrinsic factor is absorbed. In malabsorption, e.g. caused by Crohn's disease, vitamin B12 is not absorbed with or without IF.

Treatment and prognosis

Intramuscular vitamin B12 (daily for 5 days, then every 3 months for life) should be given. Surprisingly, perhaps, B12 replacement can also be given by mouth but it remains much commoner to use the IM injections. Potassium deficiency can occur within the first few days of starting treatment so potassium supplements are advisable. Iron deficiency can develop because the patient responds to the vitamin B12 with a huge increase in red cell production. The prognosis for treated patients is excellent, although there is a slightly higher incidence of gastric cancer.

Folate deficiency

Folate deficiency is a common cause of a macrocytic anaemia. Folate occurs in abundant quantities in green vegetables and is mainly absorbed in the upper part of the small intestine. Folate deficiency may be the result of:

• Dietary deficiency
• Malabsorption, such as in coeliac disease
• Excessive requirement, e.g. haemolytic anaemia
• Increased requirement, i.e. pregnancy
• Folate antagonist drugs, such as methotrexate.

Diagnosis

A macrocytic anaemia associated with a low serum and red cell folate establishes the diagnosis. The marrow will be megaloblastic.

Treatment

Treatment is with folic acid 5 mg/day. The underlying cause should be investigated and treated.

Hormonal and cytokine causes of anaemia

Erythropoietin deficiency (renal failure), hypothyroidism and chronic disease are all common causes of anaemia (see figure).

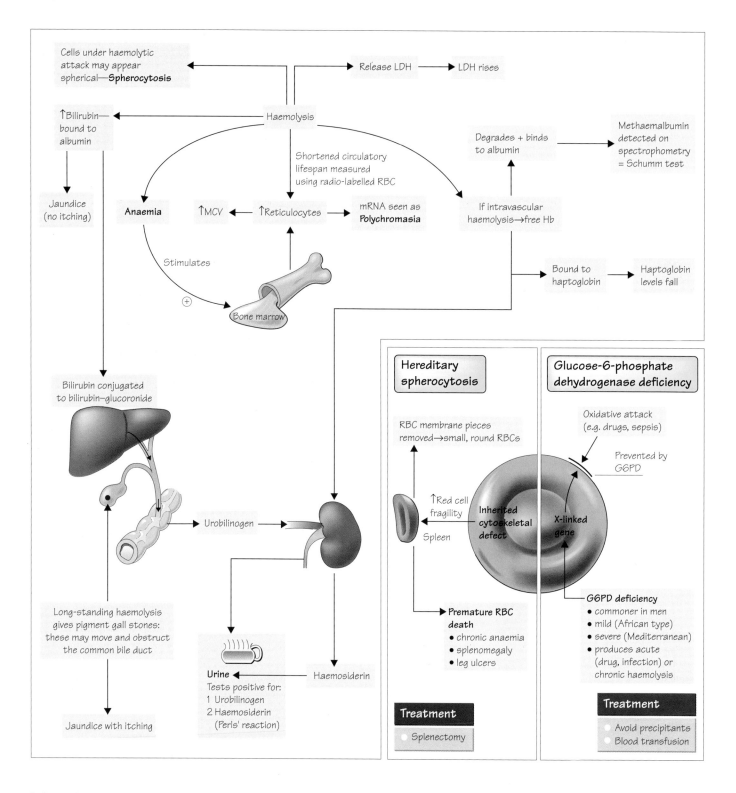

In haemolytic anaemia, the red cell life span is significantly shorter than the normal 120 days. Although the bone marrow can increase red cell production to seven times the normal level, this is inadequate and anaemia results. Such an increase in red cell production increases folate requirements, which if unmet can provoke folate deficiency. Haemolysis may be congenital or acquired (Table 162.1). General clinical features include pallor, jaundice and variably splenomegaly. Pigment gall stones can occur in those who are chronically hyperbilirubinaemic and may lead to obstructive jaundice.

Table 162.1 Common causes of haemolytic anaemia.

Congenital
Hereditary spherocytosis
Glucose-6-phosphate dehydrogenase deficiency
Pyruvate kinase deficiency
Sickle-cell disease
Thalassaemia

Acquired
Infection
Autoimmune
Drug induced
Cardiac (typically across a prosthetic heart valve)
Haemolytic transfusion reaction
Microangiopathic (e.g. haemolytic uraemic syndrome, thrombotic thrombocytopenic purpura)
Paroxysmal nocturnal haemoglobinuria

General laboratory abnormalities in haemolysis

Laboratory tests show evidence of increased red cell breakdown:
• Increased unconjugated plasma bilirubin (a breakdown product of haem).
• Raised plasma lactate dehydrogenase (LDH), released from damaged red cells.
• Low or absent plasma haptoglobin (binds avidly to free plasma haemoglobin).
• Radio-isotope studies (seldom performed) show a shortened red cell life span.

Blood film examination shows polychromasia (resulting from the residual RNA found in young but not old red cells) and a raised reticulocyte count, both indicative of increased red cell production.

Hereditary haemolytic anaemias
Hereditary spherocytosis

This autosomal dominant inherited illness results in an abnormal red cell membrane, and typically presents in childhood with pallor and attacks of jaundice. There is usually, but not always, a family history of hereditary spherocytosis (HS). Splenomegaly is very common. The diagnosis is made from the history, physical findings (splenomegaly), and the general laboratory features of haemolysis and finding spherocytes (small, spherical, darkly staining red cells with no central area of pallor) on the blood film. Many patients do not need treatment but, if anaemia is severe and symptomatic, it can be very successfully treated by splenectomy. As those without a spleen are at increased risk of infection by encapsulated bacteria, immunization with Pneumovax, HiB (*Haemophilus influenzae* B) and the meningococcus vaccines should occur beforehand. After surgery life-long prophylactic penicillin is often given.

Red cell enzyme deficiency

The deficiency of almost any enzyme involved in red cell glucose metabolism can result in a haemolytic anaemia. The most important (and common) are glucose-6-phosphate dehydrogenase (G6PD) deficiency and pyruvate kinase deficiency.

Glucose-6-phosphate dehydrogenase deficiency
NADPH (reduced nicotinamide adenine dinucleotide phosphate), essential to the maintenance of functional haemoglobin, is generated by the catalysis of glucose 6-phosphate by G6PD. A deficiency of G6PD leads to a haemolytic anaemia. G6PD deficiency results from a variety of mutant alleles of its structural gene, and is very common in the subtropics and tropical regions; because of migrations, it is increasingly found in northern Europe and the USA. The gene for G6PD is X-linked, so G6PD deficiency is much more common in males. Most people with G6PD deficiency are asymptomatic until an acute haemolytic episode occurs, triggered by infection, some drugs (e.g. sulphonamides and primaquine) and the ingestion of fava beans. An acute haemolytic attack is usually self-limiting and supportive care only is required. A chronic haemolytic anaemia is rare.

Diagnosis and treatment of G6PD deficiency
The general features of haemolysis are found. Heinz bodies (caused by denaturation of unstable haemoglobin) are detected in the red blood cells. Red cell G6PD activity is low (< 20% of normal). Treatment is by transfusion if needed and by avoidance of triggers.

Pyruvate kinase deficiency
Pyruvate kinase (PK) deficiency is a rare autosomal recessive disease with a prevalence of 1 : 10 000. The clinical features vary but most present in childhood with anaemia and jaundice. Typically the haemoglobin is 4.5–10.0 g/dL. Splenomegaly is usually only mild. Interestingly, the patient's exercise tolerance is better than expected for the degree of anaemia because PK deficiency increases red cell 2,3-diphosphoglycerate concentrations, thus lowering haemoglobin oxygen affinity and enhancing tissue oxygen delivery. The diagnosis is made by finding a haemolytic anaemia (often with a very marked reticulocytosis), bizarre 'prickle cells' in the blood and a significantly reduced red cell PK activity. Treatment is usually fairly conservative. Folic acid is recommended. Many patients need blood transfusion on occasions, but there is no benefit from regular transfusion. Splenectomy improves the haemoglobin in most anaemic patients.

Acquired haemolytic anaemias
Thrombotic thrombocytopenic purpura (TTP)

This uncommon acquired disorder is characterized by a pentad of haemolytic anaemia with red cell fragments in the blood film (microangiopathic haemolytic anaemia), thrombocytopenia, neurological abnormalities, renal impairment and fever. The onset is often abrupt and the disease is usually fatal without treatment. An antibody occurs against a metalloprotease, which cleaves the high-molecular-weight polymers of von Willebrand's factor, which normally cause platelet aggregation and adhesion to the endothelial cell surface. Endothelial cell injury and the platelet aggregation have both been implicated in the pathogenesis of thrombotic thrombocytopenic purpura (TTP). Plasmapheresis, which removes antibody, and infusion of fresh frozen plasma (FFP), which contains the metalloprotease, are the mainstays of treatment. Most patients recover, although there is a 20% mortality rate. Occasional patients have a relapsing/remitting course, caused by an inherited deficiency of the metalloprotease enzyme.

Haemolytic uraemic syndrome (HUS)

This is characterized by a microangiopathic haemolytic anaemia, thrombocytopenia and renal impairment. The aetiology is often obscure but infection with *Escherichia coli* 0157 is sometimes responsible and may cause small epidemics. HUS is associated with a deficiency of complement factor H. Although most clinical and laboratory features

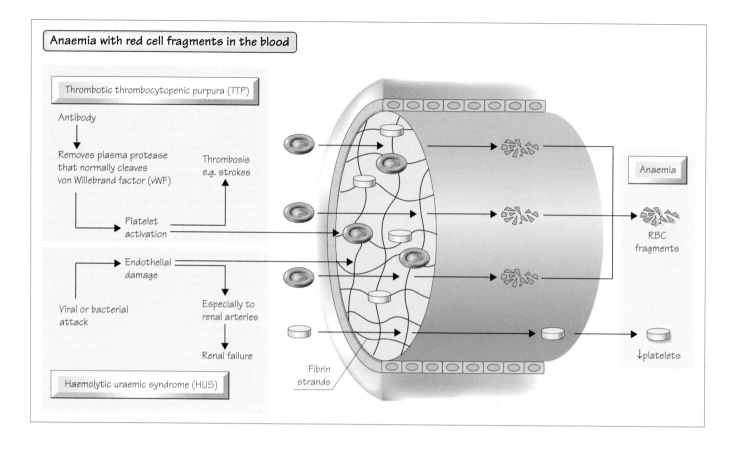

Anaemia with red cell fragments in the blood

Thrombotic thrombocytopenic purpura (TTP)

Antibody

Removes plasma protease that normally cleaves von Willebrand factor (vWF) → Thrombosis e.g. strokes

Platelet activation

Endothelial damage

Viral or bacterial attack → Especially to renal arteries → Renal failure

Haemolytic uraemic syndrome (HUS)

Fibrin strands

Anaemia

RBC fragments

↓platelets

---

of TTP and haemolytic uraemic syndrome (HUS) are similar, neurological injury is unique to TTP, and no antibody against the metalloprotease has been detected in HUS. The treatment involves supportive care. Dialysis may be required. Childhood HUS often does not need specific treatment; plasmapheresis is the mainstay of treatment in adult HUS, although the response is usually less good than for patients with TTP. Most patients recover, although there is a mortality rate of 10–30%. Some patients are left with persistent renal impairment.

Cardiac haemolysis

This usually occurs only after prosthetic heart valve replacement and is caused by a small leak around the valve. The patients are anaemic and found to have red cell fragments in the blood film. The haemolysis is usually mild but re-operation is sometimes needed. Other causes of haemolysis need to be excluded.

Autoimmune haemolytic anaemia

Autoimmune haemolytic anaemia (AIHA) may be warm or cold antibody mediated. The clinical features include fatigue and lethargy and occasionally heart failure. Splenomegaly is common. In addition to the general features of haemolysis the blood film is characterized by spherocytes (warm antibodies only) and, in some cases, by red cell agglutination.

Warm antibody-mediated haemolysis

This is usually caused by IgG binding to red cells, resulting in splenic phagocytosis, either complete or partial (the latter leads to rounder red cells—spherocytes). Some complement-mediated cell death also occurs. Causes include:

- Idiopathic.
- Lymphoproliferative diseases (e.g. chronic lymphocytic leukaemia [CLL], non-Hodgkin's lymphoma).
- Autoimmune disease (e.g. systemic lupus erythematosus [SLE]).
- Inflammatory bowel disease.
- Drugs (e.g. methyl-dopa, mefenamic acid, penicillin).

The direct antiglobulin test (Coombs' test, which detects the presence of antibody and complement on the red cell surface) is usually positive. Most patients respond to prednisolone. Blood transfusions are helpful for severe, symptomatic anaemia while waiting for steroids to work. Splenectomy is often effective at relieving haemolysis if steroids fail.

Cold-antibody-mediated haemolysis

The antibody (usually IgM) may be polyclonal and arises as a consequence of infection or monoclonal secondary to a lymphoproliferative disorder or an idiopathic disorder—cold haemagglutinin disease (CHAD).

- **Cold antibody-mediated haemolysis and infection**: polyclonal IgM antibodies causing haemolysis sometimes occur 1–2 weeks after infection, usually with either *Mycoplasma pneumoniae* or infectious mononucleosis. The disorder is usually self-limiting. Avoidance of the cold and, where needed, blood transfusion (given through a blood warmer) are appropriate measures.
- **Cold haemagglutin disease**: here, an occult clone of lymphocytes produces an IgM antibody, which binds to red blood cells *in the cold*, activates complement and destroys red cells. Typically pallor, mild jaundice and occasionally mild splenomegaly occur. Acrocyanosis of the extremities (purplish discoloration from red cell agglutination

Diseases and Treatments at a Glance

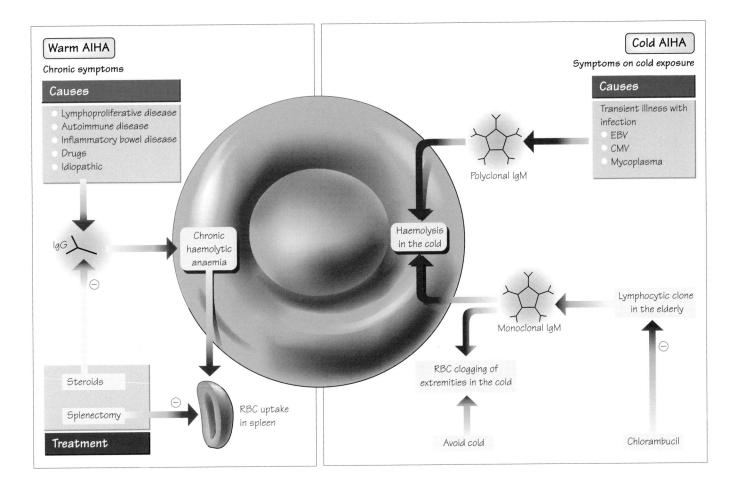

in small distal vessels) is common. Diagnosis is by finding a mild-to-moderate anaemia, red cell agglutination in the blood film and a positive Coombs' test for complement, but not for antibody (IgM antibodies elute from the red cell into the serum *in vitro*). The concentration of IgM antibodies is too low for detection by serum electrophoresis—they are instead found because of their ability to agglutinate red cells in the cold (cold agglutinins). Avoidance of the cold, folic acid supplements and alkylating agents (e.g. chlorambucil) are the mainstays of treatment. Prednisolone is often ineffective. A very similar illness to CHAD occa-

sionally complicates the clinical course of overt lymphoproliferative disorders. The management is as for CHAD.

Paroxysmal cold haemoglobinuria

This rare disorder, usually self-limiting, is most common in children, and is often preceded by a viral illness. Very rarely it may be associated with syphilis. It is caused by a polyclonal IgG cold antibody (the Donath–Landsteiner antibody).

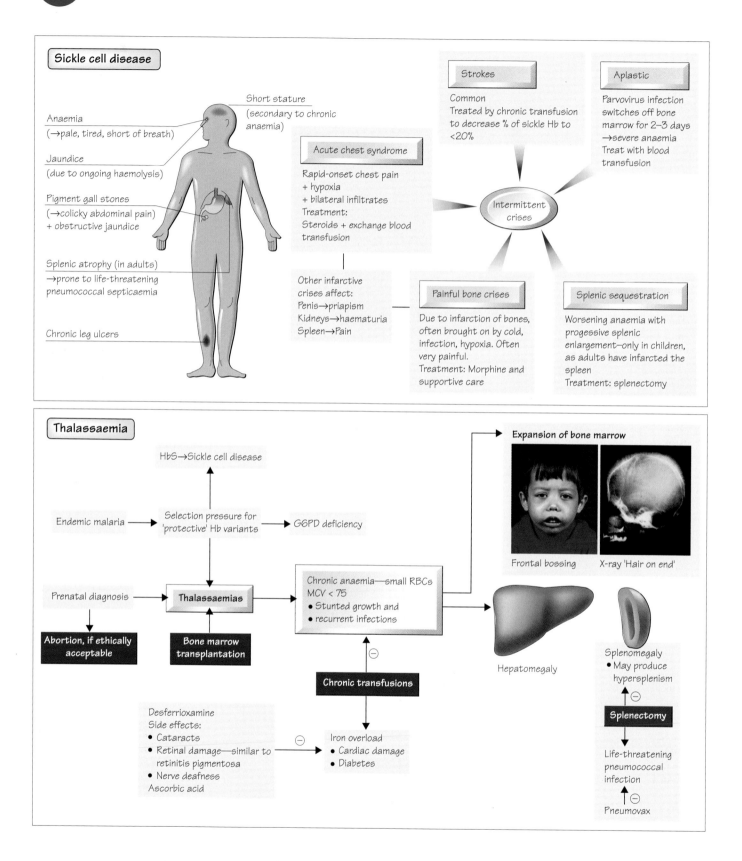

Sickle cell disease

Anaemia
(→pale, tired, short of breath)

Short stature
(secondary to chronic anaemia)

Jaundice
(due to ongoing haemolysis)

Pigment gall stones
(→colicky abdominal pain)
+ obstructive jaundice

Splenic atrophy (in adults)
→prone to life-threatening
pneumococcal septicaemia

Chronic leg ulcers

Acute chest syndrome

Rapid-onset chest pain
+ hypoxia
+ bilateral infiltrates
Treatment:
Steroids + exchange blood
transfusion

Other infarctive
crises affect:
Penis→priapism
Kidneys→haematuria
Spleen→Pain

Strokes

Common
Treated by chronic transfusion
to decrease % of sickle Hb to
<20%

Aplastic

Parvovirus infection
switches off bone
marrow for 2–3 days
→severe anaemia
Treat with blood
transfusion

Intermittent crises

Painful bone crises

Due to infarction of bones,
often brought on by cold,
infection, hypoxia. Often
very painful.
Treatment: Morphine and
supportive care

Splenic sequestration

Worsening anaemia with
progessive splenic
enlargement—only in children,
as adults have infarcted the
spleen
Treatment: splenectomy

Thalassaemia

HbS→Sickle cell disease

Endemic malaria → Selection pressure for
'protective' Hb variants → G6PD deficiency

Prenatal diagnosis → Thalassaemias

Abortion, if ethically acceptable

Bone marrow transplantation

Chronic anaemia—small RBCs
MCV < 75
• Stunted growth and
• recurrent infections

Expansion of bone marrow

Frontal bossing   X-ray 'Hair on end'

Hepatomegaly

Splenomegaly
• May produce
  hypersplenism

⊖

Splenectomy

Life-threatening
pneumococcal
infection

⊖

Pneumovax

Chronic transfusions

Desferrioxamine
Side effects:
• Cataracts
• Retinal damage—similar to
  retinitis pigmentosa
• Nerve deafness
Ascorbic acid

⊖ Iron overload
• Cardiac damage
• Diabetes

Diseases and Treatments at a Glance

These genetic disorders of haemoglobin synthesis are classified by whether α- (α-thalassaemia) or β-globin chain (β-thalassaemia) production is defective. The carrier state protects against *falciparum* malaria, explaining the disease geography. Thalassaemias are sub-divided into thalassaemia trait or thalassaemia major.

Thalassaemia

Thalassaemia trait

In β-thalassaemia trait one normal and one abnormal β-globin gene occur. Haemoglobin (Hb) electrophoresis is normal but haemoglobin A2 (a vestigial haemoglobin with no known function) is increased from 2% to 4–6%.

In α-thalassaemia trait Hb electrophoresis and HbA2 levels are normal. The diagnosis is made by excluding β-thalassaemia trait and iron deficiency (see p. 318).

Both traits have mild anaemia (Hb 10.0–12.0 g/dL) and low mean cell volume (MCV = 65–70 fL). Partners of those with thalassaemia trait should be tested, because trait carriage by both partners can lead to offspring with thalassaemia major.

Thalassaemia major

Thalassaemia major is a life-threatening illness.

β-Thalassaemia major caused by point mutations (occasionally dele-tion) in both β-globin genes, results in symptomatic anaemia at 6–12 months, as fetal haemoglobin levels fall. Untreated children are wasted, have skull bossing, splenomegaly and leg ulcers, with the patho-gnomonic 'hair on end' skull X-ray appearance (see figure). Laboratory tests show a severe microcytic anaemia, target and nucleated red cells in the peripheral blood and no HbA. Blood transfusion, to maintain a normal haemoglobin level and suppress abnormal red cell production, results in normal physical development. Iron overload from frequent transfusions causes serious disability and death by 25 years, unless prevented by chelation with desferrioxamine. Most well-treated thalas-saemic patients survive into their 30s and 40s. Bone marrow transplan-tation can be considered if a suitable sibling donor is found.

α-Thalassaemia major (hydrops fetalis) often ends in intrauterine death and is caused by deletion of all four α-globin genes. Rarely, the diagnosis is made early, when intrauterine blood transfusions are life saving. Life-long transfusion is necessary as in β-thalassaemia.

Thalassaemia intermedia

The severity of thalassaemia intermedia lies between thalassaemia trait and thalassaemia major. Several different genetic disorders underlie this condition. The most common is homozygous β-thalassaemia where one or both genes still produce small amounts of HbA. Deletion of three of the four α-globin genes (HbH disease) causes a similar picture, with a moderately severe anaemia of 7–9 g/dL and splenomegaly. *By definition* they are not transfusion dependent. Splenectomy may be used to lessen anaemia.

Sickle-cell disease

Sickle-cell haemoglobin results from a point mutation (βS). It is com-mon in Africa, the Arabian peninsula and southern Europe. Heterozygous carriers have one normal β and one βS globin gene—sickle-cell trait (AS).

Sickle-cell trait is usually asymptomatic, although haematuria and sudden death may occur more commonly. The blood count and film are normal. The diagnosis is made on finding a positive sickle solubility test and one band of haemoglobin A (normal adult haemoglobin) and one of haemoglobin S on electrophoresis. General anaesthesia requires no special precautions.

Sickle-cell disease occurs in those homozygous for haemoglobin S (SS). Sickle cells are more rigid than normal red cells and obstruct blood flow, particularly in small blood vessels. Deoxygenation of sickle haemoglobin causes the characteristic shape change. Blood examina-tion shows sickle-shaped cells, even when not in crisis, features of splenic atrophy (Howell-Jolly bodies in red blood cells) and moderate anaemia (Hb 7–9 g/dL). Electrophoresis shows the haemoglobin S band. The sickle solubility test is positive. Reasonable health inter-spersed with crises occurs:

• Painful bone crisis is the most common and may be precipitated by cold, infection or hypoxia—often no cause is found. Treatment is with simple or opiate-based analgesia (morphine, because pethidine may cause seizures). Intravenous or oral fluids, oxygen and antibiotics may be given. Most episodes settle within a few days.

• Acute chest syndrome may be fatal and is characterized by the rapid onset and progression of chest pain associated with hypoxia, cough and bilateral lung infiltrates. Exchange blood transfusion is the treatment of choice.

• Splenic sequestration is more common in children than in adults, because splenic atrophy from auto-infarction occurs by the age of 5–6 years. Typical features are a rapidly worsening anaemia and pro-gressive splenomegaly. Blood transfusion is used as necessary. The condition is usually short-lived. If patients have recurrent attacks splenectomy is undertaken.

• Aplastic crisis are caused by parvovirus infection, which switches off red cell production for 2–3 days. This does not matter in normal individuals. In haemolytic anaemias, where the red cell life span is very short, temporary cessation of red cell production causes an abrupt, life-threatening fall in haemoglobin. Red cell transfusion is life saving.

• Strokes are common in children and adults with sickle-cell disease. Blood transfusions to maintain the haemoglobin S concentration at < 20% should be given for at least 1–2 years after a stroke.

Treatment

Most patients with sickle-cell disease are treated conservatively with specific treatment for crises (as above). Hyposplenism from splenic infarction is common, so prophylaxis against encapsulated bacteria with penicillin is given. Folic acid is often prescribed. Disease severity is very variable: those with the highest concentration of haemoglobin F have the mildest clinical course. Hydroxyurea is used in severe disease to increase HbF concentration and decrease painful crises. Bone marrow transplantation may be used in young people with severe disease.

Other haemoglobin variants

Other haemoglobin variants include haemoglobins C, D and E. Hetero-zygous patients are asymptomatic. In combination with haemoglobin S or β-thalassaemia trait, a far more serious disorder occurs, e.g. the com-bination of haemoglobins S and C—haemoglobin SC disease. The clin-ical course is milder than SS, although avascular necrosis of the femoral head is just as common as in SS, and proliferative retinopathy much more common.

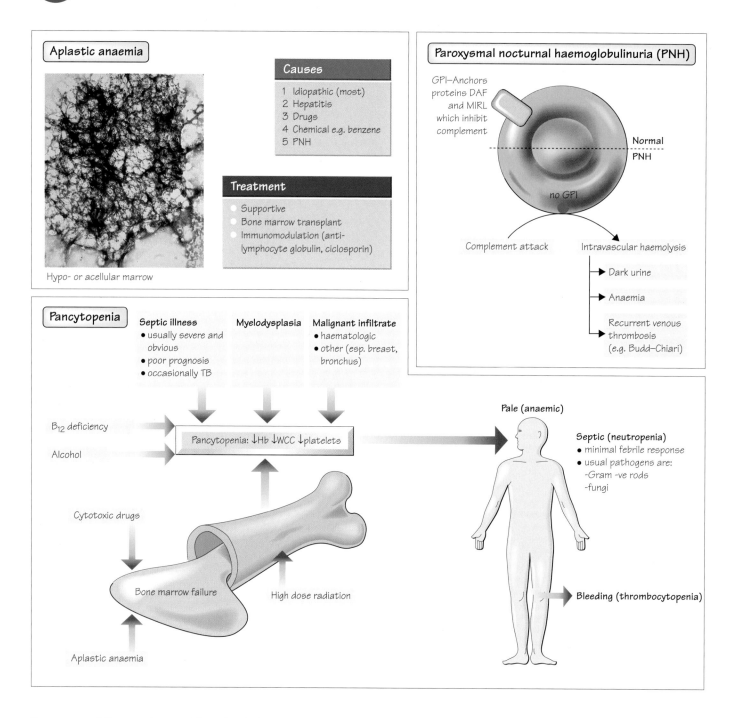

Aplastic anaemia

Hypo- or acellular marrow

Causes

1 Idiopathic (most)
2 Hepatitis
3 Drugs
4 Chemical e.g. benzene
5 PNH

Treatment

- Supportive
- Bone marrow transplant
- Immunomodulation (anti-lymphocyte globulin, ciclosporin)

Paroxysmal nocturnal haemoglobulinuria (PNH)

GPI–Anchors proteins DAF and MIRL which inhibit complement

no GPI

Normal
PNH

Complement attack — Intravascular haemolysis

- Dark urine
- Anaemia
- Recurrent venous thrombosis (e.g. Budd–Chiari)

Pancytopenia

Septic illness
- usually severe and obvious
- poor prognosis
- occasionally TB

Myelodysplasia

Malignant infiltrate
- haematologic
- other (esp. breast, bronchus)

B₁₂ deficiency

Alcohol

Pancytopenia: ↓Hb ↓WCC ↓platelets

Cytotoxic drugs

Bone marrow failure

High dose radiation

Aplastic anaemia

Pale (anaemic)

Septic (neutropenia)
- minimal febrile response
- usual pathogens are:
  -Gram -ve rods
  -fungi

Bleeding (thrombocytopenia)

Bone marrow failure may be caused intentionally by anticancer chemotherapy or radiotherapy, or may develop unexpectedly from both congenital and acquired causes. The clinical features of bone marrow failure relate to absence of:

- Haemoglobin (symptoms of anaemia)
- Neutrophils (bacterial sepsis)
- Platelets (initially a purpuric rash, later on bleeding).

Although one cell line may be more severely affected than another, the peripheral blood film shows variable depression of all three cell lines, i.e. of haemoglobin, white and platelet cell count—a pancytopenia. It is

important to realize that a peripheral blood pancytopenia does not necessarily mean that there is an underlying marrow failure caused by an aplastic anaemia. Thus, the differential diagnosis of a peripheral blood pancytopenia includes:

- Sepsis—usually clinically obvious and severe.
- Vitamin B12 deficiency (see p. 318).
- Myelodysplasia (p. 337) or acute leukaemia (p. 328). Paroxysmal nocturnal haemoglobinuria (see later) can present as a pancytopenia.
- Bone marrow failure as a result of drug toxicity, deliberate or as a unwelcome side effect, or caused by aplastic anaemia.

- Myelofibrosis often results in bone marrow failure: the clinical examination shows massive splenomegaly.

The key investigation in peripheral blood pancytopenia is the bone marrow examination, which will diagnose aplastic anaemia or an underlying haematological disease process. Bone marrow is usually obtained by aspirating cells from the posterior iliac crest or the sternum, and from a biopsy, termed a 'trephine', where the architecture of the bone marrow is preserved. In pancytopenia caused by aplastic anaemia a hypocellular marrow is seen. Aplastic anaemia may be idiopathic (primary) or secondary to another disease process or drugs.

Acquired aplastic anaemia
Epidemiology
This is a rare disorder occurring in 3 per million people per year, defined as a peripheral blood pancytopenia in conjunction with a hypocellular bone marrow in which there are no malignant cells.

Aetiology
In most patients (70–80%), no cause is found. In the rest, causes include:
- Viral infections (hepatitis C is the most common)
- An idiosyncratic reaction to some drugs (e.g. gold, chloramphenicol)
- Chemicals such as benzene
- Paroxysmal nocturnal haemoglobinuria (PNH)—see below.

Clinical features
Most patients present with bleeding as a result of thrombocytopenia, bacterial infection because of neutropenia and symptoms of anaemia. Splenomegaly is not a feature.

Diagnosis
The blood count will show a decrease in haemoglobin, platelet and white cell count, i.e. a pancytopenia of variable severity. A bone marrow aspirate and trephine biopsy show a hypocellular marrow.

Treatment and prognosis
Patients should be given supportive care with blood products (red cells, platelets) and antibiotics in the first instance, and then withdrawal of any relevant drug, or specific treatment for hepatitis C. In primary aplastic anaemia, immunosuppressive treatment with antilymphocyte globulin and ciclosporin is effective in improving the blood counts in most patients. Bone marrow transplantation is used for younger patients with severe disease who have an appropriate donor. Survival rate of patients with severe aplastic anaemia is 50–80% 5 years after diagnosis, and depends on the initial severity of disease. Unfortunately, about 50% of patients treated with immunosuppressives will develop a clonal haematopoietic illness such as leukaemia or PNH some years after treatment.

Paroxysmal nocturnal haemoglobinuria
This is a rare, acquired, clonal disease of bone marrow, which may arise during the course of aplastic anaemia. The abnormal blood cells lack a series of proteins (glycosyl-phosphatidylinositol-anchored proteins), which normally anchor complement regulatory proteins on to the cell. The absence of such proteins encourages complement attack on red cells, with the net result being complement-mediated haemolysis. The clinical features are the result of an intravascular haemolytic anaemia —with characteristic haemoglobinuria. Haemolysis is worse with sepsis, even when minor, e.g. colds and surgical trauma. Patients develop insidious symptoms of anaemia and many (although not all) have intermittently dark urine. Large vessel thrombosis is a feature and abdominal pain as a result of bowel ischaemia or infarction may occur. Occasionally Budd-Chiari syndrome occurs. The physical signs are pallor (from anaemia), mild jaundice (from intravascular haemolysis), minor splenomegaly and dark red/black urine. Urine testing reveals iron (from haemosiderin). The blood film shows a pancytopenia, with the red cells having a normal or high mean cell volume (MCV)—a low MCV suggests complicating iron deficiency from urinary iron loss. The diagnosis is made by demonstrating an increased sensitivity of red cells to complement-mediated attack. Treatment is supportive with blood products; rarely bone marrow transplantations are given. The median survival is 8 years, although 10–15% recover spontaneously.

Congenital aplastic anaemia
These disorders are rare and include conditions such as Fanconi's anaemia and dyskeratosis congenita. Fanconi's anaemia is an autosomal recessive disease in which, in addition to aplastic anaemia, which usually develops in the first few years of life, there may be other abnormalities such as small stature, skeletal defects and hyperpigmentation. In dyskeratosis congenital, learning disorders, skin, nail and hair abnormalities, and growth failure may complicate the aplastic anaemia.

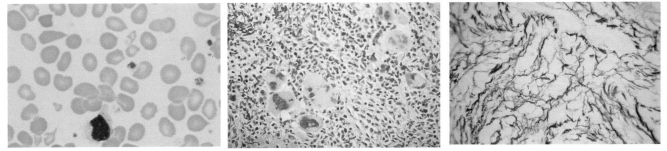

Myelofibrosis: peripheral blood film showing aniso-poikolocytosis, teardrop forms and giant platelets

Myelofibrosis: bone marrow biopsy showing increased cellularity and large numbers of megakaryocytes

Myelofibrosis: bone marrow biopsy (reticulin stain) showing increased reticulin

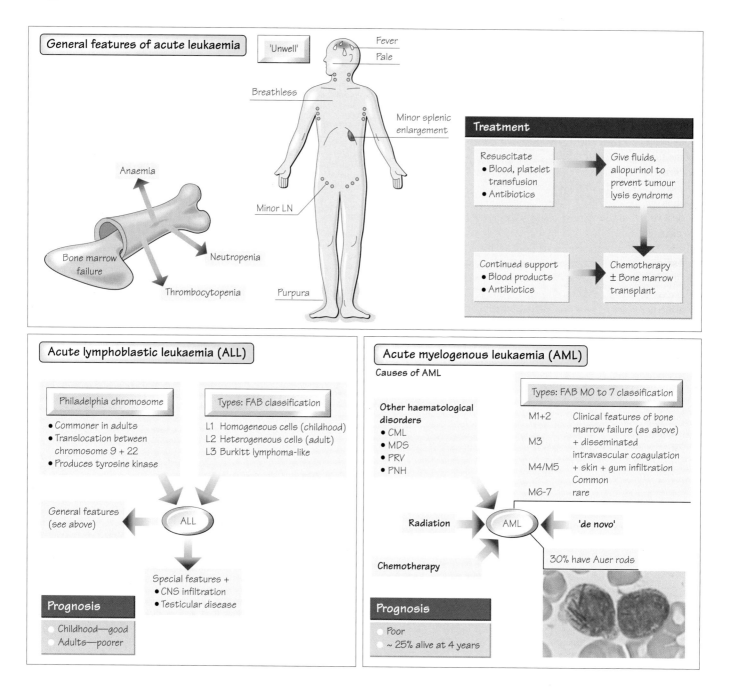

Leukaemia is a malignancy of the bone marrow. There are two main types: acute and chronic.

Acute leukaemia

Acute leukaemia is serious, progresses quickly and, in the absence of treatment, results in the death of the patient within a few weeks or months. Acute leukaemia may affect the lymphoid cell line (acute lymphoblastic leukaemia or ALL) or the myeloid cell line (acute myeloid leukaemia or AML).

Epidemiology

ALL is more common in children, with a peak age of onset of 4 years. In contrast, AML occurs more commonly with increasing age, with a peak age of onset of 70 years. For most patients the cause of acute leukaemia cannot be determined, although infection may play a role in childhood ALL. Exposure to cytotoxic drugs, radiation and some chemicals such as benzene increases the likelihood of acute leukaemia developing. Some chronic haematological diseases, such as myelodysplasia, myelofibrosis and paroxysmal nocturnal haemoglobinuria (PNH), have a high likelihood of transforming to AML.

Symptoms and signs

Symptoms of acute leukaemia usually develop over several weeks and can be divided into three types:

1 Bone marrow failure symptoms are the most common presentation complaints. Leukaemia suppresses normal bone marrow function, causing any combination of anaemia, leukopenia (shortage of white cells) and thrombocytopenia (low platelet count). Typical symptoms are fatigue and breathlessness (from anaemia), bacterial infection (from leukopenia) and bleeding (from thrombocytopenia and sometimes from disseminated intravascular coagulation [DIC]). Examination often reveals pallor, some bruising and bleeding. Fever suggests infection, although in some it may be caused by the leukaemia itself. It is, however, dangerous to assume this (see Management below). Lymphadenopathy, when present, is usually small volume and more typical of ALL than AML.

2 Systemic symptoms of malaise, weight loss, sweats and anorexia are common.

3 Local symptoms: occasional patients present with symptoms or signs of leukaemic infiltration of skin, gums or central nervous system.

Investigation

- Full blood count (FBC) usually shows anaemia and thrombocytopenia. Normal white blood cells are usually decreased and the total white blood count may be low, normal or raised. When normal or raised, most of the cells are primitive white cells (blasts).
- Biochemistry may show renal dysfunction, hypokalaemia and high bilirubin levels.
- Coagulation profile may show prolonged prothrombin time and activated partial thromoplastin time because DIC often occurs.
- Blood cultures because of the risk of infection.
- Chest X-ray: patients with ALL of T-cell lineage often have a mediastinal mass seen on the chest X-ray.
- Blood group because transfusion of blood and platelets is needed sooner or later.

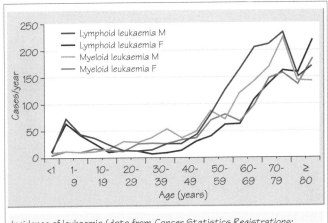

Incidence of leukaemia (data from *Cancer Statistics Registrations: registrations of cancers diagnosed in 2001 England*, Office for National Statistics, Crown copyright 2004)

- Specific diagnostic investigations include a bone marrow aspirate and trephine biopsy, and cell marker and cytogenetic studies for accurate distinction of ALL from AML. Auer rods in the cytoplasm of blast cells are pathognomonic for AML, but are found in only 30%. Cell marker studies can help distinguish B- from T-lineage ALL and the different subtypes of AML (see table in figure). This is useful for the haematologist in planning treatment and prognosis. Chromosome analysis of leukaemic cells is useful in distinguishing ALL from AML, and most importantly gives prognostic information.

Management

Resuscitation A newly diagnosed patient with acute leukaemia is often very ill and certainly vulnerable to severe infection and/or bleeding. The priority is resuscitation using broad-spectrum intravenous antibiotics for infection, platelets and fresh frozen plasma for bleeding, and blood transfusion to correct anaemia. Antibiotic usage in this situation will never be criticized even if the patient's fever turns out to be induced by disease rather than infection. It is easier to stop antibiotics later on than to salvage a septicaemic, shocked patient who has been left without antibiotic treatment.

Chemotherapy The definitive treatment of acute leukaemia is with cytotoxic chemotherapy using multiple drugs given in combination. The precise protocols differ for ALL and AML. Cytotoxic drugs work in differing ways but all kill leukaemic cells. Unfortunately, some normal cells get damaged or killed as well and this causes the side effects such as hair loss, nausea and vomiting, a sore mouth (from damage to the oral mucosa) and bone marrow failure as a result of killing bone marrow cells. One of the major consequences of chemotherapy-induced neutropenia is severe infection. Patients are treated for months (AML) or for 2–3 years (ALL).

Bone marrow transplantation This is a treatment option after very-high-dose chemotherapy and radiotherapy for some but not all patients with acute leukaemia. The bone marrow cells may be obtained either from the patient before the high-dose treatment, stored and then re-infused (autologous transplantation) or from an HLA-matched donor (allogeneic transplantation). The very-high-dose treatment kills off the patient's bone marrow, which will not recover. The infused bone marrow will restore bone marrow function. Patients receiving allogeneic transplants have a lower risk of disease recurrence than those receiving autologous transplants, because re-infused tumour cells may contribute to relapse. In allogeneic transplantations there is good evidence that the transplanted marrow exerts a powerful anti-tumour effect (graft versus leukaemia) mediated by transplanted T lymphocytes. Recent work shows that allogeneic transplantations using low-dose conditioning are possible with possible cure being produced by an immunological mechanism.

Prognosis

The prognosis gets worse with increasing age and if the leukaemia cells contain certain chromosome abnormalities. For a child with ALL, 70% will be cured. For adults less than 50 years old with ALL or AML, around 30% will be cured.

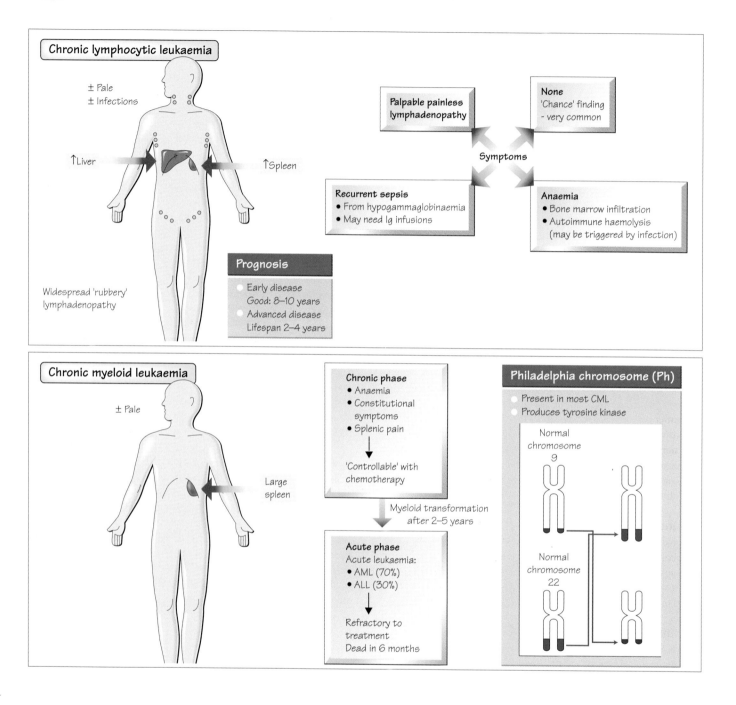

There are two important types of chronic leukaemia: chronic lymphocytic leukaemia (CLL) and chronic myeloid leukaemia (CML).

Chronic lymphatic leukaemia

Incidence of CLL rises with age. Males are affected twice as often as females and there is a slightly higher incidence of the disease in families where one family member has either CLL or acute lymphoblastic leukaemia (ALL). The genetic basis is unclear. CLL occurs less commonly in Asian individuals.

Pathophysiology

CLL is a malignant illness of B lymphocytes, of unknown cause. The cells look quite mature but functionally are immature.

Symptoms and signs

Half of the patients with CLL are diagnosed by chance when a blood count is performed for another reason. The remainder are symptomatic to some extent, such as with lymphadenopathy and/or systemic symptoms, e.g. fever, weight loss or night sweats. Infection (bacterial or viral)

Table 166.1 Binet staging of chronic lymphoblastic leukaemia.

Stage	Organ enlargement*	Haemoglobin (g/dL)	Platelets ($\times 10^9$/L)
A	0, 1 or 2 areas		
B	3, 4 or 5 areas		
C		< 10.0	< 100

*Involved areas include cervical, axillary or inguinal nodes, spleen or liver.

is common and is often the presenting feature. Symptoms of anaemia or, more rarely, thrombocytopenia may be present at diagnosis, but more commonly occur later in the course of the illness. In patients with early stage disease (Table 166.1) palpable lymphadenopathy is often absent. With more advanced disease, generalized lymph node enlargement occurs and the spleen and liver may become palpable.

Investigation

The full blood count (FBC) is the single most important test. By definition the lymphocyte count is $\geq 5 \times 10^9$/L in the absence of viral infection and is often much higher—levels of $100–300 \times 10^9$/L are common. The haemoglobin and platelet count are usually normal, although mild anaemia and thrombocytopenia may be present. The blood film confirms the characteristic lymphocytosis.

Cell marker studies demonstrate clonality and differentiate CLL from other chronic lymphoproliferative diseases such as hairy cell leukaemia, follicular or mantle cell lymphoma.

The biochemistry profile is usually normal although lactate dehydrogenase (LDH) and alkaline phosphatase may be modestly elevated.

Immunology

B cells mature into immunoglobulin-producing plasma cells. In CLL, this normal maturation process is disrupted and hypogammaglobulinaemia occurs frequently. Abnormalities of T cells are also found that contribute to the high incidence of autoimmune haemolysis and thrombocytopenia.

Prognostic markers

Prognosis depends on tumour stage, the length of time it takes for the lymphocyte count to double, the β_2-microglobulin level and certain chromosome abnormalities. The Binet stage relates to prognosis, and is best with stage A (median survival 10 years) and worst with stage C (median survival < 5 years).

Treatment

CLL is a chronic, incurable condition in most patients. As a result of its indolent nature many patients die from causes other than CLL. Treatment is only given to patients who are symptomatic. In those who are, the mainstay of treatment is oral chlorambucil; newer drugs such as purine analogues (e.g. Fludarabine) and monoclonal antibodies are increasingly used. Autologous or allogeneic bone marrow transplantation has been used in young patients.

Chronic myeloid leukaemia
Epidemiology

CML has an incidence of 1/100 000 per year and is most common in middle age. Children are rarely affected. Ionizing radiation and ben-

zene exposure have been cited as causative, although few patients have known exposure to these agents.

Pathophysiology

CML is a clonal disorder arising in a pluripotential stem cell. The cells contain the Philadelphia chromosome (see below).

Clinical features

Systemic symptoms of weight loss, sweating and anorexia are common at presentation. Abdominal pain as a result of splenomegaly is frequent and symptoms from anaemia may occur.

Investigation

The blood count shows a leukocytosis (white cell count often > 100 $\times$ 10^9/L), the haemoglobin is usually a little low and the platelet count is either normal or high. The blood film shows both mature and immature granulocytes. The bone marrow is hypercellular and the leukaemic cells contain a translocation between chromosome 9 and 22—the Philadelphia chromosome.

Treatment and prognosis

Most patients are treated initially with oral hydroxyurea, which is effective at disease control. Most patients feel well on such treatment and are able to live a normal life. However, this chronic indolent phase of disease is eventually replaced by a more aggressive acute leukaemic phase, which is usually resistant to intensive chemotherapy. The patient then dies from the disease. Median life expectancy from diagnosis is around 5 years. Interferon-α prolongs life by, on average, 1–2 years compared with hydroxyurea. A few (5–10%) of the patients treated with interferon obtain an excellent response, with a return to normal in their blood counts and a complete disappearance of the Philadelphia chromosome. These patients live much longer than the average.

Glivec, which inhibits the abnormal tyrosine kinase produced by the *BCR-ABL* gene found on the derived chromosome 22, is a new, apparently safe and effective way to control disease in most patients. Over 90% of patients develop a completely normal peripheral blood on Glivec, and most also have a reduction in the percentage of Philadelphia (leukaemic)-positive cells in the bone marrow. There is a lot of optimism, but still no certainty, that it will prolong life expectancy in patients with CML. Whether it will result in cure remains very uncertain

The only reliable curative treatment for CML is bone marrow transplantation using a matched sibling or unrelated donor. This treatment is restricted to younger patients (< 60 years) and cures about half the patients. The remainder will either die from a complication of the transplantation or relapse after the transplantation.

Treatment of relapse after bone marrow transplantation

Donor marrow exerts a powerful antileukaemia effect, mediated by T lymphocytes. Patients with CML who relapse after the transplantation are treated by collecting lymphocytes from the original donor and giving them intravenously to the patient. Of the patients, 75% will go back into a sustained remission with such treatment. This is the most powerful example of immunotherapy currently available. Such an approach has been tried in other forms of leukaemia relapsing after transplantation, but it has proved less effective in acute leukaemia than in patients with CML.

Hodgkin's disease

- Genes
- Environment (e.g. viruses)

Hodgkin's lymphoma - characterized by Reed–Sternberg cells

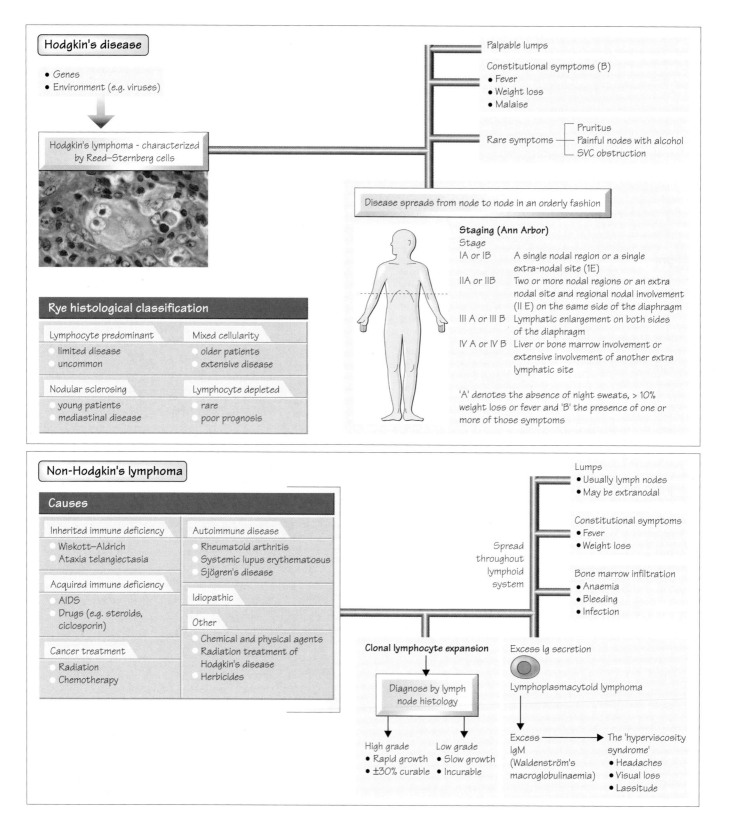

Palpable lumps

Constitutional symptoms (B)
- Fever
- Weight loss
- Malaise

Rare symptoms
- Pruritus
- Painful nodes with alcohol
- SVC obstruction

Disease spreads from node to node in an orderly fashion

Staging (Ann Arbor)

Stage	
IA or IB	A single nodal region or a single extra-nodal site (1E)
IIA or IIB	Two or more nodal regions or an extra nodal site and regional nodal involvement (II E) on the same side of the diaphragm
III A or III B	Lymphatic enlargement on both sides of the diaphragm
IV A or IV B	Liver or bone marrow involvement or extensive involvement of another extra lymphatic site

'A' denotes the absence of night sweats, > 10% weight loss or fever and 'B' the presence of one or more of those symptoms

Rye histological classification

Lymphocyte predominant	Mixed cellularity
• limited disease	• older patients
• uncommon	• extensive disease

Nodular sclerosing	Lymphocyte depleted
• young patients	• rare
• mediastinal disease	• poor prognosis

Non-Hodgkin's lymphoma

Causes

Inherited immune deficiency	Autoimmune disease
• Wiskott–Aldrich	• Rheumatoid arthritis
• Ataxia telangiectasia	• Systemic lupus erythematosus
	• Sjögren's disease

Acquired immune deficiency	
• AIDS	Idiopathic
• Drugs (e.g. steroids, ciclosporin)	

	Other
Cancer treatment	• Chemical and physical agents
• Radiation	• Radiation treatment of Hodgkin's disease
• Chemotherapy	• Herbicides

Lumps
- Usually lymph nodes
- May be extranodal

Constitutional symptoms
- Fever
- Weight loss

Bone marrow infiltration
- Anaemia
- Bleeding
- Infection

Spread throughout lymphoid system

Clonal lymphocyte expansion

Diagnose by lymph node histology

High grade
- Rapid growth
- ±30% curable

Low grade
- Slow growth
- Incurable

Excess Ig secretion

Lymphoplasmacytoid lymphoma

Excess IgM (Waldenström's macroglobulinaemia)

The 'hyperviscosity syndrome'
- Headaches
- Visual loss
- Lassitude

Diseases and Treatments at a Glance

There are two types of lymphoma: Hodgkin's disease and non-Hodgkin's lymphoma (NHL).

Non-Hodgkin's lymphoma

The non-Hodgkin's lymphomas are a heterogeneous collection of malignancies affecting the lymphoid system; 80% are of B-cell origin with the remainder derived from T cells. The incidence of NHL is slowly increasing. Some, but not all, of this increase can be attributed to NHL associated with AIDS. Other known causes of NHL are shown in the figure, though in most cases no cause is found. Cytogenetic abnormalities are seen in 85% of patients, most involving translocations of antigen receptor genes.

There are more than 20 different classification schemes for NHL. Most recently the World Health Organization classification has been widely adopted. This classification scheme defines distinct entities based on morphological, immunological and genetic features. However, most oncologists still classify the NHLs into broad groups termed 'low-grade' and 'high-grade' disease.

Low-grade NHL

This includes diseases such as follicular lymphoma and Waldenström's macroglobulinaemia. These are usually indolent disorders, with slow progression, which are generally readily controlled with simple oral chemotherapy. They are incurable in most patients, with median survival of 3–10 years.

High-grade NHL

These are aggressive diseases of rapid onset and progression. Examples include diffuse large B-cell NHL (intermediate grade) and Burkitt's NHL (high grade). Using intensive chemotherapy, 20–40% of patients < 60 years are cured. The rest die from their disease. *Staging* means to define the extent of spread of the NHL within the body. The Ann Arbor system, which relates to prognosis, is commonly used to define stage.

Low-grade NHL

Follicular lymphoma is a low-grade B-cell lymphoma, mainly found in elderly people. A translocation between chromosome 14 and 18 [t(14;18)] occurs which over-expresses *bcl-2*, thus inhibiting apoptosis and prolonging survival of lymphoma cells. Most patients present with lymphadenopathy and have stage 3 or 4 disease; one-third have B symptoms at diagnosis. Asymptomatic patients do not require treatment until symptoms or disease progression occurs. Treatment is then with oral agents such as chlorambucil. Multi-agent treatment and the use of new drugs such as fludarabine and monoclonal antibodies such as rituximab are, however, increasingly common. Bone marrow transplantation is occasionally used. This is an incurable illness for most, with a median survival of 9 years.

Waldenström's macroglobulinaemia

This is a low-grade lymphoma, most common in elderly people, in which abnormal lymphocytes have plasma cell features (lymphoplasmacytoid lymphoma) and which produce a monoclonal IgM paraprotein. Patients present either with features of lymphoma (lymphadenopathy or B symptoms) or, more commonly, with the hyperviscosity syndrome, caused by high levels of the IgM paraprotein, which comprises: lethargy; confusion; headache; light-headedness; and visual disturbance.

Plasmapheresis rapidly reduces the concentration of IgM and decreases plasma viscosity. The effect is then maintained with chemo-therapy. Oral chlorambucil or purine analogues such as fludarabine are most frequently used. Median survival is 4–5 years.

Intermediate-grade NHL

Diffuse large cell lymphoma. These B-cell tumours are of rapid onset and, if untreated, of rapid progression. Patients present with lymphadenopathy and/or systemic symptoms such as fever or weight loss (B symptoms). Of the patients 30% can be cured using multi-agent chemotherapy. The addition of a monoclonal antibody (rituximab) directed against a B cell antigen (CD 20) to standard chemotherapy has improved the prognosis for this group of patients. High-dose treatment with bone marrow or peripheral blood stem cell support cures a small number of patients whose disease relapses. The remaining patients die from their disease.

High-grade NHL

Burkitt's lymphoma. This is a very malignant B-cell tumour. Endemic African Burkitt's lymphoma is strongly linked with infection with Epstein–Barr virus (EBV), whereas in non-endemic Burkitt's EBV proteins are found in tumour cells in less than half of the patients. Children with the endemic tumour present with a tumour involving the jaw and facial bones—those with non-endemic Burkitt's often have extensive extranodal abdominal disease. In both disease types, the tumour cells contain a chromosome translocation t(8;14). Intensive chemotherapy may cure patients with both types of disease. The non-endemic form occurs commonly in patients with HIV infection and other immuno-compromised states and has a poor prognosis.

Hodgkin's disease

This lymphoma has a bimodal distribution with a peak in young adults and another peak in elderly people. The hallmark of the disease is the Reed–Sternberg cell. The cause is unknown. Epidemiology/serological studies suggest that the EBV is relevant. The EBV viral genome is found in 80% of biopsy specimens. There is a small increased risk in family members of an affected person. Most patients present with lymphadenopathy in the neck or, less commonly, elsewhere. B symptoms may occur. Occasional patients present with the effects of massive lymphadenopathy such as superior vena caval obstruction. The diagnosis is made by biopsy of an affected lymph node.

Types and staging

Four main types of Hodgkin's disease are recognized. Nodular sclerosing and the mixed cellularity types account between them for 80% of all cases. Patients are staged in the same way as for NHL. The Ann Arbor system (see figure) or variants from it are widely used.

Treatment

Patients with Hodgkin's disease are treated with radiotherapy (early stage disease) or chemotherapy (later stage disease). Some patients receive both modalities of treatment. High-dose treatment with bone marrow or peripheral blood stem cell support may be effective in curing some patients who have relapsed after standard chemotherapy.

Prognosis

The cure rate varies from 50% for patients with advanced stage disease to 70–80% for patients with early stage disease. Unfortunately, complications of the treatment are noticed more frequently as patients survive for longer periods. Secondary malignancies are a problem occurring in 5–10% of patients by 10–15 years after treatment for their Hodgkin's disease.

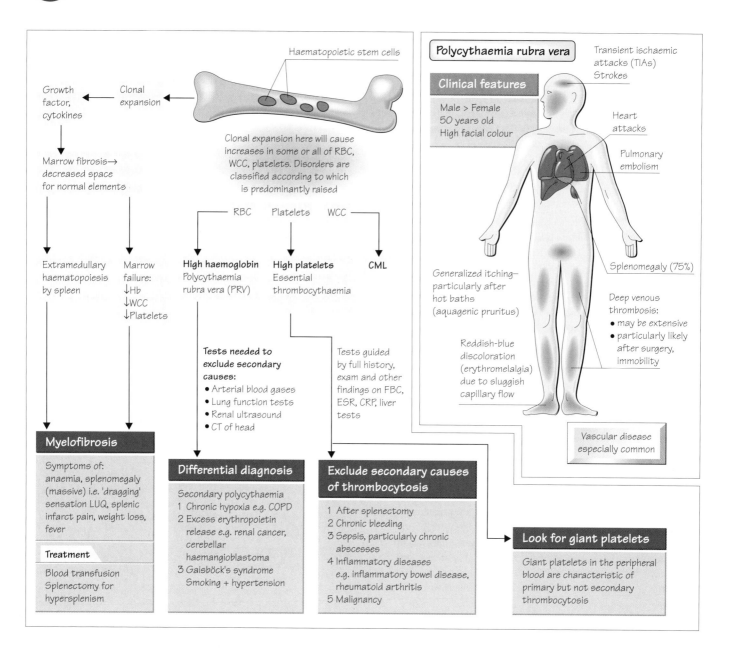

Polycythaemia rubra vera

Clinical features

Male > Female
50 years old
High facial colour

Transient ischaemic attacks (TIAs)
Strokes

Heart attacks

Pulmonary embolism

Generalized itching–particularly after hot baths (aquagenic pruritus)

Reddish-blue discoloration (erythromelalgia) due to sluggish capillary flow

Splenomegaly (75%)

Deep venous thrombosis:
• may be extensive
• particularly likely after surgery, immobility

Vascular disease especially common

Haematopoietic stem cells

Growth factor, cytokines ← Clonal expansion ←

Clonal expansion here will cause increases in some or all of RBC, WCC, platelets. Disorders are classified according to which is predominantly raised

Marrow fibrosis→ decreased space for normal elements

RBC   Platelets   WCC

Extramedullary haematopoiesis by spleen

Marrow failure:
↓Hb
↓WCC
↓Platelets

High haemoglobin
Polycythaemia rubra vera (PRV)

High platelets
Essential thrombocythaemia

CML

Tests needed to exclude secondary causes:
• Arterial blood gases
• Lung function tests
• Renal ultrasound
• CT of head

Tests guided by full history, exam and other findings on FBC, ESR, CRP, liver tests

Myelofibrosis

Symptoms of: anaemia, splenomegaly (massive) i.e. 'dragging' sensation LUQ, splenic infarct pain, weight loss, fever

Treatment

Blood transfusion
Splenectomy for hypersplenism

Differential diagnosis

Secondary polycythaemia
1 Chronic hypoxia e.g. COPD
2 Excess erythropoietin release e.g. renal cancer, cerebellar haemangioblastoma
3 Gaisböck's syndrome Smoking + hypertension

Exclude secondary causes of thrombocytosis

1 After splenectomy
2 Chronic bleeding
3 Sepsis, particularly chronic abscesses
4 Inflammatory diseases e.g. inflammatory bowel disease, rheumatoid arthritis
5 Malignancy

Look for giant platelets

Giant platelets in the peripheral blood are characteristic of primary but not secondary thrombocytosis

The myeloproliferative disorders are a group of four diseases caused by clonal proliferation of haematopoietic stem cells:
1 Chronic myeloid leukaemia (see p. 331)
2 Myelofibrosis
3 Polycythaemia rubra vera
4 Essential thrombocythaemia

Myelofibrosis

Myelofibrosis is caused by a clonal proliferation of haematopoietic stem cells—these release growth factors, particularly platelet-derived growth factor and cytokines, resulting in a characteristic polyclonal marrow fibrotic reaction, which gives the disease its name. The mean age of presentation is 60 years. Typical clinical features include anaemia, splenomegaly (often massive and causing pain), and systemic symptoms such as weight loss and fever.

The diagnostic tests are a blood count and film, and examination of the bone marrow. The blood count usually reveals anaemia. The white cell and platelet counts are usually high at diagnosis but can be normal or low. The blood film shows immature white and red blood cells (leukoerythroblastic change) and tear-drop red blood cells. The bone marrow is often inaspirable as a result of the fibrosis. The trephine biopsy is hypercellular with increased marrow fibrosis.

Treatment is unsatisfactory. With disease progression anaemia occurs and is corrected by blood transfusion or by alternative approaches (anabolic steroids and erythropoietin), although neither is very effective. Splenectomy is useful in painful splenomegaly or to reduce transfusion requirements. As disseminated intravascular coagulation (DIC) may complicate myelofibrosis, a coagulation profile should be checked before surgery. Hydroxyurea can be used to control a high white count and to try to reduce spleen size, but it has no impact on the marrow fibrosis. Poor prognostic factors include increasing age, anaemia, leukopenia and an abnormal marrow karyotype. Median survival is 4 years.

Polycythaemia rubra vera
Epidemiology and pathophysiology
This disorder is most common in the 50s. Men are affected slightly more commonly than women. Young adults are occasionally affected. Polycythaemia rubra vera (PRV) is a clonal stem cell disorder. The red cell mass is high and half of patients have an increased platelet and/or white cell count; 40% have a marrow karyotypic abnormality.

Clinical features
The common complications of PRV are vascular; they occur in 30–50%, and include transient ischaemic attacks (TIAs), strokes, myocardial infarction, deep venous thrombosis and pulmonary emboli. Such events are more common in those with other risk factors for vascular disease. Other common features are facial plethora, itching, particularly after a hot bath or shower (aquagenic pruritus), and a burning discomfort usually occurring in the fingers or toes associated with a reddish/blue discoloration (erythromelalgia), caused by sluggish blood flow and platelet aggregation in small arterioles; this may lead to gangrenous digits. There is a small increased risk of haemorrhage, as a result of abnormal platelet function. Bruising is common but more serious gastrointestinal or central nervous system (CNS) bleeding may occur. Splenomegaly occurs in 75% of patients.

Investigations
The haemoglobin and red cell count are high. The white count and platelets are often raised. Isotopic measurement shows an increased red cell mass. The plasma volume may be high. PRV must be distinguished from other causes of polycythaemia: secondary polycythaemia caused by hypoxaemia (e.g. lung disease, cyanotic heart disease, high altitude), tumours releasing erythropoietin, e.g. renal, cerebellar haemangioblastoma, etc., or polycythaemia in which the red cell mass is normal, but the plasma volume reduced (e.g. apparent polycythaemia more commonly found in hypertensive men who are heavy smokers—Gaisböck's syndrome). Criteria for the diagnosis of PRV are given in Table 168.1. A mutation in the JAK2 gene has been described in most patients with PRV. This single nucleotide mutation results in the stimulation of erythropoiesis independent of erythropoietin.

Treatment and prognosis
Venesection to reduce the haematocrit to < 45% is a simple and usually a safe treatment. Cytotoxic treatment with hydroxyurea is very effective, where adequate control of the red cell count cannot be achieved by venesection or in those with high platelet counts. Excellent control of the red cell mass and the platelet count will reduce the risk of vascular events. Antiplatelet drugs such as aspirin are widely used in those with previous vascular occlusion.

The prognosis for well-treated patients with PRV is good. The median survival is 10 years. Some patients' PRV transforms into myelofibrosis and a few patients develop acute leukaemia.

Essential thrombocythaemia
Epidemiology, aetiology and pathogenesis
Most patients will be elderly—typical age 50–80 years. The sex distribution is equal. The cause is unknown but must be distinguished from a reactive thrombocytosis (see figure). The peripheral blood platelet count will be $> 600 \times 10^9/L$ and often $> 1000 \times 10^9/L$. The differential diagnosis includes:
- Other myeloproliferative disorders.
- Illnesses associated with a reactive thrombocytosis (see figure), where the platelet count is usually $400–1000 \times 10^9/L$, but may be higher, and where cytoreductive treatment is not needed. Prophylaxis against thrombosis with aspirin is appropriate, particularly if the patient is immobile or has other risk factors for thrombosis.

Clinical features
Most patients are diagnosed by chance. In the remainder, the most common presenting symptoms are thrombotic events from the raised platelet count, such as heart attacks, strokes and venous thrombosis. The risk of a thrombotic event is increased by coincidental risk factors such as hypertension, diabetes and cigarette smoking. There is also an increased risk of bleeding in these patients because of impaired platelet function.

Investigations
There is no diagnostic test for essential thrombocythaemia. Exclusion of other myeloproliferative diseases such as polycythaemia and of a reactive cause is important.

Treatment and prognosis
Elderly patients with a platelet count $> 1000 \times 10^9/L$, other risk factors for thrombosis or a previous thrombotic event are at high risk of further vascular occlusive events and require treatment. Young patients with a platelet count $< 1000 \times 10^9/L$ and no additional risk factors might just be observed or given aspirin. If treatment is needed, hydroxyurea or anegrelide is used. Interferon-α is occasionally used.

If the platelet count is maintained within the normal range the risk of vascular events drops to close to normal. Of the patients 70% survive more than 10 years. A few (5%) develop acute myeloid leukaemia.

Table 168.1 Criteria for the diagnosis of PRV.

A1	Raised red cell mass (> 25% above predicted)	B1	Thrombocytosis (platelets $> 400 \times 10^9/L$)
A2	Absence of secondary polycythaemia	B2	Neutrophil leukocytosis ($> 10 \times 10^9/L$)
A3	Palpable splenomegaly	B3	Splenomegaly on ultrasonography
A4	Acquired cytogenetic abnormality	B4	Spontaneous growth of red cell abnormality precursors *in vitro* without added erythropoietin

A1+A2+A3 or A4 establishes the diagnosis of PRV. A1+A2+ two of B establishes the diagnosis of PRV

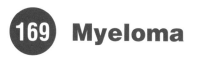
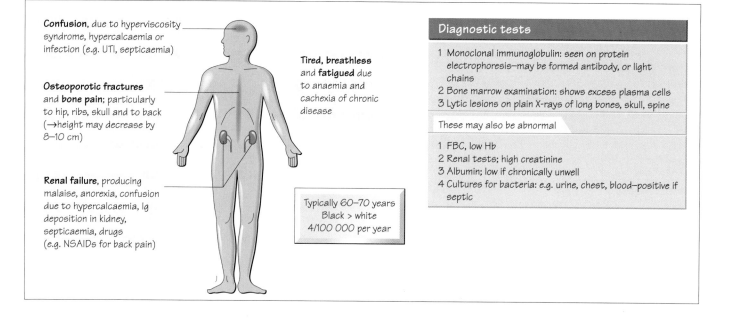

Confusion, due to hyperviscosity syndrome, hypercalcaemia or infection (e.g. UTI, septicaemia)

Osteoporotic fractures and bone pain; particularly to hip, ribs, skull and to back (→height may decrease by 8–10 cm)

Renal failure, producing malaise, anorexia, confusion due to hypercalcaemia, Ig deposition in kidney, septicaemia, drugs (e.g. NSAIDs for back pain)

Tired, breathless and fatigued due to anaemia and cachexia of chronic disease

Typically 60–70 years
Black > white
4/100 000 per year

Diagnostic tests

1 Monoclonal immunoglobulin: seen on protein electrophoresis—may be formed antibody, or light chains
2 Bone marrow examination: shows excess plasma cells
3 Lytic lesions on plain X-rays of long bones, skull, spine

These may also be abnormal

1 FBC, low Hb
2 Renal tests; high creatinine
3 Albumin; low if chronically unwell
4 Cultures for bacteria: e.g. urine, chest, blood—positive if septic

Myeloma is a malignancy of plasma cells in the bone marrow, with an incidence of 4/100 000. It is more common in elderly people and in American black populations.

Pathophysiology

In myeloma, a clone of cancerous plasma cells forms, filling the bone marrow, and producing just a single (monoclonal) immunoglobulin type, known as an M band or a paraprotein. Normal immunoglobulin production is suppressed, i.e. immunoparesis occurs, responsible for the increased risk of infection. Anaemia is common from tumour infiltration, a cytokine-mediated anaemia of chronic disease, and often coexistent renal impairment. Kidney failure affects 50% of patients at some time during their illness and is most frequently the result of the renal deposition of Bence-Jones protein (i.e. the light chains of an immunoglobulin molecule), although it can be the result of hypercalcaemia, sepsis or drugs. Usually plasma cells produce a near 1 : 1 ratio of heavy : light chains (which together make up the normal immunoglobulin molecule), but in myeloma this finely tuned cell regulation is disturbed and it is common for an excess of light chains to be produced (Bence-Jones protein), which are then deposited in the kidney and interfere with its function. Other factors contributing to renal failure are dehydration, infection, drugs (e.g. non-steroidal anti-inflammatory drugs [NSAIDs]) and hypercalcaemia. The latter is found in 25% of patients at diagnosis, and is caused by myeloma cells releasing cytokines, which stimulate osteoclasts to erode cortical bone. Calcium is then released into the blood stream, causing hypercalcaemia.

Investigations

Diagnosis depends on demonstrating a monoclonal immunoglobulin band, with depression of the other immunoglobulins, finding Bence-Jones protein in the urine, and either generalized osteoporosis or lytic lesions on a radiological skeletal survey. The bone marrow aspirate shows excess plasma cells. Renal function, the blood count and plasma calcium should be checked as they may be abnormal.

Clinical features

The mean age of presentation is 65–70 years. Common complications are bacterial infection (from hypogammaglobulinaemia), bone pain and fractures resulting from lysis and resorption of cortical bone, hypercalcaemia (which causes nausea, thirst, polyuria, constipation and confusion), anaemia and renal impairment.

Treatment and prognosis

The standard treatment is with melphalan with or without prednisolone, which provides disease control in half the patients. Disease control usually lasts only a few months, although it can occasionally be much longer. The median survival is 3 years. Combination chemotherapy does not improve the prognosis compared with melphalan alone, but very-high-dose treatment with autologous peripheral blood stem cell support does, achieving a median survival of 4–5 years in younger patients. Newer treatments such as thalidomide and the proteasome inhibitor bortezomib may help to improve outcomes for these patients. Allogeneic bone marrow transplantation has been used in a few young patients and cures around 25%. Supportive care is very important in patients with myeloma. The regular use of bisphosphonates has been shown to reduce the progression of bone disease.

Monoclonal gammopathy of uncertain significance

This condition, increasingly common with increasing age, is sometimes referred to as benign paraproteinaemia although monoclonal gammopathy of uncertain significance (MGUS) is more correct. Patients have a monoclonal paraprotein but no other features of myeloma, e.g. bone lesions, anaemia or renal impairment. Of the patients, 20% develop myeloma in the years after diagnosis.

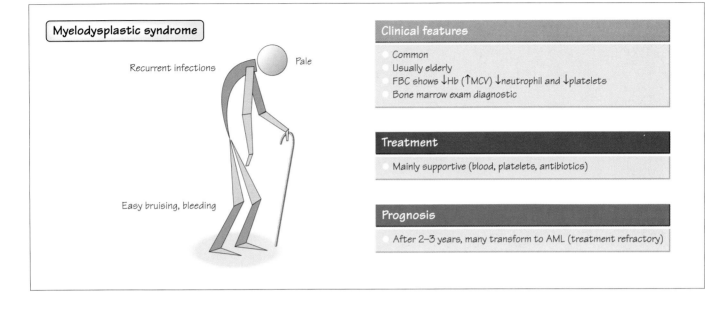

Myelodysplastic syndrome

Recurrent infections

Pale

Easy bruising, bleeding

Clinical features
- Common
- Usually elderly
- FBC shows ↓Hb (↑MCV) ↓neutrophil and ↓platelets
- Bone marrow exam diagnostic

Treatment
- Mainly supportive (blood, platelets, antibiotics)

Prognosis
- After 2–3 years, many transform to AML (treatment refractory)

Myelodysplasia is a clonal disorder of the bone marrow in which morphologically and functionally abnormal blood cells are produced. It occurs with increasing frequency with increasing age. Most patients have a macrocytic anaemia; leukopenia and thrombocytopenia are also very common. In most, no cause can be identified. In some, myelodysplasia develops after exposure to cytotoxic drugs or radiotherapy.

Clinical features

The clinical features can be predicted from the pathological findings. Symptoms of anaemia are common. There is an increased risk of bacterial infection resulting from the leukopenia and because the neutrophils are functionally abnormal. Haemorrhagic complications are common as a result of thrombocytopenia and because platelet function is usually abnormal. The previous French-American-British classification defined five types:

1 Refractory anaemia (RA): anaemia with < 5% blasts in the marrow.
2 Refractory anaemia with ring sideroblasts (RARS): sideroblastic anaemia.
3 Refractory anaemia with excess blasts (RAEB): marrow containing 5–20% blasts.
4 Refractory anaemia with excess blasts in transformation (RAEB-t) marrow, containing 21–29% blasts.
5 Chronic myelomonocytic leukaemia (CMML); there are dysplastic white cells and the absolute monocyte count exceeds 1.0×10^9/L.

These were arbitrary definitions and took no account of the presence or absence of leukopenia or thrombocytopenia, or of the fact that the patient may not be anaemic at the time of diagnosis. Accordingly, myelodysplasia is now subclassified into many types depending on the degree of dysplasia, the number of blasts in the bone marrow and cytogenetic abnormalities.

Diagnosis

Most patients have a macrocytic anaemia without vitamin B12 or folate deficiency. Abnormal looking cells (dysplastic) in the blood film are commonly found. The bone marrow is hypercellular and dysplastic.

Treatment and prognosis

There is no satisfactory treatment for myelodysplasia and care is usually supportive only:

• **Blood transfusion** is used for anaemia, and infections should be promptly treated with antibiotics. Platelet transfusions help in haemorrhage caused by thrombocytopenia, but are not recommended for uncomplicated low platelet counts because platelet antibodies may develop and lessen the effectiveness of future platelet transfusions. Transfused platelets have a life span of 24–48 h.

• **Allogeneic bone marrow transplantation** can be curative in young patients when a donor can be found. Patients with an increased blast count may benefit from anti-AML-type chemotherapy regimens, although the remission rate and survival is worse than in *de novo* acute myeloid leukaemia (AML).

• **Myelodysplasia and surgery**: the risks of bleeding and infection make any surgery more hazardous. Platelet transfusions are recommended *pre-* or *peroperatively* for those with even mild thrombocytopenia, because platelet function is abnormal. Postoperative infection should be rigorously sought and treated.

The median survival is 3 years. Patients with RA and RARS fare better than those with the other subtypes. Prognosis worsens in patients with more than one cytopenia, with increasing number of blasts and certain chromosomal abnormalities. Most patients die from either infection or haemorrhage. One-third of patients will develop AML, which is often chemotherapy resistant. For this reason, most patients with myelodysplasia who progress to AML are managed just with supportive and palliative care.

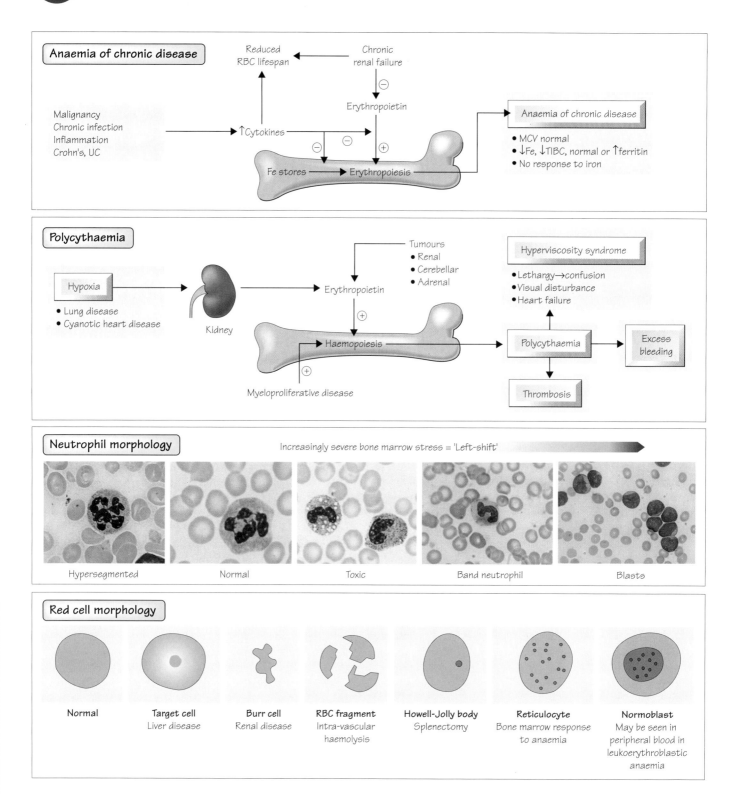

Anaemia of chronic disease

Reduced RBC lifespan ← Chronic renal failure

Chronic renal failure → (−) Erythropoietin

Malignancy
Chronic infection
Inflammation
Crohn's, UC

→ ↑Cytokines

Erythropoietin

Anaemia of chronic disease
- MCV normal
- ↓Fe, ↓TIBC, normal or ↑ferritin
- No response to iron

Fe stores → Erythropoiesis

Polycythaemia

Hypoxia
- Lung disease
- Cyanotic heart disease

→ Kidney → Erythropoietin

Tumours
- Renal
- Cerebellar
- Adrenal

Haemopoiesis

Myeloproliferative disease

Hyperviscosity syndrome
- Lethargy→confusion
- Visual disturbance
- Heart failure

Polycythaemia → Excess bleeding

Thrombosis

Neutrophil morphology

Increasingly severe bone marrow stress = 'Left-shift'

| Hypersegmented | Normal | Toxic | Band neutrophil | Blasts |

Red cell morphology

| Normal | Target cell Liver disease | Burr cell Renal disease | RBC fragment Intra-vascular haemolysis | Howell-Jolly body Splenectomy | Reticulocyte Bone marrow response to anaemia | Normoblast May be seen in peripheral blood in leukoerythroblastic anaemia |

The blood is commonly affected by systemic disease.

Anaemia of chronic disease

Many chronic disease processes produce inflammatory cytokines, which depress haematopoiesis, by reducing iron transfer to developing red cells and diminishing the effects of erythropoietin on the bone marrow. Red cell survival is also shortened. Underlying disease processes include: (i) chronic infection: infective endocarditis, abscesses, particularly in the lung, osteomyelitis; (ii) chronic inflammation, e.g. rheumatoid arthritis, temporal arteritis and other vasculitides (e.g. systemic lupus erythematosus [SLE], polyarteritis nodosa); (iii) inflammatory bowel disease causes both chronic disease and iron deficiency anaemia; (iv) malignancy; and (v) chronic renal failure causes anaemia principally by impairing production of erythropoietin, although other mechanisms are also implicated.

The anaemia is usually mild (Hb usually ≥ 8 g/dL), and the mean cell volume (MCV) is normal (80–90 fL). Serum iron is low, as are iron transfer proteins (as measured by the total iron-binding capacity [TIBC]). Bone marrow examination, indicated when iron deficiency cannot be excluded non-invasively, shows plentiful supplies of iron. The anaemia does not respond to iron supplementation, but does to treatment of the underlying disease. Erythropoietin helps in renal failure and in some other diseases, e.g. anaemia of malignancy. Blood transfusions may help symptomatic patients.

Anaemia of acute disease

Anaemia can occur within a few days in severe acute illnesses:
• Acute severe infection pneumonia, septicaemia, etc.
• Acute renal failure from any cause although especially from vasculitis.

It is vital to actively exclude acute gastrointestinal haemorrhage, a common cause of anaemia in sick patients. In addition to treating the underlying disease blood transfusion has a role.

Leukoerythroblastic anaemia

Leukoerythroblastic anaemia is anaemia with immature white and red blood cells found in the blood film. Leukoerythroblastic anaemia is a common reaction to severe bone marrow stress in:
• Severe gastrointestinal haemorrhage
• Severe haemolytic anaemia
• Overwhelming sepsis
• Bone marrow malignancy, commonly metastatic, although also intrinsic haematological malignancy, such as myelofibrosis and myeloma.

If the underlying diagnosis is unclear bone marrow examination is usually diagnostic. The treatment is of the underlying condition and blood transfusion.

Polycythaemia

Polycythaemia is an increase in haemoglobin level by ≥ 2 standard deviations from the mean. Increased haemoglobin occurs in myeloproliferative disease (see p. 334), though these are rare. Much more common is polycythaemia secondary to:
• Chronic hypoxaemia from lung disease, usually chronic obstructive pulmonary disease (COPD).
• Heavy cigarette smoking associated with systemic hypertension (Gaisböck's syndrome); occurs mainly in men. Premature death from coronary or lung disease is common.

• Cyanotic heart disease.
• Rare causes include excess erythropoietin-secreting tumours in the kidney or, rarer still, cerebellar haemangioblastomas, uterine fibroids and other tumours.
• Spurious causes: dehydration is a common cause of a transient polycythaemia.

Polycythaemia may be asymptomatic or produce a hyperviscosity syndrome (tiredness, effort intolerance, headaches and visual disturbance). Thrombosis, usually venous and occasionally arterial, may occur. As most polycythaemia is secondary or relative, investigation should include blood gases and lung function tests. Other tests include estimation of red cell mass using radioactive chromium and occasionally bone marrow biopsy. Renal, abdominal and cerebellar imaging may demonstrate a tumour. Treatment is of the underlying disease.

Leukocytosis

A neutrophil leukocytosis most commonly occurs in patients with bacterial infection and a lymphocytosis in those with a viral infection. A neutrophil leukocytosis also occurs in: (i) tissue necrosis, e.g. myocardial or pulmonary infarction, associated with a mild fever; (ii) malignancy; (iii) non-infectious inflammatory causes, including connective tissue disease; (iv) corticosteroid usage; and (v) diabetic ketoacidosis.

Investigations to exclude infection, vasculitis and malignancy may be needed if the cause is not obvious. Rarely neutrophil or lymphocytic leukocytosis is leukaemic in origin.

An increase in the eosinophil count is defined as $> 0.5 \times 10^9$ eosinophils/L. It is uncommon and occurs in:
• Drug allergy: a common cause.
• Skin diseases: atopic eczema, urticaria.
• Asthma: complicating allergic bronchopulmonary aspergillosis should be considered.
• Parasitic infection, often intestinal, although infection elsewhere may be responsible, such as in the skin (cutaneous larva migrans).
• Vasculitis, especially polyarteritis nodosa.
• Malignancy such as Hodgkin's disease.
• More rarely found in the hypereosinophilic syndrome.

Patients usually do not have symptoms from the excess eosinophils, and treatment is of the underlying condition. Occasionally very high eosinophil counts occur, usually with tropical infections (tropical eosinophilia), causing myocardial and endocardial damage (restrictive cardiomyopathy).

Thrombocytosis

Although increases in platelet counts occur in myeloproliferative diseases (see p. 334), most increases are secondary to:
• Bleeding, especially chronic blood loss anaemia
• Infection
• Post-surgery, especially after splenectomy
• Malignancy
• Inflammatory disease, including vasculitis.

Mild increases ($400-700 \times 10^9$/L) are usually asymptomatic, but the higher the platelet count the more likely is thrombosis, both arterial and venous. Treatment is of the underlying cause; if this is not possible, aspirin is used for thrombosis prophylaxis.

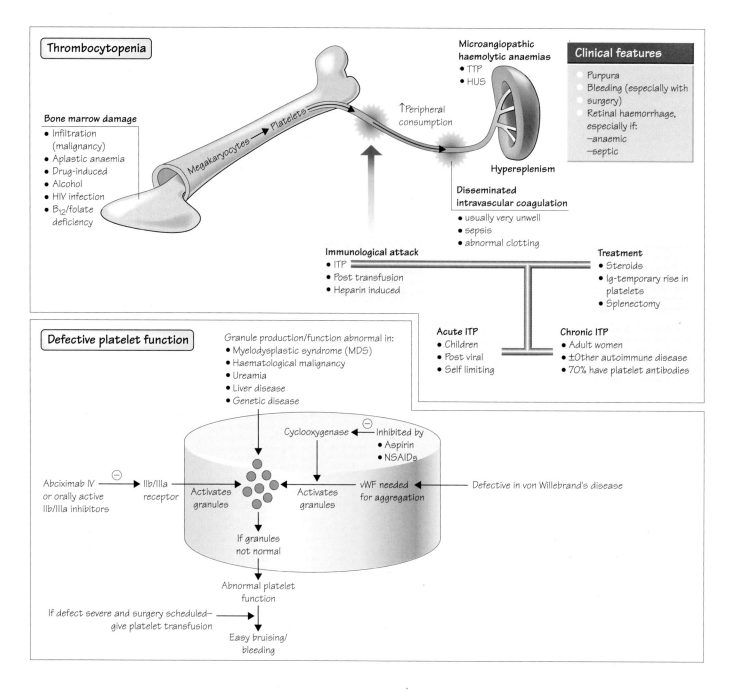

Physiology of haemostasis

When there is injury to a blood vessel, a series of five events are initiated to control haemostasis. The first three processes are: (1) local vasoconstriction, (2) adhesion and aggregation of platelets and (3) activation of the clotting cascade to create a fibrin clot. Coagulation inhibitors are then activated (4) to restrict coagulation to the site of injury and (5) fibrinolysis occurs later to restore vessel patency. Step 2 (platelet adhesion/aggregation) requires that platelets adhere to the exposed collagen in damaged blood vessels via von Willebrand's factor (vWF), a large polymeric molecule, individual subunits of which possess collagen- and platelet-binding sites (for platelet glycoprotein Ib).

The platelets aggregate to each other by cross-linking with fibrinogen, which binds to specific fibrinogen-binding sites on the platelet surface (glycoprotein IIb/IIIa). Upon activation, platelets release agents (including ADP) from their dense granules to recruit other platelets to the site and thromboxane, a potent platelet agonist, which provides positive feedback.

Platelet disorders

Platelet disorders are quantitative or qualitative. They present clinically with purpura, petechiae, mucosal bleeding, epistaxis and menorrhagia.

Table 172.1 Causes of thrombocytopenia.

Decreased production
Marrow aplasia or infiltration
Megaloblastic anaemia

Increased consumption
Immune
    Immune thrombocytopenic purpura
    Thrombotic thrombocytopenic purpura
    Post-transfusion purpura
    Heparin-induced thrombocytopenia
Non-immune
    Disseminated intravascular coagulation
    Haemolytic uraemic syndrome
    Hypersplenism

Thrombocytopenia

The causes of thrombocytopenia are summarized in Table 172.1.

Immune thrombocytopenic purpura

Immune thrombocytopenic purpura (ITP) is an autoimmune disorder where antibodies are directed against antigens on the platelet surface, causing platelet removal from the circulation by reticuloendothelial cells, largely in the spleen. An acute self-limiting form occurs in children typically after a viral infection and often not needing treatment. In adults ITP is a chronic disorder that is most common in middle-aged women. The diagnosis is largely one of exclusion, the bone marrow being normal or having an increased number of normal megakaryocytes. Treatment with steroids is only given to maintain the platelet count at safe levels and there is no need for therapy if the platelet count is above 30×10^9/L. Splenectomy is used if steroids fail or if too high a dose is needed. Intravenous IgG gives a good, rapid, albeit temporary, response and is useful for emergencies and before splenectomy or other operations.

Thrombotic thrombocytopenic purpura

Thrombotic thrombocytopenic purpura (TTP) has a classic pentad of thrombocytopenia, microangiopathic haemolytic anaemia, neurological disturbance, fever and renal failure. The defect is the absence of a vWF-cleaving protease (ADAMTS-13) normally present in plasma. This results in abnormally large vWF polymers in the circulation, which induce platelet microthrombi, resulting in end-organ ischaemia. The common sporadic form is the result of cleaving protease-directed autoantibodies. The rare autosomal recessive familial form of TTP is caused by an inherited deficiency. Treatment is with steroids and plasma, which replaces the enzyme. Plasma exchange is most effective probably because it also removes antibody.

Disseminated intravascular coagulation (DIC) (see p. 342)

Bone marrow infiltration

Bone marrow infiltration (by tumour) or aplasia (particularly chemotherapy induced) may cause thrombocytopenia.

Post-transfusion purpura

Post-transfusion purpura (PTP) is suspected if thrombocytopenia occurs about 10 days after a blood transfusion. The patient's own platelets lack the HPA-1a antigen, which is present on the platelets in 98% of the population. When transfused with HPA-1a-positive platelets the recipient makes antibodies against HPA-1a and these, bizarrely, cross-react with the recipient's own HPA-1a-negative platelets, resulting in thrombocytopenia. Treatment is with intravenous immunoglobulin and the avoidance of HPA-1a-positive platelets.

Heparin-induced thrombocytopenia

Heparin-induced thrombocytopenia (HIT) is a rare but serious adverse reaction to heparin. The patient makes IgG antibodies to heparin–platelet factor 4 complexes; this antibody then interacts with the platelet Fcγ receptor, resulting in platelet activation, thrombocytopenia, and arterial and venous thrombosis. Heparin must be stopped and an alternative such as hirudin or danaparoid substituted.

Haemolytic uraemic syndrome

Haemolytic uraemic syndrome (HUS) presents with thrombocytopenia, renal failure and microangiopathic haemolytic anaemia. Although clinically similar to TTP, the pathology is different and is the result of endothelial damage with subsequent platelet activation. It is often seen in children after infection with verotoxin-producing strains of *Escherichia coli*. Treatment is supportive.

Qualitative platelet defects

Disorders of platelet function (Table 172.2) are rare other than those caused by drugs:

Aspirin irreversibly and **non-steroidal anti-inflammatory drugs** (NSAIDs) reversibly inhibit the cyclo-oxygenase 1 (COX 1) enzyme in platelets, preventing thromboxane synthesis and so ameliorating platelet aggregation.

Myelodysplastic platelets have major functional defects, as do those from uraemic patients.

Bernard–Soulier disease and Glanzmann's thrombasthenia are rare, inherited, autosomal recessive disorders caused by the absence of platelet glycoproteins (Gp Ib and Gp IIb/IIIa, respectively). Bleeding can be severe and treatment is with platelet transfusions as required.

Storage pool disease is generally a mild disorder resulting from an inherited defect in the platelets' storage granules. The inability to release ADP and other agents from the granules reduces platelets activation and recruitment.

Table 172.2 Disorders of platelet function.

Inherited
Storage pool disease
Glycoprotein (Gp) Ib deficiency—Bernard–Soulier disease
Gp IIb/IIIa deficiency—Glanzmann's thrombasthenia

Acquired
Drugs—aspirin and NSAIDs
Hypergammaglobulinaemia
Myeloproliferative disorders
Uraemia

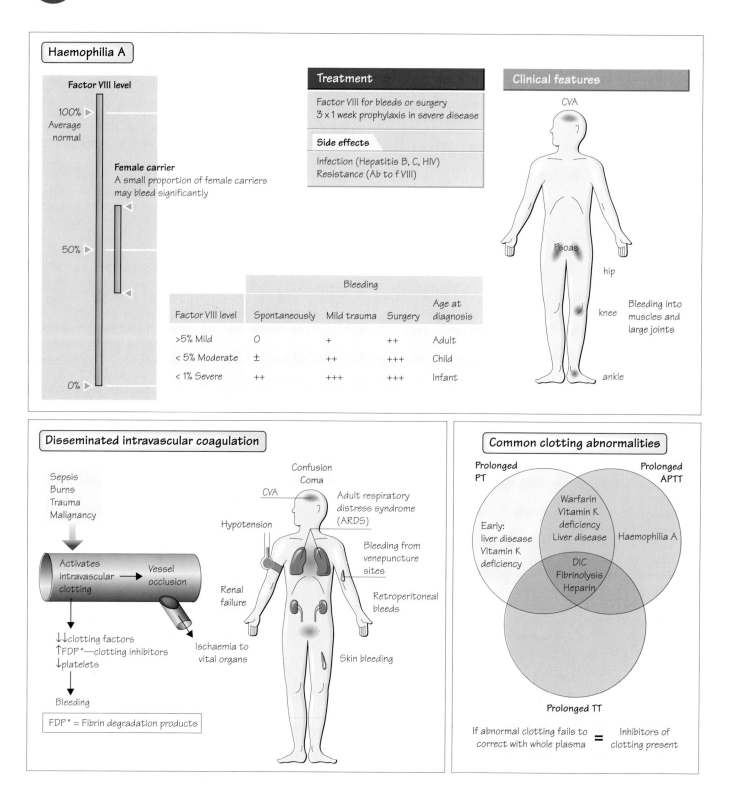

Haemophilia A

Factor VIII level

100% Average normal

Female carrier
A small proportion of female carriers may bleed significantly

50%

0%

Factor VIII level	Spontaneously	Mild trauma	Surgery	Age at diagnosis
	Bleeding			
>5% Mild	0	+	++	Adult
< 5% Moderate	±	++	+++	Child
< 1% Severe	++	+++	+++	Infant

Treatment

Factor VIII for bleeds or surgery
3 x 1 week prophylaxis in severe disease

Side effects

Infection (Hepatitis B, C, HIV)
Resistance (Ab to f VIII)

Clinical features

CVA

Psoas

hip

knee

Bleeding into muscles and large joints

ankle

Disseminated intravascular coagulation

Sepsis
Burns
Trauma
Malignancy

Activates intravascular clotting → Vessel occlusion

↓↓clotting factors
↑FDP*—clotting inhibitors
↓platelets

Bleeding

FDP* = Fibrin degradation products

Confusion
Coma

CVA

Hypotension

Adult respiratory distress syndrome (ARDS)

Bleeding from venepuncture sites

Renal failure

Retroperitoneal bleeds

Ischaemia to vital organs

Skin bleeding

Common clotting abnormalities

Prolonged PT

Prolonged APTT

Warfarin
Vitamin K deficiency
Liver disease

Early: liver disease
Vitamin K deficiency

Haemophilia A

DIC
Fibrinolysis
Heparin

Prolonged TT

If abnormal clotting fails to correct with whole plasma = Inhibitors of clotting present

In vitro tests of clotting

The coagulation cascade has classically been divided into the intrinsic pathway, which was thought to be initiated by contact between denuded endothelium and coagulation factors (contact activation) and the ex-trinsic pathway initiated by the tissue factor/factor VII (TF/VII) complex. Both pathways activate factor X, which cleaves prothrombin (II) to release thrombin. This simplified version is still the most useful for interpreting routine coagulation tests, which comprise the activated partial thromboplastin time (APTT), the prothrombin time (PT) and occasionally the thrombin time (TT) (exogenous bovine thrombin added to patient's plasma—the time taken to clot is the TT). Characteristic abnormalities in PT, APTT and PT occur in different diseases:

- PT prolonged, APTT normal: factor VII deficiency (early liver disease or vitamin K deficiency).
- PT normal, APTT prolonged: factor VIII, IX, XI (contact factor) deficiency.
- PT prolonged, APTT prolonged: interpretation depends on whether or not the thrombin time is abnormal.
  - Normal TT—factor II, V, X deficiency; frank vitamin K deficiency or warfarin therapy; liver disease.
  - Prolonged TT—deficiency of fibrinogen, disseminated intravascular coagulation (DIC), especially as a result of fibrin degradation products (FDPs) interfering with fibrin polymerization; fibrinolysis; heparin.

In vivo coagulation

In vivo it is the tissue factor/factor VII (TF/VII) pathway that initiates coagulation—largely by activation of factor IX (see figure), producing activated factor IX (factor IXa). Factor IXa in conjunction with its co-factor, factor VIII, then activates factor X. The centrality of factors VIII and IX to clotting explains why haemophilia A (deficient factor VIII) and haemophilia B (deficient factor IX) are such severe coagulation disorders. This clotting cascade also explains why patients deficient in contact factors do not bleed abnormally. Factor XI is activated by thrombin, which then activates more factor IX in a positive feedback loop. Patients with factor XI deficiency exhibit a variable bleeding disorder.

Inherited disorders of coagulation

Deficiency of coagulation factors presents with haemarthroses and muscle haematomas (in contrast with platelet disorders which present principally with skin bleeds) although gastrointestinal, genitourinary and intracranial bleeds can occur. The most common inherited deficiencies are of factors VIII and IX and von Willebrand's factor (vWF); other inherited coagulation disorders are rare.

Haemophilia A is caused by a deficiency of factor VIII. It is an X-linked recessive disorder affecting 1 in 5000 males. In severe disease (< 1% factor VIII), spontaneous bleeding into large joints and muscles (for example psoas) occurs, unless regular prophylactic treatment with factor VIII concentrate is given. Moderate (factor VIII level 1–5%) and mild (factor VIII 5–40%) disease is associated with bleeding on mild or moderate trauma. Factor VIII is given here only in response to trauma or in anticipation of surgery. Previously plasma-derived concentrates resulted in infection with hepatitis C and HIV. Recombinant factor VIII, uncontaminated with viruses, is now available.

Haemophilia B is caused by a deficiency of factor IX. Factor IX acts with factor VIII to activate factor X, and like factor VIII is encoded on the X chromosome. Haemophilia A and haemophilia B (which is only one-fifth as common) are clinically indistinguishable.

Von Willebrand's disease (vWD) is the most common inherited bleeding disorder—mild autosomal dominant forms may affect up to 1% of the population. The vWF is either deficient (partial: type 1 vWD, complete: type 3 vWD) or defective (type 2 vWD). The vWF circulates as large polymers and serves two functions. Its principal function is to form the bridge that allows platelets to adhere to damaged endothelial surfaces. Thus, in vWD clinical presentation is with the same pattern of bleeding as in patients with platelet disorders, e.g. skin bruising, epistaxis and menorrhagia. A secondary function of vWF is to stabilize circulating factor VIII. Plasma factor VIII levels therefore parallel those of vWF—although severe factor VIII deficiency occurs only in the rare type 3 disease. Treatment is with desmopressin (which raises vWF) in mild disease, and a factor VIII/VWF concentrate in more severe disease.

Acquired disorders of coagulation

The most common acquired coagulation disorders are DIC, liver disease, and vitamin K deficiency. Rarely men or women can develop autoantibodies to factor VIII and so develop an acquired haemophilia.

Disseminated intravascular coagulation describes pathological activation of coagulation resulting in widespread microvascular thrombosis. Although consumption of coagulation factors often results in bleeding, it is the end-organ damage from thrombosis, rather than the bleeding itself, that leads to the very high mortality. Many insults can trigger DIC, e.g. septicaemia, malignancy and obstetric emergencies. The key to management is to treat the underlying disease. Blood product support, with fresh frozen plasma (FFP) and platelets, is given simply to buy time.

Liver disease: coagulation factors are synthesized in the liver and deficiency occurs as liver disease progresses. The situation is often compounded by thrombocytopenia—caused by splenic uptake in the large spleen occurring in portal hypertension. As a result of the short half-life of factor VII, the PT is a sensitive marker of liver damage.

Vitamin K deficiency: vitamin K is required as a coenzyme for the γ-carboxylation of the coagulation factors II, VII, IX and X. This post-translational modification is necessary to enable these factors to bind Ca^{2+} and so phospholipid surfaces. Vitamin K deficiency may present with easy bruising and occurs in malnutrition, and especially in the malabsorption resulting from obstructive jaundice. All patients with obstructive jaundice should receive vitamin K before any surgical procedure, including endoscopic retrograde cholangiopancreatography (ERCP).

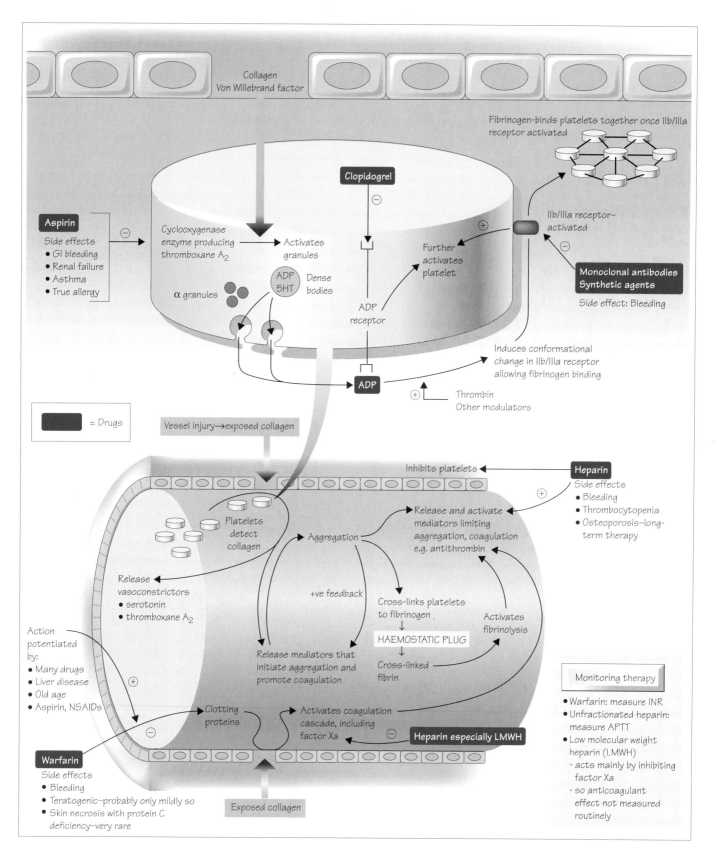

Diseases and Treatments at a Glance

Anticoagulant drugs are frequently used to prevent/treat abnormal clotting. Which anticoagulant is chosen depends on whether the mechanism underlying the clotting process is platelet or clotting protein dependent.

Antiplatelet agents

Diseases primarily involving platelet activation include most *in situ* arterial thrombosis, i.e. acute coronary syndromes (unstable angina, acute myocardial infarction [MI]), transient ischaemic attacks (TIAs) and most thrombotic strokes. Drugs with antiplatelet action include:

- **Aspirin**, powerful and cheap: inhibits platelet function by irreversibly acetylating platelet cyclooxygenase. Duration of action is several days, until new platelets are produced. Effective in stable angina (reduces MI rates), unstable angina (reduces MI and death rates), MI (reduces death rate by 15%), TIAs (reduces stroke rate) and thrombotic strokes (reduces early and late recurrence rates). If immediate action is required, e.g. MI or stroke, 300 mg should be chewed (absorbed from the mouth). Otherwise, it is given orally in a daily dose of 75–150 mg. Side effects include upper gastrointestinal ulceration and bleeding, renal dysfunction (especially if there is pre-existing renal impairment). True allergy (rash or frank anaphylaxis) is very rare and is found more frequently in those with recurrent nasal polyps.

- **Clopidogrel** irreversibly inhibits the platelet ADP receptor; expensive; expanding role in acute coronary syndromes, and after implantation of intracoronary stents (until stent endothelialization occurs after 1 month) as add-on therapy to aspirin. Used as monotherapy in aspirin allergy/intolerance. Expanding role in primary prevention of acute MI in high-risk patients. Side effects are rare and include allergy and thrombotic thrombocytopenic purpura.

- **Platelet IIb/IIIa receptor inhibitors**: the platelet glycoprotein Gp IIb/IIIa fibrinogen receptor acts as a final common pathway when fibrinogen links platelets, resulting in platelet activation. Inhibition of this receptor powerfully inhibits platelet activation. Two classes of inhibitors:
  - Abciximab: monoclonal antibody to the IIb/IIIa receptor, given intravenously, is useful in percutaneous coronary intervention (percutaneous coronary angioplasty [PTCA], intracoronary stenting), reducing MI rate and increasing procedural success rates. It is very expensive. Side effects are of bleeding around the groin (the entry site for the catheter to the arterial circulation) and retroperitoneally. Abciximab irreversibly damages the IIb/IIIa receptor: in severe haemorrhage; fresh platelet transfusion is given to stem the bleeding.
  - Intravenous, synthetic, small molecule IIb/IIIa receptor inhibitors improve outcome in high-risk unstable angina (i.e. ongoing angina despite drug therapy, pulmonary oedema during angina, persisting major abnormalities on the resting electrocardiogram [ECG], or elevation in troponin ≥ 10 the detect limit). Side effects: excess bleeding, e.g. intracranial or retroperitoneal haemorrhage.

Anticoagulants

Most venous clotting involves clotting cascade activation, e.g. deep vein thrombosis (DVT), pulmonary embolus (PE), paradoxical right-to-left embolus, left atrial thrombosis (predisposition through atrial fibrillation) and any resulting emboli; procoagulation found in the antiphospholipid syndrome. Clotting on artificial heart valves also involves the clotting cascade. For sagittal venous sinus thrombosis—see p. 368. Drugs used to counter this include:

- **Warfarin**: a vitamin K antagonist inhibiting the γ-carboxylation of clotting factors II, VII, IX and X. Its effect is measured by the international normalized ratio (INR), which is the patient's prothrombin time (PT—see p. 342), divided by the mean normal PT, raised to the power of the ISI (the International Sensitivity Index of the reagent used):
  - INR = 2.0–3.0 is usually therapeutic; some heart valves, e.g. Starr–Edwards, require an INR of 3.0–4.0.
  - An INR ≤ 2.0 provides inadequate therapeutic action and excess thrombosis.
  - INR ≥ 3.0 is associated with an increased risk of bleeding.

Although warfarin has a quick onset of action, the clotting proteins whose production is inhibited have various half-lives. This 'buffer' delays the onset of therapeutic action (and the prolongation of the INR) by several days. Thus, if an anticoagulant is required to have immediate effect, heparin rather than (or as well as) warfarin should be used. Side effects of warfarin therapy include:

- Bleeding, usually from over-anticoagulation, i.e. an INR ≥ 3.0. Bleeding can occur anywhere, e.g. intracranially, into the gastrointestinal tract, etc. Bleeding into the urinary tract, unless the INR is very prolonged, i.e. ≥ 6.0, often indicates intrinsic urinary tract pathology, e.g. urinary epithelial tumour.
- Drug interactions are very important and can increase or decrease warfarin metabolism, or compete for warfarin's albumin-binding site, increasing the effectiveness of therapy and leading to over-anticoagulation. Antibiotics can decrease gut vitamin K production, so increasing the action of warfarin. Concomitant antiplatelet drugs may lead to bleeding. As there are so many drugs that interact with warfarin, it is recommended that before prescribing additional drugs, possible interactions are identified from the *British National Formulary* (BNF).
- Skin necrosis is an exceptionally rare side effect—often a manifestation of protein C deficiency.

- **Heparin** is a powerful naturally occurring anticoagulant, which potentiates the action of anti-thrombin. It has an immediate onset of action, unlike warfarin.
  - Unfractionated heparins (UFHs) are a mixture of different molecular weights (5000–35 000, average 13 000), which inhibit activated serine protease coagulation factors by promoting their irreversible union with anti-thrombin. They are usually given by continual intravenous infusion, with the dose titrated against the activated partial thromboplastin time (APTT—see p. 342). It is difficult to obtain ideal anticoagulation. Side effects: bleeding, thrombocytopenia, and osteoporosis in long-term therapy.
  - Low-molecular-weight heparins (LMWHs) are unfractionated heparins chemically reduced in size to a molecular weight of 2000–8000. Their principal action is also via anti-thrombin, although they have a higher anti-Xa:IIa ratio. LMWHs have a much more predictable anticoagulant effect in an individual and are are given subcutaneously as a body weight-adjusted dose once/twice a day. APTT does not satisfactorily measure factor Xa inhibition, but fortunately anticoagulant action does not need to be monitored routinely. Easy and cheap to obtain effective anticoagulation. Side effects: bleeding and thrombocytopenia, both rarer than with UFHs.

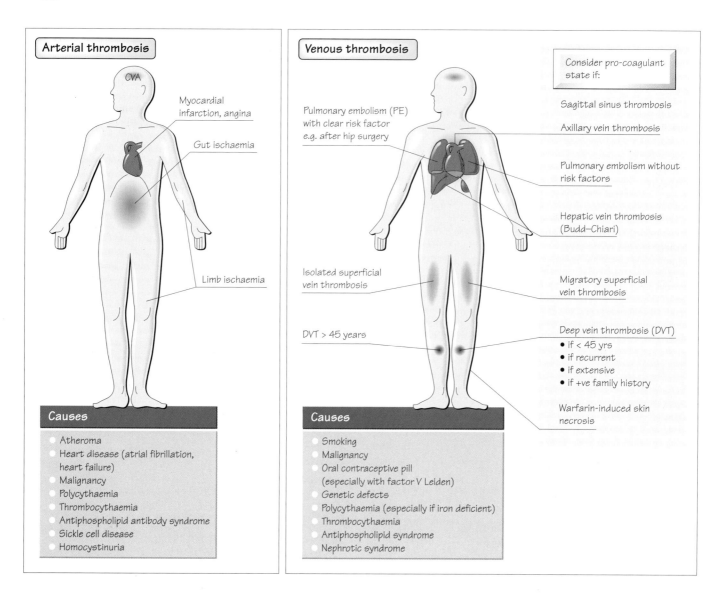

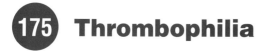

Two natural anticoagulant pathways prevent excess thrombus forming *in vivo*:

• Anti-thrombin is a serine protease inhibitor or serpin. Many coagulation proteins are serine proteases and anti-thrombin, through the formation of a 1 : 1 stoichiometric complex, has substantial inhibitory activity against such proteases. Anti-thrombin's main effect is to neutralize thrombin, although it does also have inhibitory activity against factor Xa.

• Protein C pathway: the zymogen protein C is activated by thrombin in the presence of an endothelial cell cofactor, thrombomodulin. Activated protein C is a serine protease, which acts as a natural anticoagulant by cleaving the two cofactors in the coagulation pathway, factors V and VIII, for which it needs its own cofactor, protein S. Both protein C and protein S are vitamin K-dependent proteins.

Inherited thrombophilia

Inherited mutations increasing the risk of thrombosis are common, affecting 5–7% of the population (Table 175.1). The inherited forms of thrombophilia are associated only with venous thrombosis not (in adults) with arterial disease.

Deficiencies of anti-thrombin, protein C or protein S predispose to thrombosis. Heterozygotes for these deficiencies with < 50% of normal levels are at risk, so the thrombotic tendency is inherited in an autosomal dominant fashion. Homozygous anti-thrombin deficiency is not seen and is presumably fatal *in utero*, whereas homozygosity for pro-

Table 175.1 Prevalence of inherited thrombophilia.

Deficiency/abnormality	Population prevalence
Factor V Leiden	1 in 20
Prothrombin G20210A	1 in 50–100
Protein C	1 in 300
Protein S	1 in 300
Anti-thrombin	1 in 3000

tein C or protein S deficiency leads to the very rare condition of neo-natal purpura fulminans. Until 1993, these three deficiencies were the only well-characterized forms of inherited thrombophilia.

Factor V Leiden

In 1993 the phenomenon of resistance to activated protein C (APC) was described and 1 year later the defect identified as a point mutation in factor V (G to A substitution at nucleotide position 1691), resulting in the arginine at position 506 being replaced by a glutamine. The abnormal factor is referred to as factor V Leiden. This substitution occurs at the site where protein C inactivates factor V. Normally factor V is inactivated by an initial cleavage of the peptide bond on the carboxyl side of arginine 506. Thus, the mutation here renders factor V resistant to activated protein C. Factor V Leiden is present in 5% of the population—in heterozygotes it increases the risk of venous thrombosis sevenfold, whereas in homozygotes (1 in 1600 of the population) there is a 50–100-fold increase in risk.

Prothrombin mutations

Recently a mutation in the 3′-untranslated region of the prothrombin gene has been identified, present in 1–2% of the population and associ-ated with a fourfold increased risk of venous thromboembolism. The mechanism seems to be higher prothrombin levels in individuals with the mutation.

Investigation of inherited thrombophilia

Not all cases of venous thromboembolism are investigated for genetic thrombophilia—studies are confined to those in whom testing will affect management or usefully inform relatives.

Consider testing:
• Patients with unprovoked venous thromboembolism who have a positive family history or are young with children/siblings (especially daughters/sisters).
• Relatives (especially females of child-bearing age) of a patient with proven venous thromboembolism and an identified heritable thrombophilia.

In addition to testing for the five causes of inherited thrombophilia discussed above, patients should also be tested for antiphospholipid antibodies which are acquired risk factors for both venous and arterial disease (see figure below).

Acquired thrombophilia (see figure opposite)

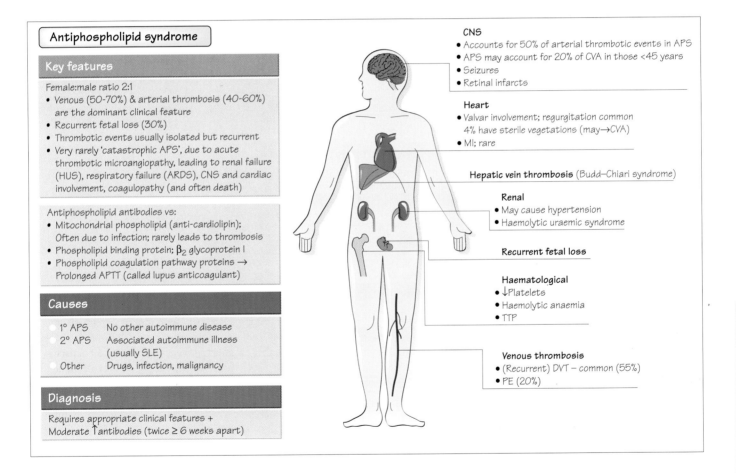

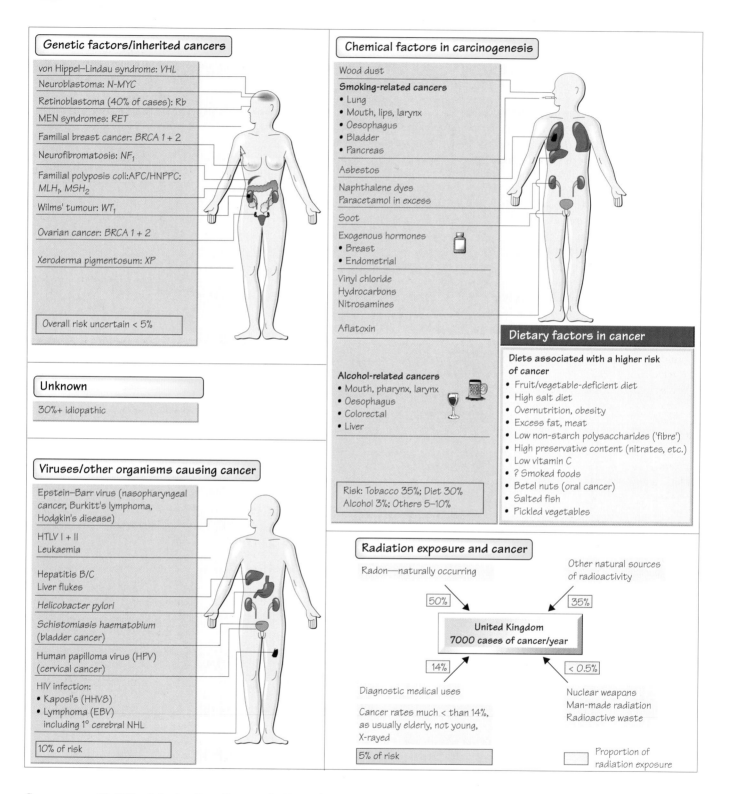

Genetic factors/inherited cancers

von Hippel–Lindau syndrome: VHL
Neuroblastoma: N-MYC
Retinoblastoma (40% of cases): Rb
MEN syndromes: RET
Familial breast cancer: BRCA 1 + 2
Neurofibromatosis: NF_1
Familial polyposis coli:APC/HNPPC: MLH_1, MSH_2
Wilms' tumour: WT_1
Ovarian cancer: BRCA 1 + 2
Xeroderma pigmentosum: XP

Overall risk uncertain < 5%

Unknown

30%+ idiopathic

Viruses/other organisms causing cancer

Epstein–Barr virus (nasopharyngeal cancer, Burkitt's lymphoma, Hodgkin's disease)
HTLV I + II Leukaemia
Hepatitis B/C Liver flukes
Helicobacter pylori
Schistomiasis haematobium (bladder cancer)
Human papilloma virus (HPV) (cervical cancer)
HIV infection:
• Kaposi's (HHV8)
• Lymphoma (EBV) including 1° cerebral NHL

10% of risk

Chemical factors in carcinogenesis

Wood dust
Smoking-related cancers
• Lung
• Mouth, lips, larynx
• Oesophagus
• Bladder
• Pancreas

Asbestos

Naphthalene dyes
Paracetamol in excess

Soot

Exogenous hormones
• Breast
• Endometrial

Vinyl chloride
Hydrocarbons
Nitrosamines

Aflatoxin

Alcohol-related cancers
• Mouth, pharynx, larynx
• Oesophagus
• Colorectal
• Liver

Risk: Tobacco 35%; Diet 30%
Alcohol 3%; Others 5–10%

Dietary factors in cancer

Diets associated with a higher risk of cancer
• Fruit/vegetable-deficient diet
• High salt diet
• Overnutrition, obesity
• Excess fat, meat
• Low non-starch polysaccharides ('fibre')
• High preservative content (nitrates, etc.)
• Low vitamin C
• ? Smoked foods
• Betel nuts (oral cancer)
• Salted fish
• Pickled vegetables

Radiation exposure and cancer

Radon—naturally occurring
Other natural sources of radioactivity

50%
35%

United Kingdom
7000 cases of cancer/year

14%
< 0.5%

Diagnostic medical uses

Cancer rates much < than 14%, as usually elderly, not young, X-rayed

Nuclear weapons
Man-made radiation
Radioactive waste

5% of risk

Proportion of radiation exposure

Cancer causes 20–25% of deaths. Overall cancer incidence is age related, reflecting the accumulation of genetic damage. Carcinogenesis is the genetic events producing malignant transformation and metastasis. There are four main aetiologies in cancer:
• **Chemical carcinogenesis**: there are two stages to chemical carcino-

genesis—tumour initiation and tumour promotion. Initiation means permanent, potentially inheritable (passed in the germline, i.e. gonadal) DNA damage from carcinogens (direct) or metabolites (indirect). Promotion can produce malignancy only in previously initiated cells and reflects increased cellular proliferation rather than direct effects on DNA (mitogenic as opposed to mutagenic). Common carcinogens include aromatic hydrocarbons and amines and nitrosamines. Aflatoxin B$_1$ induces a point mutation in *p53* (G to T transversion in codon 249) and causes hepatocellular carcinoma. Although the mechanisms are less clear, carcinogens in tobacco smoke are overwhelmingly the most important, probably causing 30% of cancers.

- **Radiation carcinogenesis**: ultraviolet irradiation, mainly UVB, produces pyrimidine dimers in DNA, normally repaired by the nucleotide excision-repair system. Excess UVB exposure overwhelms this pathway, resulting in DNA damage. Mutations in this repair pathway in xeroderma pigmentosa result in high rates of skin malignancy. UVB also causes mutations in oncogenes or tumour suppressor genes, e.g. *p53*. Ionizing radiation damages DNA by directly ionizing or through the production of highly reactive free radicals from ionization of adjacent water.

- **Viral carcinogenesis**: viruses may cause cancer by integrating genetic material into the host cell genome, which then activates oncogenes or inactivates tumour suppressor genes. RNA viruses may cause malignancy by insertion of proviral DNA near a proto-oncogene, inducing a structural change, and so conversion to a cellular oncogene (*c-onc*). This is termed 'insertional mutagenesis'. Epidemiologically the most important viruses are human papilloma virus (HPV) (cervical cancer) and hepatitis B (hepatoma).

- **Hereditable factors**: an inherited predisposition occurs in 5–10% of cancers. Inheritance of a single mutant gene in germ cells (e.g. disrupting a tumour suppressor gene) increases the risk of tumour development (e.g. retinoblastoma). Subsequent mutation of the remaining tumour suppressor gene in somatic cells causes transformation. There are several well-characterized familial cancer syndromes linked to a specific inherited mutant gene, e.g. familial breast and ovarian cancer (*BRCA-1*), and familial adenomatous polyposis (*FAP*). Although these are autosomal dominantly inherited, there are autosomal recessive syndromes (e.g. xeroderma pigmentosa). Subtle inherited variations in enzyme activity (genetic polymorphisms) alter carcinogen metabolism so increasing cancer rates.

Genetic mechanisms underlying carcinogenesis

The genetic mechanisms underlying carcinogenesis are crucial to tumour development and growth. Most human tumours so far studied show activation of several oncogenes and loss of two or more tumour suppressor genes. The four most important gene groups are:

- **Oncogenes** (cancer-causing genes) are derived from proto-oncogenes, normal cellular genes that promote and control normal growth and differentiation. They are classified as viral or cellular oncogenes (*v-onc* and *c-onc*). Each *v-onc* is named after the virus from which it was isolated, e.g. *v-fes* from the *fe*line *s*arcoma virus. The *c-onc* oncogenes are similarly named, e.g. *c-ras* from the *ra*t *s*arcoma virus or *c-myc* from murine (mouse) *my*elocytoma virus. Viral oncogenes (unique sequences within the genome of tumour-forming retroviruses) are almost identical to sequences found in normal cellular DNA. They may have become integrated into the genome during evolution by chance recombination with the DNA of the infected host cell. Cellular oncogenes are normal cellular genes that have become oncogenic through structural changes inducing altered *in situ* behaviour. Typically changes in the gene sequence produce an abnormal gene product with an aberrant function. Alternatively, changes in gene expression (protein production) by gene amplification (multiple copies) or over-expression cause high levels of normal growth-promoting proteins (often recep-

tors). Oncoproteins (proteins encoded by oncogenes) include growth factors and their receptors, signal transduction proteins, nuclear transcription factors (regulating gene expression), cyclins and cyclin-dependent kinases (regulating cell cycle progression from synthesis of new DNA to mitosis).

- **Tumour suppressor gene products** regulate cell growth by inhibition of cellular proliferation. Their loss is the key event in most, if not all, human cancers. Mutated tumour suppressor genes are mostly recessive, i.e. carcinogenesis requires inactivation of both normal alleles, e.g. the *p*rotein product of the retinoblastoma gene (*pRb*), which controls cell cycle progression, and *p53*, which monitors for genetic damage, halting cell cycle progression and triggering apoptosis if damage is not repaired.

- **Genes regulating apoptosis**: apoptosis or programmed cell death is the orchestrated involution of redundant cells. Many genes regulate apoptosis. If these genes are damaged, there is a steady inappropriate accumulation of cells, e.g. over-expression of *bcl-2* in lymphoma, mutations in *bax* associated with failure of apoptosis in several solid tumours.

- **Genes regulating DNA repair** are not themselves oncogenic when defective, but allow mutations in other genes to develop during replication, thereby increasing the likelihood of tumour development, e.g. the defective mismatch repair genes in hereditary non-polyposis colon cancer (HNPCC), the breast and ovarian cancer predisposition genes, *BRCA-1* and *-2*, and the defective DNA-repair mechanism in xeroderma pigmentosum.

- **Aging telomerase**; it is increasingly clear that cancer is a correlate of aging and the regulation of cellular longevity through telomere length has an important anti-cancer role.

Factors underlying growth and spread of tumours

Key processes in cancer are growth and metastasis:

- **Growth**: clonal expansion of a transformed cell. Cellular accumulation in cancer reflects less necrosis and apoptosis, rather than a shortened cell cycle time. Speed of growth is determined by the balance between cycle time and cell apoptosis, and by the proportion of tumour cells progressing through the cell cycle (growth fraction).

- **Invasion**: malignant cells invade locally (using collagenases and metalloproteases) or metastasize, by invading lymphatic channels and blood vessels, from where they embolize to distant sites. Adhesion molecules, vascular supply, vessel calibre, tumour cell size and target tissue characteristics determine distribution of metastases. Initial metastatic growth relates to tumour angiogenesis, which in turn depends on the production of various cytokines, including vascular endothelium growth factor (VEGF).

- **Host immunity**: host cellular immunity is effective against only a limited number of malignancies, immune surveillance typically being tolerant to the presence of cancer.

- **Cellular immortality**: malignant cells have (express) the enzyme telomerase which allows the ends of the chromosomes (telomeres – the cellular clock) to be elongated and so avoid the senescence (crisis death) of typical cellular aging.

- **Angiogenesis**: tumours need to develop a blood supply to grow beyond 1–2 mm. Angiogenesis is an important part of embryology and healing, is disordered in malignancy and driven by VEGF (Vascular Endothelial Growth Factor), inhibition of which by the monoclonal antibody bevacizumab confers a significant survival advantage in a number of tumours.

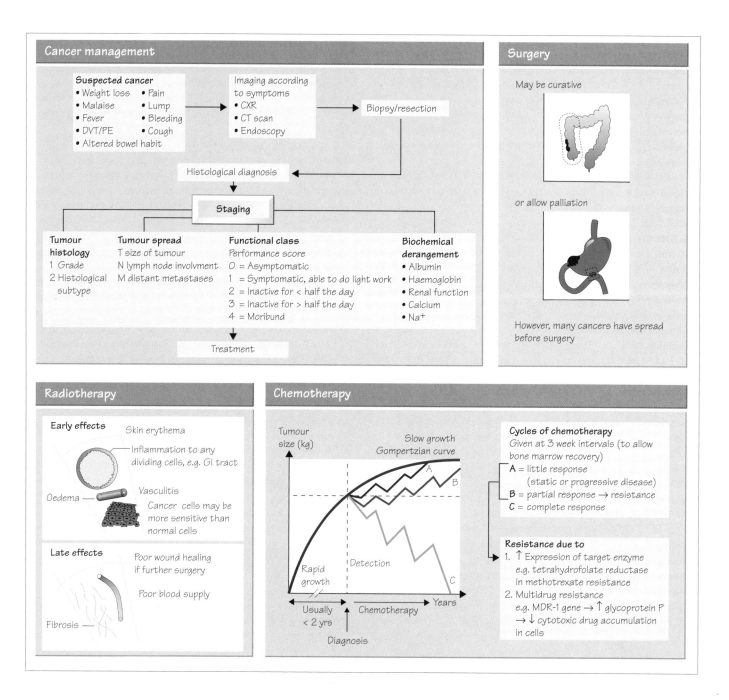

Important diagnostic strategies

Cancer needs to be diagnosed, staged, and then the effects of treatment monitored:

• Diagnosis is made by histological (tissue) or cytological (cells) examination. Cells (fine needle aspiration) or small tissue samples (needle biopsy) are usually sufficient, although in lymphomas the architectural pattern (lymph node) should be examined.

• Staging reflects the mechanisms of spread of the tumour (local invasion, lymph or blood spread), determines treatment and, along with histological subtype and grade, is the most powerful determinant of outcome. Tumour staging is occasionally done surgically, but more often radiologically and by bone marrow examination/scan. Histological characteristics, define the 'aggressiveness' of the tumour, based on mitotic rate, nuclear pleomorphism, tubule formation, etc. and on growth factor receptors, e.g. oestrogen and HER-2/neu receptors.

• Increasingly tumour markers, particularly in ovarian cancer (CA-125), germ cell tumours (α-fetoprotein [α-FP], β-human chorionic gonadotrophin (β-hCG) and lymphoma (lactate dehydrogenase [LDH]) are used in evaluating treatment and surveillance, and relate to tumour burden. The polymerase chain reaction (PCR) amplifies specific molecular markers of malignant cells and detects residual disease in chronic myeloid leukaemia (CML) and follicular lymphoma.

• Measures of age, performance score, activity and physiological function are important determinants of the response to treatment, as are laboratory measures (e.g. Na$^+$ or albumin relate to outcome).

Principles of surgical oncology

Surgery is used for both diagnosis and staging of the tumour. Historically, radical surgery gave optimal chance of cure and remains appropriate for ovarian cancer, some sarcomas, melanomas, head and neck tumours, and resection of oligo- (one or few) metastasis. However, with modern adjuvant therapies (radiation or chemotherapy), to complement surgery more conservative surgical operations with their reduced morbidities offer comparable local control. Surgical resection should, for local control, extend to a clear (cancer free) margin of 1 cm in most cancers.

Basic principles of radiotherapy

Radiotherapy plays an essential role in the treatment of many cancers. Ionizing radiation induces DNA damage, which triggers apoptosis (programmed cell death). Radiation doses are divided (fractionated) to allow for recovery of normal tissue and thus reduce side effects. Certain tissues (e.g. the lens, nervous and cardiac tissue) are particularly radiosensitive and mandate careful radiation planning. Hypoxic tissues are notoriously refractory to radiation. The concurrent use of chemotherapy is increasingly improving the outcome of radiation, as in cervical carcinoma, with encouraging results in oesophageal and lung cancer.

Increasingly computed tomography (CT) planning and conformal (shaped beam) radiotherapy enable tailored radiotherapy with minimal irradiation of adjacent tissues and brachytherapy (the use of seeds, wires or implants); monoclonal radioimmunotherapy and stereotactic radiotherapy take this advantage yet further.

Basic principles of chemotherapy

Chemotherapy works by:
• Damaging the DNA of rapidly dividing cells, which is detected by the *p53/Rb* pathway, thus triggering apoptosis.
• Damaging cellular spindle apparatus, preventing cell division.
• Inhibiting DNA synthesis.

Chemotherapy can lead to cure, either when given alone (choriocarcinoma, childhood acute lymphoblastic leukaemia [ALL], some lymphomas and leukaemias, and germ cell tumours) or in combination with surgery (osteosarcoma, adenocarcinoma of the breast and ovary, colorectal cancer and squamous cell carcinoma of the upper gastrointestinal tract). It may prolong life without producing cure, as in AML, small cell carcinoma of the lung (SCLC) and ovarian cancer. Increased understanding of cancer cell biology has improved current treatments and will lead to more innovative ones, including immunotherapy or gene therapy, oligonucleotides or monoclonal antibodies. The different classes of chemotherapy are:
• Folate antagonists, purine and pyrimidine analogues: these drugs (methotrexate, 5-fluorouracil and hydroxyurea) inhibit DNA synthesis.
• Alkylating agents damage DNA. They include cyclophosphamide (breast cancer, lymphoma), melphalan (myeloma) and platinum (testicular cancer, lymphoma, squamous cell carcinoma, ovarian and bladder cancer). Drug resistance can occur.
• Topoisomerase I and II-interacting drugs intercalate double-stranded DNA and form a cleavable complex with topoisomerase II, an essential nuclear enzyme that causes double-stranded DNA breaks. Examples include the anthracyclines (breast cancer, lymphoma) and etoposide (teratoma, lung cancer). Related drugs, including topotecan and irinotecan, associate with topoisomerase I to cause reversible single-stranded DNA breaks.
• Alkaloids and taxanes inhibit microtubule function and disrupt mitosis. Examples include the vinca alkaloids (leukaemia, lymphoma, bladder cancer) and the taxanes (ovarian cancer, breast cancer).

Side effects of chemotherapy

Chemotherapy causes myelosuppression and so risks infection (neutropenia) and bleeding (thrombocytopenia). Damage to mucous membranes causes a sore mouth; diarrhoea and stimulation of the chemotactic trigger zone produce nausea and vomiting. Any rapidly dividing tissues, such as the hair follicles (alopecia) and germinal epithelium (infertility), are vulnerable to the effects of chemotherapy and late effects such as secondary malignancies are increasingly recognized. All are teratogenic. Some drugs cause specific organ toxicity, such as to the kidney (cisplatin) and nerves (vincristine). Supportive care with the 5-hydroxytryptamine (serotonin) 5HT$_3$ antagonists and steroids has improved the control of nausea. Several recombinant human proteins are in routine use to support the effects of myelosuppression: granulocyte-colony-stimulating factor (G-CSF) reduces the depth and duration of neutropenia and erythropoietin improves chemotherapy-related anaemia.

Novel therapies

Interleukin-2 (IL2) induces a small (< 5%) complete remission rate in young patients with advanced renal cell carcinoma or melanoma. Several monoclonal antibodies are used successfully, including trastuzumab (breast cancer—anti-HER-2/neu) and rituximab (lymphoma—anti-CD20). Gene therapy, tumour vaccines and antiangiogenic therapy are all investigational. Imatinib (Glivec®), an oral tyrosine kinase (bcr/Abl gene product) inhibitor, has revolutionized the treatment of chronic myeloid leukaemia. Gefitinib (Iressa®) is another tyrosine kinase inhibitor that targets the epidermal growth factor receptor (EGFR) and has recently been approved for use in non-small cell lung cancer.

Basic principles of hormonal therapy

Some tumours (breast, endometrial, prostate and thyroid cancer) are hormone responsive, and the removal of endogenous hormones improves prognosis, e.g. one-third of premenopausal women with advanced breast cancer have a remission with oophorectomy. Drugs interfere with hormone action within cancer cells, e.g. tamoxifen, a competitive inhibitor of the oestrogen receptor, with some oestrogenic activity, is used in breast cancer. The progesterone receptor, stimulation of which alters transcription, is often present on breast cancer and endometrial cancer cells. 5α-Reductase inhibitors prevent the generation of active testosterone metabolites within cells and are useful options for treatment in metastatic prostate cancer as are gonadotrophin-releasing hormone (GnRH) analogues, steroidal and non-steroidal antiandrogens. Corticosteroids are potent agents in lymphoma and myeloma.

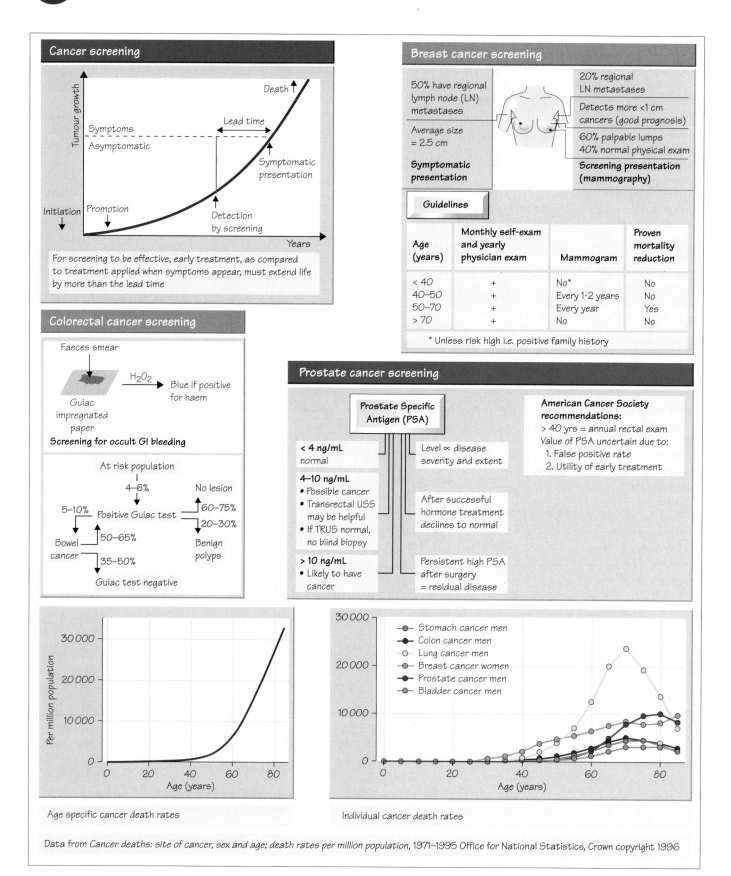

Cancer screening

For screening to be effective, early treatment, as compared to treatment applied when symptoms appear, must extend life by more than the lead time

Breast cancer screening

50% have regional lymph node (LN) metastases

Average size = 2.5 cm

Symptomatic presentation

20% regional LN metastases

Detects more <1 cm cancers (good prognosis)

60% palpable lumps
40% normal physical exam

Screening presentation (mammography)

Guidelines

Age (years)	Monthly self-exam and yearly physician exam	Mammogram	Proven mortality reduction
< 40	+	No*	No
40–50	+	Every 1-2 years	No
50–70	+	Every year	Yes
> 70	+	No	No

* Unless risk high i.e. positive family history

Colorectal cancer screening

Faeces smear

Guiac impregnated paper

H_2O_2 → Blue if positive for haem

Screening for occult GI bleeding

At risk population
4–6%
5–10% — Positive Guiac test
Bowel cancer — 50–65%
35–50%
Guiac test negative

No lesion
60–75%
20–30%
Benign polyps

Prostate cancer screening

Prostate Specific Antigen (PSA)

< 4 ng/mL normal

4–10 ng/mL
• Possible cancer
• Transrectal USS may be helpful
• If TRUS normal, no blind biopsy

> 10 ng/mL
• Likely to have cancer

Level ∝ disease severity and extent

After successful hormone treatment declines to normal

Persistent high PSA after surgery = residual disease

American Cancer Society recommendations:
> 40 yrs = annual rectal exam
Value of PSA uncertain due to:
1. False positive rate
2. Utility of early treatment

Age specific cancer death rates

Individual cancer death rates

Legend:
- Stomach cancer men
- Colon cancer men
- Lung cancer men
- Breast cancer women
- Prostate cancer men
- Bladder cancer men

Data from *Cancer deaths: site of cancer, sex and age; death rates per million population, 1971–1995* Office for National Statistics, Crown copyright 1996

Early disease detection offers the best hope for cure with the least intervention. Treatment success is often dependent on the spread (stage) and biology (grade and behaviour) of disease, both of which worsen with time. Successful screening strategies should:
• Address a common and dangerous disease.
• Use a simple, safe, inexpensive and valid screening test.
• Enable curative treatment, which when instituted earlier has a significant impact on survival.

Although observational, cohort and randomized controlled trials have shown the advantage of some screening programmes, there are problems:
• Screening can provoke anxiety.
• Screening may only increase lead time (time before development of symptoms).
• Screening may only increase the detection of more indolent cancers, which may never become clinically apparent. When added to the clinically relevant cancers, these apparently increase the percentage of early cases and overall survival. In screening, one of the earliest indicators of a future decrease in mortality is a decrease in the absolute rate (not percentage) of cases of advanced disease.

The impact of screening has been limited by the huge size of target populations, the difficulty of follow-up, poor compliance and poor test sensitivity with high false-positive rates.

Breast cancer

In 1963, the first randomized cancer-screening trial investigating mammography in breast cancer was undertaken, using mortality as an endpoint. Subsequently several studies have supported this approach. It is clear that screening 50- to 69-year-old women with mammography decreases the breast cancer mortality rate by 30%. There is controversy about women aged 40–49 because:
• Although breast cancer is the leading cause of death in such women, breast cancer incidence and mortality rates are lower in this age group.
• To date the randomized controlled trials have been too small to be statistically unambiguous.
• Sensitivity of mammography is lower in denser breast tissue.
• There is a higher relative rate of ductal carcinoma in situ (DCIS).

Two-view mammography diagnoses twice as many patients with benign breast disease as with cancer. Wire localization and conservative surgery detect more node-negative breast cancers with a good prognosis that are < 1 cm in size (5-year survival rate of 80–90%). The current guidelines state that:
• Women should be 'breast aware'.
• Clinicians should perform opportunistic breast examination.
• Mammography should occur every 1–3 years, and yearly in those with previous breast cancer, atypical ductal hyperplasia or a strong family history of breast cancer.

The finding that some breast cancer is genetically inherited has opened the question of genetic screening. At present assays of *BRCA-1* and *-2* may be offered to young women with a strong family history of breast and ovarian cancer occurring early in life. The best management of those found to carry these genes is unclear although prophylactic surgery (mastectomy and oophorectomy) and tamoxifen look promising.

Colorectal cancer

Colorectal cancer is the second leading cause of cancer death. For localized disease the 5-year survival rate is 90%, for node-positive (Dukes' stage C) disease it is 60%, and for patients presenting with metastatic disease it is < 10%. Many screening studies show an increase in the proportion of early cases detected by colonoscopy, sigmoidoscopy or digital rectal examination and faecal blood examination. Of asymptomatic patients aged > 50 years, 1–5% have positive faecal occult bloods, of whom 10% have cancer and 20–30% have adenomas—annual faecal occult blood and flexible sigmoidoscopy every 5 years thus have the potential to reduce mortality significantly, although this has not yet been unequivocally shown. The current guidelines for colorectal screening suggest that:
• Those with a very high incidence of colon and/or rectal cancer, e.g. familial polyposis coli, hereditary non-polyposis coli, cancer family syndrome or ulcerative pan-colitis should have yearly faecal occult bloods ± colonoscopy.
• Rectal examination should be included in routine check-ups (especially those with a personal history of adenoma, colon cancer or ulcerative colitis. or a strong family history of colon cancer).
• Some cancer societies recommend sigmoidoscopy or colonoscopy at age 50 years, regardless of symptom status or whether occult blood positive or not. This is not routine practice in the UK.

Prostate cancer

In the last 10 years the incidence of prostate cancer has soared in the USA. The average age of presentation with prostate cancer is 70 years, close to life expectancy, and competing causes of death influence the epidemiology and management of the disease. Furthermore, the negative impact of treatment (impotence/incontinence) limits their utility. Finally, no study has yet shown a survival advantage for screening, although ongoing studies are under way investigating the role of transrectal ultrasonography, prostate-specific antigen (PSA) and digital rectal examination in screening. It may be appropriate to screen high-risk patients (black men and men with a family history of prostate cancer).

Cervical cancer

The mortality rate for cervical cancer has decreased in several countries, following the introduction of screening programmes based on Papanicolaou's (Pap) smears. Although there are no randomized controlled trials, the introduction of Pap smear screening in Finland and Iceland were associated with a 50% and 80% reduced mortality rate over a 20-year period. The guidelines recommend that:
• A Pap smear should be done on all sexually active women > 18 years every 3 years.
• After three consecutive normal Pap smears, the Pap test may be performed less frequently.
• There is no clear upper age when screening can be discontinued.

Education and awareness

There are two tumours where the principal screener should be the patient:
• Testicular tumours are typically detected by accident or self-examination, and although rare are the most common tumour in young men. Education and increased awareness reduces delays in diagnosis.
• Skin tumours: education about the dangers of excess sun (UV) exposure, especially for fair-skinned individuals and those with a personal/family history of melanoma or dysplastic naevi syndrome, has decreased the incidence of sun-related cancers and improved early diagnosis, e.g. a high-profile public education programme in Scotland decreased the proportion of thick, poor prognosis lesions from 34% to 15%.

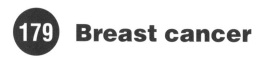

(179) Breast cancer

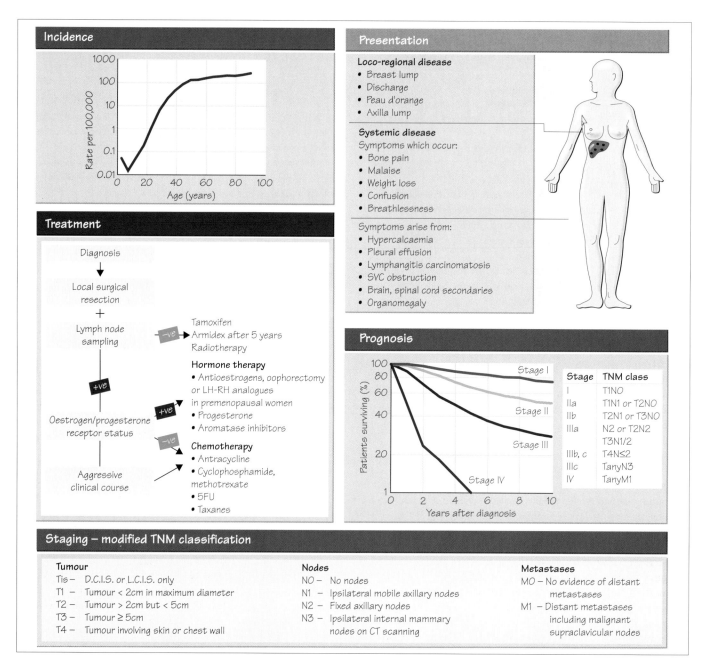

Incidence

Rate per 100,000 vs Age (years)

Presentation

Loco-regional disease
- Breast lump
- Discharge
- Peau d'orange
- Axilla lump

Systemic disease
Symptoms which occur:
- Bone pain
- Malaise
- Weight loss
- Confusion
- Breathlessness

Symptoms arise from:
- Hypercalcaemia
- Pleural effusion
- Lymphangitis carcinomatosis
- SVC obstruction
- Brain, spinal cord secondaries
- Organomegaly

Treatment

Diagnosis
↓
Local surgical resection
+
Lymph node sampling

—ve → Tamoxifen
Armidex after 5 years
Radiotherapy

+ve

Oestrogen/progesterone receptor status

+ve

Hormone therapy
- Antioestrogens, oophorectomy or LH-RH analogues in premenopausal women
- Progesterone
- Aromatase inhibitors

—ve

Chemotherapy
- Antracycline
- Cyclophosphamide, methotrexate
- 5FU
- Taxanes

Aggressive clinical course

Prognosis

Patients surviving (%) vs Years after diagnosis

Stage I
Stage II
Stage III
Stage IV

Stage	TNM class
I	T1N0
IIa	T1N1 or T2N0
IIb	T2N1 or T3N0
IIIa	N2 or T2N2
	T3N1/2
IIIb, c	T4N≤2
IIIc	TanyN3
IV	TanyM1

Staging – modified TNM classification

Tumour
Tis – D.C.I.S. or L.C.I.S. only
T1 – Tumour < 2cm in maximum diameter
T2 – Tumour > 2cm but < 5cm
T3 – Tumour ≥ 5cm
T4 – Tumour involving skin or chest wall

Nodes
N0 – No nodes
N1 – Ipsilateral mobile axillary nodes
N2 – Fixed axillary nodes
N3 – Ipsilateral internal mammary nodes on CT scanning

Metastases
M0 – No evidence of distant metastases
M1 – Distant metastases including malignant supraclavicular nodes

Epidemiology

Breast cancer is the second most common tumour in women, with 24 000 women diagnosed in the UK each year and 15 000 dying of the disease. By 80 years of age the lifetime risk to a woman is 1 in 9.

Aetiology

Most breast cancer occurs without an obvious cause, although several predisposing factors are recognized, including:
- Oestrogen exposure: particularly unopposed by progestogens, explaining the association with early menarche, late menopause and nulliparity.
- Family and personal history: 10% of breast cancer is genetically

determined with links to the genes *BRCA-1*, *BRCA-2*, *p53* and *A-T*. A previous history of breast, endometrial or ovarian cancer indicates a genetically determined increased risk. Previous benign breast disease and chest irradiation are also risk factors.
- High fat consumption and socioeconomic status.

Molecular genetics

The autosomal dominant *BRCA-1* or *BRCA-2* genes occur in 2% of all breast cancer but in 50–80% of young patients aged < 40 years with a strong family history (i.e. more than one affected first degree relative) of breast and ovarian cancer. Of breast cancer patients, 10% are heterozygotes for the ataxia-telangiectasia (A-T) gene, an autosomal recessive DNA repair gene found in 0.5–1% of the general population.

Pathology

Adenocarcinoma is most commonly infiltrating ductal. Lobular, medullary, mucinous, papillary or tubular carcinomas are rarer. It can also present as Paget's disease of the nipple (tumour of main excretory ducts involving overlying nipple and skin), and rarely lymphoma, sarcoma, squamous or clear cell carcinomas.

Breast adenocarcinomas are graded histologically using the 'modified Bloom and Richardson' scheme to categorize aggressiveness and probable behaviour, on the basis of tubule formation, nuclear pleomorphism and mitotic rate. Other important histological findings are:
• Receptor status: breast cancer cells may express oestrogen and/or progestogen receptors. Their presence or absence affects treatment.
• Ductal carcinoma *in situ* (DCIS): malignant cell proliferation within the ducts without stromal invasion, usually unilateral, occasionally multifocal. Often detectable on mammography. Without treatment, 14–30% of patients develop invasive breast cancer.
• Lobular carcinoma *in situ* (LCIS): proliferation of malignant cells within breast lobules. Rarely palpable or visible on mammography. Usually multicentric and often bilateral. Not premalignant, but rather an indicator of increased breast cancer risk.
• 25% of breast cancers express HER-2/neu and these have a worse prognosis.

Investigations

Initial diagnosis

• Two-view mammography (oblique/craniocaudal): rarely useful in women < 40 years old (breasts are radiodense).
• Breast ultrasonography—useful if a palpable mass. Malignant lesions have indistinct edges. Not useful for screening.
• Fine needle or Tru-Cut biopsy: manual or stereotactic.

Staging (Table 179.1)

(i) Routine haematological and biochemical screening (including liver function tests and serum calcium); (ii) chest radiograph; (iii) ultrasonography of liver; and (iv) isotope bone scan.

Treatment

Surgery

For most patients the primary surgical treatment aims to remove the tumour (minimizes the risk of local recurrence) and to obtain staging and prognostic information from the tumour and axillary nodes. Surgery may be modified radical mastectomy or breast conserving (lumpectomy with postoperative radiotherapy). Local excision of the tumour (with a histologically confirmed margin of normal tissue), combined with postoperative radical radiotherapy, achieves as good local control as total mastectomy, though the latter is indicated for large (> 4 cm), multicentric tumours, or if there is extensive DCIS or skin involvement. Extensive axillary dissection reduces the risk of axillary recurrence:
• Axillary node sampling: no benefit in local axillary control unless combined with postoperative axillary radiotherapy.
• Axillary node clearance/dissection: removal of all axillary nodes. Good local control, no radiotherapy required and maximum prognostic information obtained about number of lymph nodes with metastases.

Radiotherapy

Adjuvant radiotherapy to the breast remnant reduces the risk of local tumour recurrence following breast-conserving surgery. Radiotherapy to the axilla is given if axillary node sampling has revealed positive nodes, although not if full axillary dissection has been performed, because it adds little to local control and has an unacceptably high incidence of lymphoedema.
• **Adjuvant systemic therapy**: 30–50% of patients with apparently resectable breast cancer subsequently die of their disease, suggesting that micrometastases were present at diagnosis. Systemic adjuvant therapy reduces the risk of disease relapse.
• **Endocrine therapy**: tamoxifen, an antioestrogen, reduces the risk of disease relapse in all women. It is given for 5 years, after which modest risks of continuing use outweigh any benefit. Similar hormonal manipulation can also be obtained with luteinizing hormone-releasing hormone (LHRH) agonists or by oophorectomy.
• **Chemotherapy**: most patients (not small—< 1 cm, low-grade, node-negative disease) with moderate- to high-risk disease benefit from adjuvant chemotherapy. Equivalent relative benefit is seen in post- and premenopausal women. Combination chemotherapy is used (doxorubicin and cyclophosphamide in combination with or followed by a taxane).

Follow-up

Follow-up is used to detect disease recurrence, manage treatment-related toxicity, and screen for a new primary lesion and for psychological support, but it does not improve survival. The cancer risk to the second breast is increased fourfold. Mammography should be performed on a yearly basis, bilaterally if the patient had breast-conserving treatment.

Locally advanced breast cancer

This is defined as tumours > 5 cm in size or showing evidence of skin or chest wall invasion (i.e. 'fixed') or inflammatory breast cancer (erythematous with lymphatic permeation). A response to primary treatment with endocrine therapy and chemotherapy may facilitate surgery and radiotherapy and may allow breast-conserving surgery.

Metastatic breast cancer

Endocrine therapy with tamoxifen is the first treatment choice. Second-line therapies include aromatase inhibitors (e.g. anastrozole) or progestogens. Oestrogen suppression can be obtained with surgical or radiation-induced ovarian ablation or with LHRH antagonists.

Chemotherapy should be considered in young, healthy patients with rapidly progressive, oestrogen receptor (ER)-negative, visceral disease, particularly if relapse has occurred early after surgery or in ER-negative disease that is unlikely to respond to hormonal therapy. The same regimens used in the adjuvant setting are given. The taxanes (docetaxel and paclitaxel) are particularly active and are given as second-line agents.

Hormone replacement therapy

Hormone replacement therapy (HRT) slightly increases the risk of breast cancer and should be avoided in patients with node-positive breast cancer, but this remains controversial.

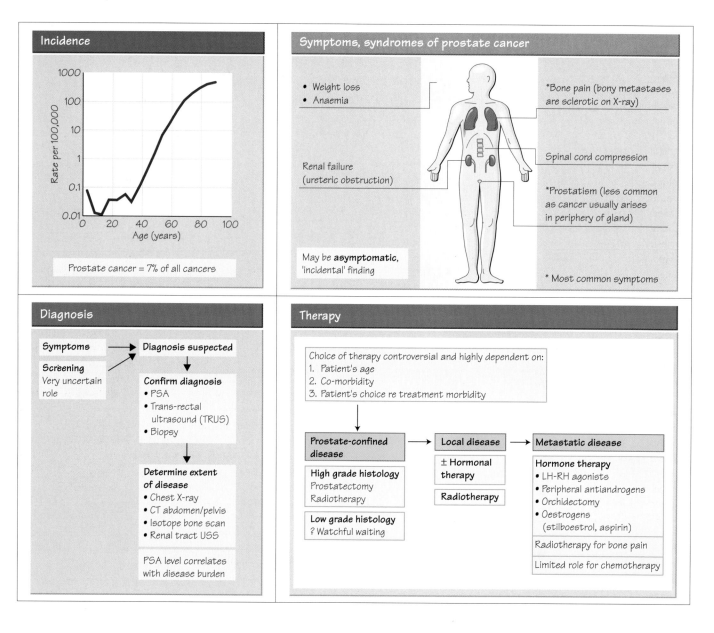

Incidence

Rate per 100,000 vs Age (years)

Prostate cancer = 7% of all cancers

Symptoms, syndromes of prostate cancer

- Weight loss
- Anaemia

Renal failure
(ureteric obstruction)

*Bone pain (bony metastases
are sclerotic on X-ray)

Spinal cord compression

*Prostatism (less common
as cancer usually arises
in periphery of gland)

May be **asymptomatic**,
'incidental' finding

* Most common symptoms

Diagnosis

Symptoms → Diagnosis suspected

Screening
Very uncertain
role

↓

Confirm diagnosis
- PSA
- Trans-rectal
  ultrasound (TRUS)
- Biopsy

↓

Determine extent
of disease
- Chest X-ray
- CT abdomen/pelvis
- Isotope bone scan
- Renal tract USS

PSA level correlates
with disease burden

Therapy

Choice of therapy controversial and highly dependent on:
1. Patient's age
2. Co-morbidity
3. Patient's choice re treatment morbidity

Prostate-confined disease → Local disease → Metastatic disease

Prostate-confined disease

High grade histology
Prostatectomy
Radiotherapy

Low grade histology
? Watchful waiting

Local disease
± Hormonal therapy

Radiotherapy

Metastatic disease

Hormone therapy
- LH-RH agonists
- Peripheral antiandrogens
- Orchidectomy
- Oestrogens
  (stilboestrol, aspirin)

Radiotherapy for bone pain

Limited role for chemotherapy

Prostate cancer is the most common malignancy in men and it may soon exceed lung cancer as the most frequent cause of cancer death. Many patients have metastatic disease at diagnosis. Prostate cancer is highly sensitive to androgen ablation. The incidence rises exponentially with age and the older age of patients and co-morbidity make screening with prostate-specific antigen (PSA) and treatment decisions about early stage disease particularly controversial.

Aetiology

Most prostate cancer occurs without obvious cause. Family history, radiation exposure and environmental pollutants contribute to the risk.

Pathology

A number of tumour cell types arise in the prostate gland:

- Adenocarcinoma is the most common. It arises in the acinar epithelium in the peripheral region of the gland. Cells stain for acid phosphatase and PSA. Various grading systems predict the biological behaviour of the tumour. The most commonly used of these is the Gleason system, where the tumour is graded (both predominant and highest grade) histologically between grade I (well-differentiated, uniform gland formation) and grade V (very poorly differentiated, minimal gland formation) for a total score out of 10.
- Rarer subtypes (< 2%): transitional cell carcinoma arises in the ductal epithelium. Stromal sarcomas: lymphoma; small cell carcinoma.

Clinical presentation

Unfortunately, early prostatic cancer is usually asymptomatic and may be detectable clinically only by the presence of a rectally palpable mass or induration of the gland. The tumour usually arises peripherally in the gland, so obstructive symptoms ('prostatism') are late unless secondary to associated benign prostatic hypertrophy. Haematuria and perineal pain sometimes occur. Many patients have metastatic disease at diagnosis, and present with symptoms related to these, such as the constitutional symptoms of weight loss or anaemia, bone pain, lymphadenopathy or neurological complications.

Staging

Prostate cancer most typically metastasizes to bone. It may, however, spread through the lymphatics to regional pelvic nodes and then to abdominal nodes. Visceral metastases may also occur.

Clinical approach

Investigations in suspected prostate cancer aim to confirm the diagnosis histologically and determine whether metastases are present. If disease is confined to the prostate, local therapy with radiotherapy or radical prostatectomy may be appropriate. These treatments may have similar outcomes (> 30% incontinence and impotence), although this has not been tested in an adequately powered clinical trial. However, they may both reduce local complications and may be better than watchful waiting.

Investigations

Examination under anaesthesia with clinical staging (Table 180.1) and needle biopsy:

- Transrectal ultrasonography to identify small peripherally sited lesions, with sextant biopsy.
- Transurethral resection of the prostate (TURP) if there is prostatism.
- Biochemistry: serum PSA: levels > 10 IU suggest metastatic disease. Alkaline and acid phosphatase.
- Radiology: computed tomography of abdomen and pelvis may identify pelvic or abdominal nodes. Magnetic resonance imaging (MRI) of the pelvis defines the tumour and the degree of local extension better if radical (curative) treatment is an option. Chest X-ray and isotope bone scan needed for metastases.

Screening for prostate cancer remains controversial. The use of serum PSA analysis combined with digital rectal examination is quite effective in terms of early disease detection. It remains unclear whether early detection and treatment saves lives.

Treatment

- Localized prostatic carcinoma: the principal treatment approaches are surgery, radiotherapy and watchful waiting. There is no consensus about the benefit of intervention in early prostatic cancer.
- Surgery is recommended for poorly differentiated tumours confined to the prostate, although this has never been tested against radiotherapy in a randomized clinical trial. Patients with well or moderately well-differentiated tumours survive equally long (5-year survival rate is 85%) whether they receive radical radiotherapy or they are simply kept under observation (watchful waiting).
- Radical radiotherapy has similar survival figures, new initiatives are investigating increasing the radiation dose using more targeted (conformal) radiotherapy, or combining radiotherapy with hormonal therapy.
- Brachytherapy using radioactive palladium or iodine seeds implanted directly into the prostate gland can be performed on an outpatient basis, and is used for small low-grade tumours with excellent results in selected patients.
- Hormone treatment (androgen ablation): prostate cancer cell growth shows a striking dependence on androgens. Hormonal therapy directed at interfering with this association typically produces disease response in both metastatic and locoregional disease. Bilateral orchidectomy or gonadotrophin-releasing hormone agonists, such as goserelin or buserelin, can mediate this. They only block pituitary-driven testicular androgen production. Complete androgen blockade requires the concomitant use of a peripheral antiandrogen (flutamide, bicalutamide or cyproterone acetate). Oestrogens such as diethylstilboestrol produce similar effects but are associated with significant cardiovascular morbidity. Hormone therapy before radiotherapy can reduce the size of the prostate gland, hence also reducing the radiation treatment volume and lowering toxicity; there is also improved local control and disease-free survival. Overall survival may not be prolonged, although this is an area of active clinical research. Antiandrogen side effects include hot flushes, weakness, impotence and loss of sexual drive.

Metastatic prostate cancer

Widespread metastatic disease is often initially very responsive to hormone therapy; it is the first line of therapy in most cases, and is associated with a considerable symptomatic improvement and clinical response. The response may be followed closely and accurately by regular assessment of PSA levels. Patients may continue to respond to hormone therapy for several years, but on average the disease escapes hormonal control after about 18 months. Radiotherapy has a role to play in the palliation of symptoms either from the primary tumour or from troublesome sites of metastases. The response rates of chemotherapy in prostate cancer are disappointingly low and generally chemotherapy does not form part of standard therapy, although there has been considerable interest in improvements in quality of life in younger patients using mitozantrone and estramustine. Finally, bone-seeking radioisotopes (strontium) have an experimental role in some patients with bony metastases. Bisphosphates decrease the skeletal morbidity of androgen deprivation.

Table 180.1 TNM staging of prostate cancer.

T1	Tumour neither palpable nor imageable, identified only in resected specimens or by needle biopsy
T2	Tumour confined to the prostate
T3	Tumour extending through the prostate capsule including seminal vesicle invasion
T4	Tumour is fixed or invading adjacent structures other than the seminal vesicles (e.g. bladder, rectum or pelvic side wall, etc.)
N1	Single metastatic lymph node measuring < 2 cm
N2	Single node 2–5 cm or multiple notes < 5 cm
N3	Nodes > 5 cm
M0	No evidence of distant metastases
M1	Distant metastases present

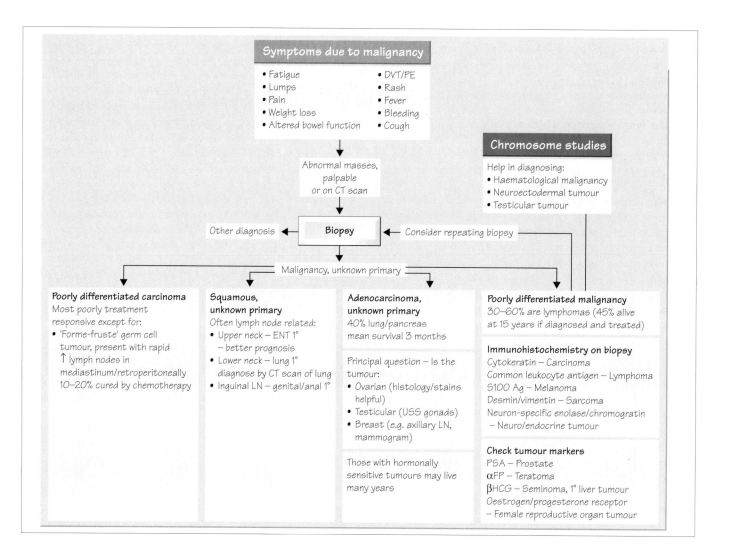

Incidence

Cancer is present without a clear primary source in 5% of all cases. This is a heterogeneous group of cancers that contains treatable and indeed curable subgroups. In this situation, therapeutic nihilism is inappropriate and a treatable cancer should be actively sought. There are four light microscopic diagnoses that typically describe the spectrum of neoplasms of unknown primary site:

1 Poorly differentiated malignancy
2 Adenocarcinoma
3 Squamous carcinoma
4 Poorly differentiated carcinoma

Poorly differentiated malignancy

These are less commonly seen now that advanced immunohisto-chemistry techniques are widely used.

Of the poorly differentiated neoplasms that are hard to identify histologically, the most important of the non-epithelial cancers are lymphoma, melanoma, and sarcoma. Between 30% and 60% of totally undifferentiated neoplasms are lymphomas and eminently treatable

with chemotherapy, with some 45% alive and disease free after 15 years.

The most common cause for uncertainty is an inadequate biopsy, particularly with fine-needle aspiration of accessible but unrepresentative areas of abnormality. Other than repeat biopsy, the most helpful investigation is immunohistochemistry (see figure). Chromosome translocations can be helpful in terms of suggesting a specific diagnosis for a number of haematological diagnoses, but they are also increasingly useful in diagnosing solid tumours such as peripheral neuroectodermal tumours or testicular tumours.

Adenocarcinoma of unknown primary

Adenocarcinoma of unknown primary is the most common type of cancer presenting with an unknown primary and has the poorest prognosis. Of these cases, 40% are the result of lung and pancreatic cancer with a median survival of approximately 3 months. The diagnosis is achieved by elucidating certain histological features, e.g.:

• Papillary formation suggests an ovarian or thyroid primary.
• Mucinous signet rings suggest a gastric primary.

The history and examination (including rectal and vaginal examination) should be reviewed. It is appropriate to measure a number of simple tumour-specific antigens and carry out basic imaging:

• Mammography and computed tomography (CT) of the abdomen, which finds a primary in 10–30% of patients.

• Upper or lower gastrointestinal endoscopy has a very low sensitivity in patients without relevant symptoms.

• In male patients testicular ultrasonography is important.

Certain diagnoses are important to establish, because these cancers are treatable:

• **Papillary ovarian cancer**, suggested by psammoma body formation in women with malignant ascites and a pelvic mass. Serum CA-125 antigen levels may be raised. Surgical cytoreduction and platinum-based chemotherapy prolongs median survival to > 20 months, with some long-term survivors.

• **Occult breast cancer**: serum CA-15.3 antigen levels may be raised. Women with axillary node metastasis usually (40–80% of cases) have a locally advanced breast primary that should be treated surgically. Metastatic disease can be treated by tamoxifen (if oestrogen receptor positive) or chemotherapy.

• **Prostate cancer** in men can present with osteoblastic bone metastases and hormone therapy may provide excellent palliation. Serum prostate-specific antigen (PSA) levels are usually raised. Other cancers that commonly spread to bone are lung, breast, thyroid and renal cancer. Patients with hormonally sensitive cancers typically have a median survival measured in years.

Squamous carcinoma

Patients with squamous cell histology typically present with lymphadenopathy. It is the site of the lymphadenopathy that suggests the location of the underlying primary:

• Upper cervical lymphadenopathy is commonly the result of an ENT (ear, nose, throat) primary, whereas involvement of lower cervical nodes more commonly represents metastases from lung cancer. In young patients with lymphadenopathy and poorly differentiated squamous carcinoma, it is important to determine whether tissue polymerase chain reaction (PCR) reveals Epstein–Barr virus (EBV), because this suggests a nasopharyngeal carcinoma that has a much better prognosis with chemoradiation treatment than other subtypes.

• Inguinal nodes containing squamous cell carcinoma (SCC) typically arise from a genital or an anal primary.

• Skin SCC is rarely metastatic except in immunocompromised patients.

Poorly differentiated carcinoma

It is important to determine whether a poorly differentiated tumour is a variant of germ cell tumour, because these are responsive to chemotherapy. These typically present as rapidly progressing tumours in young adults with lymphadenopathy and involvement of the mediastinum or retroperitoneum. There may be chromosomal abnormalities (i12p), or some staining of histological samples for α-fetoprotein (α-FP). These patients have a 10–20% long-term disease-free survival rate when treated with bleomycin, etoposide and cisplatin (BEP) chemotherapy.

Neuroendocrine carcinoma

Lastly, there is a continuum between carcinoid, low-grade neuroendocrine carcinoma and small cell carcinoma. The first is typically treated with octreotide (and chemotherapy such as temozolomide) with or without interferon, and can be very indolent. The last is similar to small cell carcinoma of the lung, which initially responds to platinum-based chemotherapy.

The decision to treat relates to both the disease and the patient. Palliative chemotherapy is appropriate for fitter and younger patients. Referral to an oncologist is appropriate for every patient who has cancer. In all patients with cancer, or indeed any terminal illness, compassion and support, both emotional and physical (e.g. planning terminal care in conjunction with the local hospice), are vital and are the measure of the physician (see p. 362).

General approach to management

Modern approaches to the management of cancer change rapidly and caring for patients with life threatening diseases is challenging. Patients with more difficult cancers should be referred to multidisciplinary care in cancer centres, as these usually offer not only better care, but more compassionate care.

Paraneoplastic syndromes and hormone-producing cancers

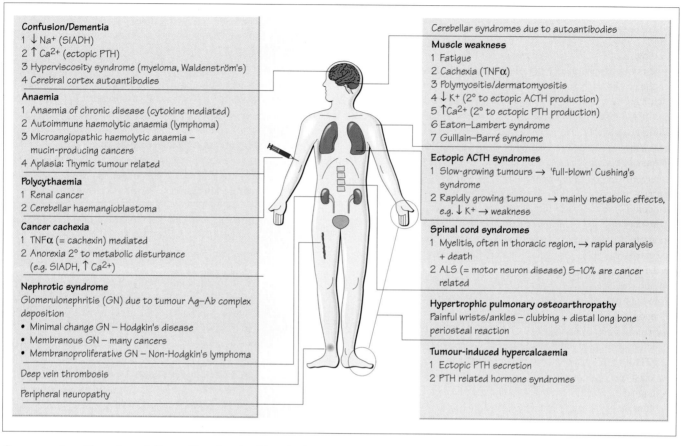

Confusion/Dementia
1 ↓ Na⁺ (SIADH)
2 ↑ Ca²⁺ (ectopic PTH)
3 Hyperviscosity syndrome (myeloma, Waldenström's)
4 Cerebral cortex autoantibodies

Anaemia
1 Anaemia of chronic disease (cytokine mediated)
2 Autoimmune haemolytic anaemia (lymphoma)
3 Microangiopathic haemolytic anaemia – mucin-producing cancers
4 Aplasia: Thymic tumour related

Polycythaemia
1 Renal cancer
2 Cerebellar haemangioblastoma

Cancer cachexia
1 TNFα (= cachexin) mediated
2 Anorexia 2° to metabolic disturbance (e.g. SIADH, ↑ Ca²⁺)

Nephrotic syndrome
Glomerulonephritis (GN) due to tumour Ag–Ab complex deposition
• Minimal change GN – Hodgkin's disease
• Membranous GN – many cancers
• Membranoproliferative GN – Non-Hodgkin's lymphoma

Deep vein thrombosis

Peripheral neuropathy

Cerebellar syndromes due to autoantibodies

Muscle weakness
1 Fatigue
2 Cachexia (TNFα)
3 Polymyositis/dermatomyositis
4 ↓ K⁺ (2° to ectopic ACTH production)
5 ↑Ca²⁺ (2° to ectopic PTH production)
6 Eaton–Lambert syndrome
7 Guillain–Barré syndrome

Ectopic ACTH syndromes
1 Slow-growing tumours → 'full-blown' Cushing's syndrome
2 Rapidly growing tumours → mainly metabolic effects, e.g. ↓ K⁺ → weakness

Spinal cord syndromes
1 Myelitis, often in thoracic region, → rapid paralysis + death
2 ALS (= motor neuron disease) 5–10% are cancer related

Hypertrophic pulmonary osteoarthropathy
Painful wrists/ankles – clubbing + distal long bone periosteal reaction

Tumour-induced hypercalcaemia
1 Ectopic PTH secretion
2 PTH related hormone syndromes

Cancers produce illness through direct effects (e.g. local invasion) and the release of biologically active substances. Diseases produced by the latter are termed 'paraneoplastic syndromes', the most common of which are: anaemia, cachexia and fatigue, tumour-induced hypercalcaemia, syndrome of inappropriate antidiuretic hormone production (SIADH), cushing's syndrome from ectopic ACTH, hypoglycaemia associated with the production of insulin-like growth factors (IGFs)

Pathogenesis

Paraneoplastic syndromes arise from a variety of mechanisms, many of which are still unknown: 1) Through the release of normal cellular proteins, in increased amounts (e.g. ectopic hormone production). 2) Through cytokine production. 3) Via autoantibody production, which typically results in neurological disorders. 4) Via abnormal metabolism of steroids, the production of enzymes or the expression of fetal proteins.

Anaemia

Anaemia in cancer can relate to many factors, including iron deficiency (especially in GI tumours), and folate deficiency (in malnourished patients, and those with very rapidly dividing tumours). However, much anaemia relates to 'the anaemia of chronic disease', whereby the inflammatory response associated with malignancy leads to the production of a number of cytokines that suppress the bone marrow. These include: 1) Disturbance of normal iron metabolism by transforming

growth factor-beta, interleukin (IL)-1, IL-6, and interferon-gamma. These may act through increasing the levels of hepcidin, which suppresses iron uptake and utilization. 2) TNFα (whose levels can be greatly increased in patients with cancer) antagonizing the effects of erythropoietin on the bone marrow. Satisfactory haemoglobin levels can be achieved in about 50% of such patients by giving synthetic recombinant erythropoietin. 3) In rare patients malignancy induces an auto-immune haemolytic anaemia. 4) Rarer still, malignancy can induce red cell aplasia.

Cachexia

The weight loss and malaise associated with cancer relate to the tumour burden, but also, importantly, to the production of cytokines such as TNF or cachexin. Thalidomide, a TNFα antagonist, and progesterones may have a useful symptomatic role.

Syndrome of inappropriate ADH secretion

The inappropriate secretion of vasopressin (ADH) results in hyponatraemia, renal sodium loss, hypervolaemia and inappropriately high urine osmolality. Clinically this may only produce biochemical disease, but it may also produce symptoms relating to the hyponatraemia: tiredness, mental clouding, delirium and coma. The mechanism for the syndrome of inappropriate secretion of ADH (SIADH) in cancer is twofold: 1) Reflex release, by central nervous system (CNS) tumours, drugs or coexisting lung disease. 2) Ectopic hormone release by the tumour, as in SCLC, and more rarely tumours of the duodenum, pancreas, thymus and lymphomas. A precursor molecule is split to produce ADH and neurophysin.

The underlying disease should be aggressively treated; fluid restriction is the mainstay of management. Refractory cases may respond to demeclocycline, which induces nephrogenic diabetes insipidus.

Hypercalcaemia

The most common clinical presentation of an ectopic hormone syndrome is tumour-induced hypercalcaemia (TIH), typically associated with the production of parathyroid hormone-related protein (PTHrP), which has homologues at 8 of its 13 amino acids to parathyroid hormone (PTH) and may activate the PTH receptor. The solid tumours causing ectopic PTH-like secretion are those of squamous cell (e.g. lung), genitourinary or gynaecological origin. The differential diagnosis is hypercalcaemia from bony metastases, usually from lung, breast, prostate, thyroid or renal cell primaries, which develop in 10–20% of patients with disseminated malignancy. Bony metastases, which are the most common cause of malignancy-associated hypercalcaemia, cause hypercalcaemia by causing the release of tumour necrosis factor (TNF), various prostaglandins and other paracrine agents that activate local osteoclasts. Multiple myeloma and T-cell HTLV-associated lymphoma are the most common haematological malignancies associated with TIH, the latter being, in part, the result of the production of vitamin D within the tumour.

Treatment involves correcting the volume depletion that all hypercalcaemic individuals have (caused by calcium-induced diabetes insipidus). Bisphosphonates have revolutionized management of TIH but PTHrP-related hypercalcaemia is often refractory. They inhibit osteoclast function, reduce raised levels of calcium quickly, slow the development of bone metastases, and reduce both the associated symptoms and complications. Steroids are used for steroid-responsive tumours, e.g. multiple myeloma and lymphoma.

Cushing's syndrome

Tumours can produce bizarre syndromes of metabolic upset related to ectopic hormone production. The most common of these is Cushing's syndrome in small cell lung cancer (SCLC), caused by ectopic ACTH production, first reported by Brown in 1928. Overall, 40% of patients with SCLC secrete polypeptides, most of which are not functional, e.g. the precursor molecule to ACTH (pro-opiomelanocortin) is often present in these tumours but only possesses 4% of the biological activity of ACTH. Overall only 2–3% of patients with SCLC have Cushing's syndrome. When the syndrome is acute and prominent, it is typically associated with hirsutism, acne and hypokalaemia, and warrants medical control (see p. 291) both in its own right and because it increases the toxicity of chemotherapeutic regimens.

Hypoglycaemia

Hypoglycaemia in cancer occurs through three mechanisms:

1 Massive size of a slow growing tumour, e.g. mesenchymal sarcomas, lymphomas or mesotheliomas.

2 IGF typically from hepatic or adrenal carcinomas.

3 Insulin secretion by insulinomas, with the rare but classic presentation of fasting hypoglycaemia, commonly associated with neuropsychiatric sequelae and relentless weight gain.

Neurological paraneoplastic syndromes

There are a number of paraneoplastic syndromes affecting the nervous system (see Table 182.1):

• Cerebellar syndrome: anti-Purkinje antibodies (anti-Yo) are associated with this syndrome of cerebellar–cortical degeneration, most commonly seen with carcinoma of the lung, breast or ovary. The cerebellar syndrome has prominent involvement of eye movements, is extremely disabling and precedes the diagnosis of the underlying cancer. The prognosis is poor and is not reversible with successful treatment of the malignancy. Magnetic resonance imaging (MRI) is typically normal and the diagnosis is often one of exclusion.

• The Lambert–Eaton myasthenic syndrome (LEMS): characterized by symmetrical muscle weakness, hyporeflexia and autonomic dysfunction, with improvement in strength on reinforcement. Eye involvement (unlike in myasthenia gravis) is rare. Nerve-evoked acetylcholine release at the neuromuscular junction is reduced. Serum antibodies against voltage-gated calcium channels occur.

• Encephalomyelitis is commonly limbic and associated with dementia or acute behavioural disturbance with hallucination and delusions.

• A subacute sensory neuropathy producing a sensory ataxia is associated with lymphoma, SCLC and the presence of anti-Hu antibodies.

Dermatological

There are many dermatological paraneoplastic syndromes, all of which are associated with stomach or other intra-abdominal malignancies:

• Trousseau's sign of superficial migratory thrombophlebitis.

• The sign of Leser-Trelat (prominent seborrhoeic keratosis).

• Acanthosis nigricans: hyperpigmented velvety plaques found in the axillae and flexural areas.

After the age of 50 half of dermatomyositis cases are associated with an occult malignancy. Pemphigus is associated with malignancy. Gynaecomastia is associated with the production of βhCG by hepatomas or germ-cell tumours.

Rare syndromes

Polymyositis, glomerulonephritis, thrombocytosis, erythrocytosis, pseudo-obstruction.

Table 182.1 Characteristics of paraneoplastic neurological degeneration associated tumours.

* Tumours are often difficult to detect
* Tumours are histologically identical to tumours that develop in patients without paraneoplastic neurological degeneration (PND), except that many tumours have evidence of immune infiltration
* Patients often have improved prognosis relative to those with comparable but non-immunogenic tumours (anti-Hu paraneoplastic syndrome, Lambert-Eaton myasthenic syndrome and some paraneoplastic cerebellar degeneration)
* Rare instances of spontaneous regression have been documented (anti-Hu paraneoplastic syndrome and others)
* Prospective analysis of surrogate of antitumour immune responses predict cancer patient populations with improved prognosis (Hu syndrome)
* Tumours are associated with circulating PND-antigen-specific killer T-cells (paraneoplastic cerebellar degeneration)

From *Nat Rev Cancer* **4**(1):36–44, 2004. © 2004 Nature Publishing Group.

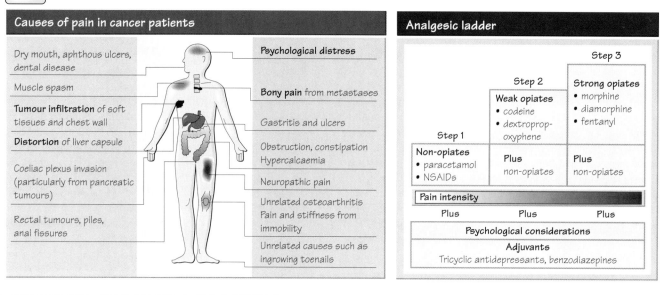

The management of patients with terminal malignant illness is challenging—there are many physical and psychological symptoms to relieve and there are important ethical issues surrounding withholding and withdrawing treatment. The last phase of a terminal illness should be managed meticulously because this dramatically improves the quality of life for the patient and his or her family. Patients require:
• Physical support (symptom control); these can be assessed from the acronym OPQRST 'O – onset or origin; P – palliate or provoke; Q – quality and quantity; R – radiation; S – severity or significance; T – timing.
• Psychological support
• Social, financial and spiritual support.
  Underlying terminal illness care is clear and empathic communication with the patient and his or her family.

Pain

Multiple factors moderate pain appreciation, including psychological factors, e.g. *anxiety, fear and cultural beliefs*. Social factors and interpersonal relationships influence pain appreciation in positive or negative ways. A critically important factor is the quality and quantity of sleep; tiredness makes any pain worse. Mechanisms underlying pain in malignancy include:
• Direct causes: neuropathic pain (nerve damage), bony pain (malignant infiltration), visceral and soft tissue pain (pressure effects or direct obstruction).
• Treatment-related pain: from radiotherapy, surgery or drug side effects.
• Cancer-related causes: patients with advanced cancer are debilitated and immobile. This may cause joint pains, pressure sores and constipation.
• Causes unrelated to cancer: cancer patients are prone to all the diseases that those without cancer experience, e.g. arthritis.

Clinical evaluation of pain

A careful history and examination are vital, both to diagnose the problem and to build trust and develop empathy with the patient. Site, severity, nature, duration, timing, and precipitating and relieving factors should be noted. As those with cancer often have more than one pain, all the different pains should be discussed. Examination allows accurate determination of exactly where the pain is and its severity (see figure opposite).

General approach to treating pain

Reassurance, a calm confident manner and empathy are critically important. The fears of the patient need to be identified and addressed, and this is best done when rapport has been established.
• Local heat is useful for most types of pain, especially muscular pain.
• Non-traditional measures such as acupuncture, massage and reflexology are all helpful in many patients regardless of causation of the pain.
• Lifestyle modification, such as avoiding painful activity, if necessary using aids or wheelchairs, may be helpful.
• Specific therapies: radio- or chemotherapy and surgery all have important roles, both at the site of the primary and the metastasis.
• Surgery is also used for anticipated complications such as imminent bowel obstruction.
• Medical therapies: the standard approach to pain management is 'the analgesic ladder'—non-opioid drugs (paracetamol, etc.), weak opioids (codeine, etc.), strong opioids (morphine, etc.). Opiates should be given regularly in sufficient doses; it is easier to prevent than treat breakthrough pain. The pain ladder is *not* a substitute for a careful clinical assessment of the pain, and it is important to realize that some pains respond better to adjuvant treatment rather than to one specified on the ladder.
• Anaesthetic interventions: nerve infiltration/block relieve well-localized pain with fewer side effects than drugs. Occasionally epidurals

Diseases and Treatments at a Glance

are used. TENS (transcutaneous electrical nerve stimulation) may also be very helpful.

Treatment of specific forms of pain

Neuropathic pains are burning, stinging, stabbing or shooting in nature, have a deep aching component and prevent sleep. Pain follows a dermatomal distribution, although in sympathetically mediated pain an arterial distribution occurs. Important clues to the presence of neuropathic pain are: altered or absent sensation in the area where the pain is perceived; allodynia—a normally painless stimulus experienced as a painful one; and opiate-resistant pain. Neuropathic pain arises from:
- Tumour infiltration of nerves: steroids or radiotherapy help.
- Neural damage from treatment (particularly radiotherapy to the brachial plexus or neurotoxic chemotherapy).
- Other causes (e.g. post-herpetic neuralgia).

In all cases a good night's sleep helps (night sedation), as do tricyclic antidepressants ± anticonvulsants (e.g. gabapentin). If these are ineffective, class I agents (e.g. flecainide) or low-dose ketamine may help.

Bone pain: tenderness over bone is the main diagnostic feature. Exclude pathological fractures and spinal cord compression. Non-steroidal anti-inflammatory drugs (NSAIDs) are first-line treatment, and radiotherapy if these fail. Bisphosphonates work in metastatic pain caused by myeloma or breast cancer. Occasionally surgical fixation/resection is necessary.

Abdominal discomfort/pain arises from:
- Constipation, from drug side effects, poor diet (anorexia) and immobility, treated with laxatives. Obstruction (see p. 36) and impaction must be excluded, because these require specific treatments.
- Gastritis: proton pump inhibitors and stopping NSAIDs.
- Liver capsule pain from hepatic secondaries may respond to steroids.
- Bladder spasm responds to oxybutynin.

- Hypercalcaemia can cause abdominal pain and responds to rehydration, bisphosphonates and steroids.

Rectal pain mainly relates to constipation and its complications or direct tumour invasion. Laxatives, local (topical) steroids, anaesthetics (e.g. lidocaine or lignocaine) and radiotherapy all have therapeutic roles.

Muscle spasm usually responds to simple measures or benzodiazepines.

Other symptoms

Nausea and vomiting have many of the same causes as abdominal discomfort, although there are additional aetiological factors:
- Local causes, e.g. bowel obstruction or raised intracranial pressure.
- Unrelated, e.g. alcoholic gastritis, coincidental renal failure, etc.
- Full examination and 'basic' tests (renal and liver function, calcium, chest or abdominal X-rays) usually elucidate the mechanism and direct therapy. Otherwise, good oral hygiene, antiemetics, haloperidol, metoclopramide and odansetron may all prove useful; if not dexamethasone may ease symptoms.
- Mouth care: mouth discomfort relates to a dry mouth (anorexia, dehydration, opiates, tricyclics). Sucking ice cubes or fruit, regular mouthwash and antifungal therapy (fluconazole) all help.
- Respiratory distress: an accurate diagnosis is needed and specific therapy may help (antibiotics for infection, radiotherapy for bronchial obstruction). Opiates are given for irremediable pathology. Home oxygen may help.
- Night sweats and anorexia, if not related to infection, may relate to 'cachexin' (TNFα) and respond to steroids ± thalidomide.
- Psychological distress and depression: empathy, active listening and realistic encouragement ± antidepressants.

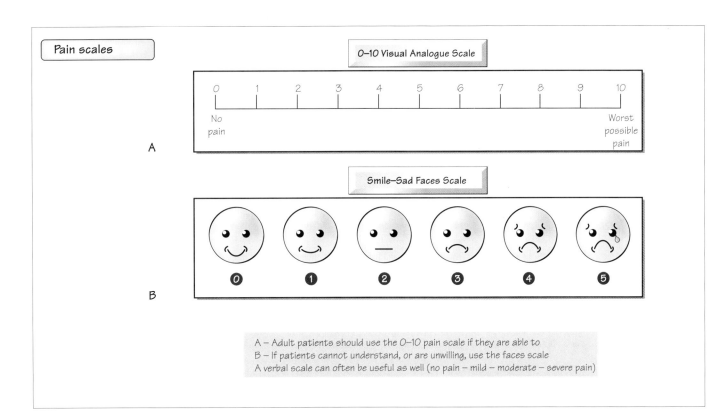

Pain scales

0–10 Visual Analogue Scale

0 1 2 3 4 5 6 7 8 9 10

No pain — Worst possible pain

A

Smile–Sad Faces Scale

0 1 2 3 4 5

B

A – Adult patients should use the 0–10 pain scale if they are able to
B – If patients cannot understand, or are unwilling, use the faces scale
A verbal scale can often be useful as well (no pain – mild – moderate – severe pain)

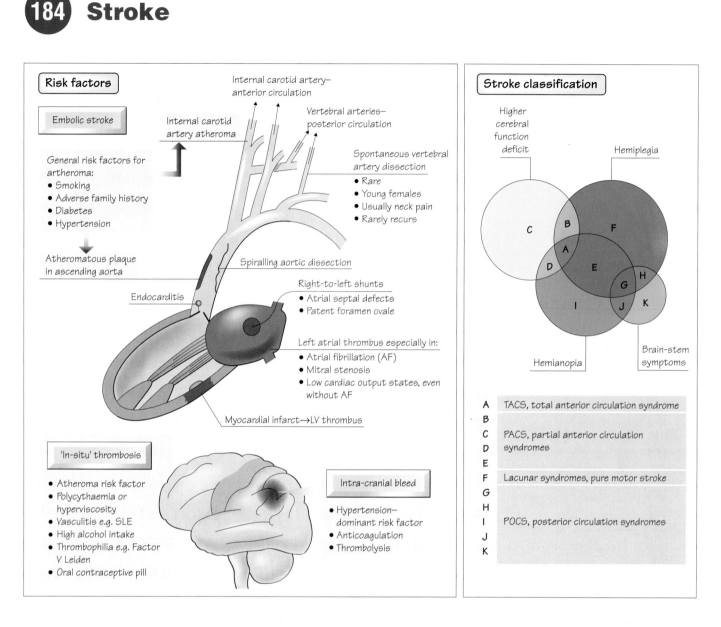

Risk factors

Embolic stroke

Internal carotid artery–anterior circulation

Vertebral arteries–posterior circulation

Internal carotid artery atheroma

General risk factors for artheroma:
- Smoking
- Adverse family history
- Diabetes
- Hypertension

Spontaneous vertebral artery dissection
- Rare
- Young females
- Usually neck pain
- Rarely recurs

Atheromatous plaque in ascending aorta

Spiralling aortic dissection

Right-to-left shunts
- Atrial septal defects
- Patent foramen ovale

Endocarditis

Left atrial thrombus especially in:
- Atrial fibrillation (AF)
- Mitral stenosis
- Low cardiac output states, even without AF

Myocardial infarct→LV thrombus

'In-situ' thrombosis

- Atheroma risk factor
- Polycythaemia or hyperviscosity
- Vasculitis e.g. SLE
- High alcohol intake
- Thrombophilia e.g. Factor V Leiden
- Oral contraceptive pill

Intra-cranial bleed

- Hypertension—dominant risk factor
- Anticoagulation
- Thrombolysis

Stroke classification

Higher cerebral function deficit

Hemiplegia

Hemianopia

Brain-stem symptoms

A	TACS, total anterior circulation syndrome
B	
C	PACS, partial anterior circulation
D	syndromes
E	
F	Lacunar syndromes, pure motor stroke
G	
H	
I	POCS, posterior circulation syndromes
J	
K	

Stroke is the most common condition affecting the brain, with 100 000 new strokes/year in the UK.

Key features
Neurological symptoms resulting from cerebrovascular disease are:
- Of sudden onset: very occasionally other neurological diseases present suddenly, e.g. brain tumours, demyelination and hypoglycaemia. Evolving neurological signs are not usually the result of vascular pathology, although occasionally major vessel occlusion (e.g. internal carotid artery) presents as a stuttering stroke.
- Usually vaso-occlusive, either thromboembolic (emboli from the heart in 20% of cases, or from atheromatous plaques in the aorta, extra- or intracranial circulation in the remaining 80%) leading to major vessel occlusion or *in situ* vascular blockage, usually small vessel and leading to lacunar syndromes.
- Occasionally caused by haemorrhage, which should be considered in those with marked hypertension, on anticoagulants or with prominent headache.

There are a small number of very common stroke syndromes and a very large number of rare stroke syndromes.

Time course of strokes
- Transient ischaemic attacks (TIAs) by definition can last up to 24 h although usually they last less than a few minutes.
  - Types: TIAs affect all vascular territories, causing any pattern of neurological dysfunction. The most characteristic is amaurosis fugax, where embolic atherogenic debris from the carotid artery travels to the ophthalmic branch of the internal carotid, causing unilateral blindness, lasting less than a few minutes. Transient global amnesia, is where patients are transiently (a few hours or more) unable to lay down memory. Of uncertain pathology, it may be a migrainous phenomenon or an unusual form of TIA.
  - Significance: TIAs imply an active intravascular plaque, i.e. one on which thrombosis is actively occurring and embolizing distally. They are a major risk factor for subsequent disabling stroke.
  - Investigation: urgent investigation (carotid ultrasonography), to

Table 184.1 Stroke prognosis.

	TAC	PAC	LAC	POC
30 day				
Dead	40	5	5	5
Dependent	55	40	30	30
Independent	5	55	65	65
1 year				
Dead	60	15	10	20
Dependent	35	30	30	20
Independent	5	55	60	60

LAC, lacunar infarction; PAC, partial anterior circulation; POC, posterior circulation; TAC, total anterior circulation.

determine whether a high-grade lesion, i.e. > 7 stenosis in the internal carotid artery is present, should be undertaken because surgical resection ('carotid endarterectomy') significantly reduces the rate of disabling stroke.

• Minor strokes have small neurological deficits. Their importance is the same as TIAs—they may be a harbinger of more severe strokes. Sufferers have established vascular disease and need vigorous anti-atherogenic therapy.

• Completed stroke implies that the deficit is major, persistent and does not subsequently deteriorate. Unless recovery is good, 'the horse has bolted' and investigations as a prelude to carotid endarterectomy are not indicated.

Anatomy of strokes

An important distinction is between stroke in the anterior (carotid) or the posterior (vertebrobasilar) circulation, because this relates to prognosis (see Table 184.1) and determines the nature of the investigations. Constitutional differences in the cerebral circulation, and the effects of diffuse atheroma on the circle of Willis, mean that it is not always possible to give an accurate clinical determination of the site of occlusion.

Anatomy of stroke 'syndromes'

Carotid territory stroke presents with a combination of hemiplegia and language dysfunction (dominant hemisphere) or dyspraxia (inability to carry out complex tasks not caused by motor deficits) or denial of the existence (neglect) of the left side (non-dominant hemisphere). Middle cerebral artery (MCA) occlusion has in addition hemianaesthesia and hemianopia. An MCA infarct is often large and extensive brain damage may occur, resulting in coma and even death. Recovery is often very poor.

Vertebrobasilar: there are many eponymous brain-stem vascular syndromes of dubious relevance. The combination of any of the following with sudden onset suggests a posterior circulation stroke:

• Diplopia
• Dysarthria
• Unsteadiness
• Dysphagia
• Unilateral weakness with contralateral facial weakness
• Bilateral visual loss
• Amnesia.

Posterior strokes, unlike anterior circulation ones, may have a stuttering evolution. Basilar artery occlusion is frequently catastrophic and fatal. Pontine strokes cause coma, pinpoint pupils, paresis, pyrexia and frequently death.

Lacunar syndromes are by definition small (< 1.5 cm^3). They may cause internal capsule strokes which are usually either pure motor or pure sensory. Neither of these has an ocular field defect. Recovery is typically more complete than in MCA occlusive syndromes.

Summary of causes of hemiplegia (see p. 96)

• **MCA cortical infarct** (hemiplegia + hemianaesthesia + hemianopia). Haemorrhage into the internal capsule produces a similar triad of signs.

• **Internal capsule lesions**: usually produce rather discrete neurological deficits, such as a 'pure' motor hemiplegia/monoplegia or 'pure' sensory hemianaesthesia.

• **Basis pontis**: dysarthria but not dysphasia may occur, i.e. clumsy hand dysarthria.

• **Brain-stem lesions**: associated with nystagmus, ocular palsies, cerebellar signs.

Risk factors for stroke

These are as for arterial disease, i.e. increasing age, male sex, adverse genes (i.e. family history of vascular disease), hypertension, smoking and diabetes. Structural heart disease predisposes to stroke, especially recent myocardial infarction (MI) (± 1% of patients have a stroke during an MI) or atrial fibrillation (especially in those > 65 years or with left ventricular dysfunction). Excess alcohol is a substantial risk factor, particularly in young men. Polycythaemia underlies a few strokes. It has not been established that high cholesterol is a strong primary risk factor for stroke, though lowering cholesterol is an important measure in secondary prevention. With neurosyphilis 45% of cases present as a stroke. For intracerebral haemorrhage, the strongest risk factor is hypertension or vascular abnormality, e.g. arteriovenous malformation (AVM) or aneurysm, a bleeding diathesis or thrombolytic therapy.

'Young stroke'

Most people aged over 40 years who have had a stroke have the same risk factors as older patients. A few additional conditions should also be considered:

• Infective endocarditis.
• Antiphospholipid syndrome.
• Syphilis.
• Cerebral vasculitis (including systemic lupus erythematosus [SLE]).
• Carotid/vertebral dissection.
• Mitochondrial diseases such as MELAS (**m**itochondrial **e**ncephalopathy, **l**actic **a**cidosis, **s**troke-like episodes).
• Inherited thrombophilias, such as protein C and S deficiency, usually produce venous thrombosis in the deep veins of the calf, but occasionally cause stroke, particularly venous sinus thrombosis.
• Structural abnormalities of the extracranial vessels (e.g. moya moya disease, angiographic diagnosis of bilateral distal occlusion/multiple stenosis of the internal carotid artery, with net-like collaterals around the brain base).
• Drug induced, e.g. cocaine.

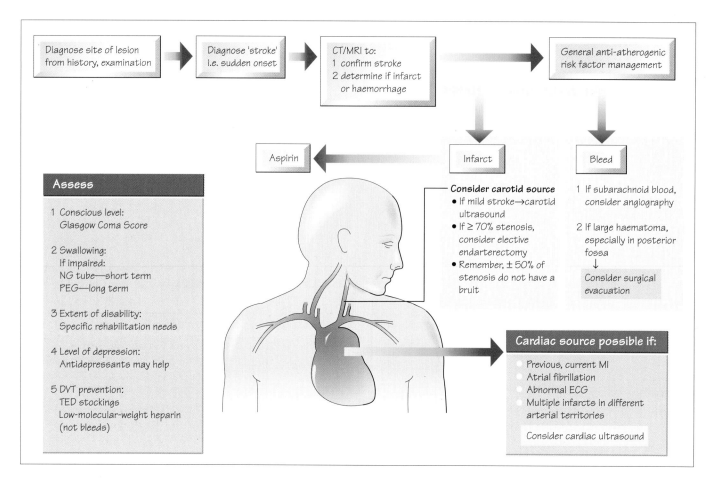

Diagnose site of lesion from history, examination → Diagnose 'stroke' i.e. sudden onset → CT/MRI to: 1 confirm stroke 2 determine if infarct or haemorrhage → General anti-atherogenic risk factor management

Aspirin ← Infarct   Bleed

Assess

1 Conscious level: Glasgow Coma Score

2 Swallowing: If impaired: NG tube—short term PEG—long term

3 Extent of disability: Specific rehabilitation needs

4 Level of depression: Antidepressants may help

5 DVT prevention: TED stockings Low-molecular-weight heparin (not bleeds)

Consider carotid source
- If mild stroke→carotid ultrasound
- If ≥ 70% stenosis, consider elective endarterectomy
- Remember, ± 50% of stenosis do not have a bruit

1 If subarachnoid blood, consider angiography

2 If large haematoma, especially in posterior fossa ↓ Consider surgical evacuation

Cardiac source possible if:
- Previous, current MI
- Atrial fibrillation
- Abnormal ECG
- Multiple infarcts in different arterial territories

Consider cardiac ultrasound

General approach

The mechanism of stroke (infarct or bleed) must be determined by computed tomography (CT) or magnetic resonance imaging (MRI):
- Infarct: the origin of thrombus must be worked out, i.e. from *in situ* thrombosis or emboli originating more proximally, either from the heart or atheromatous plaques in the:
  - carotid artery, which are diagnosed by ultrasonography
  - aortic arch found by transoesophageal echocardiography; management is unclear.
- Haemorrhage: if the clinical condition of the patient is not poor, and especially if there is any suggestion that the bleed is the result of a subarachnoid haemorrhage (see below), it may be appropriate to undertake angiography (conventional or MR) to exclude an aneurysm/ arteriovenous malformation (AVM) that might benefit from surgery/ intervention.

Acute management

A realistic assessment of prognosis should be sympathetically communicated to relatives. Patients should, if possible, be nursed in dedicated stroke units because these improve outcome.

Cerebral infarcts

- Blood pressure in the long term should be low, but should not be decreased acutely because this may provoke watershed infarcts.

- Aspirin and other antiplatelet agents are used to decrease the incidence of further strokes. Thrombolytics continue to undergo evaluation. Current evidence suggests that disability is reduced if given < 3 h from symptom onset.

Intracerebral haemorrhage

- Blood pressure should probably be lowered more rapidly in cerebral haemorrhage.
- Posterior fossa bleeds may need neurosurgical evacuation to prevent coning of the brain. Likewise, large intracerebral bleeds with mass effects in young people may benefit from evacuation.

All strokes

- Swallowing dysfunction should be assessed. If the risk of aspiration is not low, feeding should be by nasogastric tube or, in the longer term, by percutaneous enterogastrostomy (PEG) feeding tube.
- Prevention of deep venous thrombosis: using thromboembolic (TED) stockings, or possibly low-dose heparin (not cerebral bleeds).
- Good nursing care is the most important factor in outcome.
- Physiotherapy to prevent contractures and help in mobilization.
- Depression occurs in 50–75% of patients. Antidepressants may help.

Long-term management (see Table 185.1)

- General vascular risk protection: the annual stroke recurrence rate of

10% is reduced by meticulous control of vascular risk factors (secondary prevention), especially smoking, diabetes and blood pressure (aim for ≤ 140/85). Cholesterol reduction reduces the rate of further strokes, despite an elevated cholesterol not being a major risk factor for stroke in epidemiological studies.

• Carotid endarterectomy: most patients ≤ 75 years with small anterior circulation stroke syndromes should have carotid imaging. Those with high-grade lesions (≥ 70% stenosis) may benefit from carotid endarterectomy.

• Management and prevention of disability: 25–50% after a first stroke do not re-achieve independence and require extensive nursing support. Financial and physical aids help.

• Multidisciplinary management of home environment can restore independence.

Table 185.1 The management of stroke.

Problem	Frequency	Importance	Preventive measures	Interventions for established problem
Fever	Common	Associated with worse outcome	Routine antipyretics	Fanning, antipyretics, treat underlying cause
Low PO_2	Common	↑ Brain ischaemia	Positioning to avoid cardio-respiratory problems	Supplementary O_2
Low BP	Uncommon—may reflect dehydration	May ↑ brain ischaemia	Avoid cause	Treat cause
High BP	Very common	May reflect long-standing ↑ BP, or reaction to CVA; may ↑ brain oedema/bleeding		BP lowering—but these may ↑ brain ischaemia
↑ Blood glucose	20–40%	Associated with ↓ outcome	Avoid dextrose infusions	Insulin
↑ Intracranial pressure	↓ Consciousness in most CVAs reflects ↑ ICP	Commonest cause of death ≤ 1 week	Raising end of bed; avoid over-hydration	Anti-oedema drugs, ventilation, decompressive surgery
Sleep disordered breathing	65% of patients	Unknown	Avoid sedatives	CPAP
Dysphagia	50% of patients	Prevents oral feeding; increases risk of chest infection	Routine screening (SALT)	Nil by mouth, parenteral or enteral feeding
Epileptic seizures	5% of patients	Leads to neurological deterioration	None	Anticonvulsants
Spasticity and contractures	Depends on preventative measures	Limits function and predisposes to bed sores	Positioning, relief muscle tone (anxiety, pain, overuse)	Physiotherapy, splinting, tone modifying drugs, botulinum toxin
Emotionalism	20%	Interrupts therapy, social isolation		Antidepressants
Urinary infection	25% in first month	Unwell →↓ functional level	Maintain hydration, avoid catheters	Antibiotics, fluids
Chest infection	25% in first month	↓ PO_2; → ↓ functional level	Early mobilization, chest physiotherapy, SALT	Antibiotics, chest physiotherapy
Undernutrition	20%	Associated with worse outcome	Nutritional screening; oral supplementation	Oral supplementation, enteral-tube feeding
Electrolyte imbalance	Common	May → confusion, seizures	Monitor biochemistry	Supplements etc.
DVT	50%	May progress to lethal PE; pain, fever	Early mobilization, good hydration, antiplatelet drugs, TED stockings	Anticoagulation
PE	5%	May → death	As above	As above
Urinary, faecal incontinence	50%	Demeaning, bed sores	Avoid exacerbating factors, e.g. diuretics	Treat cause if found; bladder retraining, pads, catheters
Pressure sores	< 3% with good nursing	Painful, distressing, can → death	Good nursing	Relieve pressure, antibiotics, vitamins
Falls and fractures	Falls common in 35%; fractures rare	Pain, ↓ functional level	Careful supervision; anti-osteoporosis drugs	Standard orthopaedic care for fractures
Painful shoulder	Common	↓ Function and mood	Avoid traction injury	Physiotherapy, analgesics, local steroid injections
Low mood	Very common	Associated with worse outcome	Positive attitude in stroke unit staff	Antidepressants, cognitive behavioural therapy

Adapted from Charles Warlow et al., Stroke, *Lancet* 2003; 362: 1211–24 with permission from Elsevier © 2003

Diseases and Treatments at a Glance

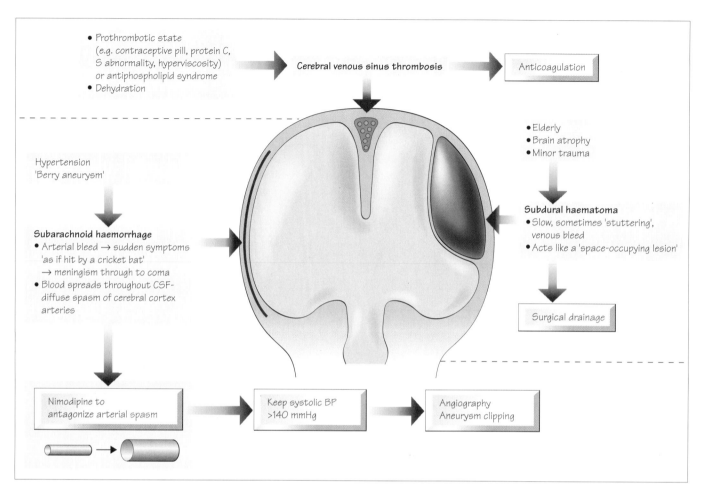

Subarachnoid haemorrhage

Subarachnoid haemorrhage (SAH) is an arterial bleed from a ruptured berry aneurysm (70% of cases) or arteriovenous malformation (AVM) (10% of cases). There are 3000 cases/year in the UK.

Clinical features and diagnosis

Classic presentation is with a thunderclap headache, often in the occiput. The signs range from none (headache only), through mild meningism to coma. Focal neurological signs are uncommon. Thirty per cent of patients die of the acute bleed: if a re-bleed occurs the mortality rate is ≥ 60%. A computed tomography (CT) scan should be performed in all suspected cased of SAH. If this is not diagnostic then a delayed (≥ 12 h after symptom onset) lumbar puncture, looking for xanthochromia (bilirubin on spectrophotometry) should be undertaken.

Treatment

Acutely, blood pressure (BP) should be maintained at 150 mmHg (with intravenous fluids/inotropes if BP too low), although more chronically BP should be lowered to < 140/85. Subarachnoid blood induces damaging cerebral artery spasm, which can be antagonized by nimodipine to improve outcome. The responsible aneurysms can be detected by angiography and treated by surgical clipping (open craniotomy) or by endovascular occlusion with platinum coils.

Prognosis

Prognosis is poor once coma or major neurological defect has developed —intervention should therefore occur early on. Overall < 40% of cases have a good outcome.

Subdural haemorrhage

Subdural haemorrhage (SHD) is a venous bleed, often occurring in the context of brain shrinkage (from age, dementia, chronic alcoholism, etc.). Blood slowly oozes into the subdural space. As this breaks down, osmotically active degradation products are formed, sucking in fluid from the extracellular space. Thus SHDs act as space-occupying lesions, expanding slowly over several weeks. Clinically there may be a history of trauma, although this is often absent. Subsequently, there is the slow (a few weeks or more) progression of a focal neurological deficit; equally, elderly patients may present rather non-specifically with decreased mobility ('off-legs') or decreased mental agility. There are usually focal neurological signs, although these are not always present. CT scanning is diagnostic, although a diagnostic trap for the unwary is that 'old' blood (i.e. of the age of many SDHs) may be isodense with the brain. Surgical evacuation should be considered in all affected patients, however, elderly.

Venous sinus thrombosis

Cerebral venous sinus thrombosis (CVT) is a life-threatening condition with an extremely broad range of clinical neurological presentations and a large differential diagnosis.

Demographics

Cerebral vein thrombosis is a rare event, there being estimated to be only some 250–500 cases/year in the UK (60 in peri/postpartum women). Seventy-five per cent of patients are female and younger ages predominate.

Clinical features

CVT must be considered in acute or subacute headache, seizures, and disorders of consciousness or papilloedema. The condition can mimic stroke, abscess, tumour, encephalitis or idiopathic intracranial hypertension.

The presenting symptoms depend on which vein occluded (see below). The pathophysiology can be traced to one of the following two causes:

1 Due to local cerebral vein occlusion → local effects (→ focal signs e.g. cortical signs—weakness etc.; or from deep structures e.g. thalamus → confusion, amnesia, mutism; brain stem → coma). Seizures occur in 40% due to local brain tissue damage.

2 Due to occlusion of cerebral sinuses, leading to intra-cranial hypertension (→ headache, found in 90%; the only symptom in 20%, 80% have focal defects).

Aetiology

There is a wide range of underlying aetiologies including inherited thrombophilias, oral contraception, pregnancy, local intracranial sepsis and systemic inflammatory diseases, such as sarcoidosis and Behçet's disease. It occurs very rarely following lumbar puncture. A predisposing illness is found in 85% of patients.

Diagnosis

The diagnosis can usually be reliably made with magnetic resonance imaging (MRI with contrast angiography—shows the thrombus, the veinous infarct with, in 40%, haemorrhagic transformation), although the 'gold' standard is conventional angiography.

Treatment

Treatment with heparin may improve survival and disability, and patients who continue to deteriorate may be suitable for local thrombolysis. If the intracranial pressure is high, mannitol, ± acetazolamide are sometimes used. Surgical removal of the brain infarct has been recommended by some for high intracranial pressures with deteriorating neurological condition.

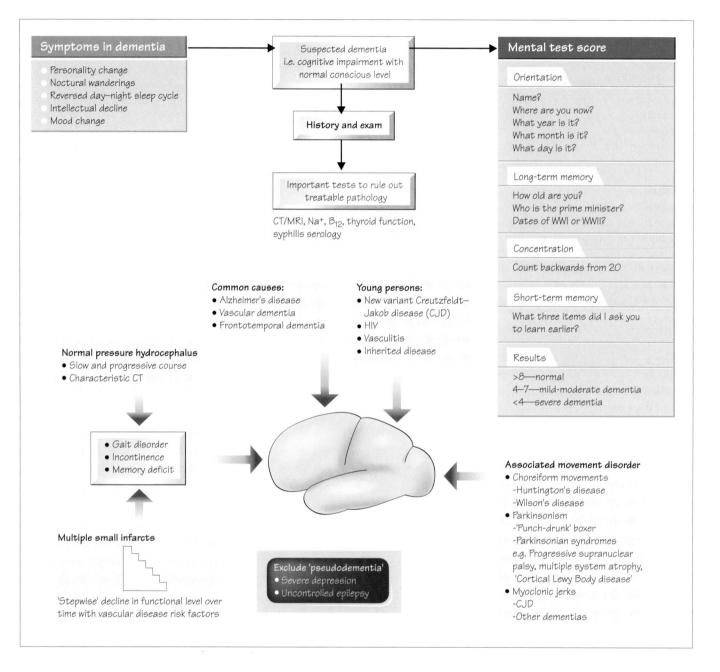

Symptoms in dementia

- Personality change
- Noctural wanderings
- Reversed day–night sleep cycle
- Intellectual decline
- Mood change

Suspected dementia
i.e. cognitive impairment with
normal conscious level

History and exam

Important tests to rule out
treatable pathology

CT/MRI, Na$^+$, B$_{12}$, thyroid function,
syphilis serology

Mental test score

Orientation

Name?
Where are you now?
What year is it?
What month is it?
What day is it?

Long-term memory

How old are you?
Who is the prime minister?
Dates of WWI or WWII?

Concentration

Count backwards from 20

Short-term memory

What three items did I ask you
to learn earlier?

Results

>8—normal
4–7—mild-moderate dementia
<4—severe dementia

Common causes:
- Alzheimer's disease
- Vascular dementia
- Frontotemporal dementia

Young persons:
- New variant Creutzfeldt–Jakob disease (CJD)
- HIV
- Vasculitis
- Inherited disease

Normal pressure hydrocephalus
- Slow and progressive course
- Characteristic CT

- Gait disorder
- Incontinence
- Memory deficit

Multiple small infarcts

'Stepwise' decline in functional level over
time with vascular disease risk factors

Exclude 'pseudodementia'
- Severe depression
- Uncontrolled epilepsy

Associated movement disorder
- Choreiform movements
  -Huntington's disease
  -Wilson's disease
- Parkinsonism
  -'Punch-drunk' boxer
  -Parkinsonian syndromes
  e.g. Progressive supranuclear
  palsy, multiple system atrophy,
  'Cortical Lewy Body disease'
- Myoclonic jerks
  -CJD
  -Other dementias

Dementia is 'the global impairment of cognition with normal levels of consciousness', in contrast to an acute confusional state, in which conscious level is impaired. The incidence is 5% in those aged ≥ 65 years and 20% in those aged ≥ 85 years. With emerging therapies, it is important to attempt a specific diagnosis, although this is not easy because clinical tools are not accurate. Many people labelled as having Alzheimer's disease have a different postmortem diagnosis. Patients who complain of memory disturbance are far more likely to be suffering from anxiety, because those with genuine dementia usually have no insight. Potentially treatable causes of cognitive impairment include:

- Depression: all patients with dementia should have a mental state examination to exclude depressive pseudo-dementia. However, it

should be remembered that depressive symptomatology is a feature of all dementias.

- Normal pressure hydrocephalus may be the result of a diffuse abnormality affecting cerebrospinal fluid (CSF) uptake; it causes ventricular dilatation, and is suggested by the triad of dementia, incontinence and gait disturbance. Therapeutic lumbar puncture can lead to overt improvement and is used to select patients suitable for shunting.

- Subdural haematoma may present without any antecedent history of trauma as a subacute change in cognitive function with gait disturbance.

- Intracranial tumours are a common cause of sub-acute cognitive decline. Focal symptoms/signs are usually present.

- Hypothyroidism may produce mild-to-moderate cognitive impairment.

- Chronic severe hyponatraemia
- Vitamin B12 deficiency.
- Neurosyphilis or general paralysis of the insane (GPI).
- Vasculitis.
- Paraneoplastic syndromes (see p. 360) rarely cause pure dementia, e.g. tumour-associated limbic encephalitis can present with personality changes.
- Whipple's disease is associated with cognitive impairment, which may improve with antibiotics.

All patients should therefore have CT head scans, and vitamin B12, thyroid function and syphilis serology checked, as well as a full blood count, biochemical tests of renal and hepatic function and an erythrocyte sedimentation rate (ESR) to look for systemic diseases producing cognitive impairment.

Alzheimer's disease

Alzheimer's disease begins most frequently with gradual impairment of episodic memory, but eventually produces global cognitive decline, i.e. early on new memory cannot be laid down, although childhood memories remain accessible. Later on, no memory can be recalled. Although it may be normal early in the disease, volumetric MRI shows specific atrophy of the temporal lobes. Of the cases of Alzheimer's disease, 5% are familial and usually of earlier onset. Mutations have been identified in the Presenilin 1 and 2 genes and in the amyloid precursor protein gene (APP). Certain apolipoprotein E polymorphisms, specifically ε4, predispose to Alzheimer's disease. Pathologically, there is cortical neuron loss, including loss of cholinergic neurons, which form the basis of the usage of acetylcholinesterase inhibitors, which have small but definite beneficial effects. The disease progresses relentlessly, causing death from pneumonia or inanition after 8–10 years. The key to management is to care for the sufferer on a 'symptom-by-symptom' basis and to provide good support and relief for the caregiver.

Frontotemporal dementia (Pick's disease)

In frontotemporal dementia (FTD), there is prominent personality change and a dysexecutive syndrome develops, i.e. sufferers are reluctant to initiate any actions or they may be frankly disinhibited. Preserved areas of ability such as memory are key diagnostic features. Onset is usually at age 65 years or older. MRI shows frontal and/or temporal atrophy. The FTDs are heterogeneous in aetiology and include Pick's disease, in which characteristic neuropathology occurs. Other FTDs are the result of mutations in the microtubule-associated tau protein. Of patients with motor neuron disease, 30% develop a mild dysexecutive syndrome and occasionally (3–4%) frank frontotemporal dementia is the predominant clinical finding, with denervation atrophy and fasciculations appearing later.

Vascular dementia

The history is of stepwise evolution of cognitive impairment and focal neurological signs, in someone with the appropriate risk factors. A small stepping gait is characteristic. Memory may be less impaired in relation to defects in visuoperceptual tasking. MRI shows atrophy with diffuse white and grey matter vascular lesions (Binswanger's encephalopathy is CT evidence of white matter infarction, with dementia, in hypertensive patients with a stroke). The diagnostic accuracy is often hampered by finding cerebrovascular disease in Alzheimer's disease patients. Treating vascular disease risk factors and aspirin may slow progression.

Lewy body dementia

This causes parkinsonism (see p. 386). Typical features are fluctuating cognition, nocturnal visual hallucinations and disordered rapid eye movement (REM) sleep. Imaging is normal or shows diffuse atrophy. L-Dopa may dramatically exacerbate the psychiatric symptoms, while treatment with antipsychotics can lead to a catastrophic and potentially fatal decline in motor performance.

Prion diseases

Prions are mutated proteins that induce a conformational change in certain constitutive brain proteins, so producing non-functional, non-metabolizable forms. These gradually build up, producing brain dysfunction. Sporadic and inherited forms of Creutzfeldt–Jakob disease (CJD) cause a rapidly progressive dementia with myoclonus, ataxia and cortical blindness progressing over months. The EEG shows characteristic repetitive complexes. New variant CJD (transmitted from cattle infected with the bovine spongiform encephalopathy agent) seems to occur in younger patients, has a slower evolution and is associated with psychiatric symptoms as the earliest feature.

Cognitive impairment in younger patients

The distinction between young and old in terms of causation is potentially artificial, and consideration of the conditions listed below should be driven by the presence of specific neurological symptoms and signs, such as dystonia, and the presence of specific risk factors:

- 'Recreational' drugs, especially alcohol, and also glue.
- HIV-related dementia occurs as a late feature. Infections and structural lesions must be ruled out (lymphoma, toxoplasmosis, progressive multi-focal leukoencephalopathy [PML]).
- Cerebral vasculitis.
- End-stage multiple sclerosis.
- Adrenoleukodystrophies resulting from fatty acid dysmetabolism cause a 'multiple sclerosis-type' pattern with prominent dementia.
- CADASIL: a white matter disease associated with mutations in the notch-3 gene—presents as hemiplegic migraine or a progressive dementia.
- Wilson's disease.
- Uncontrolled epilepsy may produce a 'twilight' state, in which seizures are so frequent as to disallow full recovery in between. Rarely, so-called 'non-convulsive status', in which patients appear vacant and are seen to perform repetitive movements, may be misinterpreted as a rapidly progressive dementia. The EEG is diagnostic.

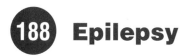

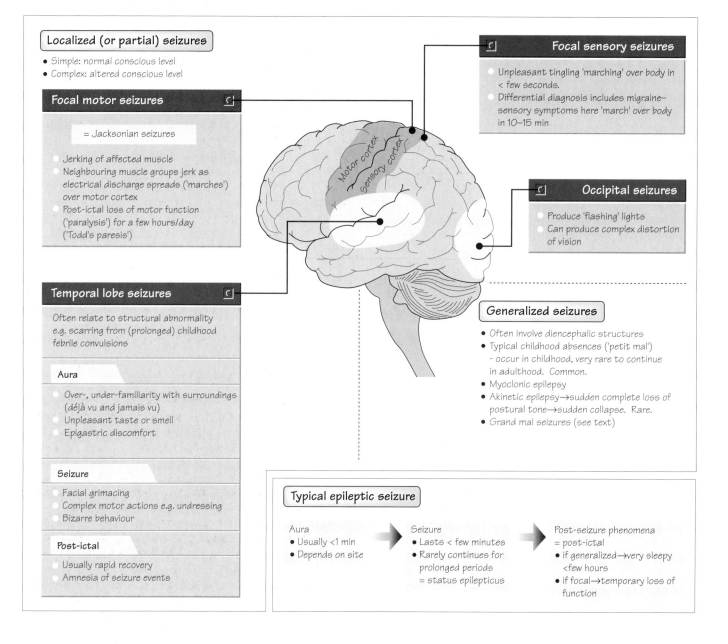

Localized (or partial) seizures

- Simple: normal conscious level
- Complex: altered conscious level

Focal motor seizures [C]

= Jacksonian seizures

- Jerking of affected muscle
- Neighbouring muscle groups jerk as electrical discharge spreads ('marches') over motor cortex
- Post-ictal loss of motor function ('paralysis') for a few hours/day ('Todd's paresis')

Temporal lobe seizures [C]

Often relate to structural abnormality e.g. scarring from (prolonged) childhood febrile convulsions

Aura

- Over-, under-familiarity with surroundings (déjà vu and jamais vu)
- Unpleasant taste or smell
- Epigastric discomfort

Seizure

- Facial grimacing
- Complex motor actions e.g. undressing
- Bizarre behaviour

Post-ictal

- Usually rapid recovery
- Amnesia of seizure events

Focal sensory seizures

- Unpleasant tingling 'marching' over body in < few seconds.
- Differential diagnosis includes migraine— sensory symptoms here 'march' over body in 10–15 min

Occipital seizures [C]

- Produce 'flashing' lights
- Can produce complex distortion of vision

Generalized seizures

- Often involve diencephalic structures
- Typical childhood absences ('petit mal') - occur in childhood, very rare to continue in adulthood. Common.
- Myoclonic epilepsy
- Akinetic epilepsy→sudden complete loss of postural tone→sudden collapse. Rare.
- Grand mal seizures (see text)

Typical epileptic seizure

Aura
- Usually <1 min
- Depends on site

Seizure
- Lasts < few minutes
- Rarely continues for prolonged periods = status epilepticus

Post-seizure phenomena = post-ictal
- if generalized→very sleepy <few hours
- if focal→temporary loss of function

Epilepsy is 'the recurrent tendency to spontaneous, disordered electrical discharge in the brain manifesting as alteration in motor, sensory or psychological function'. Generalized seizures arise in the brain of anyone subjected to the appropriate stimulus, e.g. hypoxia or electroconvulsive therapy. Therefore a single seizure does not make the diagnosis of epilepsy.

Causes of seizures
Metabolic, especially ↓ Na⁺ or ↓ glucose; liver failure, renal failure. **Drugs**, especially alcohol (especially chronic alcohol excess and alcohol withdrawal), 'street' drugs, penicillins, anti-psychotics, antidepressants. **Cerebrovascular disease**. **Tumours**. **Intracranial infec-**tions, especially meningitis, encephalitis, syphilis. **Cerebral anoxia**, especially arrhythmia related. **Developmental brain abnormalities**. **Degenerative brain disease**.

Treatment of the underlying cause, if it can be identified, is the preferred management option; anticonvulsants may also be required.

Epidemiology of epilepsy
The lifetime risk of a generalized convulsion is 3–4%, with peaks at the beginning (neonatal convulsions) and end of life (tumours and stroke). The incidence is 0.7%. There are 300 000 people in the UK with active seizures; 15–20% attend hospital each year.

Simplified classification

The simplest way to divide seizures is whether on the EEG seizures are focal or generalized.

Primary generalized epilepsy

This refers to electrical seizure activity on the EEG arising in both hemispheres simultaneously. It usually begins in childhood or adolescence. There may be a family history. Brain imaging (computed tomography [CT] or magnetic resonance imaging [MRI]) is normal. Often photosensitive (triggered by flashing lights). Three common manifestations:

1 Typical childhood absences ('petit mal')
2 Myoclonic jerks
3 Generalized tonic–clonic seizures: a brief tonic stiffening of the limbs associated with sudden loss of consciousness followed by a variable period of clonic jerking.

Differential diagnosis of generalized tonic-clonic seizures

- All causes of seizures (see above).
- Loss of cardiac output, e.g. arrhythmias, vasovagal, postural hypotension, etc.
- Psychogenic: seizures usually occur in public places, often hospitals; eyes are held tightly shut; bizarre movements common, often in those with genuine epilepsy.

Localization-related epilepsy

There is a clear electrical focus on the EEG from which the seizure activity arises. Often an abnormality is identified on imaging (hippocampal sclerosis, benign tumours, arteriovenous malformations, cortical dysplasia). There is no family history. The common forms are:
- Simple partial seizures.
- Complex partial seizures (the term 'complex' denotes altered awareness).
- If electrical activity spreads a secondary generalized seizure occurs.

Diagnosis: The diagnosis of epilepsy is clinical, based on the history from the patient and reliable observers. The EEG supports the clinical diagnosis and differentiates between primary generalized seizures (3-Hz spike and wave discharge triggered by flashing lights) and localization-related seizures (focal spike discharges). Of patients with true seizures, 50% have a normal interictal EEG, emphasizing the importance of the history in making the diagnosis. Similarly, imaging findings must be interpreted in the context of the appropriate history of seizures.

Specific syndromes
Typical childhood absences

This was previously called 'petit mal' epilepsy. Onset is at age 3–6 years. It is associated with brief interruptions of 3–5 s in awareness, with minimal or no motor manifestation. Attacks can be provoked by hyperventilation. There is a characteristic EEG pattern of 3-Hz spike and wave activity. Responds to sodium valproate or ethosuximide. It is likely to remit fully by adolescence.

Juvenile myoclonic epilepsy

This develops later in childhood. It is associated with early morning myoclonic jerks, which may be reported as clumsiness. Generalized tonic–clonic seizures occur in most. The epilepsy responds to sodium valproate. In many, the tendency to seizures is life-long.

Complex partial seizures with secondary generalization

These are common. Seizures arising from the temporal lobes are typically heralded by an aura, which can take the form of abdominal rising sensations, altered taste and, more rarely, visual and auditory hallucinations. Patients appear 'blank' during an attack and may make repetitive movements, e.g. lip smacking. Of cases, 70% are controlled on monotherapy, although a significant number have drug-resistant seizures and are socially and economically handicapped. Approximately 30% of complex partial seizures arise outside of the temporal lobe, usually from the frontal lobe.

Frontal lobe seizures

These present a diagnostic challenge because the EEG is often normal, even during an attack, and the seizure semiology may be bizarre. Patients may appear to remain awake, but to thrash their limbs about uncontrollably and yell. Instantaneous recovery often occurs and patients may be labelled as having non-epileptic attacks.

Jacksonian seizures

These are simple partial seizures arising in the motor cortex. The onset is with rhythmical twitching of the face which spreads down through the arms and into the legs in a characteristic march-like fashion. There is a high likelihood of a finding a structural lesion, so imaging is mandatory.

Treatment

Primary generalized epilepsy responds well to sodium valproate or lamotrigine; it may be worse on carbamazepine. There is little evidence for any other anticonvulsant specificity by seizure type, so drugs are selected on patient characteristics and cost:
- Side-effect profile: phenytoin is avoided in young people because it causes gingival hyperplasia and androgenizes the face.
- Potential for teratogenicity: all the older drugs are teratogenic and so may the newer agents be. Pre-conception counselling is vital.
- Effect on other drugs, particularly the oral contraceptive pill.

Monotherapy is preferred. Any changes should be made gradually and in the context of an overall seizure pattern, not in response to single seizures.

Status epilepticus (common causes: poor compliance in a known epileptic, sudden anticonvulsant withdrawal, alcohol withdrawal, drug overdose, hypoglycaemia) is defined as continuous seizure activity (arbitrarily for 30 min) or frequent seizures without recovery. This is a medical emergency with a high morbidity. Continuous seizure activity eventually results in cerebral oedema and cardiorespiratory arrest. Management involves:
- **A**irway, **b**reathing and **c**irculation.
- Urgent glucose (fingerprick testing), electrolytes and toxicology screen.
- 10 mg diazepam i.v.: terminates most seizures and can be repeated once.
- Phenytoin or fosphenytoin intravenous infusion.
- Intubation and transfer to the intensive care unit for thiopental (thiopentone) or propofol infusion.

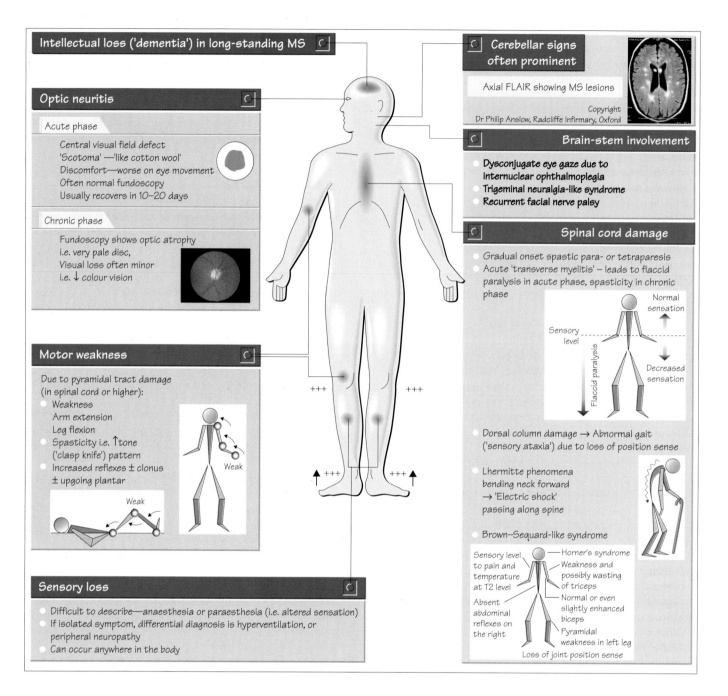

Intellectual loss ('dementia') in long-standing MS

Cerebellar signs often prominent

Axial FLAIR showing MS lesions

Copyright
Dr Philip Anslow, Radcliffe Infirmary, Oxford

Optic neuritis

Acute phase

- Central visual field defect
  'Scotoma' —'like cotton wool'
  Discomfort—worse on eye movement
  Often normal fundoscopy
  Usually recovers in 10–20 days

Chronic phase

- Fundoscopy shows optic atrophy
  i.e. very pale disc,
  Visual loss often minor
  i.e. ↓ colour vision

Brain-stem involvement

- Dysconjugate eye gaze due to internuclear ophthalmoplegia
- Trigeminal neuralgia-like syndrome
- Recurrent facial nerve palsy

Spinal cord damage

- Gradual onset spastic para- or tetraparesis
- Acute 'transverse myelitis' – leads to flaccid paralysis in acute phase, spasticity in chronic phase

Normal sensation

Sensory level

Flaccid paralysis

Decreased sensation

Motor weakness

Due to pyramidal tract damage (in spinal cord or higher):
- Weakness
  Arm extension
  Leg flexion
- Spasticity i.e. ↑tone ('clasp knife') pattern
- Increased reflexes ± clonus ± upgoing plantar

Weak

Weak

- Dorsal column damage → Abnormal gait ('sensory ataxia') due to loss of position sense
- Lhermitte phenomena bending neck forward → 'Electric shock' passing along spine
- Brown–Sequard-like syndrome

Sensory level to pain and temperature at T2 level

Absent abdominal reflexes on the right

Horner's syndrome

Weakness and possibly wasting of triceps

Normal or even slightly enhanced biceps

Pyramidal weakness in left leg

Loss of joint position sense

Sensory loss

- Difficult to describe—anaesthesia or paraesthesia (i.e. altered sensation)
- If isolated symptom, differential diagnosis is hyperventilation, or peripheral neuropathy
- Can occur anywhere in the body

+++   +++

+++   +++

Multiple sclerosis (MS) is the most common of a group of inflammatory conditions in which the basic pathological process is one of loss of myelin in the brain and spinal cord. This leads initially to a relapsing and remitting neurological disturbance, but ultimately, in all but a few patients, to permanent and progressive disability as a result of loss of axons. It is a common disease (50 000 sufferers in the UK) affecting young people, for which currently there is no proven treatment. It is presumed to be a disorder of altered immune responsiveness to targets in the central nervous system (CNS), in which there is a genetic susceptibility and a series of environmentally determined triggers, the nature of which (viral, toxic, etc.) remains obscure.

Clinical spectrum

There are a number of typical patterns of disease (see figure).
- **Relapsing and remitting**: initially the patient presents with episodes of monophasic neurological disturbance with return to normal function in between attacks. Thereafter, the patient may not return to normality, so there is a background of progressive dysfunction with superimposed relapses (termed secondary progressive MS). This accounts for most patients with MS.
- **Relapsing progressive**: there is a progressive course with superimposed relapses but no recovery in between episodes.
- **Primary progressive**: there is relentless progression from the outset.

This subtype is associated with males, later onset and a paucity of imaging changes, a presentation with progressive spastic paraparesis and an overall poorer prognosis. There is rarely any response to steroids.

The most common clinical features are:
• Optic neuritis and subsequent optic atrophy: patients experience blurring of vision through to more profound visual loss, with restoration of eye sight over several months. Colour vision may be permanently lost.
• Cerebellar ataxia (see p. 104).
• Spastic paraparesis (see p. 380).
• Internuclear ophthalmoplegia: the internuclear tracts are nerve fibres linking the nuclei of the nerves controlling the external ocular muscles. MS plaques commonly disrupt them. There is failure of conjugate eye movements, with slow abduction in the ipsilateral eye usually associated with contralateral nystagmus.
• Patchy sensory disturbance.

The clinical signs most commonly associated with MS are shown in the figure.

Diagnosis

Magnetic resonance imaging (MRI) shows typical changes in most patients (with white matter hyperintensities usually around the ventricles or in the brain stem) although a spinal cord presentation can be associated with normal imaging. Visual evoked potentials (VEPs) to document slowing of optic nerve conduction caused by demyelination are a useful adjunct if the MRI cannot distinguish the changes of vascular disease. Lumbar puncture to look for oligoclonal bands is much less frequently performed than in the past but is of use when the MRI changes are not diagnostic, particularly where there is early disease or it is confined to the spinal cord. Oligoclonal bands in the cerebrospinal fluid (CSF) occur in 97% of MS patients, but also in other conditions: Paraneoplastic cerebellar degeneration, Behçet's disease, neurosarcoid and CNS infections.

Differential diagnosis

A first attack of demyelination can be caused by parainfectious immune-mediated damage (acute disseminated encephalomyelitis or ADEM). Strictly speaking, it is not possible to establish the diagnosis of MS after one attack but, if the MRI shows lesions not referable to the site of clinical involvement, there is at least an 80% chance of going on to develop MS. A number of rarer conditions can look like MS:
• Progressive cerebrovascular disease can occasionally be difficult to distinguish on clinical and imaging grounds, but is associated with negative oligoclonal bands and usually normal VEPs.
• Cerebral vasculitis.
• Similar white matter changes to those seen in MS can occur in Sjögren's syndrome, sarcoidosis and Behçet's disease of the nervous system, and occasionally in cerebral lymphoma.

Prognosis

Occasional patients run a relentlessly progressive course from the beginning of the disease and may die within a few years of the first symptoms. In most patients, however, MS does not significantly shorten life. The disease runs a course over decades, during which time there will in most patients be an increasing burden of disability. However, some patients experience a relapsing and remitting course with good functional recovery for many years.

Treatment

The overall approach is vital: 'par excellence' this disease allows a physician to demonstrate his or her humanity. The patient requires psychological empathy and support, with accurate advice about work, home life (and adaptations) and prognosis, and a balanced view on therapy —the last sometimes being particularly difficult. A multidisciplinary approach involving general practitioners, social workers, relatives, physiotherapists, occupational therapists and sometimes psychiatrists is crucial. Such a 'humanistic' approach is true for all disease, but is particularly important in multiple sclerosis.

Acute relapses: corticosteroids (high dose intravenously or orally) have been shown to reduce the severity and duration of acute relapses, although not in every patient. There is no effect on relapse rate or long-term disability. In general, steroids become less effective after repeated attacks.

Disease process and progression: there continues to be debate about the effectiveness of interferon-β. It appears to reduce the number of clinical relapses in selected patients and the number of new lesions on MRI. However, there appears to be no effect on disability.

Symptomatic treatment

• Unpleasant sensory phenomena such as shooting pains and paraesthesiae can be treated with anticonvulsants such as carbamazepine and gabapentin.
• Bladder spasticity can be treated with oxybutynin or intermittent self-catheterization—although this risks frequent urinary tract infections (UTIs). Such infections are common in MS; fever may (temporarily) dramatically worsen weakness.
• Sexual dysfunction in men may respond to sildenafil (Viagra).
• Constipation is common and requires laxatives, and sometimes manual evacuation.
• Muscle spasticity can be treated with baclofen.
• Depression severe enough to require medication occurs in 30% of patients.

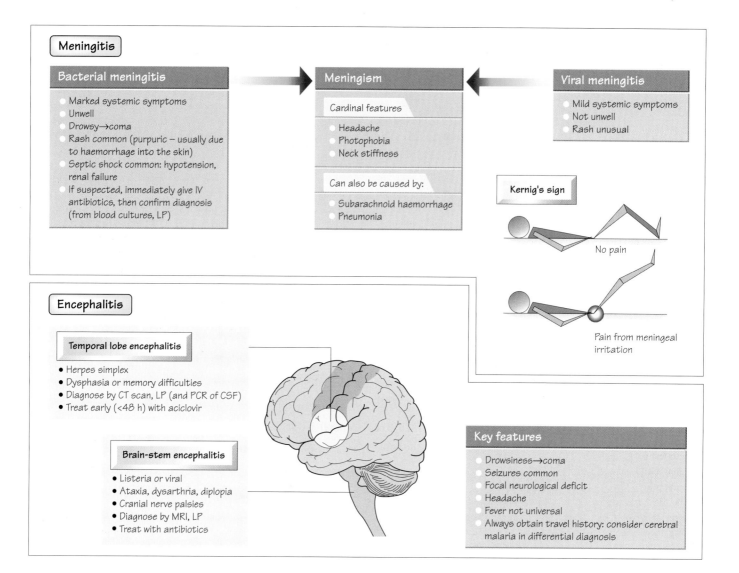

Meningitis

Bacterial meningitis
- Marked systemic symptoms
- Unwell
- Drowsy→coma
- Rash common (purpuric – usually due to haemorrhage into the skin)
- Septic shock common: hypotension, renal failure
- If suspected, immediately give IV antibiotics, then confirm diagnosis (from blood cultures, LP)

Meningism

Cardinal features
- Headache
- Photophobia
- Neck stiffness

Can also be caused by:
- Subarachnoid haemorrhage
- Pneumonia

Viral meningitis
- Mild systemic symptoms
- Not unwell
- Rash unusual

Kernig's sign
No pain

Pain from meningeal irritation

Encephalitis

Temporal lobe encephalitis
- Herpes simplex
- Dysphasia or memory difficulties
- Diagnose by CT scan, LP (and PCR of CSF)
- Treat early (<48 h) with aciclovir

Brain-stem encephalitis
- Listeria or viral
- Ataxia, dysarthria, diplopia
- Cranial nerve palsies
- Diagnose by MRI, LP
- Treat with antibiotics

Key features
- Drowsiness→coma
- Seizures common
- Focal neurological deficit
- Headache
- Fever not universal
- Always obtain travel history: consider cerebral malaria in differential diagnosis

Several infective processes affect the central nervous system (CNS): meningitis, encephalitis, cerebral abscess, prior diseases, and neurological consequences of HIV.

Meningitis

Meningitis presents with fever, headache, stiff neck and photophobia, and can be caused by bacteria or viruses:

• Bacterial meningitis is often associated with a septic syndrome (fever, tachycardia, hypotension or shock—see p. 296), complicated by septicaemia-induced disseminated intravascular coagulation (DIC—see p. 342). Meningitis is usually secondary to bacteraemia caused by *Neisseria meningitidis*, although *Streptococcus pneumoniae* occurs in those with pneumococcal pneumonia (more common in elderly people and those who abuse alcohol) or damaged dura (skull fracture, ear sepsis or sinus disease). Once bacterial meningitis is suspected, broad-spectrum antibiotics (e.g. high-dose cefotaxime) must be given immediately (i.e. in the community if necessary). The diagnosis is confirmed by identifying the organism (blood culture, cerebrospinal fluid [CSF; see Table 190.1] microscopy, culture and polymerase chain reaction [PCR], or blood serology). The prognosis is variable. In meningococcal meningitis, 5–10% die, and a significant proportion have permanent sequelae, including loss of digits (infarction secondary to hypotension), deafness, blindness and intellectual impairment. Immunization against meningococcal serotype A and C is effective (but serotype B, against which there is no vaccine, underlies ± 50% of cases).

• *Listeria monocytogenes* causes meningitis in susceptible individuals (pregnant women, people with alcohol problems and immunocompromised individuals), and a rapidly progressive picture resembling brain-stem encephalitis with focal signs and meningism.

• Viral meningitis presents with prominent headache and less obvious signs of meningeal irritation than in bacterial infections. The responsible organism is identified (CSF, PCR or serology) in only 50% of cases, and is often an enterovirus. Many of the common exanthemata of childhood, including measles and chickenpox, are accompanied by a meningitic illness which, although usually mild, can rarely be life threatening. Management is symptomatic with rehydration and analgesia.

Diseases and Treatments at a Glance

Table 190.1 CSF findings in different infections.

Disease	CSF pressure	Protein	Cell count	Glucose
Bacterial meningitis	Raised	Moderately to severely elevated	> 50 polymorphs	Low
Viral meningitis	Normal	Mildly elevated or normal	Lymphocytes	Normal
TB meningitis	Raised Normal	Moderately elevated	Pleocytosis or lymphocytosis	Low
Encephalitis	Raised or normal	Mildly elevated or normal	Lymphocytosis	Normal
Malignant meningitis	Mildly raised or normal	Raised	Raised: either reactive lymphocytes or malignant cells	Low

• Unusual infections include syphilis, fungi and cryptococci (immuno-compromised individuals). Tubercular meningitis is rare in the West but increasing in frequency (see p. 309).

• Non-infectious causes of meningism (i.e. headache, photophobia and stiff neck) include subarachnoid haemorrhage and migraine (although this requires exclusion of more serious diagnoses). Malignant meningitis from cancer usually presents with sequential cranial nerve palsies, initially painless, later painful, rather than meningism. Spinal nerve root involvement also occurs.

• Meningoencephalitis is meningitis plus some parenchymal involvement.

Encephalitis

Encephalitis implies infection of the brain substance itself. This is rare. The clinical picture is of fever, headache and a diffuse (i.e. confusion, drowsiness up to coma) rather than focal disturbance of cerebral function. The onset may be very dramatic over just a few hours, although more usually the history extends back several days. Other features include:

• Seizures
• Wandering
• Behavioural change
• Frank psychiatric syndromes.

The diagnosis is made from the combination of suggestive clinical features and a lymphocytosis in the CSF. Supportive data come from finding focal inflammation on CT/MRI, focal slow wave activity on EEG and detection of the organism (culture, PCR, serology). There are a large number of viruses responsible, with a marked geographical variation (e.g. Japanese B in the Far East, Western Equine in the USA) so a travel history is vital. However, in only 30% of cases is a cause identified. The prognosis is variable. The principal treatable cause is herpes simplex encephalitis, which has the following features:

• Rare: causes 20% of viral encephalitis.
• Presents with viral prodrome followed by behavioural change with amnesia and sometimes dysphasia.
• Rapid evolution to coma may occur.
• EEG shows repetitive epileptic discharges localized to the temporal lobes. CT/MRI shows necrotizing inflammation in the temporal lobes.
• Treatment: immediate high-dose aciclovir. The prognosis is poor and long-term sequelae are common: 10% die acutely, 10% are so severely impaired as to be rendered institutionalized, 20% are left dependent, 60% recover but in the majority formal neuropsychological testing reveals residual deficits and most do not function at their premorbid occupational level.

Cerebral abscess

Cerebral abscess is rare and presents with headache, fever and focal neurological signs. Infection arises from direct spread (e.g. infected ears, sinuses) or from infected emboli (endocarditis or cyanotic congenital heart disease). First-line investigation is CT/MRI. Lumbar puncture must not be performed because the risk of 'coning' (i.e. herniation of the brain through the foramen magnum, precipitating coma and death) is high. Organisms are cultured from the blood or pus aspirated from the abscess. Echocardiography to exclude cardiac infection (see p. 166) should be undertaken. Treatment is with prolonged antibiotics and sometimes neurosurgical drainage. The mortality rate is 25%.

Prion diseases

The biologically unique features of these diseases are that they can be simultaneously inherited and infectious. The agent of transmission is thought to be a protein (a 'prion') only, rather than an 'organism' containing DNA or RNA. Prion diseases principally result in dementia (see p. 370) and include:

• Sporadic Creutzfeldt-Jakob disease (CJD): rare ($1/10^6$), causes rapid dementia with myoclonus and a characteristic EEG.
• Variant CJD (vCJD): ≤ 150 cases in total in UK to date, and the incidence appears to be declining. Occurs in younger people with a slower course than sporadic CJD. Characteristic pathological features. Psychiatric presentation (depression, personality changes) frequently seen.
• Autosomal dominant CJD: familial form of classic CJD.
• Gerstmann-Straussler-Scheinker syndrome (GSS): familial spongiform encephalopathy with prominent ataxia.
• Fatal familial insomnia.
• Kuru: endemic in New Guinea Highlanders who performed ritual cannibalism. Now very rare.

Neurological consequences of HIV disease

These are multiple, and include the consequences of direct viral infection of the CNS (AIDS dementia, seroconversion meningitis, Guillain–Barré syndrome-like polyneuropathy), opportunistic infections (toxoplasmosis, cryptococcal meningitis, progressive multifocal leukoencephalopathy), primary cerebral lymphoma and drug toxicity (antiretrovirals: nucleoside analogues and protease inhibitors).

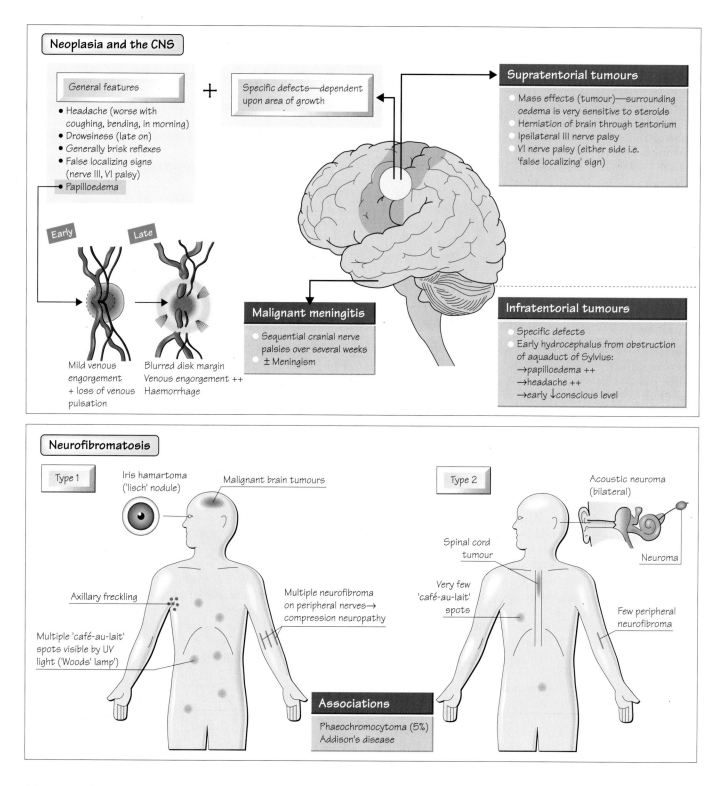

Neoplasia and the CNS

Neoplasia and the CNS

General features

+ **Specific defects—dependent upon area of growth**

- Headache (worse with coughing, bending, in morning)
- Drowsiness (late on)
- Generally brisk reflexes
- False localizing signs (nerve III, VI palsy)
- Papilloedema

Supratentorial tumours

- Mass effects (tumour)—surrounding oedema is very sensitive to steroids
- Herniation of brain through tentorium
- Ipsilateral III nerve palsy
- VI nerve palsy (either side i.e. 'false localizing' sign)

Early

Late

Mild venous engorgement + loss of venous pulsation

Blurred disk margin Venous engorgement ++ Haemorrhage

Malignant meningitis

- Sequential cranial nerve palsies over several weeks
- ± Meningism

Infratentorial tumours

- Specific defects
- Early hydrocephalus from obstruction of aquaduct of Sylvius:
  → papilloedema ++
  → headache ++
  → early ↓ conscious level

Neurofibromatosis

Type 1

Iris hamartoma ('lisch' nodule)

Malignant brain tumours

Axillary freckling

Multiple neurofibroma on peripheral nerves → compression neuropathy

Multiple 'café-au-lait' spots visible by UV light ('Woods' lamp)

Type 2

Acoustic neuroma (bilateral)

Neuroma

Spinal cord tumour

Very few 'café-au-lait' spots

Few peripheral neurofibroma

Associations

Phaeochromocytoma (5%)
Addison's disease

Neoplasia and the central nervous system

CNS neoplasia may present with:
- Epilepsy.
- Symptoms of raised intracranial pressure (headache, intellectual deterioration, vomiting) with papilloedema. Posterior fossa (e.g. cere-bellar) metastases produce a rapid rise in intracranial pressure and rapid onset of symptoms.
- Focal deficits, the onset of which is often slow, but occasionally sudden (i.e. stroke-like). The deficit relates to damage caused by the expansion of the tumour (which acts as a space-occupying lesion

[SOL]) and the surrounding oedema. Focal signs usually reflect the site of the tumour, but occasionally false localizing signs occur from the tumour shifting brain contents and damaging distant nervous structures (e.g. nerve VI palsy). These false localizing signs are rare but important because they indicate that the tumour is extensive enough to damage distant brain tissue, i.e. death is imminent unless urgent intervention occurs.

Diagnosis is usually straightforward, using computed tomography (CT) or magnetic resonance imaging (MRI) and stereotactic guided biopsy. Occasionally tumours are difficult to see on an unenhanced CT scan—accordingly once a tumour is suspected CT scanning must be contrast enhanced. EEG, although not indicated, may during the course of epilepsy investigations suggest an underlying neoplasm (focal slow wave activity). Lumbar puncture must not be undertaken because of the risk of 'coning' the brain into the foramen magnum.

Specific tumours

Of CNS tumours, 50% are secondary deposits from extracranial malignancies, commonly breast, lung, kidney, thyroid, stomach, prostate and melanoma. Accordingly, many patients with brain tumours should be investigated for an extracranial primary (breast examination, chest X-ray, prostate-specific antigen [PSA], abdominal imaging). A quarter of patients with carcinomatosis have brain involvement.

Primary tumours may be malignant or benign. However, the clinical effects of histologically non-malignant tumours may not be benign because pressure effects from expansion within the cranial cavity may lead to disability and death.

Astrocytoma is the most common primary brain tumour, prevalent in the 50–60-year age range. They are divided into four types (I–IV) depending on the degree of malignancy. Glioblastoma multiforme is so undifferentiated as to make the cell of origin impossible to define. Growth is rapid and attempts at surgical excision result in disability and do not improve survival. Dexamethasone results in rapid reduction in neurological deficit as a result of reduction in oedema. Radiotherapy improves quality of life in selected cases and may extend survival by a few months.

Oligodendroglioma is a slow-growing tumour, which may thus show calcification on CT scanning. Oligodendrogliomas occur in a younger population than astrocytomas. Ependymomas occur anywhere throughout the ventricular system and infiltrate into surrounding tissues.

Primary CNS lymphoma may be single or multifocal and is more common in immunocompromised patients, such as those with HIV, where the Epstein–Barr virus drives tumour growth. Metastatic spread from systemic lymphoma is uncommon and is usually meningeal rather than parenchymal. Primary CNS lymphoma may be exquisitely sensitive to steroids.

Meningiomas account for 20% of intracranial tumours; they arise from the arachnoid granulations and are usually closely related to the venous sinuses. They exert their clinical effects by direct compression of the brain and, although presentation is usually slow, it may be surprisingly acute, leading to the view that there is an inflammatory component. A reactive hyperostosis may occur in overlying bone. The aim of treatment is complete surgical excision, but the recurrence rate is 30% at 10 years.

Acoustic neuroma/schwannoma is the most common infratentorial tumour. They arise from the vestibular portion of nerve VIII and lie in the cerebellopontine angle, giving rise to symptoms referable to cranial nerves VIII, VII and VI.

Malignant meningitis

Spread of tumours to the nervous system may be via the blood stream to the meninges. This can cause a diffuse subacute meningitis with headache, stiff neck and vomiting, or a multifocal neurological syndrome of deafness and other, typically lower, cranial nerve palsies. Examination of the cerebrospinal fluid (CSF) reveals a reactive lymphocytosis, a low glucose and a high protein. CSF cytology may reveal tumour cells. Occasionally severe limb weakness, mimicking motor neuron disease, can result from diffuse infiltration of nerve root with tumour. Treatment is usually unsuccessful, except in the case of lymphoma.

Paraneoplastic disorders

The loss of genetic regulation in malignant tumours may lead to the cell surface expression of proteins normally only found in neurons (onconeuronal antigens). These may initiate an immune response, provoking damage of the nervous system. Antineuronal antibodies can be detected but these may not be pathogenic. Each of the syndromes has in common:
• An evolution over weeks to months.
• A relentlessly progressive course.
• A failure to respond to treatment of the primary tumour or of the immune response (steroids, intravenous immunoglobulin [IVIG] or plasma exchange).
• Oligoclonal bands in the CSF.
• Relatively normal CNS imaging.
   Specific syndromes are described on p. 360.

Neurocutaneous syndromes

These are dominantly inherited and are the result of mutations in tumour suppressor genes. They lead to benign and malignant tumours:
   Neurofibromatosis has an incidence of 1 in 3000, occurs in several patterns and may have an associated phaeochromocytoma (which should be suspected if hypertension occurs):
• Type I (peripheral type) characterized by multiple neurofibromas, café-au-lait patches, axillary freckling, Lisch nodule in the iris, meningiomas and malignant brain tumours, usually astrocytomas of the optic pathway. It is caused by mutations in the neurofibromin gene and has a very high new mutation rate.
• Type II (central type) is the result of mutations in a gene called *Merlin*. Although the hallmark of this disease is bilateral vestibular schwannomas, most patients develop benign or malignant tumours in the spinal cord and elsewhere in the brain. There are also cutaneous manifestations.
   Von Hippel–Lindau disease involves tumours in multiple organ systems. As well as cerebellar and spinal cord haemangioblastomas and ocular angiomas, von Hippel–Lindau disease causes renal angiolipomatosis and renal cell carcinoma, phaeochromocytoma and islet cell tumours.

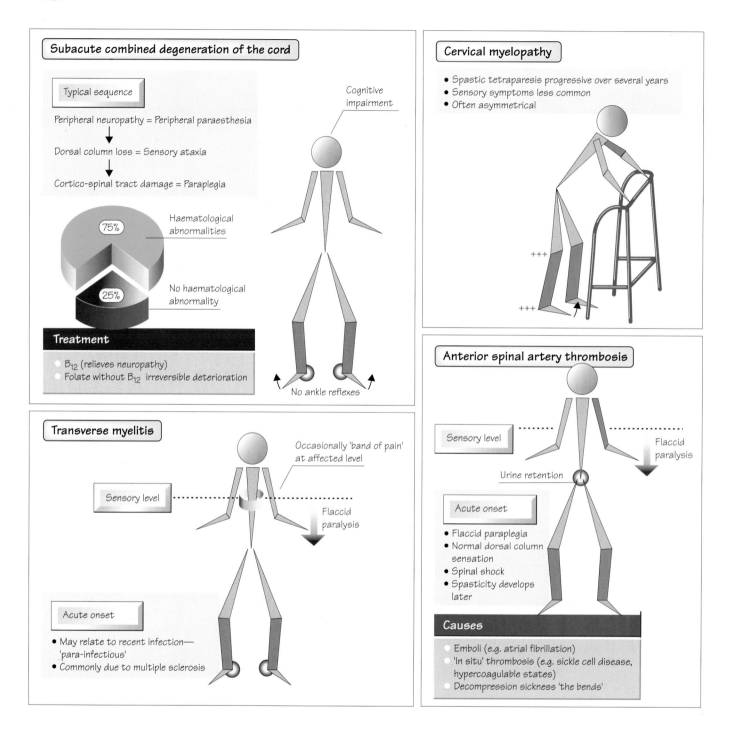

Subacute combined degeneration of the cord

Typical sequence

Peripheral neuropathy = Peripheral paraesthesia

↓

Dorsal column loss = Sensory ataxia

↓

Cortico-spinal tract damage = Paraplegia

75% — Haematological abnormalities

25% — No haematological abnormality

Treatment
- B₁₂ (relieves neuropathy)
- Folate without B₁₂ irreversible deterioration

Cognitive impairment

No ankle reflexes

Cervical myelopathy
- Spastic tetraparesis progressive over several years
- Sensory symptoms less common
- Often asymmetrical

+++

+++

Transverse myelitis

Occasionally 'band of pain' at affected level

Sensory level

Flaccid paralysis

Acute onset
- May relate to recent infection— 'para-infectious'
- Commonly due to multiple sclerosis

Anterior spinal artery thrombosis

Sensory level

Flaccid paralysis

Urine retention

Acute onset
- Flaccid paraplegia
- Normal dorsal column sensation
- Spinal shock
- Spasticity develops later

Causes
- Emboli (e.g. atrial fibrillation)
- 'In situ' thrombosis (e.g. sickle cell disease, hypercoagulable states)
- Decompression sickness 'the bends'

Acute spinal cord compression

Spinal cord compression presents with motor dysfunction predominantly affecting the lower limb, *whatever the level of the lesion*. This is associated with a sensory level and upper motor neuron signs below the level of the lesion. Abdominal reflexes are lost when the lesion is above T9. This is a medical emergency whatever the cause—urgent magnetic resonance imaging (MRI) is mandatory, and the results of such imaging dictate management. The spinal cord is most often compressed by:

- Secondary tumours from breast, prostate and lung.
- Prolapsed intervertebral discs, which usually herniate laterally causing asymmetrical signs, although central disc prolapse can also occur.

Abscess and other inflammatory lesions can also compress the spinal cord. The treatment usually involves surgical decompression or radiotherapy for malignant tumours.

Diseases and Treatments at a Glance

Progressive spastic paraparesis

Bilateral weakness with marked spasticity of the lower limbs and extensor plantar responses can be subacute or chronic; it is always investigated by MRI of the spine, and has a number of important causes:

• Vitamin B12 deficiency causes corticospinal tract damage (spastic paraparesis) associated with a peripheral neuropathy (absent ankle jerks) and dorsal column dysfunction (a high stepping gait, rombergism and pseudo-athetosis of the outstretched fingers). This syndrome complex is termed subacute combined degeneration of the cord (SACD). It is important to appreciate that neurological dysfunction in isolation can occur before a rise in mean cell volume (MCV) or anaemia (see also p. 318). In SACD, folic acid alone may exacerbate the neurological deficit. Accordingly, it is crucial to measure vitamin B12, and replace if deficient, in megaloblastic anaemias with any suggestion of spinal cord involvement.

• Cervical spondylotic myelopathy: this is a condition of middle-aged and elderly people, in which degenerative changes in the vertebrae cause slowly progressive constriction of the cervical cord and sometimes the nerve roots at the exit foramina, producing a 'radiculopathy' (wasting, weakness, sensory loss and decreased reflexes). It can present with various combinations of neck pain, tingling of the upper limbs, sphincter dysfunction and gait disturbance. Reflexes in the arms and legs (except those supplied by compressed nerve roots) are very brisk, and often show clonus. Diagnosis is by MRI. The aim of surgery is to prevent worsening because only rarely does it improve symptoms.

• Hereditary spastic paraparesis is a genetically heterogeneous disease which is usually autosomal dominant. It selectively affects long motor tracts and characteristically produces more spasticity than weakness. It is very slowly progressive and typically comes on in early adult life, although cases may present into the 50s.

• Of cases of motor neuron disease, 1% present with a indolent form called primary lateral sclerosis, in which upper motor neuron signs predominate until late in the illness. Survival may be prolonged (10–15 years as opposed to 2–3 years for amyotrophic lateral sclerosis [ALS]).

• Primary progressive multiple sclerosis.

Transverse myelitis

This is an inflammatory illness localized to the middle of the spinal cord, which presents as acute weakness with an ascending sensory level, i.e. rather similar to acute cord compression (which must be excluded by urgent MRI). A proportion of patients have had a recent flu-like illness and this condition may occur as a parainfectious complication of *Mycoplasma* or *Legionella* spp., Epstein–Barr virus infections, herpes simplex and zoster, and others. Imaging may show a focal lesion in the spinal cord or be normal. In a proportion of patients, transverse myelitis is the first manifestation of multiple sclerosis.

Anterior spinal artery thrombosis

The particular anatomical arrangement of the blood supply to the spinal cord makes the mid and upper thoracic regions vulnerable to vascular insufficiency. Two posterior spinal arteries, which provide good collateral circulation, supply the posterior portion of the spinal cord. The anterior part of the cord, however (spinothalamic tracts and corticospinal tracts), is supplied by a solitary anterior spinal artery formed by the anastomosis of a branch from each vertebral artery at the level of the medulla. At a variable level (typically T4) there is a paucity of collateral circulation. If the blood supply here is compromised (e.g. by *in situ* thrombosis or an embolus), this leads to ischaemia in the anterior spinal artery territory which presents as a sudden (maximally over a few hours) flaccid paraparesis and loss of bladder function. Dorsal column function is preserved. Autonomic instability from spinal shock may ensue. Imaging is often normal acutely. There is no treatment and the prognosis for recovery is poor. An embolic source should be looked for (e.g. atrial fibrillation, recent myocardial infarction), vasculitis excluded, and general antiatherogenic measures undertaken (see Chapters 70 and 71).

Disc prolapse

The prolapse may be central (see above) or lateral, so compressing the exit foramina of nerves, producing radicular pain. The most common example of this is of a L4/5 or L5/S1 disc prolapse, resulting in pain radiating down the buttock and lower limb (sciatica). The signs are of decreased straight leg raising and diminished reflexes. Recovery is usually spontaneous—occasionally laminectomy is required.

Syringomyelia

This is an exceptionally rare illness, in which the central canal in the cervical spinal cord enlarges into a large fluid-filled cavity (the syrinx). This is predisposed to by mild (or more severe) herniation of the cerebellar tonsils into (or beyond) the foramen magnum (the Arnold–Chiari malformation) or previous trauma. The expanding syrinx damages local structures, especially the decussating spinothalamic tracts (producing loss of pain and temperature sensation and, distressingly, severe pain in the same distribution), the corticospinal tracts (spastic weakness) and anterior horn cells (muscle wasting). Cranial nerve signs follow extension of the syrinx into the medulla. Diagnosis is by MRI. Neurosurgical drainage may have a role.

Spinal shock

Sudden transsection of the spinal cord at a cervical or upper thoracic level (often traumatic) can lead to loss of autonomic vasomotor control of blood pressure, which leads to catastrophic hypotension. Substantial fluid replacement is needed.

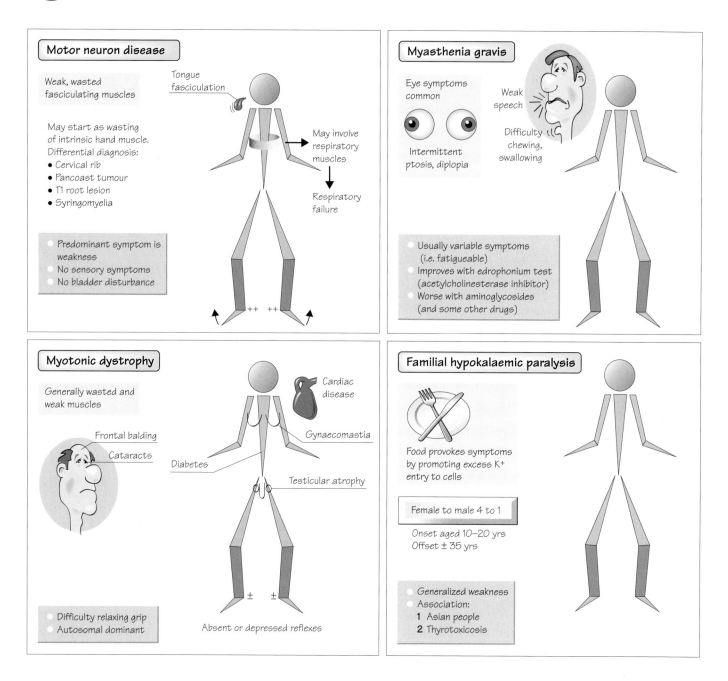

Motor neuron disease

Weak, wasted fasciculating muscles

Tongue fasciculation

May start as wasting of intrinsic hand muscle. Differential diagnosis:
- Cervical rib
- Pancoast tumour
- T1 root lesion
- Syringomyelia

May involve respiratory muscles

Respiratory failure

- Predominant symptom is weakness
- No sensory symptoms
- No bladder disturbance

++ ++

Myasthenia gravis

Eye symptoms common

Weak speech

Intermittent ptosis, diplopia

Difficulty chewing, swallowing

- Usually variable symptoms (i.e. fatigueable)
- Improves with edrophonium test (acetylcholinesterase inhibitor)
- Worse with aminoglycosides (and some other drugs)

Myotonic dystrophy

Generally wasted and weak muscles

Frontal balding

Cataracts

Diabetes

Cardiac disease

Gynaecomastia

Testicular atrophy

± ±

- Difficulty relaxing grip
- Autosomal dominant

Absent or depressed reflexes

Familial hypokalaemic paralysis

Food provokes symptoms by promoting excess K+ entry to cells

Female to male 4 to 1

Onset aged 10–20 yrs
Offset ± 35 yrs

- Generalized weakness
- Association:
  1 Asian people
  2 Thyrotoxicosis

The motor unit

There are four possible locations for pathological processes of the neuromuscular unit to act:

1 The anterior horn cell or lower motor neuron
2 The peripheral nerve
3 The neuromuscular junction
4 The muscle.

Peripheral neuropathies are dealt with on p. 384.

Motor neuron disease

Motor neuron disease (MND) is a disorder of obscure aetiology, which leads to selective, but not exclusive, degeneration of upper and lower motor neurons. It is rare (2/100 000 per year) and malignant in behaviour—the average time from diagnosis to death is 2.5 years. Of cases of MND, 5% are genetic in origin (autosomal dominant inheritance) and some are the result of mutations in the gene for superoxide dismutase-1. The genetic identity of the other cases is as yet unknown.

The most common presentation (70%) is with wasting and weakness of one limb. Examination shows mixed upper and lower motor signs in several limbs—a combination of fasciculation, wasting, weakness, extensor plantar responses and brisk reflexes (amyotrophic lateral sclerosis). Tongue fasciculation is a useful sign because it makes a compressive lesion of the spinal cord unlikely.

Other patients (20%) present with prominent bulbar symptoms before developing signs in the limbs (progressive bulbar palsy) or a pure lower motor neuron picture of symmetrical weakness, wasting and areflexia (progressive muscular atrophy). Similarly the disease may appear to be restricted to the upper motor neuron and present a picture of progressive spastic paraparesis. This variant, known as primary lateral sclerosis, is more indolent and survival may be prolonged.

Diagnosis is clinical but supported by electromyographic demonstration of denervation in all four limbs. There are no specific treatments and management aims to preserve nutritional status and provide supportive and terminal care. The glutamate antagonist riluzole prolongs time to ventilation and tracheostomy by 3 months.

Poliomyelitis

Poliomyelitis is rarely seen in countries with effective immunization programmes. It produces asymmetrical motor weakness with bulbar and respiratory compromise in the context of an acute febrile illness. Some patients undergo late deterioration in function decades after the acute illness (post-polio syndrome).

Myasthenia gravis

Myasthenia gravis is an autoimmune disease—antibodies are directed against the acetylcholine receptor at the neuromuscular junction. The clinical features are variable, but include:
• Symmetrical proximal muscle weakness, which fatigues on exertion.
• Prominent involvement of the extraocular muscles, producing diplopia and ptosis. Significant limb weakness without eye involvement is rare. In contrast, myasthenia confined to the eyes (ocular myasthenia) is a distinct condition in which many patients do not have acetylcholine receptor antibodies and whose course is more benign.
• Bulbar involvement with dysphagia, dysarthria and a risk of aspiration.
• Myasthenic crises with a rapid evolution of neuromuscular weakness, leading to emergency ventilation.
• An association with thymoma in older patients, and thymic hyperplasia in younger patients.

Treatment is with immunomodulatory therapy (corticosteroids, azathioprine, plasma exchange), thymectomy and drugs that prolong the action of acetylcholine in the neuromuscular junction.

Inflammatory myopathies

Inflammatory myopathies are of presumed autoimmune aetiology, although usually without specific antibodies, where muscle is involved in isolation or in the context of a more diffuse connective tissue disease. They are typically painless. The creatine phosphokinase level is elevated by several thousand. There is a clinical and pathological spectrum from polymyositis to dermatomyositis (see p. 413). The latter is associated in elderly people with malignancy and more often involves swallowing dysfunction. Therapy is with steroids, intravenous immunoglobulin (IVIG) and occasionally plasma exchange. Inclusion body myositis affects elderly people and presents with the insidious onset of slowly progressive, asymmetrical, painless wasting and weakness of muscles, especially quadriceps. There is no effective treatment.

Muscular dystrophies

Muscular dystrophies are inherited diseases leading to progressive wasting and weakness. The nosology of the dystrophies is being redefined according to specific genetic mutations and associated molecular deficits:
• Dystrophinopathies are caused by mutations in the gene encoding the very large membrane-associated protein dystrophin, thought to have a function in anchoring the muscle cytoskeleton to the extracellular matrix. Duchenne muscular dystrophy is caused by mutations that lead to complete loss of functional protein and a severe muscle disease, with onset in early childhood, loss of ambulation by adolescence and death in the 20s or 30s from cardiorespiratory failure. Becker dystrophy is caused by mutations in dystrophin, which produce a truncated and partially functional protein. Onset can be at any time from infancy to late adult life and the prognosis is much more favourable.
• Sarcoglycanopathies are rarer disorders resulting from mutations in genes encoding a variety of other membrane-associated proteins.
• Limb girdle muscular dystrophies.
• Facioscapulohumeral muscular dystrophy.
• Oculopharyngeal muscular dystrophy.

Myotonic dystrophy

Myotonic dystrophy is a multisystem disorder characterized by distal weakness and wasting, male pattern balding, an increased incidence of diabetes mellitus, cardiac conduction defects, cataract and excessive daytime somnolence. It is caused by mutations in the non-coding part of the myotonin protein kinase gene, which contains a triplet repeat (CTG) and undergoes dynamic expansion. Successive generations are progressively more severely affected (genetic anticipation). In one pedigree the phenotype may range from cataract to congenital myotonic dystrophy with death in infancy. Genetic testing usually makes diagnosis by electromyography (EMG) unnecessary.

Metabolic myopathies

Metabolic myopathies are rare disorders caused by specific enzyme defects in pathways important for muscle function. There is a wide spectrum of clinical presentation, but suggestive features are exertional muscle pain and myoglobinuria:
• Mitochondrial diseases: myopathy is associated with a variable phenotype, including glucose intolerance, pigmentary retinopathy, seizures, stroke-like episodes and deafness. One form is chronic progressive external ophthalmoplegia.
• Disorders of fatty acid metabolism, e.g. carnitine palmitoyl transferase deficiency.
• Disorders of carbohydrate metabolism, e.g. glycogen storage diseases such as acid maltase deficiency.
• Periodic paralysis occurs in a hypokalaemic and a rarer hyperkalaemic form. These are the result of mutations in ion channels (channelopathies). Patients present with attacks of generalized weakness lasting for several hours. Precipitants include large meals, alcohol and cold weather.

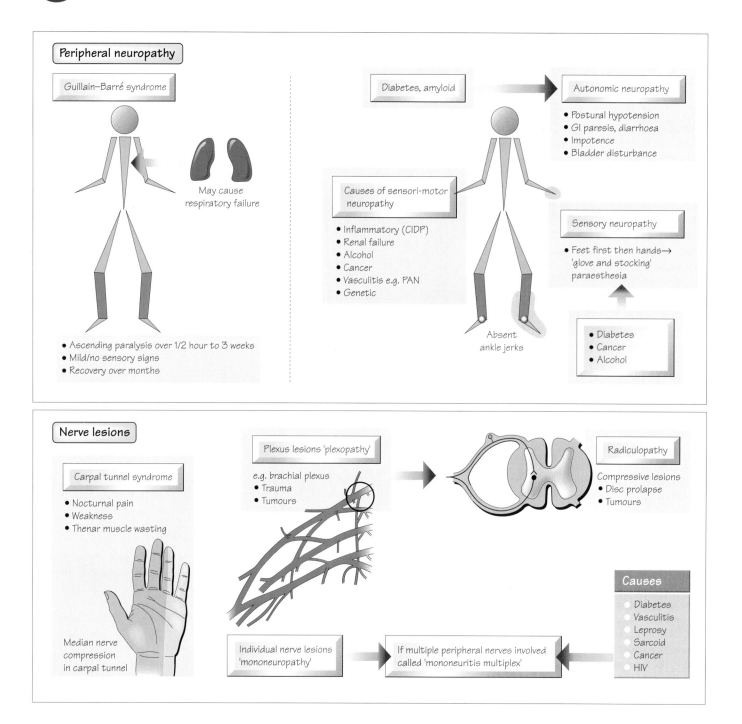

Peripheral neuropathy

Guillain–Barré syndrome

May cause respiratory failure

- Ascending paralysis over 1/2 hour to 3 weeks
- Mild/no sensory signs
- Recovery over months

Diabetes, amyloid

Autonomic neuropathy
- Postural hypotension
- GI paresis, diarrhoea
- Impotence
- Bladder disturbance

Causes of sensori-motor neuropathy
- Inflammatory (CIDP)
- Renal failure
- Alcohol
- Cancer
- Vasculitis e.g. PAN
- Genetic

Sensory neuropathy
- Feet first then hands→ 'glove and stocking' paraesthesia

Absent ankle jerks

- Diabetes
- Cancer
- Alcohol

Nerve lesions

Carpal tunnel syndrome
- Nocturnal pain
- Weakness
- Thenar muscle wasting

Median nerve compression in carpal tunnel

Plexus lesions 'plexopathy'

e.g. brachial plexus
- Trauma
- Tumours

Radiculopathy

Compressive lesions
- Disc prolapse
- Tumours

Individual nerve lesions 'mononeuropathy'

If multiple peripheral nerves involved called 'mononeuritis multiplex'

Causes
- Diabetes
- Vasculitis
- Leprosy
- Sarcoid
- Cancer
- HIV

Clinical approach

Accurate diagnosis of a peripheral neuropathy requires an understanding of neuropathy classification and the speed of onset of symptoms, and a knowledge of which diseases commonly cause neuropathy.

Neuropathy classification

• Polyneuropathies: diffuse damage to peripheral nerves. The longest nerves (i.e. supplying the hand and foot) are most vulnerable to damage and are usually affected earliest. Polyneuropathies may be:

• Pure motor or pure sensory.

• Sensorimotor: the most common pattern. Damage is symmetrical. Paraesthesiae and dysaesthesiae are early symptoms. Cramps and spasms commonly occur later. Examination shows diminution of reflexes, weakness, variable wasting and sensory loss. Sensory ataxia is manifest by rombergism and pseudo-athetosis. Trophic changes such as ulcers and joint deformity are found in long-standing neuropathies.

• Autonomic.

- Radiculopathy is a disorder of the nerve roots—if present at multiple levels it is termed a polyradiculopathy.
- Plexopathy affecting the nerves of the brachial or lumbosacral plexus.
- Mononeuropathy: isolated to a single peripheral nerve or if a number of anatomically discrete nerves are affected mononeuritis multiplex.

Consider the evolution of the problem:
- Acute: vascular, inflammatory, toxic.
- Subacute: toxic, nutritional, systemic illness.
- Chronic: hereditary, metabolic.

Investigation of peripheral nerve disease

Neuropathy is confirmed and classified (i.e. demyelinating versus axonal) by nerve conduction studies and electromyography (EMG). Parameters measured include: (i) nerve conduction velocity; (ii) the amplitude of nerve and muscle response to stimulation; (iii) denervation of muscle, i.e. spontaneous electrical activity (fibrillation).

In demyelinating neuropathies (e.g. Guillain–Barré syndrome), there is slowing of conduction velocity and little evidence of denervation. In axonal neuropathy (e.g. caused by drugs such as vincristine), there is normal motor conduction velocity with decreased compound muscle action potential and evidence of denervation on EMG.

Nerve biopsy is not performed frequently. It is most useful to confirm vasculitis before commencing therapy. Other common aetiologies are looked for using: blood glucose, vitamin B12, thyroid function, serum electrophoresis (for a paraprotein) and autoantibodies (especially anti-neutrophil cytoplasmic antibody and antinuclear antibody).

Polyneuropathies

Inherited

Peripheral neuropathy occurs as part of many complex neurogenetic disorders. The most common cause of inherited isolated peripheral neuropathy is hereditary motor and sensory neuropathy (HMSN) or Charcot–Marie–Tooth disease. The most common genetic subtype is a duplication of part of the short arm of chromosome 17, which causes a demyelinating neuropathy with wasting below the knees, pes cavus and hand involvement.

Metabolic derangement

- Diabetes mellitus is the most common cause of peripheral neuropathy in the developed world. The usual picture is a progressive, predominantly sensory neuropathy. Loss of vibration sense is the earliest sign. Over time, if diabetes is poorly controlled, autonomic involvement becomes universal. Pain can be difficult to manage.
- Vitamin deficiencies (vitamin B12, thiamine and vitamin E) all cause neuropathy as part of a broader neurological syndrome.
- Chronic renal failure and liver failure can produce peripheral neuropathy.
- Hyperthyroidism is a rare cause.

Toxic and drug induced

- Alcohol is a very common cause, as are drugs: amiodarone, metronidazole, cytotoxics, pyridoxine, isoniazid, dapsone, lithium.

Inflammatory/Immune polyneuropathy

- Guillain–Barré syndrome: incidence 1–2 per 100 000. Autoimmune response to an infection (sometimes with *Campylobacter* sp.) occurring

2–3 weeks earlier. The illness starts with weak distal muscles, i.e. the feet. Mild sensory symptoms are often present. Weakness ascends proximally over a few days. Respiratory failure requiring ventilation may occur (vital capacity should be frequently measured). Spontaneous recovery, sometimes full, occasionally incomplete is usual, although 5% die. Autonomic imbalance can produce cardiac arrhythmias. Illness duration is shortened with γ-globulin or plasma exchange.
- Chronic idiopathic demyelinating polyneuropathy (CIDP) runs a waxing–waning course. Nerve conduction studies are diagnostic. Steroids or γ-globulin help.
- Other neuropathies: vasculitis, critical illness polyneuropathy, infective (leprosy, Lyme disease, HIV, diphtheria), traumatic (entrapment or crush injuries), paraneoplastic.

Common mononeuropathies

Nerve entrapment is generally the result of local factors, but in some conditions it is much more common and sometimes multiple: (i) hypothyroidism; (ii) acromegaly; (iii) Paget's disease; (iv) rheumatoid disease; and (v) hereditary neuropathy with liability to pressure palsies (HLPP) caused by deletion of the *PMP*-22 gene.

In mononeuropathies it is important to consider the possibility that the apparently isolated nerve lesion is part of a mononeuritis multiplex syndrome.

Median nerve: by far the most common mononeuropathy is carpal tunnel syndrome. Lifetime incidence is 6% in women, 0.6% in men (usually manual workers using vibrating machinery). Typical symptoms are of pain, discomfort and tingling in the hand radiating to the forearm and occasionally the shoulder. These commonly wake the patient from sleep and are relieved by shaking the wrist. Symptoms are also precipitated by repetitive flexion at the wrist, e.g. when steering a car. Treatment is by surgical release. Wrist splints are occasionally helpful.

The **ulnar nerve** is vulnerable to compression and injury at the elbow (e.g. arthritis, fracture) where it is superficially located. Patients present with numbness of the little and ring fingers and ulnar border of the hand, wasting and weakness of the first dorsal interosseous, and weakness of abductor digit minimi.

Lateral popliteal (common peroneal) nerve is very vulnerable to compressive injury at the head of the fibula (e.g. by a plaster cast). Lesions cause painless foot drop as a result of weakness of tibialis anterior. The ankle jerk is retained.

Rarer mononeuropathies

Radial nerve damage is the result of nerve compression in the axilla (e.g. by a chair, 'Saturday night' palsy), or as the nerve winds round the head of the humerus. Patients present with wrist drop.

Femoral nerve damage relate to diabetes, pelvic lesions, particularly inflammation or haematoma (in anticoagulated patients), iliopsoas pathology or, more rarely, lesions in the femoral canal. The quadriceps wastes, extension at the knee is weak, and there is variable sensory loss over the anterior thigh occurs.

Mononeuritis multiplex

Occurs in diabetes, systemic vasculitis, leprosy, sarcoidosis, non-metastatic manifestation of malignancy and HIV. Investigation and treatment are of the underlying disease.

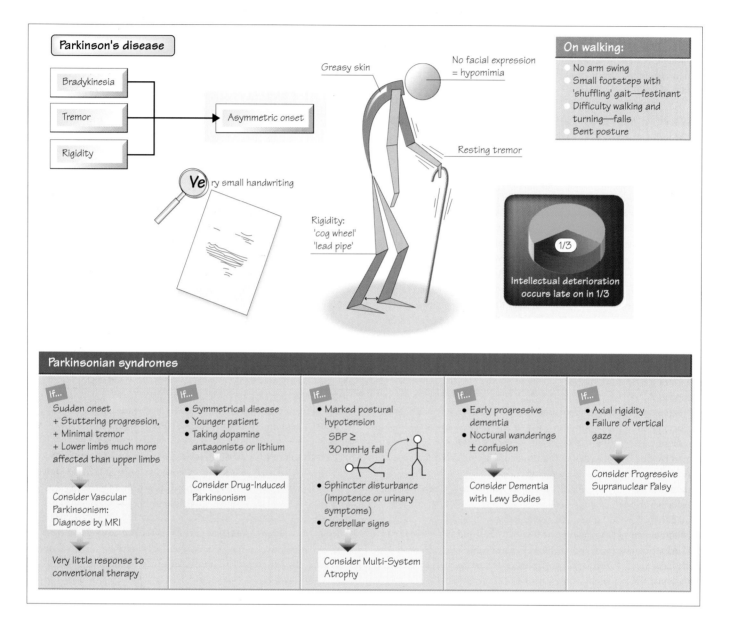

Parkinsonism

The term 'parkinsonism' describes a syndrome of poverty of movement, resting tremor, rigidity and varying degrees of postural instability.

Idiopathic Parkinson's disease (PD) is characterized by asymmetrical onset, slow progression and good response to L-dopa therapy. Only 60% develop tremor. The pathology is loss of dopamine-producing cells of the substantia nigra and Lewy bodies (intraneuronal inclusions). The aetiology is poorly understood. Most Parkinson's disease is probably not genetic, although onset at the age of 30 years or less is associated with a mutation in the *parkin* gene.

The diagnosis is clinical—structural imaging is normal. Helpful signs are loss of arm swing, micrographia (small handwriting) and facial hypomimia, and the more 'classic' signs of 'cogwheel' stiffness, 4–7 Hz resting tremor. Other neurodegenerative conditions (see below) are included in the differential diagnosis and are suspected if there are:

- Early falls
- Early cognitive impairment
- Symmetrical onset
- Prominent autonomic disturbance including sphincter involvement
- Pyramidal tract or cerebellar signs.

Treatment and prognosis

Parkinson's disease is progressive and pharmacological manipulation changes as the condition advances. At onset it is usually a problem of poverty of movement. Later on, troublesome dyskinesia, unpredictable freezing and on–off phenomena dominate the picture. Of patients with Parkinson's disease, 10% develop these problems for each year from diagnosis. Drug therapy involves increasing dopamine levels in the central nervous system (CNS), by giving either L-dopa with a peripheral decarboxylase inhibitor, or drugs that stimulate CNS dopamine receptors (apomorphine, bromocriptine, pergolide) or inhibit the breakdown of CNS dopamine. Drug side effects are common and include dyskinesias and 'on–off' phenomena. In advanced disease ablation of structures in the basal ganglia is increasingly used, as is deep brain stimulation.

Drug-induced parkinsonism: neuroleptics, antiemetics and occasionally lithium can all produce parkinsonism. This is typically an early side effect and more common with ageing. In contrast to Parkinson's disease, it is symmetrical in onset, tremor is less prominent and improvement occurs on withdrawal of the offending agent. Sometimes drugs unmask idiopathic PD.

Vascular parkinsonism: this rare disorder is characterized by bradykinesia and rigidity of the lower limbs, with marked sparing of the upper limbs. There will usually be a history of stuttering evolution, vascular risk factors and an abnormal magnetic resonance image.

Neurodegenerative akinetic–rigid syndromes mimicking Parkinson's disease

- **Multiple system atrophy** (MSA): formally known as Shy–Drager syndrome, nigrostriatal degeneration or olivopontocerebellar atrophy, depending on the predominant clinical features, until it was realized that all these conditions are linked by the same pathology (specific glial inclusions that stain for α-synuclein) and that they overlap clinically. Current classification divides the condition into MSA-P if parkinsonian features predominate or MSA-C if cerebellar features dominate. Patients have the insidious onset of parkinsonism with sphincter disturbance, postural hypotension, cerebellar signs and, characteristically, stridor. Cognition is unaffected. The prognosis is poor and the response to L-dopa is absent or rapidly wanes.
- **Progressive supranuclear palsy** is characterized by prominent axial rigidity, progressive loss of downgaze and upgaze, apraxia of eyelid opening and facial dystonia, imparting a characteristic expression to the face of frowning and surprise. Cognitive impairment occurs later in the condition, which leads to death within 5–7 years.
- **Dementia with Lewy bodies**: parkinsonism with prominent nocturnal wanderings and hallucinations, early and progressive cognitive impairment and myoclonus. Poor response to L-dopa.
- **Corticobasal degeneration**: the picture is of a stuttering evolution of parkinsonism plus parietal lobe abnormalities, including, characteristically, an alien limb abnormality of the arm, dysphasia, extensor plantars, myoclonus and dystonia; dementia; rare. Death in 5–7 years.

Dystonia (see p. 105)

Focal dystonias such as writer's cramp and hemifacial spasm can be treated with injections of botulinum toxin. It is a presynaptic blocker of neuromuscular transmission, causing weakness of the injected muscles for up to 3 months, relieving the symptoms over that period.

Huntington's disease

Huntington's disease is caused by an expanded trinucleotide repeat mutation in the *Huntingtin* gene and is inherited as an autosomal dominant. This is a disorder of insidious onset and inexorable progression, in which the first changes are often in personality (poor impulse control, irritability) and the subsequent development of chorea, dementia and immobility occurs over 10–15 years.

Drug-induced movement disorders

The neuroleptic class of drugs (e.g. haloperidol), including antiemetics (e.g. prochlorperazine), are dopamine receptor antagonists and, in addition to parkinsonism, can induce acute dystonias, including oculogyric crisis, akathisia (motor restlessness) and tardive dyskinesias. The last are involuntary writhing movements of the face (especially mouth) and limbs, commonly seen in patients treated for schizophrenia.

Movement disorders in young people

The main condition to consider is Wilson's disease because it is treatable. This is an autosomal recessive disease caused by mutations in a gene coding for a copper-transporting protein. It can present as:
- Fulminant hepatic failure in childhood
- Progressive neuropsychiatric disturbance in adolescence
- Focal dystonia, dysarthria and drooling.

Diagnosis is by finding a low level of ceruloplasmin and free copper in serum. Patients with neurological Wilson's disease all have Kayser–Fleischer rings visible on slit-lamp examination of the cornea. The condition is treated by copper chelation therapy, usually with penicillamine.

Gilles de la Tourette syndrome presents with a combination of multiple motor and vocal tics (i.e. involuntary vocalizations) both of varying complexity, with onset in childhood usually between 7 and 11 years of age. The prevalence is 1/2000 with a very wide range of severity. Involuntary swearing (coprolalia) is a feature in a minority of cases. Obsessive–compulsive disorder is often also present. The tics can be treated with neuroleptics, e.g. sulpiride, or clomipramine.

Dopa-responsive dystonia is another rare but treatable genetic disorder caused by mutations in a gene in the pathway of dopa synthesis. It presents with lower limb dystonia, which fluctuates throughout the day. Treatment with L-dopa can result in dramatic improvement.

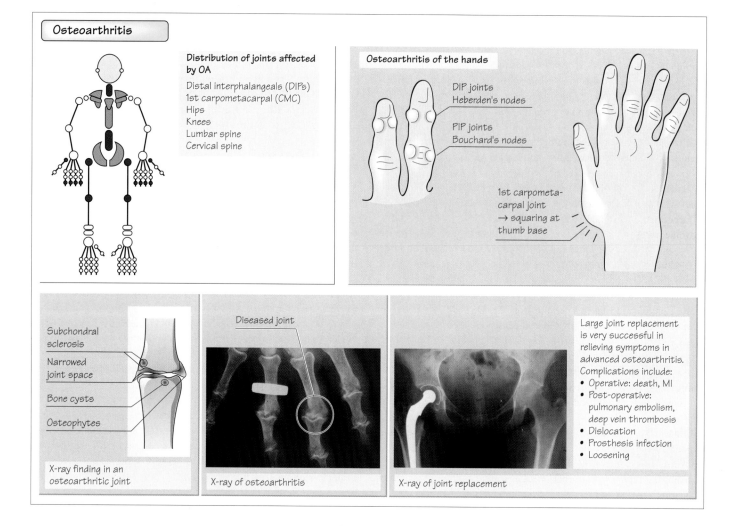

Distribution of joints affected by OA

Distal interphalangeals (DIPs)
1st carpometacarpal (CMC)
Hips
Knees
Lumbar spine
Cervical spine

Osteoarthritis of the hands

DIP joints
Heberden's nodes

PIP joints
Bouchard's nodes

1st carpometa-carpal joint
→ squaring at thumb base

Subchondral sclerosis

Narrowed joint space

Bone cysts

Osteophytes

X-ray finding in an osteoarthritic joint

Diseased joint

X-ray of osteoarthritis

Large joint replacement is very successful in relieving symptoms in advanced osteoarthritis. Complications include:
• Operative: death, MI
• Post-operative: pulmonary embolism, deep vein thrombosis
• Dislocation
• Prosthesis infection
• Loosening

X-ray of joint replacement

Osteoarthritis (OA) is the most common arthropathy of adults. Its aetiology is multifactorial, and it is characterized by progressive cartilage loss and hypertrophic changes in surrounding bone (osteophytosis), resulting in progressive degenerative joint disease. Inflammation is not a marked feature.

Epidemiology

The overall prevalence of OA is 12–15% in at least one joint, and is much higher in > 65 years age group. The prevalence continually increases with advancing age, such that more than 80% of > 75 years have radiographic evidence of OA. Slight female preponderance overall, particularly in interphalangeal joint disease (F/M 10 : 1).

Aetiology and pathogenesis

The cause is unknown. Idiopathic OA, particularly of the distal interphalangeal (DIP) joint (Heberden's nodes), has a strong genetic basis with a dominant pattern of inheritance in females and a recessive pattern in males. The sister of a female with DIP OA is three times as likely to develop, and their mother twice as likely to have DIP OA than those of an unaffected female. Siblings of patients undergoing major

lower limb joint replacement for OA are three times more likely than the general population to require similar surgery themselves.

Pathological features are those of progressive cartilage damage and loss. Reactive bony hypertrophy next to cartilage loss results in characteristic 'osteophyte' development. Underlying subchondral bone may remodel leading to subchondral cyst formation and sclerosis (see figure). The osteophytosis, subchondral sclerosis and cysts are clearly visible on plain X-rays (see figure).

Classification

Primary or idiopathic OA—see above.

Secondary OA arises in association with:
• Trauma, including repetitive use (proven only for occupation overuse, e.g. jackhammer use, not for athletic/sporting overuse). A late complication of a fracture that involves the cartilage of a joint is OA.
• Obesity increases the risk of knee OA, but not that of hand or hip OA.
• Congenital conditions, e.g. hip dislocation or underlying joint dysplasia.
• Inflammatory arthritis (RA, gout).
• A late complication following bacterial infection of a joint.

- Metabolic disorders (Wilson's disease, haemochromatosis, hyperparathyroidism).
- Acromegaly.
- Haemophilia.

Clinical features

Distinguishing features on history:
- Joint pain tends to be insidious in onset.
- Pain is aggravated by activity, relieved by rest, is worst at the end of the day and as the condition progresses, and becomes increasingly severe, occurring on minimal movement. Ultimately it may interfere with sleep.
- Stiffness is minor in the morning but recurs throughout the day with periods of rest, and is described as 'gelling' following inactivity.
- Bony swelling may be noted particularly in the hands (see figure) as Heberden's (DIP joint involvement) and Bouchard's (proximal interphalangeal [PIP] joint involvement) nodes. Asymmetric involvement of large joints is usual and leads to progressive decrease in range of movement at a joint, and later gait and mobility problems.

Physical findings

The distribution of joints affected in OA is shown in the figure. Examination reveals:
- Bony prominence due to a combination of marginal osteophytes and joint deformities (occasionally OA can cause effusions particularly in knees).
- Reduction in range of movement in affected joints with 'end of range' pain and limitation, with characteristic 'crepitus'.
- Instability in later stages, particularly where there is associated muscle wasting around the joint and substantial cartilage loss.

Subsets of OA

These include:
- Primary generalized OA (predominantly in middle-aged women, affecting first carpo-metacarpal (CMC) joint, PIP joint, distal DIPs joint, knee, hips and spine).
- Chondromalacia patellae (limited patellofemoral joint OA, causing pain on climbing stairs, running or squatting).
- Inflammatory OA. This is an unusual presentation of OA. Affects predominantly postmenopausal women in the distal or proximal IP joints of the hand. Episodes of pain and inflammation finally result in joint deformity, at which point the episodes are usually asymptomatic. X-rays often show erosions as well as the classical hallmarks of OA. Probably associated with crystal deposition (calcium pyrophosphate and hydroxyapatite).

Investigation

Inflammatory markers (ESR, CRP) are normal: serology for ANA and rheumatoid factor are unnecessary except in cases with symptoms suggestive of inflammation. Synovial fluid from joint aspiration is clear with normal viscosity and is non-inflammatory (low WCC) on microscopy; the fluid should be examined for calcium pyrophosphate crystals. Plain X-ray reveals characteristic features (see figure). Consider iron and calcium studies in those with atypical distribution or age of onset (to exclude haemochromatosis or hyperparathyroidism).

The differential diagnosis may include the arthropathy of psoriasis, Reiter's syndrome, or crystal deposition disease, indicating tests for these conditions where clinically indicated.

Management

The goals of therapy are to relieve pain and maintain function.

Pharmacological management

- Should rely on simple step-up analgesia such as paracetamol, and topical therapies such as ice, heat or locally applied analgesic creams, including capsaicin cream applied locally.
- Low dose non-steroidal anti-inflammatory agents if no contra-indication.
- Unresponsive or progressive pain may necessitate full dose NSAID therapy or other analgesia including opiates.
- Intra-articular injection of corticosteroid sometimes gives relief of pain. Periarticular injection of painful soft tissues may also be of benefit. In a small number of patients a course of intra-articular injections of hyaluronan (a component of synovial fluid) may be useful.

Physical therapy

- Particularly a low impact aerobic exercise regime (cycling/swimming) and weight loss programmes are associated with symptomatic improvement and may reduce progression and the requirement for surgery.
- Provision of soft collars and lumbar braces for short time periods are useful for those with cervical and lumbar OA when their symptoms flare up.

Surgical therapy

Joint replacement dramatically improves quality of life in those with advanced disease with intractable pain and significant loss of function. Outcome following hip or knee surgery is good or excellent in 95% of patients. The main benefit is loss of pain; restricted movement responds less well to joint replacement. The prostheses may be expected to function satisfactorily for 15 years. Revision surgery may subsequently be required and provides good results in 80% of cases.

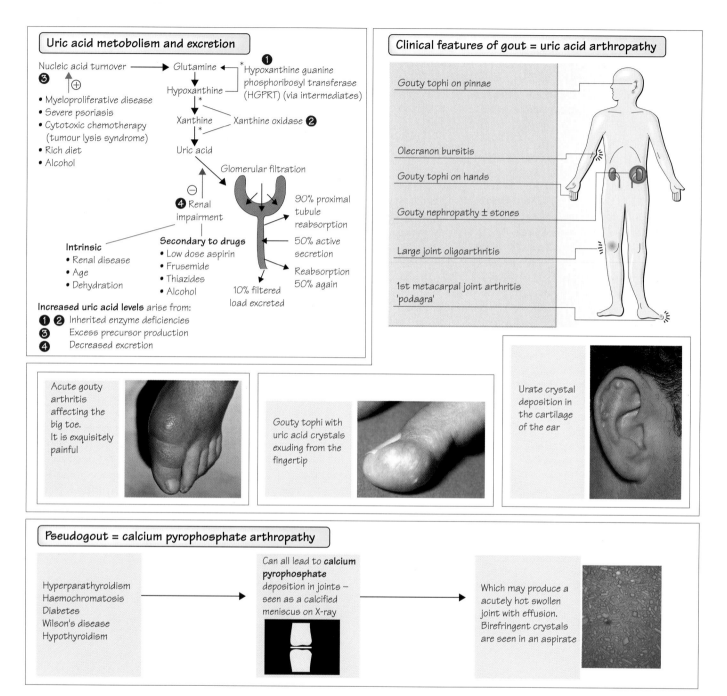

Uric acid metobolism and excretion

Nucleic acid turnover ⟶ Glutamine ⟵ *Hypoxanthine guanine **1**
phosphoribosyl transferase
Hypoxanthine ⟶ (HGPRT) (via intermediates)

3
⊕
- Myeloproliferative disease
- Severe psoriasis
- Cytotoxic chemotherapy
  (tumour lysis syndrome)
- Rich diet
- Alcohol

Xanthine ⟵ Xanthine oxidase **2**
*
Uric acid

Glomerular filtration

⊖
4 Renal
impairment

90% proximal
tubule
reabsorption

50% active
secretion

Intrinsic
- Renal disease
- Age
- Dehydration

Secondary to drugs
- Low dose aspirin
- Frusemide
- Thiazides
- Alcohol

Reabsorption
50% again

10% filtered
load excreted

Increased uric acid levels arise from:
1 **2** Inherited enzyme deficiencies
3 Excess precursor production
4 Decreased excretion

Clinical features of gout = uric acid arthropathy

Gouty tophi on pinnae

Olecranon bursitis

Gouty tophi on hands

Gouty nephropathy ± stones

Large joint oligoarthritis

1st metacarpal joint arthritis
'podagra'

Acute gouty
arthritis
affecting the
big toe.
It is exquisitely
painful

Gouty tophi with
uric acid crystals
exuding from the
fingertip

Urate crystal
deposition in
the cartilage
of the ear

Pseudogout = calcium pyrophosphate arthropathy

Hyperparathyroidism
Haemochromatosis
Diabetes
Wilson's disease
Hypothyroidism

Can all lead to **calcium
pyrophosphate**
deposition in joints –
seen as a calcified
meniscus on X-ray

Which may produce a
acutely hot swollen
joint with effusion.
Birefringent crystals
are seen in an aspirate

Crystal-related arthropathy defines a syndrome of synovitis in response
to crystal deposition/formation in the joint. Two types of crystals are
commonly implicated: monosodium urate (MSU, gout) and calcium
pyrophosphate dihydrate (CPPD, pseudogout). The resulting synovitis
may be limited to a single joint (monarticular) or become more widespread (polyarticular). Gout is the more common entity.

Gout
Epidemiology

Gout almost never occurs in premenopausal females, is of low prevalence (1–6 per 10 000) in women < 60 years and is 5–6-fold higher than
this in males aged 40–50. Environmental factors such as dietary purine
intake, alcohol consumption and the use of drugs such as diuretics con-

Diseases and Treatments at a Glance

tribute. Inherited metabolic abnormalities also contribute by causing over-production or under-excretion of uric acid.

Pathogenesis of hyperuricaemia

Uric acid is produced and excreted as shown (see figure). Any factor causing over-production or under-excretion will raise the plasma concentration of uric acid. The risk of developing acute gout increases as plasma uric acid increases:

- Levels < 420 μmol/L are associated with an incidence of 0.8/1000.
- Levels of > 540 μmol/L increase this to 49/1000.

Clinical features

The spectrum of clinical features of hyperuricaemia and gout are shown in the figure.

- Hyperuricaemia in isolation may not require treatment.
- Classic gout gives rise to a monoarthritis: 50% start in the first metatarsophalangeal joint (MTP). Ten per cent of first episodes are poly-articular. Attacks are agonizing and last 7–10 days.
- Acute episodes of gout may be triggered by trauma, exercise, alcohol excess or starvation.
- Crystals may also precipitate in the renal parenchyma, giving rise to gouty nephropathy and renal stones.
- Acute gout may progress to chronic gout, associated with characteristic subcutaneous deposits of urate (tophi) and may become polyarticular in nature.
- Chronic gout usually requires uric acid lowering therapy.

Differential diagnosis

The differential diagnosis of monoarticular gout includes septic arthritis, trauma, and cellulitis, as there is often significant swelling and erythema of the surrounding tissues. The patient may also be febrile. The differential of asymmetric large joint polyarticular gout includes the seronegative arthropathies and OA.

Investigations

- Demonstration of intracellular crystals in synovial fluid neutrophils aspirated from the inflamed joint is diagnostic.
- Measurement of serum uric acid is helpful, but not diagnostic. Uric acid levels may be normal in 20% of acute attacks.
- Patients without clear risk factors (e.g. young males with no family history) should have a full blood count to rule out an occult myeloproliferative disorder, as the increased DNA turnover that occurs here can give rise to gout. Likewise patients undergoing cancer chemotherapy should be pretreated with allopurinol (or occasionally recombinant uricase), to prevent gout (particularly with renal deposition of crystals) occurring with tumour cell lysis.

- Plain radiographs in established gout show punched out cortical erosions (often away from the joint margin), unlike the erosions found in rheumatoid arthritis.
- Plain radiographs in pseudogout sometimes show calcification of fibrocartilage (e.g. knee menisci, triangular cartilage in wrist), and of hyaline cartilage (knee, glenohumeral joint). The structural changes are similar to those of OA with cartilage loss, sclerosis, cysts and osteophytes, which may be prominent and exuberant.

Management

NSAIDs are indicated during the acute attack, and if inadequately effective/poorly tolerated, colchicine is an alternative. Intra-articular steroids are also highly effective. Therapy to lower uric acid formation (allopurinol) or promote excretion (probenicid or sulphinpyrazone) may be given in those with recurrent attacks, high urate levels or early disease involvement. This treatment should ideally be deferred until 4–6 weeks after the acute attack has settled (otherwise the attack may be prolonged). NSAIDs/colchicine are continued for the first 3 months of hypouricaemic therapy, because the risk of further attacks remains until normal urate levels have been achieved. Diet and alcohol intake may need to be adjusted.

Pseudogout

Calcium pyrophosphate deposits in joint cartilage are a common age-related phenomenon which may be present in one-quarter of those > 60 years old. Rarely it is related to a familial predisposition (activating mutations in Ank, a transmembrane transporter of inorganic pyrophosphate), hyperparathyroidism or haemochromatosis. When crystals are released into the joint cavity they produce an acute monoarthritis, diagnosed by finding characteristic rhomboidal crystals in the joint fluid. Treatment is with non-steroidal anti-inflammatory agents, or intra-articular steroids. Pyrophosphate arthropathy often has a chronic course, which may mimic rheumatoid or osteoarthritis. Fifty per cent of such cases are punctuated by episodes of acute pseudogout. Pseudogout is the commonest cause of monoarthritis in the elderly.

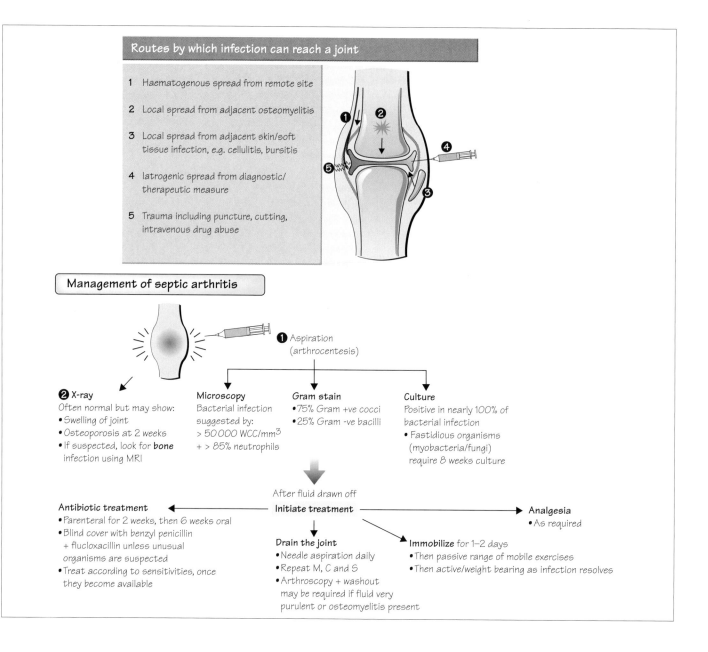

Routes by which infection can reach a joint

1 Haematogenous spread from remote site

2 Local spread from adjacent osteomyelitis

3 Local spread from adjacent skin/soft tissue infection, e.g. cellulitis, bursitis

4 Iatrogenic spread from diagnostic/ therapeutic measure

5 Trauma including puncture, cutting, intravenous drug abuse

Management of septic arthritis

❶ Aspiration (arthrocentesis)

❷ X-ray
Often normal but may show:
• Swelling of joint
• Osteoporosis at 2 weeks
• If suspected, look for **bone** infection using MRI

Microscopy
Bacterial infection suggested by:
> 50 000 WCC/mm³
+ > 85% neutrophils

Gram stain
• 75% Gram +ve cocci
• 25% Gram -ve bacilli

Culture
Positive in nearly 100% of bacterial infection
• Fastidious organisms (myobacteria/fungi) require 8 weeks culture

After fluid drawn off
Initiate treatment

Antibiotic treatment
• Parenteral for 2 weeks, then 6 weeks oral
• Blind cover with benzyl penicillin + flucloxacillin unless unusual organisms are suspected
• Treat according to sensitivities, once they become available

Drain the joint
• Needle aspiration daily
• Repeat M, C and S
• Arthroscopy + washout may be required if fluid very purulent or osteomyelitis present

Immobilize for 1–2 days
• Then passive range of mobile exercises
• Then active/weight bearing as infection resolves

Analgesia
• As required

Definitions

Joint infection gives rise to three distinct clinical patterns:
• Sepsis from colonization with pathogenic organisms.
• Arthritis as a significant clinical feature of systemic infection, e.g. rubella, parvovirus B19 infection, Lyme disease.
• Reactive arthritis: a sterile joint inflammation that develops as an immunologically mediated reaction to infection at a distant site. Triggering infections most commonly arise in the urogenital or gastrointestinal tract. Reactive arthritis is considered in Chapter 202.

Epidemiology of joint infection

Annual incidence varies widely and is related to the prevalence of underlying predisposing conditions.

Septic arthritis
Pathogenesis and aetiology

Pathogenic organisms may reach a joint by several routes (see figure). Factors which predispose an individual to septic arthritis, include:
• Impaired host defences:
  Inherited impairment of host defences, e.g. complement deficiency, hypogammaglobulinaemia.
  Immunosuppressive illness or therapy, e.g. steroids, cytotoxics, HIV
  Chronic illness, e.g. diabetes mellitus renal failure, cirrhosis
  Elderly or very young
  Neoplasia.
• The presence of a prosthetic or damaged (OA/RA/gout) joint.
  Notably, septic arthritis is usually a disease of the very young, the

elderly or those with damaged joints. Young adults with disseminated gonococcal infection may present with septic arthritis.

Clinical features

Septic arthritis affects the knee, hip, shoulder, wrist, ankle and elbow most commonly. Twenty per cent of presentations are polyarticular. The onset of symptoms is usually sudden and progressive, usually with florid systemic symptoms. The involved joint exhibits the classic features of local inflammation, being red, swollen, tender and hot. Usually held in flexion, avoiding movement and weight bearing. Disseminated gonococcal infection may feature urogenital symptoms and a pustular rash. Prosthetic joint infection in the early postoperative period is usually self evident with high fever and a wound discharging pus. Later infection is associated with low-grade fever, recurrent pain, impaired function and less impressive local signs. Infection should always be considered in those with loosening of the prosthesis.

Organisms responsible for septic arthritis

In adults the range of pathogens is narrow:
- *Staphylococcus aureus* is the most frequent joint pathogen in adults.
- About 25% of infections are due to Gram-negative bacilli.
- 15% are due to β-haemolytic streptococci.

Predisposing conditions are associated with less typical organisms such as:

- Gram-negative bacilli and *Streptococcus pneumoniae* in the debilitated patient (malignancy, alcoholism, diabetes, etc.).
- *Pseudomonas* in intravenous drug abusers.
- Under 2 years of age: high incidence of *Haemophilus influenzae* infection.

Management of septic arthritis

A management algorithm of joint sepsis is shown (see figure). Antibiotic therapy should be selected depending on joint aspirate culture and sensitivity and should continue for at least two weeks parenterally and a further six weeks orally. Close involvement of infectious disease or clinical microbiology experts is vital. Progression to chronic infection has decreased from 10–20% to < 2% of acute infections with early antibiotic therapy and appropriate surgical intervention.

Arthritis as a feature of systemic infection

Viral agents such as parvovirus B19, rubella and other acute viral syndromes may have arthritis as a predominant feature. The acute presentation of these arthropathies may be indistinguishable in joint distribution from that of acute onset rheumatoid arthritis. Characteristic features of the underlying infection are usually present, and the joint symptoms usually subside without sequelae within 6 weeks of onset. Serology is useful when the result influences management.

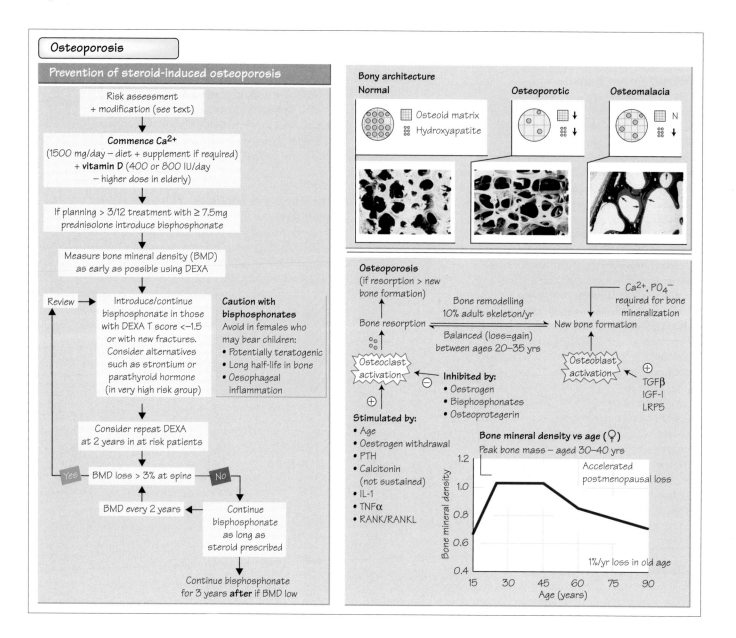

Osteoporosis

Osteoporosis is very common and predisposes to skeletal fractures from a quantitative decrease in bone matrix components (osteoid and hydroxyapatite) of bone. Fifty per cent of women and 15% of men sustain an osteoporosis related fracture by age 90. Osteoporosis may be primary or secondary to a specific disease (below). Osteoporosis is common in elderly women, especially those with a late menarche, early menopause or long history of oligomenorrhoea (e.g. athletes, anorexia nervosa). Other important risk factors include smoking, alcohol, sedentary life-style (or non-weight bearing exercise), positive family history (peak bone mass is under strong genetic control) and lean body type. Secondary osteoporosis occurs in:

• Endocrine disease: thyrotoxicosis, Cushing's disease, hypogonadism, hyperparathyroidism.

• Rheumatological disease: any inflammatory arthropathy, especially if treated with steroids.

• Gastroenterological disease: malabsorption, cirrhosis.

• Neoplasia.

• Drug therapy, especially corticosteroids, heparin, warfarin and phenytoin.

• A variety of rare genetic disorders, including osteogenesis imperfecta and hypophosphatasia.

Clinical features

The hallmarks of osteoporosis are low impact fractures (distal radius—Colles' fracture—or femoral neck) and (wedge) fractures of vertebrae in the thoracic region, causing loss of height, an exaggerated dorsal kyphosis (dowager's hump) and pain.

Diagnosis
- Plain radiographs are useful for demonstrating osteoporosis-related fractures.
- Dual emission X-ray absorptiometry (DEXA) is used to measure bone density and quantify the degree of osteopenia (mild-to-moderate bone loss) or osteoporosis (severe bone loss). Measurement is useful in those at risk (e.g. corticosteroid therapy, premature menopause) and particularly in those aged < 70 years with low impact fractures.

Management
Prevention of osteoporosis is a major public health goal and the following strategies are promoted to minimize osteoporosis and its complications:
- **Maximization of peak adult bone mass**: young women should not smoke, should minimize their alcohol and caffeine intake, and take adequate dietary calcium and weight-bearing exercise.
- **Reducing rate of bone loss**: peri/postmenopausal women, those on > 7.5 mg/day of prednisolone, and other high-risk individuals should have DEXA scans. If significant osteoporosis is found, bisphosphonates and/or calcium/vitamin D should be given. HRT and selective oestrogen receptor modulators should also be considered. However, HRT is now prescribed less commonly for osteoporosis than bisphosphonates because it is less effective and carries some concerns regarding the risk of malignancy.
- **Prevention of fractures**: those with established osteoporosis should be routinely assessed for remediable factors that may cause falls, e.g. drugs causing postural hypotension, and for padded hip protectors (which protect against hip fractures). Vitamin D deficiency is common in the elderly, and supplementation should be considered.

In symptomatic osteoporosis treatment aims to prevent further fractures. DEXA measurements are useful in identifying those at significant risk and may be useful in monitoring treatment in selected cases. Current treatment options are:
- Agents which reduce bone resorption: a combination of elemental calcium/vitamin D, a bisphosphonate and/or oestrogen therapy confers benefit. Calcitonin is useful to reduce the pain of ostoeporotic fractures.
- Other agents include strontium ranelate and recombinant parathyroid hormone.

Steroid therapy and osteoporosis
Rapid loss of bone occurs within 3 months of starting steroids, thereafter slowing to a rate 2–3 × normal loss. Osteoporosis risk is related to dose and treatment duration (total cumulative dose). Highly significant bone loss occurs with prednisolone doses > 7.5 mg/day for 3 months. However, there is no safe steroid dose for bone loss. Many conditions requiring steroids themselves result in osteoporosis, e.g. rheumatoid arthritis, SLE, inflammatory bowel disease. The figure shows the methods for preventing bone loss in those taking steroids. Current steroids use doubles the risk of fracture irrespective of bone density.

Osteomalacia/rickets
Osteomalacia results from impaired mineralization of the osteoid matrix. It causes skeletal deformity in the young (rickets) and bone pain, non-specific aches, fractures and proximal muscle weakness in adults (osteomalacia). The causes include:
- **Vitamin D deficiency**: dietary inadequacy, lack of sunshine or malabsorption are the commonest causes in clinical practice, e.g. osteomalacia is relatively common in Asian women who dress traditionally, vegetarians, and those (children and the elderly) with poor diets. Coeliac disease.
- **Vitamin D metabolic abnormality**: reduced liver 25-hydroxylation (cirrhosis), reduced renal hydroxylation (renal failure), or increased hepatic metabolism (anticonvulsants).
- **Very rare causes include vitamin D receptor mutations** causing defective vitamin D mediated calcium absorption, 1α hydroxylase deficiency and familial (X-linked) hypophosphataemic rickets.

Clinical features
Delay or deficiency in bone mineralization in childhood (rickets) leads to structural skeletal deformities, including enlargement of the ends of the long bones, widened cranial sutures and frontal bossing (in those < 1 year old) and tibial bowing, genu varum/valgum (knock or bow knees) in older children. Adults experience non-specific pains and aches, predominantly in the proximal limb girdles, and lower back. Pressure over the long bones or the rib cage may elicit tenderness. Significant osteomalacia may cause pathological fractures and results in secondary hyperparathyroidism which may complicate the picture biochemically and radiologically.

Investigation
This diagnosis must be considered in at risk individuals with musculoskeletal symptoms:
- Diagnosis is something evident from plain radiographs showing Looser's zones or pseudofractures (translucent bands occur at sites of stress, e.g. the ribs, the axillary borders of the scapulae and pubic rami).
- Histology (usually not necessary) shows decreased hydroxyapatite component with increased number of unmineralized osteoid lamellae.
- Characteristic biochemistry: low phosphate (early), low calcium (variable) and raised alkaline phosphatase (late due to secondary hyperparathyroidism).
- Low vitamin D and high PTH.

Treatment
- Treat any underlying cause (e.g. coeliac disease).
- Give oral daily vitamin D supplementation according to the degree of depletion and bony abnormality
- Malabsorption states require high doses
- Deficiency of vitamin D due to renal or hepatic disease may be overcome by using hydroxylated forms such as alfacalcidol or calcitriol.

Therapy relieves symptoms and corrects bony abnormalities within 3–4 months. Occasionally, hyperparathroidism becomes autonomous in long standing osteomalacia (tertiary hyperparathyroidism).

Parathyroid and renal bone disease
These metabolic conditions have characteristic effects on bone (pp. 270 and 288).

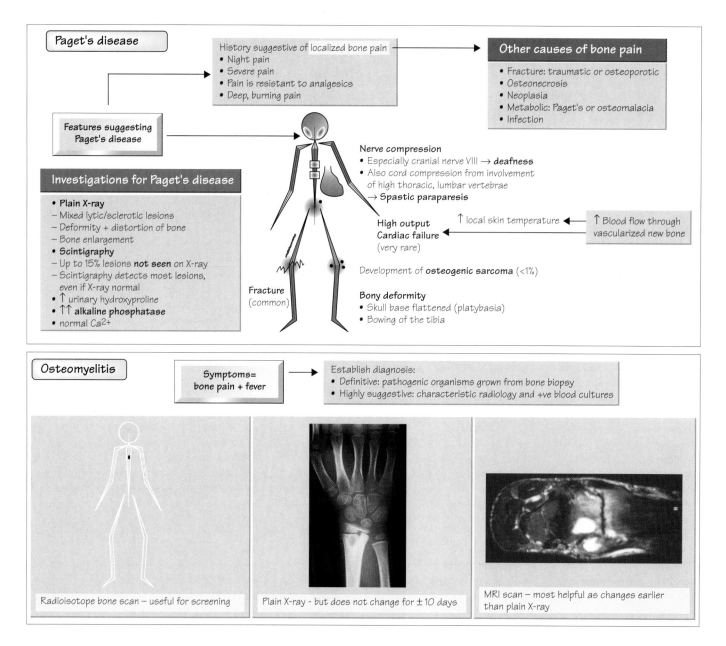

Paget's disease

History suggestive of localized bone pain
- Night pain
- Severe pain
- Pain is resistant to analgesics
- Deep, burning pain

Other causes of bone pain
- Fracture: traumatic or osteoporotic
- Osteonecrosis
- Neoplasia
- Metabolic: Paget's or osteomalacia
- Infection

Features suggesting Paget's disease

Nerve compression
- Especially cranial nerve VIII → **deafness**
- Also cord compression from involvement of high thoracic, lumbar vertebrae → **Spastic paraparesis**

Investigations for Paget's disease

- **Plain X-ray**
  – Mixed lytic/sclerotic lesions
  – Deformity + distortion of bone
  – Bone enlargement
- **Scintigraphy**
  – Up to 15% lesions **not seen** on X-ray
  – Scintigraphy detects most lesions, even if X-ray normal
- ↑ urinary hydroxyproline
- ↑↑ **alkaline phosphatase**
- normal Ca2+

High output Cardiac failure (very rare) ← ↑ local skin temperature ← ↑ Blood flow through vascularized new bone

Development of **osteogenic sarcoma** (<1%)

Fracture (common)

Bony deformity
- Skull base flattened (platybasia)
- Bowing of the tibia

Osteomyelitis

Symptoms= bone pain + fever

Establish diagnosis:
- Definitive: pathogenic organisms grown from bone biopsy
- Highly suggestive: characteristic radiology and +ve blood cultures

Radioisotope bone scan – useful for screening

Plain X-ray - but does not change for ± 10 days

MRI scan – most helpful as changes earlier than plain X-ray

Paget's disease

Associated with abnormal remodelling of bone. The aetiology is variable but about 10% of cases are familial, indicating a significant genetic contribution. It is primarily a disorder of osteoclasts, which become highly activated altering the normal homeostasis of bone remodelling:
- Early stages: increased bone resorption occurs, so producing lytic lesions (osteoporosis circumscripta).
- Later stages: disproportionate stimulation of new bone formation occurs in a disorganized fashion, resulting in areas of bone sclerosis.

Cycles of resorption and formation result in a huge increase in bone turnover and ultimately grossly disorganized bone, which is weak and prone to fracture.

Epidemiology

Paget's occurs mainly in the elderly (> 70 years). The prevalence is 10% in ≥ 80 years and < 0.3% in those ≤ 40. It is commonest in western countries and is rare in Africa and Asia. Male preponderance is 3 : 2, increased incidence in relatives. Mutations in the sequestosome gene are well described both in familial and sporadic cases and likely cause disease through their effects on osteoclast activation through the NF-κB pathway. However, no such genetic basis has been described for the majority of cases.

Clinical features

Paget's disease is often asymptomatic with the only abnormality being an isolated raised alkaline phosphatase. Between 5 and 10% develop symptoms bringing them to medical care. Symptomatic presentation depends on the sites and extent of bony involvement (see figure). Twenty per cent of patients have a single bony lesion. The pelvis, spine, long bones and the skull are most commonly affected. The common symptoms include: bone pain, bone deformities and increased warmth over an affected area. Important bony complications are: fractures (10%) and osteogenic sarcoma (rare < 1%). A sudden increase in pain, deformity or serum alkaline phosphatase should alert the clinician to one of these possibilities. Other complications are very rare, and include:

• Cardiovascular complications; a high output state exacerbating heart failure or ischaemic heart disease.
• Neurological complications; cranial nerve compression, conductive hearing loss (or sensori neural) and spinal stenosis.
• Other; including hypercalcaemia, or hypercalciuria, which in turn may lead to renal stones.

Management
Investigations
• Raised alkaline phosphatase (reflects increased osteoblastic activity).
• Increased urinary hydroxyproline excretion (derived from bone collagen). Useful in following disease activity.
• Radiology: X-rays show gross bony distortion and deformity and mixed osteolytic and sclerotic areas, with abnormal trabecular architecture and enlargement of bones. Skull involvement may lead to the 'Tam O'Shanter' appearance. Technetium-labelled bone scan delineates the extent of Pagetic involvement in bone (15% of lesions, usually early active areas, are not visible on plain film).
• Bone biopsy if imaging cannot exclude tumour.
• Calcium in Paget's disease is normal but may rise with a fracture or prolonged inactivity.

Treatment
Asymptomatic disease does not require treatment. Indications for treatment are:
• Active disease at the skull base or in the spine above L2 or any neurologic compromise (cranial or spinal nerves).
• Pain.
• Progressive deformity.
• The very rare complications of either immobilization hypercalcaemia or high output cardiac failure.

Treatment of symptomatic patients
• Analgesia.
• Agents that inhibit bone resorption, such as bisphosphonates (e.g. alendronate, pamidronate), which reduce bone turnover.
• Calcitonin is useful for severe pain or extensive lytic disease. Side-effects include troublesome flushing, nausea and hypocalcaemia. Beneficial effects are seen within 2 weeks; maximum effectiveness may not be seen for 6–12 months.
• Surgery is used to relieve compression neuropathy.

Osteonecrosis (avascular necrosis)
Avascular necrosis describes the death of cellular elements of bone, occurring in all ages and both sexes, which potentially causes structural collapse.

Aetiology and pathogenesis
Avascular necrosis is well recognized in pregnancy, corticosteroid therapy, and following radiotherapy or cytotoxic chemotherapy. It may also occur in sickle cell disease and other haemoglobinopathies and decompression sickness, though many cases are idiopathic. It commonly affects the femoral head and the scaphoid after fracture of these bones.

Clinical features
• Characteristic feature is bone pain.
• Initially on weight bearing, subsequently at rest and at night.
• Increasing severity of pain, becoming resistant to escalating analgesia.

Management
Radiographs are frequently normal early on; subsequently patchy osteopenia and osteosclerosis develop, and later still characteristic 'crescent sign' demarcates viable and dead bone. In advanced disease destruction and collapse of the articular surface. MRI is diagnostic even when X-rays are normal, and is the investigation of choice in early cases. Treatment is:
• Conservative with analgesia and muscle strengthening early in course, with reduced weight and load bearing until recovery occurs.
• Surgical 'core decompression' or arthroplasty.
• May require joint replacement if severe.

Osteomyelitis
Osteomyelitis is infection of the bone arising either from direct inoculation with infecting organisms, e.g. an 'open' fracture, or from haematogenous spread. Though common in children, it is relatively rare in adults.

Underlying conditions and responsible organisms
• Diabetes leads to Gram-negative and/or *Staphylococcus aureus* foot infection.
• 90% of adult osteomyelitis is due to *Staphylococcus* infection.
• *Staphylococcus aureus* septicaemia (e.g. a complication of intravenous cannula in hospitalized patients) is complicated by osteomyelitis in 1% of cases.
• Sickle cell disease (80% of infections are due to *Salmonella* species).
• Immunosuppression predisposes to many different infections.
• Spinal tuberculosis is relatively common in countries with a high prevalence of tuberculosis. In some areas, infection with atypical mycobacteria is common.
• Foot puncture wounds (e.g. 'drawing pin' related) can cause calcaneal osteomyelitis, which is due to *Pseudomonas aeruginosa* in 90% of cases.
• Late syphilis can cause bone infection, resulting in nocturnal pain, and a 'sabre' deformity of the tibia may occur in congenital syphilis.

Clinical features
Osteomyelitis presents with systemic symptoms (fever, malaise) and local pain. Vertebral osteomyelitis can lead to vertebral collapse and cord compression. Osteomyelitis in diabetics is often painless. Sterile and occasionally septic arthritis can complicate the picture.

Diagnosis and treatment
Standard X-rays do not show changes within 10 days. MRI is therefore the investigation of choice. Treatment is with prolonged antibiotics, debridement of dead bone, and stabilization when necessary. Occasionally it proves impossible to eradicate the infection, and life-long antibiotics are required.

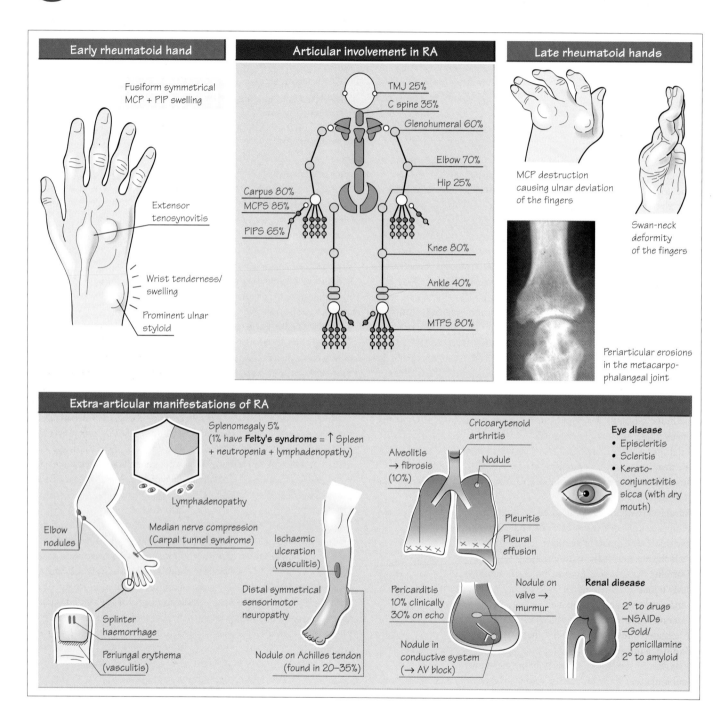

Early rheumatoid hand

Fusiform symmetrical MCP + PIP swelling

Extensor tenosynovitis

Wrist tenderness/ swelling

Prominent ulnar styloid

Articular involvement in RA

TMJ 25%
C spine 35%
Glenohumeral 60%
Elbow 70%
Hip 25%
Carpus 80%
MCPS 85%
PIPS 65%
Knee 80%
Ankle 40%
MTPS 80%

Late rheumatoid hands

MCP destruction causing ulnar deviation of the fingers

Swan-neck deformity of the fingers

Periarticular erosions in the metacarpo-phalangeal joint

Extra-articular manifestations of RA

Splenomegaly 5% (1% have **Felty's syndrome** = ↑ Spleen + neutropenia + lymphadenopathy)

Lymphadenopathy

Elbow nodules

Median nerve compression (Carpal tunnel syndrome)

Ischaemic ulceration (vasculitis)

Splinter haemorrhage

Periungal erythema (vasculitis)

Distal symmetrical sensorimotor neuropathy

Nodule on Achilles tendon (found in 20–35%)

Cricoarytenoid arthritis

Alveolitis → fibrosis (10%)

Nodule

Pleuritis

Pleural effusion

Pericarditis 10% clinically 30% on echo

Nodule in conductive system (→ AV block)

Nodule on valve → murmur

Eye disease
• Episcleritis
• Scleritis
• Kerato-conjunctivitis sicca (with dry mouth)

Renal disease

2° to drugs
—NSAIDs
—Gold/ penicillamine
2° to amyloid

Rheumatoid arthritis (RA) is a systemic autoimmune disorder characterized by a chronic, symmetric and erosive arthritis of synovial joints resulting in major disability and handicap. It is also associated with extra-articular manifestations and circulating autoantibodies to immunoglobulin, known as rheumatoid factors (RF).

Epidemiology

Worldwide prevalence is 1% and the peak age of onset early 40s, although it may present in later life. Women are 2–3 times more com-monly affected than men, but the sex ratio varies with age (at 30 years, F/M is 10 : 1, at 65 years, 1 : 1).

Aetiology and pathogenesis

RA represents an immune mediated response to an undefined antigen, in a genetically predisposed individual. This process triggers inflammation, endothelial cell activation and recruitment of specific inflammatory cells to the joint, facilitated by the up-regulation of adhesion molecules on synovial vascular endothelium and on circulating

Table 201.1 1987 Criteria for diagnosis of rheumatoid arthritis. A patient shall be said to have RA if he/she has satisfied at least four of these seven criteria. The first four criteria must have been present for at least 6 weeks.

Criterion	Definition
Morning stiffness	In and around the joints lasting at least 1 h
Arthritis of three or more joint areas	Soft-tissue swelling or fluid observed by a physician
	Possible areas are right or left PIP, MCP, wrist, elbow, knee, ankle, and MTP joints
Arthritis of hand joints	At least one area swollen in a wrist, MCP, or PIP joint
Symmetric arthritis	Simultaneous involvement of these joint areas bilaterally
Rheumatoid nodules	Subcutaneous nodules over bony prominences/extensor surfaces/in juxta-articular regions
Serum rheumatoid factor	
Radiographic changes	Typical of rheumatoid arthritis on hand and wrist radiographs (see figure)

inflammatory cells. Amplification of inflammation occurs in response to the local production of inflammatory cytokines (tumor necrosis factor-alpha [TNFα] and interleukin-1 [IL-1]).

Synovial tissue proliferates and becomes locally invasive in the joints. Pannus is the characteristic pathological lesion in RA, a thickened inflammatory granulation tissue. Cells within the pannus produce destructive collagenases and proteases. These enzymes mediate the erosion of cartilage at the subchondral bone/cartilage junction and inwards until the articular cartilage is destroyed. Cartilage destruction leads to subluxation, mechanical disarray and ultimately instability of joints resulting in the characteristic clinical and radiological destructive arthropathy of RA.

Clinical features

Initial presentation:
- Joint swelling, tenderness, pain and stiffness, particularly troublesome in the morning and improving as the day goes on, and recurring in the evening.
- Small joints of the hands and feet (see figure) tend to be affected initially asymmetrically, eventually symmetrically, followed by involvement of larger joints such as knees and elbows where clear effusions may be demonstrable.
- Onset is often insidious, and asymmetrical with fluctuating joint pain, swelling and stiffness, frequently accompanied by fatigue and lassitude. The clinical examination at onset may be normal, but more usually reveals the characteristic features of synovitis:
- Warmth, swelling and tenderness of the MCPs and PIPs, the wrists and MTP joints of the feet in a strikingly symmetric distribution.
- Tenosynovitis is a prominent early feature, often affecting the extensor tendon sheaths on the dorsum of the hand.

  Alternative presentations of RA include:
- **Explosive onset** in 5–10%.
- A **systemic onset** in 5%, usually in middle-aged men with non-articular manifestations (such as weight loss) as the dominant feature. Arthritis may be minor or even absent but elevated RF titres are usually found.
- **Palindromic onset** in 5%, comprising irregular episodes of transient though possibly severe synovitis. Attacks come on suddenly, may be debilitating and abate within 24–72 h with no residual deficit. Fifty per cent of these evolve into typical RA (typically RF positive).
- **Polymyalgic onset** in 5%: diffuse proximal limb girdle stiffness without joint inflammation. Associated with presence of rheumatoid factor. Shows a less dramatic response to steroids than classical polymyalgia and progresses to typical RA in time.

  Diagnostic criteria for RA are shown (Table 201.1). Differential diagnosis of RA includes:

- Infection-related transient arthritis, e.g. parvovirus B19, rubella infection: these typically last < 6 weeks.
- Chronic pyrophosphate arthritis (p. 391).
- Small joint arthritis associated with psoriasis (RF negative).
- Non-erosive arthritis of SLE.

Features of established/chronic RA

Established RA pursues an unpredictable clinical course characterized by acute 'flares' of involved joints and variable systemic and extra-articular symptoms. Acute flares give rise to ongoing pain, discomfort and functional impairment as a result of active synovitis (e.g. inability to grip due to MCP and PIP swelling and stiffness). These are usually responsive to anti-inflammatory therapy. This fluctuating clinical picture is usually accompanied by an underlying slowly progressive course of structural joint damage. Progressive joint damage ultimately leads to severe loss of function; within 10 years of onset only 50% of patients are able to work full time. Extra-articular manifestations contribute significantly to the morbidity and mortality of RA. Major vasculitis affects 1 in 9 men, and 1 in 30 women with RA. Infections are also at least three times more common than in the general population, particularly in those on steroids. Clinical features of established RA are shown (see figure).

Investigation

An acute inflammatory response (raised ESR, CRP, and diffuse hypergammaglobulinaemia) is found. Rheumatoid factor is present in the majority of cases (85–90%) though may not be positive early in the disease (70% at onset). Measurement of anti-cyclic citrullinated peptide [CCP] antibodies may be a more specific diagnostic test than rheumatoid factor. X-rays typically reveal only soft tissue swelling at presentation. (See Table 201.2.) Erosive changes often occur within 2 years of onset usually first in the feet.

Management (see figure)

Individual patients with rheumatoid arthritis have distinct patterns of damage and unique rehabilitation requirements. Treatment must be tailored to these needs within the framework of a multidisciplinary team. The introduction of biologic agents, including those directed against TNF, have had a major beneficial effect in the past 5 years.

Pharmacological therapy (see table in figure, p. 401)

Principles of therapy

A multidisciplinary approach involving physicians, physiotherapists, surgeons, etc. is vital. Therapy aims to minimize symptoms and improve prognosis.

Table 201.2 Assessment in RA.

	Indicating active inflammation	Indicating structural damage
Clinical	Symptoms • Prolonged early morning stiffness • Painful and swollen joints • Lassitude, fatigue Signs • Hot swollen tender joints • Inability to make a fist/reduction in grip strength • Demonstrable effusion	Symptoms • Joint deformity or instability • Functional loss due to tendon rupture or deformity Signs • Joint subluxation • Joint deformity (e.g. swan neck, boutonnière, hallux valgus)
Laboratory tests	↑ ESR, ↑ CRP, ↑ gammaglobulins Anaemia High titre RF is associated with more severe disease	
Radiological		Presence of erosion, bony malalignment, secondary osteoarthritis

1 Symptomatic relief. Simple analgesics or anti-inflammatory drugs (NSAIDs). These agents have no effect on long-term outcome measures (disability and deformity). NSAIDs with relative specificity for the COX-2 isoform of cyclooxygenase produce fewer GI complications. However, while these drugs may be useful in the elderly and in those with major risk factors for GI ulceration, there are major concerns that they may be associated with an increased thrombotic risk. They should be used only with extreme caution in those with cardiovascular risk factors.

2 Modification of underlying disease. Second-line (disease modifying antirheumatic drugs [DMARDs]) immunomodulatory agents include methotrexate, sulfasalazine, leflunomide, azathioprine, injectable gold salts, ciclosporin and antimalarials. DMARDs have been proven in clinical trials to slow the progression of erosions (deforming) disease but have very little impact on morbidity and disability in the long term. They are associated with significant side-effects and the least toxic agents (hydroxychloroquine and sulfasalazine) are often chosen in early disease. Methotrexate is often chosen as the initial agent in patients who have adverse prognostic indicators at onset (high rheumatoid factor titre, very active disease, early erosions) as it is the DMARD with most predictable benefit. Methotrexate is increasingly being used in combination with other DMARDs.

3 Adjunctive therapy with corticosteroids. For severe systemic illness, intermittent troublesome (mono- or pauci-articular) inflammation and/or vasculitis steroids may be given as intermittent 'pulses', e.g. 80–120 mg i.m. depot or 500–1000 mg i.v. methylprednisolone. Intramuscular steroids are particularly valuable for the rapid amelioration of symptoms in patients with early disease at the initiation of treatment with DMARDs, which typically require several months for effect. Low-dose oral prednisolone (7.5 mg a day) may also be useful to control symptoms, while other DMARDs are taking effect and may exert a weak effect on suppressing erosions.

4 Biological agents. The realistic goal of treatment is now complete disease remission. For those patients not responding adequately to DMARD, either as single agents or in combination, biologic therapies should be considered. These include monoclonal antibodies directed against TNFα (infliximab, adalimumab) and recombinant TNF receptor/IgG fusion protein (etanercept). These drugs are expensive compared to DMARD but result in remission of disease in 25% of patients within 3 months and 50% improvement in 40% of patients. They are also highly effective in arresting bone erosion and have a rapid onset of action. Theoretical risks of increased risk of infection demand careful monitoring and all patients should be screened for latent tuberculosis because of the observed risk of reactivation.

Prognosis and outcome

The course and outcome of RA in an individual patient is unpredictable. Poor prognostic factors are:
• Generalized polyarthritis (total involved joints > 20)
• High ESR and CRP despite therapy
• Extra-articular features, e.g. nodules/vasculitis
• Rheumatoid factor positivity
• Erosions on plain radiographs within 2 years of onset
• HLA-DR4 status.

The spectrum of severity of rheumatoid arthritis ranges from mild or subclinical to aggressive and destructive forms, which are associated with excess mortality (standardized mortality 2–2.5 times that of age- and sex-matched controls). Up to 33% of patients will leave the workforce within 5 years of disease onset, and fewer than half are able to work full-time within 10 years of disease onset. Factors contributing to excess mortality include an increase in cardiovascular infections (which accounts for the majority of the excess) and neoplastic diseases, which are increased 5–8 times over that of the general population (particularly non-Hodgkin's lymphoma, and other haematological malignancies including leukaemia and myeloma). Other long-term damage results from:
• Drug side effects, especially from long-term steroids
• Cervical myelopathy
• Cardiac involvement
• Amyloidosis (causing renal failure and the nephrotic syndrome)
• Rheumatoid lung disease.

Overall rheumatoid arthritis reduces life span by 10–15 years.

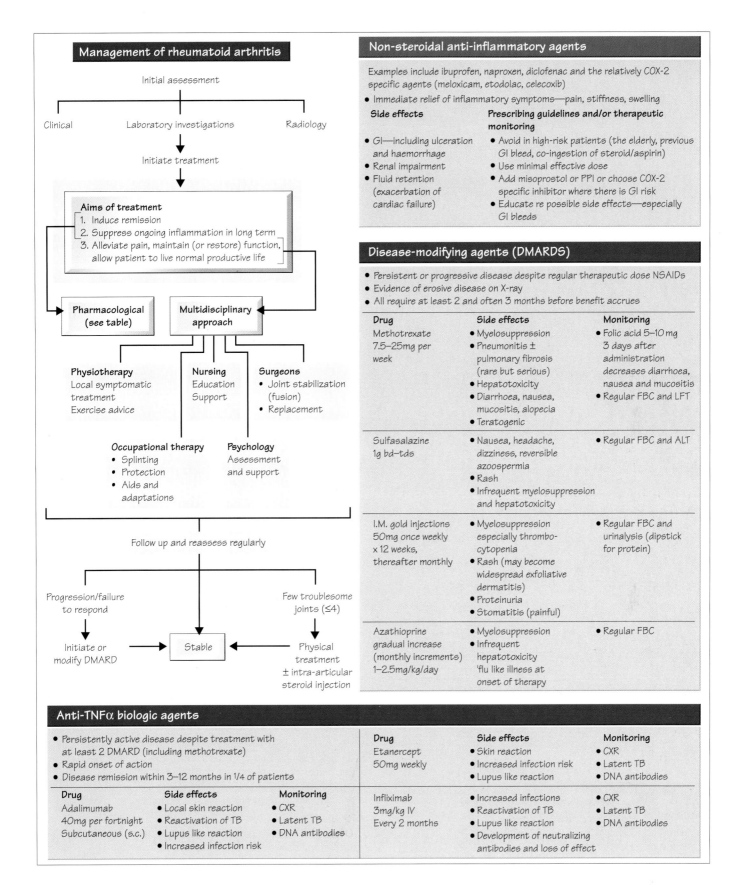

Management of rheumatoid arthritis

Initial assessment

Clinical — Laboratory investigations — Radiology

Initiate treatment

Aims of treatment
1. Induce remission
2. Suppress ongoing inflammation in long term
3. Alleviate pain, maintain (or restore) function, allow patient to live normal productive life

Pharmacological (see table) — Multidisciplinary approach

Physiotherapy
Local symptomatic treatment
Exercise advice

Nursing
Education
Support

Surgeons
• Joint stabilization (fusion)
• Replacement

Occupational therapy
• Splinting
• Protection
• Aids and adaptations

Psychology
Assessment and support

Follow up and reassess regularly

Progression/failure to respond

Few troublesome joints (≤4)

Initiate or modify DMARD — Stable — Physical treatment ± intra-articular steroid injection

Non-steroidal anti-inflammatory agents

Examples include ibuprofen, naproxen, diclofenac and the relatively COX-2 specific agents (meloxicam, etodolac, celecoxib)
• Immediate relief of inflammatory symptoms—pain, stiffness, swelling

Side effects	Prescribing guidelines and/or therapeutic monitoring
• GI—including ulceration and haemorrhage • Renal impairment • Fluid retention (exacerbation of cardiac failure)	• Avoid in high-risk patients (the elderly, previous GI bleed, co-ingestion of steroid/aspirin) • Use minimal effective dose • Add misoprostol or PPI or choose COX-2 specific inhibitor where there is GI risk • Educate re possible side effects—especially GI bleeds

Disease-modifying agents (DMARDS)

• Persistent or progressive disease despite regular therapeutic dose NSAIDs
• Evidence of erosive disease on X-ray
• All require at least 2 and often 3 months before benefit accrues

Drug	Side effects	Monitoring
Methotrexate 7.5–25mg per week	• Myelosuppression • Pneumonitis ± pulmonary fibrosis (rare but serious) • Hepatotoxicity • Diarrhoea, nausea, mucositis, alopecia • Teratogenic	• Folic acid 5–10 mg 3 days after administration decreases diarrhoea, nausea and mucositis • Regular FBC and LFT
Sulfasalazine 1g bd–tds	• Nausea, headache, dizziness, reversible azoospermia • Rash • Infrequent myelosuppression and hepatotoxicity	• Regular FBC and ALT
I.M. gold injections 50mg once weekly x 12 weeks, thereafter monthly	• Myelosuppression especially thrombo-cytopenia • Rash (may become widespread exfoliative dermatitis) • Proteinuria • Stomatitis (painful)	• Regular FBC and urinalysis (dipstick for protein)
Azathioprine gradual increase (monthly increments) 1–2.5mg/kg/day	• Myelosuppression • Infrequent hepatotoxicity 'flu like illness at onset of therapy	• Regular FBC

Anti-TNFα biologic agents

• Persistently active disease despite treatment with at least 2 DMARD (including methotrexate)
• Rapid onset of action
• Disease remission within 3–12 months in 1/4 of patients

Drug	Side effects	Monitoring
Adalimumab 40mg per fortnight Subcutaneous (s.c.)	• Local skin reaction • Reactivation of TB • Lupus like reaction • Increased infection risk	• CXR • Latent TB • DNA antibodies
Etanercept 50mg weekly	• Skin reaction • Increased infection risk • Lupus like reaction	• CXR • Latent TB • DNA antibodies
Infliximab 3mg/kg IV Every 2 months	• Increased infections • Reactivation of TB • Lupus like reaction • Development of neutralizing antibodies and loss of effect	• CXR • Latent TB • DNA antibodies

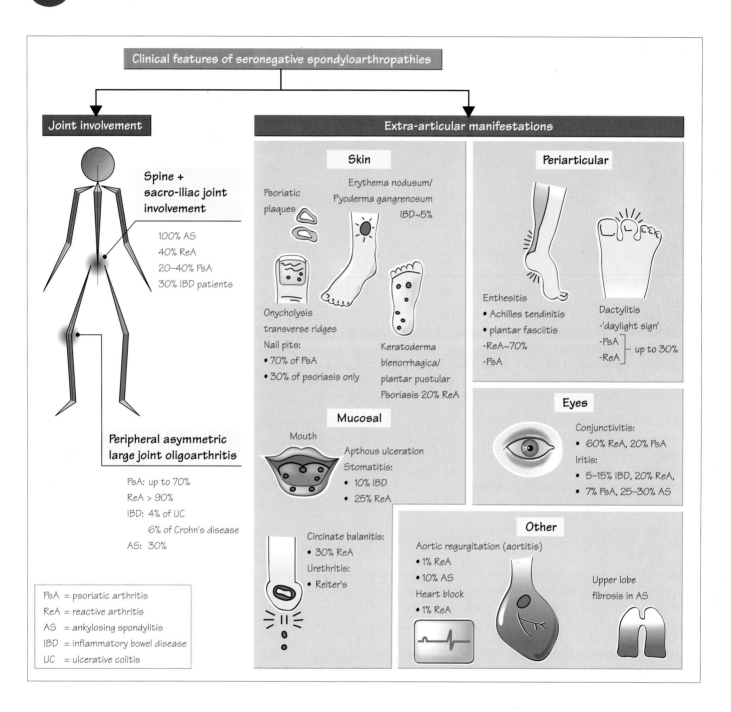

The seronegative spondyloarthropathies are a group of inflammatory arthritides, which share similar clinical features, pathological findings, the absence of rheumatoid factor and a strong association with the histocompatibility antigen HLA-B27. They comprise:

- Ankylosing spondylitis (AS).
- Psoriatic arthropathy.
- Reactive arthritis (sexually acquired reactive arthritis [SARA] follows a sexually acquired infection, enteric reactive arthritis [ERA] follows an enteric infection).
- Enteropathic arthritis (inflammatory bowel disease [IBD]).

Epidemiology

These conditions may present at any age, though they most frequently affect young adults. Males are consistently affected more commonly than females (3 : 1 for SARA, 2.5 : 1 for AS), except in the peripheral arthritis of IBD, which is more commonly found in females. In the UK, the prevalence ranges from 150/100 000 for AS to 20/100 000 for SARA/ERA. About 10% of those with psoriasis have an accompanying arthritis, making this the most common inflammatory arthritis after rheumatoid arthritis.

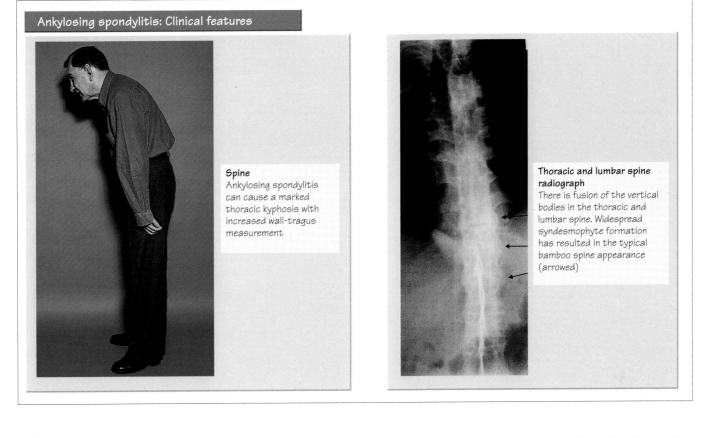

Spine
Ankylosing spondylitis can cause a marked thoracic kyphosis with increased wall-tragus measurement

Thoracic and lumbar spine radiograph
There is fusion of the vertical bodies in the thoracic and lumbar spine. Widespread syndesmophyte formation has resulted in the typical bamboo spine appearance (arrowed)

Clinical features

These conditions share many common clinical features (see figure). Spondyloarthropathies characteristically affect the spine, though peripheral arthritis is common, most frequently asymmetric, oligoarticular and predominantly of the lower limb large joints.

• Periarticular features such as enthesopathy and tendinitis are also very frequent.

• Extra-articular involvement includes the eye, skin, mucous membranes, the genitalia, lungs and proximal aorta (see figure).

The particular combination of these extra-articular features and axial/peripheral joint involvement are usually highly characteristic of particular types of seronegative spondyloarthropathy. Comparison between the various seronegative spondyloarthropathies is shown in Table 202.1.

Ankylosing spondylitis

The onset is usually in late teens or early adulthood. First-degree relatives are affected in 10% of cases. The male/female ratio is 2.5 : 1. AS usually presents with an insidious onset of inflammatory type lower back pain/buttock pain. Features of lower back pain suggesting inflammation include:

• Young age (< 40 years)
• Significant early morning stiffness (> 20 min)
• Improvement on exercise
• Localized tenderness over the sacroiliac joints.

Any level of the spine may be involved, but characteristically the lumbar spine is involved early on, and the cervical spine relatively late. Chest pain may arise from the:

• Thoracic spine itself
• Costovertebral joints
• Costochondral junction.

The lumbo-sacral spine is most frequently affected but AS may affect the spine at any level. Chest expansion (< 2.5 cm) and thoracic spine rotation are greatly reduced (see figure). Examination of the lumbar spine shows:

• Decrease in flexibility in all three planes, most consistently in lateral flexion. Reduction in forward flexion is measured by Schober's test (see figure). Sacroiliac joint stress tests (direct application of pressure or Patrick's test) produce pain but are unreliable indicators of sacroiliitis.

• Advanced disease results in bony ankylosis and the development of deformities characteristic of AS (see figure). As the disease progresses and ankylosis develops, the symptoms of active inflammation recede and those of disability predominate.

• Extraskeletal manifestations are shown (see figure).

Investigation of ankylosing spondylitis

• Inflammatory markers (ESR, CRP) are variably raised. Rheumatoid factor is negative.

• HLA-B27 is present in > 90% compared with 8% of the general population. However, only about 1 in 20 of HLA-B27 positive individuals will develop AS. HLA typing for B27 should therefore only be carried out where there is a relatively high pre-test probability on clinical grounds.

• Plain radiographs of the sacroiliac joints may show juxta-articular sclerosis, marginal erosions and eventually ankylosis (fusion), but they are insensitive to early disease. MRI is the investigation of choice for early disease, because it can detect inflammatory change as well as erosions. CT is also very sensitive at detecting small erosions.

Management of ankylosing spondylitis

Management of these conditions includes:

Table 202.1 Summary of findings in seronegative spondyloarthropathies.

	Ankylosing spondylitis	Reactive arthropathy	Inflammatory bowel disease associated	Psoriatic arthropathy
Sex	M > F	M > F	M = F	F = M
Age	< 30 years	< 30	Any age	Any age
Peripheral joints	~40%	> 90%	> 90%	> 90%
Sausage digits (dactylitis)	–	+	–	+
Axial spine	100%	20%	30%	30%
Sacroiliitis				
Enthesitis (achilles tendinitis, plantar fasciitis)	++	+++	+	+++
Extra-articular				
Uveitis	+++	++	+	+
Conjunctivitis	0	+++	+	++
Skin	0	++ (keratoderma blenorrhagica)	+ (pyoderma gangrenosum, erythema nodosum)	+++ (psoriasis)
Mucous membranes	0	+ (circinate balanitis)		
Aortic incompetence	+	+	0	0
Urethritis	0	++	0	0
Prostatitis	++	++	0	0

• Intense physiotherapy and hydrotherapy. NSAIDs for persistent symptoms.
• Methotrexate or sulfasalazine are useful for persistent peripheral joint arthritis but not for axial disease.
• Anti TNFα biologics are highly effective for patients with more severe forms of disease refractory to NSAID and some patients also respond to therapy with i.v. bisphosphonates, such as pamidronate.
• Topical corticosteroids for uveitis.
• Intra-articular steroids for localized peripheral synovitis and for refractory sacroiliitis. Local steroids also for enthesitis (e.g. plantar fasciitis).

Psoriatic arthritis

Ten per cent of those with psoriasis (plaque, guttate or pustular) develop arthritis, which may precede skin lesions or begin simultaneously (33%). It is important to enquire about a family history of psoriasis in anyone presenting with a mono- or oligoarticular arthritis. Psoriatic nail changes (pitting, onycholysis) occur in 70% of those with arthritis. Occult psoriasis may be apparent only in the scalp, natal cleft or umbilicus.

Clinical patterns of psoriasis-associated arthritis

• Asymmetric large-joint oligoarthritis in 50–70%.
• Axial arthritis/sacroiliitis—asymmetric and isolated in 5%, or with peripheral joints involvement in 20–40%.
• Peripheral small-joint arthritis indistinguishable from rheumatoid arthritis in 15–25% (negative rheumatoid factor).
• Distal interphalangeal (DIP) arthritis associated with dystrophic changes in adjacent nails in 5–10%.
• Arthritis mutilans is a destructive arthritis of the small joints of the hands that rapidly results in joint destruction of such severity as to cause the fingers to collapse and lose length or 'telescope'—so called 'opera glass hands' in < 5%.
• Dactylitis ('sausage digits') are common.

Clinical management of psoriasis-associated arthritis

Treatment is similar to ankylosing spondylitis. Many patients can be managed with NSAIDs alone. Sulfasalazine, gold salts and methotrexate have a proven role in symptom relief. Methotrexate is particularly useful where skin disease is also troublesome. Ciclosporin is more effective for skin disease than the arthritis.
• Anti-TNF biologic agents are highly effective for the skin and arthritis in resistant cases. Fifty per cent improvement can be expected within 3 months in 40% of patients.
• Systemic steroids may precipitate a skin flare if decreased too rapidly.
• Morbidity is much less than for rheumatoid arthritis. Though oligoarticular involvement is common at presentation, there is typically progressive recruitment of joints over time.

Reactive arthritis

Aseptic inflammation of the joints (typically lower limb oligoarticular) may complicate a range of infections at distant sites, typically genital tract and enteric infections are responsible. Seventy per cent of patients are HLA-B27 positive. *Chlamydia*, *Salmonella*, *Shigella*, *Yersinia* and *Campylobacter* species are well-characterized triggers, but culture is often negative by the time joint involvement occurs. Bacterial proteins and DNA can be isolated from the joints sometimes, but not viable organisms.

Reiter's syndrome refers to the triad of arthritis, conjunctivitis and urethritis originally described by Reiter in 1916, now considered a subset of reactive arthritis. The differential diagnosis includes the other seronegative arthritides and septic arthritis/trauma and gout if presenting as a monoarthritis.

Investigations in reactive arthritis

The diagnosis is clinical but the following may be useful:
• Inflammatory markers are raised and the rheumatoid factor is neg-

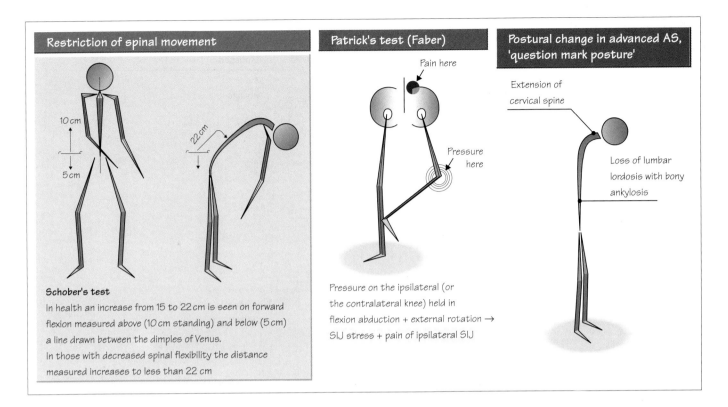

Restriction of spinal movement

10 cm

5 cm

22 cm

Schober's test

In health an increase from 15 to 22 cm is seen on forward flexion measured above (10 cm standing) and below (5 cm) a line drawn between the dimples of Venus.

In those with decreased spinal flexibility the distance measured increases to less than 22 cm

Patrick's test (Faber)

Pain here

Pressure here

Pressure on the ipsilateral (or the contralateral knee) held in flexion abduction + external rotation → SIJ stress + pain of ipsilateral SIJ

Postural change in advanced AS, 'question mark posture'

Extension of cervical spine

Loss of lumbar lordosis with bony ankylosis

ative. Synovial fluid is not diagnostic, and a diagnostic tap is indicated primarily to exclude sepsis or crystals, when a sterile leukocytosis (acute = neutrophils, chronic = lymphocytes) is found.

• Urinalysis: pyuria (usually sterile). Culture—urine/stool/synovial fluid/high urethral or vaginal swab, and serology for chlamydia, yersinia. Referral to a genitourinary clinic may be appropriate and contact tracing should be attempted.

• HLA-B27 testing may help to consolidate the diagnosis where there is a strong clinical suspicion.

Management of reactive arthritis

Establish the diagnosis and rule out sepsis. Bed rest, intra-articular steroids and splinting in the acute attack, followed by passive strengthening exercises at about 10 days. NSAIDs are usually sufficient for symptom control but some patients (< 5%) may need systemic corticosteroids.

Recurrent or chronic symptoms may require DMARD (e.g. sulfasalazine or methotrexate). Remission is usual at 2–6 months, but persistence of symptoms or recurrent flares are common (15–20%). Severe

systemic features with weight loss, fevers, and deranged liver function tests may mimic deep sepsis or malignancy in some cases. The role of antibiotic therapy in limiting arthritic complications is controversial. However, in sexually acquired forms of the disease contact tracing and eradication of chlamydia is clearly important to prevent long-term damage to the genital tract.

Enteropathic arthritis

Enteropathic arthritis is summarized in Table 202.2:

• Peripheral and spinal joint involvement may occur.

• Extra-articular/extra-intestinal manifestations occur in the eye (5–15%), the skin (pyoderma gangrenosum [< 5%], erythema nodosum [< 10%]).

• Type I peripheral enteropathic arthritis is oligoarticular, self-limiting and associated with flares of IBD.

• Type II enteropathic peripheral arthritis is polyarticular, protracted and not related to disease activity in the gut. Both types of arthropathy may respond to sulfasalazine or methotrexate. Anti-TNFα therapy is also highly effective.

Table 202.2 Peripheral arthritis vs. sacroiliitis in inflammatory bowel disease.

	Peripheral arthritis	Sacroiliitis
Frequency of involvement	Crohn's > UC 10% vs. 5%	Crohn's > UC 30% vs. 10%
Relationship to B27	25% of type I arthritis Type II unrelated	~100% of B27 positive IBD patients develop sacroiliitis
Relationship to IBD disease extent/activity	Yes (type I), no (type II) Coincident bowel/joint flares in 60–70% in type I	No May even precede bowel symptoms
Responsive to NSAIDs*	Yes	Yes
Responsive to DMARD (sulfasalazine first choice)	Yes	No
Responsive to bowel resection	UC yes, Crohn's no	Neither

*Caution—may flare IBD.

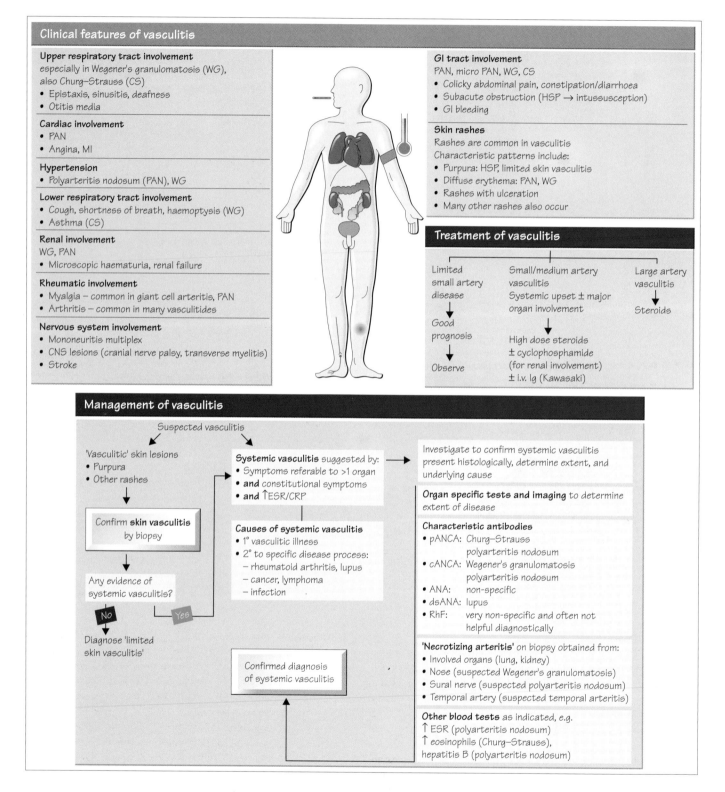

Clinical features of vasculitis

Upper respiratory tract involvement
especially in Wegener's granulomatosis (WG),
also Churg–Strauss (CS)
- Epistaxis, sinusitis, deafness
- Otitis media

Cardiac involvement
- PAN
- Angina, MI

Hypertension
- Polyarteritis nodosum (PAN), WG

Lower respiratory tract involvement
- Cough, shortness of breath, haemoptysis (WG)
- Asthma (CS)

Renal involvement
WG, PAN
- Microscopic haematuria, renal failure

Rheumatic involvement
- Myalgia – common in giant cell arteritis, PAN
- Arthritis – common in many vasculitides

Nervous system involvement
- Mononeuritis multiplex
- CNS lesions (cranial nerve palsy, transverse myelitis)
- Stroke

GI tract involvement
PAN, micro PAN, WG, CS
- Colicky abdominal pain, constipation/diarrhoea
- Subacute obstruction (HSP → intussusception)
- GI bleeding

Skin rashes
Rashes are common in vasculitis
Characteristic patterns include:
- Purpura: HSP, limited skin vasculitis
- Diffuse erythema: PAN, WG
- Rashes with ulceration
- Many other rashes also occur

Treatment of vasculitis

Limited small artery disease	Small/medium artery vasculitis Systemic upset ± major organ involvement	Large artery vasculitis
Good prognosis ↓ Observe	High dose steroids ± cyclophosphamide (for renal involvement) ± i.v. Ig (Kawasaki)	Steroids

Management of vasculitis

Suspected vasculitis

'Vasculitic' skin lesions
- Purpura
- Other rashes

Confirm **skin vasculitis** by biopsy

Any evidence of systemic vasculitis?
No → Yes

Diagnose 'limited skin vasculitis'

Systemic vasculitis suggested by:
- Symptoms referable to >1 organ
- **and** constitutional symptoms
- **and** ↑ESR/CRP

Causes of systemic vasculitis
- 1° vasculitic illness
- 2° to specific disease process:
  – rheumatoid arthritis, lupus
  – cancer, lymphoma
  – infection

Confirmed diagnosis of systemic vasculitis

Investigate to confirm systemic vasculitis present histologically, determine extent, and underlying cause

Organ specific tests and imaging to determine extent of disease

Characteristic antibodies
- pANCA: Churg–Strauss
  polyarteritis nodosum
- cANCA: Wegener's granulomatosis
  polyarteritis nodosum
- ANA: non-specific
- dsANA: lupus
- RhF: very non-specific and often not
  helpful diagnostically

'Necrotizing arteritis' on biopsy obtained from:
- Involved organs (lung, kidney)
- Nose (suspected Wegener's granulomatosis)
- Sural nerve (suspected polyarteritis nodosum)
- Temporal artery (suspected temporal arteritis)

Other blood tests as indicated, e.g.
↑ ESR (polyarteritis nodosum)
↑ eosinophils (Churg–Strauss),
hepatitis B (polyarteritis nodosum)

Definition

The vasculitides are a group of conditions characterized by inflammation of the arterial wall and are usefully classified according to the size of the vessel involved (Table 203.1). They may arise as a primary process or secondary to other conditions such as drugs, infection or neoplasia. Diagnosis is based upon clinical features, confirmation of the pathological lesion on tissue biopsy and the presence of autoantibodies found in association with certain of the vasculitides.

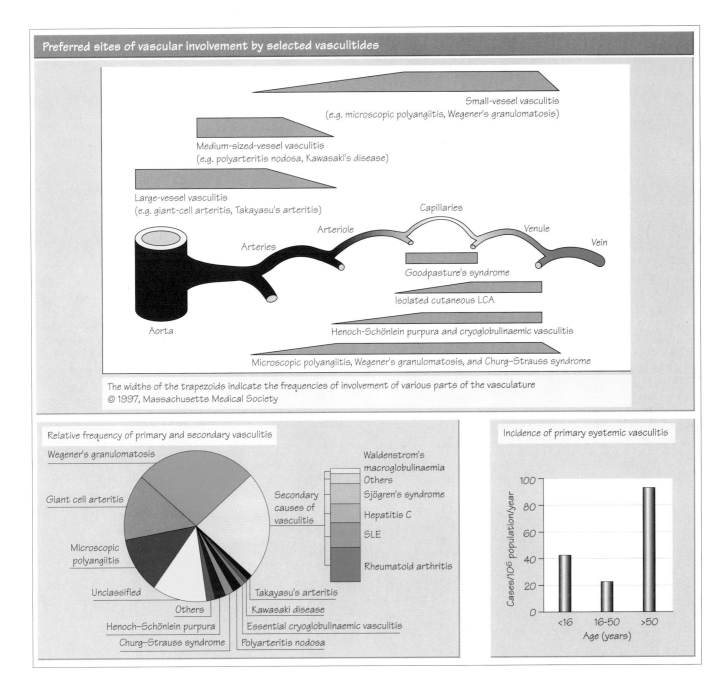

Preferred sites of vascular involvement by selected vasculitides

Small-vessel vasculitis
(e.g. microscopic polyangiitis, Wegener's granulomatosis)

Medium-sized-vessel vasculitis
(e.g. polyarteritis nodosa, Kawasaki's disease)

Large-vessel vasculitis
(e.g. giant-cell arteritis, Takayasu's arteritis)

Capillaries

Arteriole

Venule

Arteries

Vein

Goodpasture's syndrome

Aorta

Isolated cutaneous LCA

Henoch-Schönlein purpura and cryoglobulinaemic vasculitis

Microscopic polyangiitis, Wegener's granulomatosis, and Churg–Strauss syndrome

The widths of the trapezoids indicate the frequencies of involvement of various parts of the vasculature
© 1997, Massachusetts Medical Society

Relative frequency of primary and secondary vasculitis

Wegener's granulomatosis

Giant cell arteritis

Microscopic polyangiitis

Unclassified

Others

Henoch–Schönlein purpura

Churg–Strauss syndrome

Secondary causes of vasculitis

Waldenstrom's macroglobulinaemia
Others
Sjögren's syndrome
Hepatitis C
SLE
Rheumatoid arthritis

Takayasu's arteritis
Kawasaki disease
Essential cryoglobulinaemic vasculitis
Polyarteritis nodosa

Incidence of primary systemic vasculitis

Cases/10⁶ population/year

Age (years)

Key points

- Clinical features of systemic vasculitis result from ischaemic damage in the affected organ(s) and the severity of the vasculitis is reflected by the extent or amount of tissue damage. Inflammation is widespread in systemic vasculitis and several organs may be affected simultaneously.
- Systemic features (fever, weight loss, malaise and anorexia) accompanied by a rise in inflammatory markers indicate widespread inflammation.
- A thorough evaluation of organs potentially involved is necessary to determine the extent and severity of disease. This requires thorough history taking and examination of the patient, followed by laboratory investigations and imaging or biopsy of all target organs.

Epidemiology and pathogenesis

Giant cell arteritis is common with an annual incid-ence of 18 : 100 000.

Other systemic vasculitides are much less common (3 : 100 000 in the UK). Vasculitis is particularly prevalent at the extremes of age. For example, Kawasaki disease is almost exclusively paediatric whereas giant cell arteritis generally occurs after the sixth decade. There is no exclusive pathology but the following are frequently found: 1) 'Leukocytoclastic vasculitis' is a characteristic histological appearance resulting from dissolution of leukocytes, seen in small vessels. 2) Necrosis of medium and small arterial walls is found in the systemic necrotizing vasculitides (Wegener's, Churg–Strauss and polyarteritis nodosa [PAN]). Lesions are focal and segmental within vessels; hence tissue diagnosis may be elusive.

History and examination

- Systemic features often predominate; weight loss, fatigue and fever (see pyrexia of unknown origin, p. 68).

Table 203.1 Classification of the vasculitides (From Scott's *Classification of the Vasculitides* published in *ABC of Rheumatology*, BMJ Publishing, 2002).

Size of vessel affected	Primary	Secondary
Large arteries	Giant cell arteritis	Rheumatoid arthritis (aortitis) Anklyosing spondylitis, Behçet's syndrome
	Takayasu's arteritis	Infection • Syphilis
Medium arteries	Kawasaki disease Classic polyarteritis nodosa	• Hepatitis B and C
Medium and small arteries	Wegener's granulomatosis* Churg–Strauss syndrome* Microscopic polyangiitis*	RA, SLE, Sjögren's Drugs (see below) Infection, e.g. HIV
Small arteries (leukocytoclastic/hypersensitivity)	Henoch–Schönlein purpura Essential mixed cryoglobulinaemia	• Drugs, e.g. sulphonamides, penicillins, thiazides, • Infection, e.g. tuberculosis, group A streptococci • Malignancy, lymphoma • RA, SLE, Sjögren's

*Associated with ANCA antibodies, renal impairment and responsive to immuno-suppression with cyclophosphamide.
RA, rheumatoid arthritis; SLE, systemic lupus erythematosus.

• Specific symptoms and signs are dependent on the end-organs involved (see figure).
• Involvement of more than one organ in an inflammatory process is a key clue to the presence of an underlying vasculitis.

Investigations

The aims of investigation are to confirm the diagnosis and to determine the extent of disease (which organs are involved?) and severity (what is the degree of inflammation/tissue damage?).

Laboratory

Laboratory findings in vasculitic syndromes (see figure).

Immunology

• Anti-neutrophil cytoplasmic antibodies (ANCA) are circulating antibodies directed against cytoplasmic components of neutrophils. These are classified according to the pattern of neutrophil cell staining: cytoplasmic (cANCA) associated with antibodies to proteinase-3 (PR3-ANCA), which are strongly associated with Wegener's granulomatosis, and perinuclear (pANCA) directed against myeloperoxidase [MPO], associated with other primary small vessel arteritides.
• Rheumatoid factors are antibodies directed against the Fc component of immunoglobulin. They occur in many patients with rheumatoid arthritis, and are also found in many other vasculitides (SLE, cryoglobulinaemia, PAN) and chronic infections
• Anti-nuclear antibodies (ANA) are classified according to the pattern of nuclear staining. A diffuse pattern is found with anti-DNA antibodies, characteristic of SLE, though found also in other conditions. Anti-double-stranded DNA antibodies are specific for active SLE. Staining restricted to the centromere suggests systemic sclerosis. A speckled staining pattern is found with antibodies against extractable nuclear antigens (ENA). There are several different forms, common in SLE (anti-Ro, Sm) and Sjögren's syndrome (anti-Ro, La).

Radiology

Plain chest radiographs may show pulmonary infiltrates (small and medium vessel vasculitides). Computerized tomography is useful in investigation of the upper respiratory tract and sinuses (Wegener's granulomatosis). Angiography (including MR angiography) may be used to delineate the extent of involvement in large vessel vasculitis. Coeliac axis angiography may show clusters of small aneurysms 'bunches of grapes' in some vasculitides (especially PAN).

Histology

A tissue biopsy shows characteristic vessel wall inflammation, fibrinoid necrosis and 'leukocytoclasis' resulting from dissolution of leukocytes. Suitable sites for biopsy are: blood vessels (e.g. superficial temporal arteries in suspected temporal arteritis), involved skin or other organ such as kidney, muscle, nerve and lung.

Assessing other organ involvement

Screening for involvement of major organs in the small vessel vasculitides is by routine biochemical tests (kidney, liver) or radiology (lung) in the first instance. Characterization of the extent and severity of this involvement requires more invasive investigation (see figure).

Prognosis and treatment

These diseases retain a significant morbidity and mortality despite recent therapeutic advances. Immunosuppression is the mainstay of therapy. The large vessel vasculitides are generally responsive to steroid immuno-suppression with large doses of oral prednisolone (up to 1 mg/kg/day), and smaller 'maintenance' doses of steroids are often required for prolonged periods. The medium- and small-vessel vasculitides (Wegener's, Churg–Strauss and microscopic polyangiitis [mPAN]), which are associated with production of ANCA antibodies, frequently involve the kidney, and respond well to cyclophosphamide plus oral prednisolone. Primary small-vessel vasculitis is typically self limiting in nature (e.g. Henoch–Schönlein purpura). In systemic vasculitis, the prognosis is worse for those with renal or other major organ involvement. A comprehensive evaluation of the extent and severity of multi-organ involvement is vital to prevent potentially fatal complications, and to avoid unnecessary use of toxic agents in limited small-vessel vasculitis. An algorithm for management and treatment is shown in the figure on p. 406.

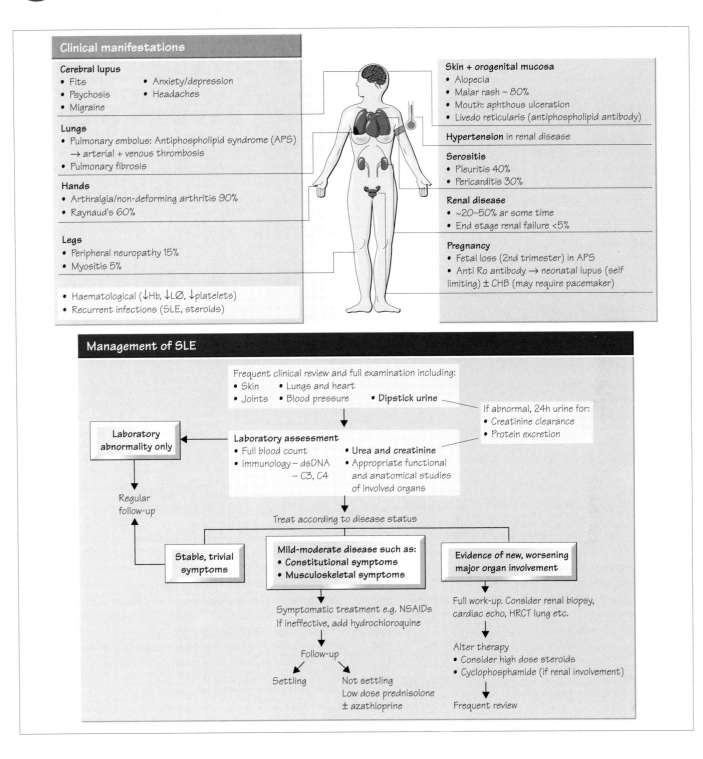

Clinical manifestations

Cerebral lupus
- Fits
- Anxiety/depression
- Psychosis
- Headaches
- Migraine

Lungs
- Pulmonary embolus: Antiphospholipid syndrome (APS) → arterial + venous thrombosis
- Pulmonary fibrosis

Hands
- Arthralgia/non-deforming arthritis 90%
- Raynaud's 60%

Legs
- Peripheral neuropathy 15%
- Myositis 5%

- Haematological (↓Hb, ↓LØ, ↓platelets)
- Recurrent infections (SLE, steroids)

Skin + orogenital mucosa
- Alopecia
- Malar rash – 80%
- Mouth: aphthous ulceration
- Livedo reticularis (antiphospholipid antibody)

Hypertension in renal disease

Serositis
- Pleuritis 40%
- Pericarditis 30%

Renal disease
- ~20–50% ar some time
- End stage renal failure <5%

Pregnancy
- Fetal loss (2nd trimester) in APS
- Anti Ro antibody → neonatal lupus (self limiting) ± CHB (may require pacemaker)

Management of SLE

Frequent clinical review and full examination including:
- Skin
- Lungs and heart
- Joints
- Blood pressure
- **Dipstick urine**

If abnormal, 24h urine for:
- Creatinine clearance
- Protein excretion

Laboratory abnormality only

Laboratory assessment
- Full blood count
- Immunology – dsDNA – C3, C4
- **Urea and creatinine**
- Appropriate functional and anatomical studies of involved organs

Regular follow-up

Treat according to disease status

Stable, trivial symptoms

Mild-moderate disease such as:
- **Constitutional symptoms**
- **Musculoskeletal symptoms**

Evidence of new, worsening major organ involvement

Symptomatic treatment e.g. NSAIDs. If ineffective, add hydrochloroquine

Full work-up. Consider renal biopsy, cardiac echo, HRCT lung etc.

Follow-up

Settling

Not settling Low dose prednisolone ± azathioprine

Alter therapy
- Consider high dose steroids
- Cyclophosphamide (if renal involvement)

Frequent review

Systemic lupus erythematosus (SLE) is a multisystem disease characterized by inflammation involving many systems, exhibits a relapsing and remitting course. It is strongly associated with autoantibodies to components of the cell nucleus (antinuclear antibodies, ANA).

Aetiology and epidemiology

The aetiology of SLE is unknown, but multiple genetic and environmental factors are probably involved. Concordance is 25% in monozygotic twins, but only 2% in non-twin siblings. HLA-B8, -DR2 and -DR3 are positively associated with SLE. It is particularly prevalent in the African-American female population of the USA (1 in 250), in contrast to the low prevalence in similar ethnic groups in West Africa. In mixed ethnicity UK populations the prevalence is 45–50 per 100 000 females. Females are 10 times more commonly affected than males. Peak age of

Diseases and Treatments at a Glance

onset is 15–40 years. A range of drugs (e.g. minocycline, procainamide, hydralazine) can induce a lupus-like syndrome, particularly in those with certain metabolic polymorphisms of the cytochrome P450 system.

Immunopathology

There is no single immunopathological feature. Vasculitis, coagulapathy, tissue inflammation and immune complex deposition may all occur. There are abnormalities in:

• Cellular and humoral immunity.
• The complement system, which may underlie abnormal clearance of immune complexes.
• Apoptosis, which may lead to the generation of characteristic antinuclear and antiphospholipid antibodies.

Renal pathology is well studied and five histological groups are recognized (in the World Health Organization criteria), from minimal change to proliferative and sclerosing glomerulonephritis. Anti DNA antibodies may be involved in the pathogenesis of lupus nephritis.

Clinical features

Non-specific constitutional features include joint pains, lethargy, weight loss and lymphadenopathy. Systemic upset (fever and extreme malaise) is usually very marked in active lupus and is often the dominant presenting feature. The best-recognized clinical feature of lupus is the 'butterfly'/malar facial rash, commonly arising following sun exposure. Other rashes, mouth ulcers and a non-deforming arthritis are common. Vital organ involvement, such as renal or CNS, determines prognosis and treatment. Renal involvement may manifest as nephrotic syndrome, or covertly with proteinuria, active renal sediment and progressive loss of renal function. CNS manifestations, such as headaches, seizures, strokes and altered behaviour are common, and occasionally are predominant. Encephalopathy occasionally occurs.

Formal diagnosis rests on finding four of a possible eleven features (eight clinical and three laboratory) as defined by the American College of Rheumatology (Table 204.1).

Immunology and other investigations in SLE

Haematology: leukopenia/lymphopenia occur in active SLE. Anaemia is due to chronic disease or Coombs-positive haemolysis. Immune thrombocytopenia can occur, and can predate lupus by many years.

Immunology: antinuclear antibodies (ANA) occur universally in SLE patients but these alone are neither sufficient nor specific for diagnosis. Double-stranded DNA (dsDNA) antibodies are specific for SLE, but titres correspond only loosely to activity (Tables 204.2 and 204.3). Antibodies to extractable nuclear antigens (ENA), e.g. Ro (SSA) and

Table 204.1 Diagnostic criteria for SLE. Four of out of eleven criteria present at any time is required for diagnosis of SLE.

Clinical	Laboratory
Malar rash	Haematological abnormalities
Photosensitive rash	(see text)
Discoid lupus rash	Immunological abnormalities
Neurological involvement	(see text)
Seizures or psychosis	ANA positive
Renal disease: Proteinuria or casts	
Serositis: Pleuritis or pericarditis	
Mucosal aphthous ulceration	
Arthritis	

Table 204.2 Immunological and other tests for SLE.

Test	% positive
Immunological	
dsDNA binding	70–85
Antinuclear antibodies (high titre, IgG class)	95
Raised serum IgG level	65
Low serum complement (C3/C4 levels)	60
Platelet autoantibodies	60
Cryoglobulinaemia	60
Antibodies to ENA	
• Sm	5–30
• RNP	35
• Ro	30
• La	15
Antibodies to phospholipids	30
Rheumatoid factor (low titre)	30
Skin biopsy of normal skin +ve for IgG, C3 & C4 deposits	75–85
Haematological	
Raised ESR	60
Leukopenia	45
Direct Coombs test +ve	40
Lupus anticoagulant	10–20
Others	
C-reactive protein	Normal unless infection present
Proteinuria	30

Table 204.3 Interpretation of changes in complement and dsDNA in SLE.

dsDNA	C3	C4	Interpretation dsDNA antibodies
↑	→	→	↑ Activity–watch for change in clinical state
↓/→	↓	↓	Renal involvement should be suspected
↑/→	↑	↑	Look for infection–measure CRP (not usually increased unless infection present)

La (SSB), are found in Sjögren's syndrome. Maternal anti-Ro antibodies are associated with neonatal lupus and fetal congenital heart block (CHB). Anti-histone antibodies are associated with drug-induced lupus. Complement components C3, C4 are typically depressed in active SLE. In contrast to other inflammatory disorders, C-reactive protein (CRP) is often (not always) normal in active SLE. A raised CRP raises the suspicion of complicating infection.

The **lupus band test** is specific for lupus, demonstrating a characteristic band of IgG and/or IgM deposition at the dermo-epidermal junction in involved and uninvolved skin.

Renal function: renal impairment (decreased GFR) or proteinuria (> 3 + dipstick, > 0.5 g/24 h) are common in SLE, and of extreme therapeutic importance. An 'active renal sediment' with red cell and/or granular casts may be the *only* indication of serious renal disease. Renal biopsy is required in those with renal dysfunction.

Clotting abnormalities: venous and arterial thromboses may occur due to autoantibodies that activate *in vivo* clotting. *In vitro* these cause a prolonged APTT. The platelet count is often slightly reduced [c. 100×10^9/L]. Testing must look for **both**:

• Lupus anti-coagulant: this can be detected with the dilute Russell Viper Venom Test (dRVVT).
• Anti-cardiolipin (phospholipid) antibodies (IgG and IgM class).

Either test may be abnormal alone, but the significance is the same, and suggests the presence of the antiphospholipid syndrome APS. SLE underlies many cases of the APS; cases can occur without SLE. Clinical features of the antiphospholipid syndrome include recurrent fetal loss, arterial and/or venous thromboses. Although clotting times are prolonged *in vitro*, there is a thrombotic tendency *in vivo*. 'False-positive' VDRL (syphilis) serology also identifies one form of the antiphospholipid antibody associated with an increased thrombotic risk.

Management and therapy

Lupus is an unpredictable disease, which relapses and remits. Management is aimed at the acute flare but also at preventive strategies such as UV protection and prompt evaluation and treatment of infection. Close clinical supervision, with regular assessment of the disease is vital to determine the need for anti-inflammatory and immunosuppressive therapy, particularly to minimize renal and CNS damage. Pharmacological options are shown below:

• NSAIDs: musculoskeletal manifestations, serositis and constitutional symptoms.
• Antimalarials: hydroxychloroquine is used for musculoskeletal, cutaneous and constitutional manifestations. Side effects include retinal toxicity.
• Corticosteroids: used topically for inflammatory rashes, orally for active disease, and sometimes intravenously for acute severe manifestations such as CNS lupus. Azathioprine, methotrexate and mycofenylate mofetil may be used as steroid-sparing agents. Long-term steroids induce osteoporosis.
• Cyclophosphamide suppresses lupus nephritis and reduces the risk of end-stage renal failure. May also benefit CNS and haematological complications. ACE inhibitors may help in SLE nephritis.
• Dapsone is useful for the cutaneous manifestations of SLE.
• Anticoagulation is used in the antiphospholipid syndrome:
  • Aspirin prophylactically.
  • Life-long warfarin in patients who have experienced thrombosis.
• Intravenous immunoglobulin or danazol may be used for immune thrombocytopenia.
• Symptomatic treatment as appropriate for depression, epilepsy, Raynaud's phenomenon and mouth ulcers.

Prognosis

Survival is 90% overall at 5 years, but there is an early excess mortality in those with severe disease. End-organ involvement differs widely between individuals but renal disease is the most important adverse prognostic indicator. At 15 years only 60% of patients with nephritis are alive compared with 85% of the rest. The main causes of death in SLE are cardiovascular, CNS lupus, infection, lupus nephritis and renal failure. Scrupulous attention should be paid to correcting adverse cardiovascular risk factors.

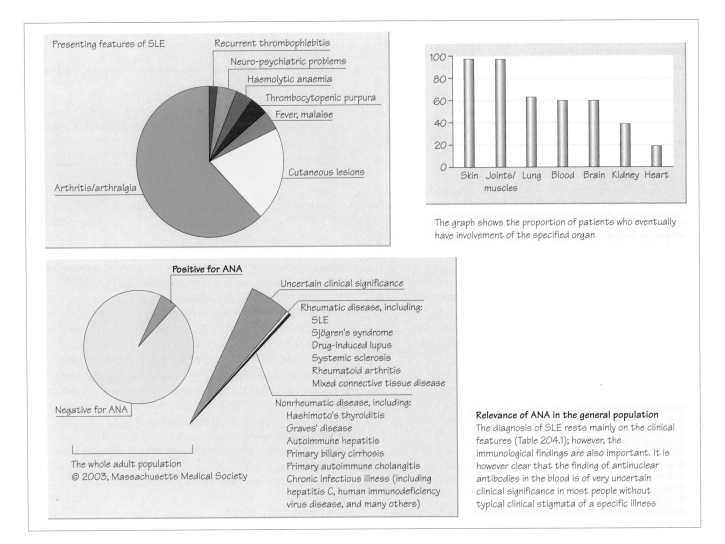

The graph shows the proportion of patients who eventually have involvement of the specified organ

Relevance of ANA in the general population
The diagnosis of SLE rests mainly on the clinical features (Table 204.1); however, the immunological findings are also important. It is however clear that the finding of antinuclear antibodies in the blood is of very uncertain clinical significance in most people without typical clinical stigmata of a specific illness

Diseases and Treatments at a Glance

Inflammatory muscle disease and other conditions

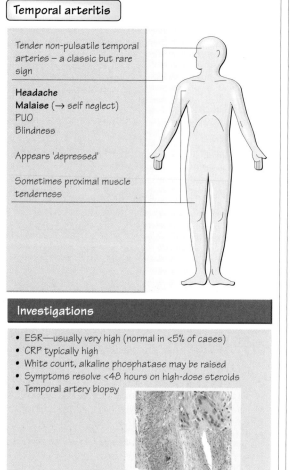

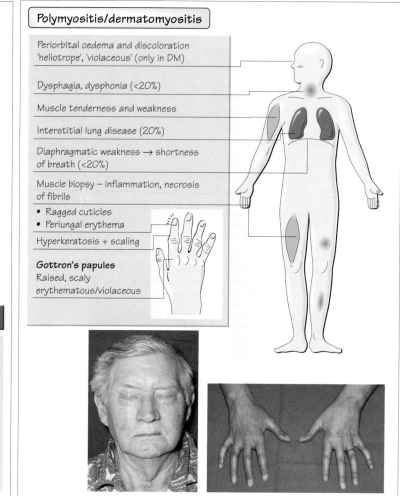

Polymyalgia rheumatica

Polymyalgia rheumatica (PMR) is an inflammatory disorder of unknown aetiology affecting older adults, resulting in pain and stiffness of the proximal muscle groups. In those > 60 years the prevalence is ~1%, and the female/male ratio is 2 : 1. The disease is uncommon in non-Caucasians. The pathophysiology is unclear and no histological lesion is diagnostic. There may be synovitis.

Clinical features

• Pronounced early morning stiffness in the limb girdles with ache and weakness, which leads to difficulty rising from squat or raising arms above head.
• Systemic features of weight loss, fatigue and lassitude may occur.
• Up to one-fifth have concurrent giant cell arteritis.

Investigations

The ESR is usually > 60. The CRP is also raised and is a more sensitive indicator of activity. Other laboratory investigations, including muscle enzymes, are usually normal. Normochromic anaemia and/or raised alkaline phosphatase may be found. There is no diagnostic radiology.

Management

• Oral prednisolone therapy gives prompt and dramatic improvement in symptoms. Doses of 15 mg are used initially (typically for 2 months), tapering slowly by 1 mg per month as symptoms resolve and inflammatory markers fall. Steroid therapy can usually be stopped after 12–18 months but up to 20% of patients require long-term low-dose maintenance.
• Relapse in symptoms are managed by increasing back to the last effective dose of prednisolone.
• Consider bone protection with calcium/vitamin D preparations or bisphosphonates.

Prognosis

Not life threatening. Morbidity in long term may arise due to steroid therapy.

Giant cell arteritis (temporal arteritis)

This is a relatively common vasculitis, mainly affecting those > 60 years old (annual incidence 10–25/100 000). The clinical presentation is often with a severe, unremitting headache associated with scalp tenderness (lying the head on a pillow is painful, as is combing hair). Transient visual disturbance (amaurosis fugax) or blindness can occur. A minority present with systemic symptoms (malaise, fever and weight loss) and minor scalp tenderness. The CRP is often very high. The diagnosis is confirmed by finding characteristic changes (including 'giant cells') on a temporal artery biopsy (70% are biopsy positive). The disease can patchily affect the temporal artery, so a negative temporal artery biopsy does not rule out temporal arteritis.

Treatment is high-dose steroids (40 mg/day), initiated immediately the diagnosis is suspected because of the risk of blindness. These relieve symptoms in < 48 h; if this does not occur the diagnosis should be re-evaluated. Steroids can be tailed over a few weeks to a lower maintenance dose, which are continued until the illness 'burns' itself out, usually within 2 years. A few patients need life-long steroids. Some patients may need additional immunosuppressive drugs to control the disease.

Complications include retinal artery inflammation, leading to sudden and irreversible blindness. It is to avoid this dreaded complication that treatment is started early and aggressively. Other much rarer complications include aortitis, which can lead to aortic dissection or aneurysm formation (in the aorta or the other large head and neck arteries). Occasional patients present with a stroke (1–2% of all strokes); accordingly an ESR or CRP should be performed in all patients with strokes.

Polymyositis and dermatomyositis

Polymyositis (PM) and dermatomyositis (DM) are inflammatory myopathies of unknown aetiology. The peak incidence of polymyositis occurs from 40 to 60 years. Dermatomyositis also occurs in childhood. Overall prevalence is 5–10 per million. Pathological findings are of inflammation in muscles (and skin in dermatomyositis) and in the vessels that supply them. There is a recognized association of these conditions with an underlying (usually undiagnosed) malignancy.

Clinical features (see figure): both are characterized by a subacute onset of proximal arm and leg weakness. Dermatomyositis is a distinct clinical entity associated with a rash, most commonly affecting the face and trunk. Rarely skin involvement occurs without myositis.

Classification

PM and DM are classified according to age, and whether or not there is an underlying disease process:

- Childhood-onset DM: not associated with malignancy, characteristically results in an inflammatory myopathy (with atrophy and contractures), with skin involvement, subcutaneous calcification and vasculitis affecting the skin, muscle and gut.
- Primary PM: there is no underlying disease process, with an insidious onset over months of a symmetrical (especially proximal) muscle weakness, which can also involve oesophageal muscles (resulting in dysphagia) and respiratory muscles (causing respiratory failure)
- Primary DM: in addition to the features of primary PM, skin involvement occurs, especially a lilac-coloured rash, and oedema, of the upper eyelids, and a scaly violaceous eruption over the extensor surfaces of joints (knuckles, elbows and knees).
- PM/DM associated with autoimmune rheumatic diseases (especially rheumatoid arthritis, systemic sclerosis and SLE).
- PM/DM associated with malignancy, of which lung, ovary, breast, GI tract, and myeloproliferative disorders are the commonest.

Investigation

The most helpful tests are markers of muscle damage, be they biochemical, electrical or histological. CK is raised in > 70% cases and the EMG is abnormal in almost all cases of polymyositis, with characteristic findings. Muscle biopsy shows inflammatory cellular infiltrate with necrosis of muscle fibres. Autoantibodies, such as ANA, are positive in 50–75%, with antisynthetase antibodies (e.g. anti Jo-1) characterizing those particularly at risk of interstitial lung disease, arthritis and florid hand rash. It is important to perform a screening history and full physical examination to search for underlying malignancy (present in 20% of those with DM, less in PM). Other investigations are dictated by these findings.

Management and outcome

Early diagnosis is important to preserve muscle function and avoid major organ involvement:

- High-dose prednisolone (1 mg/kg) initially to achieve disease control. Tapering of steroids according to symptoms and CK level.
- 10–15% may not respond to steroids. Second-line agents such as methotrexate or azathioprine are then initiated.
- Intravenous immunoglobulin can be useful.
- In the absence of underlying malignancy, up to 85% of patients have a good or partial response to steroids.

Kawasaki arteritis

This syndrome, essentially only occurring in childhood, is important in adult medicine as it may underlie cases of myocardial infarction/acute coronary syndromes presenting in teenagers and young adults. Children (75% are less than 5 years old), with a male preponderance (male : female ratio 1.6 : 1), present with a systemic illness of > 5 days duration, comprising fever, often high (without treatment this can last up to 4 weeks, though usually lasts some 11 days; with immunoglobulin the fever goes in < 2 days). A rash occurs, with erythema of the hands/feet, progressing to peeling a few days later. The conjunctiva becomes infected, and the lips and oral cavity are often inflamed. Cervical lymphadenopathy may be seen. Any other organs may be involved; a carditis is particularly common. Coronary dilatation (seen by transthoracic cardiac ultrasound) occurs early on, and in the absence of treatment up to 20% develops significant aneurysms of the coronary arteries. Though the illness is self-limiting (with a mortality of < 0.1% in the acute phase) the main therapeutic issue is to prevent the formation of such coronary aneurysms, as they can lead to myocardial ischaemia at any time after the acute illness. Intravenous immunoglobulin therapy reduces the chance of aneurysm developing, and all children with Kawasaki's arteritis should receive this. If aneurysms occur, they may regress over a few years, though they may be replaced with coronary stenosis. There remains a long-term risk of future myocardial ischaemia.

Takayasu's arteritis

This rare arteritis results in inflammation of major large arteries (e.g. the aorta, and its major branches) particularly in young Oriental females (commonly 15–35 years), resulting in a systemic illness (fever, malaise) with tenderness over any palpable arteries. Bruits occur and peripheral pulses may disappear (hence its synonym 'pulseless' disease). Renovascular hypertension may occur, as may strokes. Steroids are beneficial in the acute phase but treatment with cyclophosphamide or methotrexate may be necessary in steroid resistant patients.

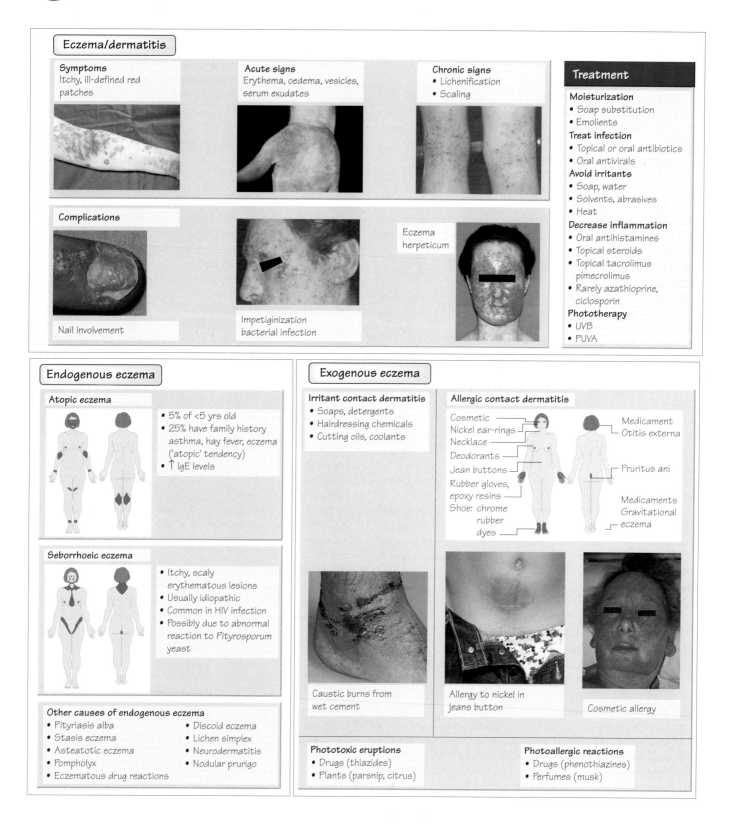

Eczema/dermatitis

Symptoms
Itchy, ill-defined red patches

Acute signs
Erythema, oedema, vesicles, serum exudates

Chronic signs
• Lichenification
• Scaling

Treatment

Moisturization
• Soap substitution
• Emolients

Treat infection
• Topical or oral antibiotics
• Oral antivirals

Avoid irritants
• Soap, water
• Solvents, abrasives
• Heat

Decrease inflammation
• Oral antihistamines
• Topical steroids
• Topical tacrolimus pimecrolimus
• Rarely azathioprine, ciclosporin

Phototherapy
• UVB
• PUVA

Complications

Nail involvement

Impetiginization bacterial infection

Eczema herpeticum

Endogenous eczema

Atopic eczema

• 5% of <5 yrs old
• 25% have family history asthma, hay fever, eczema ('atopic' tendency)
• ↑ IgE levels

Seborrhoeic eczema

• Itchy, scaly erythematous lesions
• Usually idiopathic
• Common in HIV infection
• Possibly due to abnormal reaction to *Pityrosporum* yeast

Other causes of endogenous eczema
• Pityriasis alba
• Stasis eczema
• Asteatotic eczema
• Pompholyx
• Eczematous drug reactions
• Discoid eczema
• Lichen simplex
• Neurodermatitis
• Nodular prurigo

Exogenous eczema

Irritant contact dermatitis
• Soaps, detergents
• Hairdressing chemicals
• Cutting oils, coolants

Allergic contact dermatitis

Cosmetic
Nickel ear-rings
Necklace
Deodorants
Jean buttons
Rubber gloves, epoxy resins
Shoe: chrome rubber dyes

Medicament
Otitis externa

Pruritus ani

Medicaments
Gravitational eczema

Caustic burns from wet cement

Allergy to nickel in jeans button

Cosmetic allergy

Phototoxic eruptions
• Drugs (thiazides)
• Plants (parsnip, citrus)

Photoallergic reactions
• Drugs (phenothiazines)
• Perfumes (musk)

Diseases and Treatments at a Glance

Eczema and dermatitis are practically synonymous. They are subdivided aetiologically and clinically. Lesions are very itchy, with ill-defined edges. Histologically, intercellular epidermal oedema (spongiosis) is seen.

Atopic dermatitis
Aetiology and pathogenesis
Atopic dermatitis is a relapsing condition beginning in infancy and sometimes continuing into later life. Atopy is an inherited tendency to develop an altered state of immune reactivity (type I and other hypersensitivity reactions). Patients who have a personal or first-degree family history of asthma, hay fever, conjunctivitis or eczema have the atopic diathesis (25% of the population). Atopic patients have elevated serum IgE levels.

Clinical features
Ill-defined erythematous scaly patches occur on the face and in flexural sites. Scratching and rubbing lead to infection, skin thickening and lichenification.

Investigations
Atopic dermatitis is a clinical diagnosis. Infection is common and skin swabs may be indicated. IgE may be elevated.

Management
Atopic eczema can be difficult to manage. The principles of therapy are to moisturize the skin with emollients and minimize itching with oral antihistamines. Irritants such as soap, chronic wet work, heat and solvents should be avoided. House-dust mite avoidance may be helpful. Specific treatments include topical therapy with tar, steroids or calcineurin inhibitors and antibiotics for complicating infection. A sunny dry climate is beneficial. Systemic therapy with oral/intravenous antibiotics and antiviral agents may be indicated. Phototherapy with ultraviolet light or immunosuppression using azathioprine and ciclosporin may be indicated in more severe cases.

Secondary infection with herpes simplex virus (eczema herpeticum) constitutes an emergency requiring hospitalization and treatment with systemic aciclovir.

Prognosis
The major features of the condition resolve in 40% after 5 years of age and 90% by 15–20 years of age.

Other types of endogenous eczema
- Lichen simplex is eczema in response to repeated trauma or scratching.
- Nodular prurigo is a widespread manifestation of the above.
- Stasis eczema (varicose eczema, lipodermatosclerosis) results from venous hypertension (which may relate to venous valvular damage from deep venous thrombosis [DVT], pregnancy, etc.). Blood leaks from the capillaries into the surrounding tissue, depositing fibrin and haemosiderin around the capillaries, so diminishing tissue perfusion and predisposing to skin ulceration. It occurs over the inner shin and medial malleolus, and is itchy, indurated, scaly and purpuric. It is often complicated by contact dermatitis caused by topically applied drugs, diagnosed by patch testing or by 'autosensitization' (secondary generalization of chronic stasis eczema supposedly resulting from 'sensitization' to epidermal antigens). Autosensitization affects the face, neck and extensor regions of the arms and thighs.
- Asteatotic eczema occurs on the legs of elderly patients where there

is dry skin. There is a glazed 'crazy-paving' effect. It responds to emollients and topical steroids.
- Discoid eczema is characterized by itchy, symmetrical, coin-shaped lesions on the extensor surfaces of the limbs and feet. The lesions are differentiated from those of ringworm/tinea corporis (which have an active border), psoriasis (often non-itchy with a silvery scale) and mycosis fungoides (asymmetrical and persistent). Discoid eczema is treated with emollients, topical steroids and systemic antihistamines.
- Pompholyx is acute vesicular eczema of the palms and soles. It is treated with potassium permanganate soaks, and topical or systemic steroids. Concomitant fungal infection of the foot (tinea pedis) should be sought. Pompholyx often recurs.
- Seborrhoeic dermatitis is a common, mildly itchy, scaly, red rash with a predilection for the scalp, face, chest, back, axillae and groins. It is an abnormal cutaneous reaction to commensal pityrosporum yeasts. Treatment is with topical steroids plus an anti-yeast agent (e.g. imidazole). When the scalp is affected (dandruff), ketoconazole or selenium sulphide shampoo can be helpful.

Contact dermatitis
Epidemiology, aetiology and pathogenesis
Contact dermatitis is a major industrial and occupational category of disease. It may be allergic or irritant. Almost anything in the environment may be an irritant and many substances are sensitizers, including medicaments. Allergic contact dermatitis is the archetypal type IV cell-mediated immunological reaction.

Investigation
Patch testing is the principal technique. A battery of common allergens is applied to the non-inflamed back. The patches are removed at 48 h and the reactions read. The patient is seen again at 72 h and late responses recorded. Interpretation (false-negatives, false-positives and significance of positives) requires specialist input.

Management and prognosis
Withdrawal of the offending agent is vital, but prophylaxis is important in industry because, once initiated, allergic contact dermatitis may persist despite removal of the responsible chemical.

Prevention of hand eczema
Hand eczema may be a diagnostic and management problem. Often atopic, irritant and allergic factors coexist. The use of cotton gloves inside rubber gloves for all wet and dirty tasks is recommended. Consider barrier creams prophylaxis where there is industrial/occupational risk.

Urticaria
Urticaria (hives) describes itchy red (erythematous) wheals (i.e. skin swellings resulting from leaky capillaries). Management aims to exclude an underlying cause, identify and remove precipitants or provocatants and provide effective symptomatic treatment.

Epidemiology, aetiology and pathogenesis of urticaria
Urticaria is very common and results from mast cell degranulation (a type I immunological reaction) in response to an antigen, with the release of histamine and other vasoactive mediators, leading to erythema and oedema (Table 206.1). Of patients with this condition, 70% have idiopathic urticaria (where the antigen is not known), the remainder having other forms (Table 206.2). The differential diagnosis

Table 206.1 Types of urticaria.

Type	Features
Common urticaria	Lesions last for several hours
Angioedema	Deeper dermal and subdermal involvement
Contact urticaria	Immediate response to allergens (e.g. foods)
Physical urticaria	Lesions last several minutes, but < 1 h
Dermographism	In response to scratching or trauma
Cholinergic	In response to heat/exercise
Cold/Aquagenic	In response to cold/water
Heat/Solar	In response to heat/sun
Urticarial vasculitis	Lesions last several days or longer; purpuric
Hereditary angio-oedema	C1 esterase inhibitor deficiency

Table 206.2 Causes and exacerbating factors of common urticaria (most cases are idiopathic).

Drugs	Aspirin, codeine, morphine, non-steroidal anti-inflammatory drugs
Foods	Fish and shellfish, eggs, nuts, tomatoes
Additives	Tartrazine, benzoates
Inhalants	Pollen, spores, house dust
Infections	Focal sepsis: (e.g. urinary tract infection, upper respiratory tract infection, hepatitis, *Candida* spp., protozoa, helminths)
Systemic	Systemic lupus erythematosus, reticuloses and carcinoma

includes insect bites, prodromal pemphigoid, toxic erythema and erythema multiforme.

Urticaria, when severe, can also affect subcutaneous tissues, so producing angio-oedema (swelling in the hands, lips and around the eyes, and less commonly but more importantly of the tongue or larynx). Angioedema may:

• be idiopathic;

• occur in individuals exposed to food antigens to which they have been sensitized, e.g. peanuts;

• occur in those with congenitally deficient C1 esterase levels (hereditary angioedema).

Investigations

If other than acute idiopathic urticaria is suspected (e.g. symptoms for > 2 months), a full blood count (FBC), eosinophil count and erythrocyte sedimentation rate (ESR), thyroid function, renal and liver function, and complement levels may be done, and a stool sample taken for ova, cysts and parasites.

Management

Counselling and reassurance are the mainstays of treatment. Itching may be exacerbated by psychological factors. High doses of non-sedating anti-H1-receptor histamines by day are supplemented by sedating antihistamines at night. The patient should be warned about drowsiness, alcohol and driving. Sometimes the addition of high doses of an anti-H2-receptor agent such as cimetidine is helpful. Systemic steroids are avoided, but have a role in severe cases.

Urticarial vasculitis

Urticarial vasculitis (5% of all urticarias) is a leukocytoclastic vasculitis and is suspected if urticarial lesions last > 24 h and resolve with purpura. It is associated with diseases such as systemic lupus erythematosus (SLE) and hepatitis B and C. Treatment depends on the cause, but oral corticosteroids or other immunosuppressants are sometimes needed.

Hereditary angioedema

Hereditary angioedema caused by congenital (autosomal dominant) deficiency of C1 esterase inhibitor is suspected when there is a family history and angioedema, often spontaneously, sometimes in response to minor trauma. Urticaria is NEVER present. Patients often have abdominal pain. Angioedema may affect the face, lips and neck, and threaten laryngeal patency. Finding a normal C3 and undetectable level of C4 during an attack makes the diagnosis. Total and functional C1 esterase inhibitor levels may then be measured. Modified androgens such as stanozolol and danazol or an anti-fibrinolytic such as tran-examic acid have been used successfully as prophylaxis. Purified steam-treated C1 esterase inhibitor is used before and during surgery and in an attack; if this is not available fresh frozen plasma may be used but may cause a deterioration rather than improvement in symptoms. Respiratory obstruction is managed by intubation or tracheostomy. Adrenaline and hydrocortisone are ineffective.

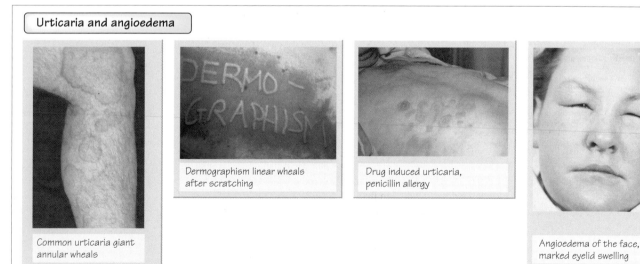

Urticaria and angioedema

Common urticaria giant annular wheals

Dermographism linear wheals after scratching

Drug induced urticaria, penicillin allergy

Angioedema of the face, marked eyelid swelling

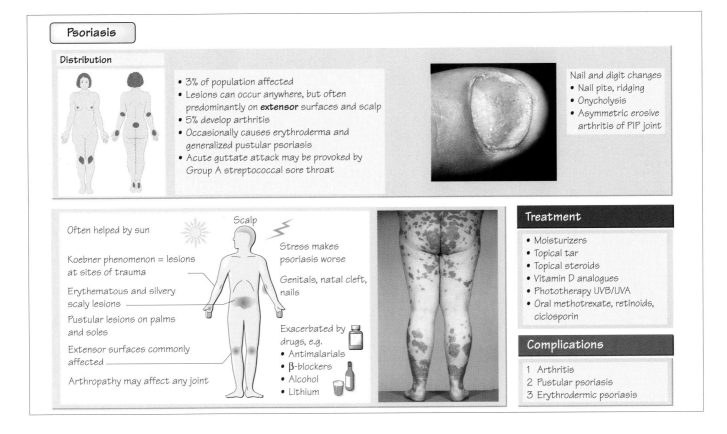

Aetiology and pathogenesis

A polygenic susceptibility exists. Some HLA types (Cw6) are associated with skin disease alone, whereas others (e.g. B27) are associated with additional joint disease. Infections, stress or drugs may precipitate attacks of psoriasis. Plaques are characterized by the dual pathological features of epidermal hyperproliferation and cutaneous inflammation.

Clinical features

Psoriasis manifests as red, silver-scaled lesions, which may be guttate or nummular, or plaques. The scalp is frequently involved, as are the nails. Pustulosis may occur, particularly in the palms and soles, and occasionally psoriasis causes erythroderma. Arthritis, which can be severe, can complicate the disease. The common subtypes of psoriasis are:

• Stable chronic plaque psoriasis.
• Guttate psoriasis: this form of psoriasis may be precipitated by streptococcal sore throat or other infection. Lesions are small (< 1 cm), scaly and widespread. Spontaneous resolution usually occurs after a few months.
• Erythrodermic psoriasis: widespread erythema occurs, with 'skin failure', which may lead to failure of thermoregulation, infection fluid and protein loss, and a high output form of heart failure. Other causes of erythroderma include eczema, mycosis fugoides (cutaneous T cell lymphoma) and drug eruption.

• Pustular psoriasis: this severe form results in a sudden crop of widespread small pustules throughout the skin, with considerable systemic upset.

The differential diagnosis includes atopic dermatitis, seborrhoeic dermatitis, mycosis fungoides, tinea or, acutely, pityriasis rosea.

Investigation

Skin biopsy, if necessary, shows irregular epidermal hyperplasia, suprapapillary thinning, clubbing of rete pegs, leukocyte infiltration and epidermal pustulosis.

Management and prognosis

Treatment is hierarchical and depends on severity, site, age, sex and occupation.

Reiter's syndrome

Reiter's syndrome (arthritis, urethritis and conjunctivitis) occurs in response to urinary or gastrointestinal tract infection in genetically predisposed individuals, and is part of the same disease continuum as psoriasis. Skin lesions in Reiter's syndrome are similar to psoriasis. In Reiter's syndrome, thickened yellow palms and soles with a cobblestone appearance, with or without pustular lesions (keratoderma blenorrhagica) and involvement of the penis (circinate balanitis), are found. Other features of psoriasis may be found.

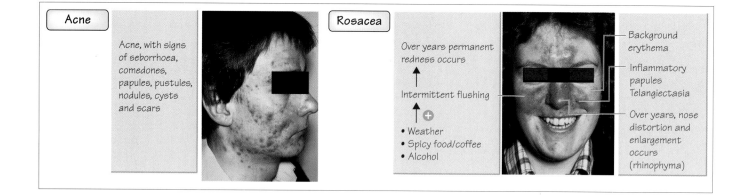

Acne vulgaris
Aetiology and pathogenesis
Acne vulgaris is universal in adolescence; 1% of men and 5% of women may require treatment up until the age of 40. Acne vulgaris is a chronic disorder of the pilosebaceous duct with increased sebum production, ductal hyper-cornification, a deranged symbiotic relationship with commensal micro-organisms (*Propionobacterium acnes*) and cutaneous inflammation. Increased sebum production is probably the fundamental abnormality.

The sebaceous glands are driven by androgens. Women with acne manifest a complex form of cutaneous androgenization. Many women with acne have polycystic ovaries on ultrasonography, although most do not have the other features of the polycystic ovary syndrome. There is no evidence for systemic endocrine abnormalities in men. Rarely, endocrine disorders, such as 'full-blown' polycystic ovary syndrome, Cushing's syndrome, virilizing neoplasms or exogenous corticosteroids/androgens, underlie the acne.

Clinical features
The clinical features of acne are seborrhoea, comedones, papules, pustules, nodules, cysts and scars distributed on the face, neck, back and chest. Pyoderma faciale is acute severe facial acne. Acne fulminans is acute severe acne with fever, arthralgia and sterile lytic lesions of bone.

Investigation
Investigations are only indicated if Cushing's syndrome or virilization is suspected. Pelvic ultrasonography can demonstrate polycystic ovaries.

Management and prognosis
Treatment depends on the severity of the condition and an objective record of severity helps follow-up. The principles of therapy are to keep the skin clean, to discourage micro-organism growth, and keratolytics to relieve comedones.
• Mild acne: topical antibiotics, keratolytics and retinoids.
• Moderate-to-severe acne: both topical and systemic therapy, with oral antibiotics (which can result in failure of the oral contraceptive pill

or teratogenicity) or antiandrogenic hormones (for women, i.e. suitable contraceptive pill).
• Severe nodulocystic (conglobate) acne or failure to respond to other treatments is an indication for the oral retinoid (vitamin A derivative) isotretinoin (13-*cis*-retinoic acid). This highly effective drug affects all four aetiological factors operating in acne and reduces sebum production by 75–90%. Treatment lasts 4–6 months. Side effects, which are essentially those of hypervitaminosis A, include teratogenesis (women must not get pregnant when on treatment), eczema, cheilitis (sore lips), conjunctivitis, benign intracranial hypertension, mood disturbance, and biochemical hepatitis and hyperlipidaemia.

Acne is usually self-limiting. With the exception of isotretinoin, treatment does not alter the natural history, and thus should continue throughout the course of the disorder. Topical therapies are needed long term and antibiotics should be given for at least 6 months. Repeated courses or long-term treatment may be necessary. Maintenance topical treatment is needed after oral therapy is stopped. Combined therapy is rational because there are several pathogenic factors.

Rosacea
Rosacea is a disorder of unknown aetiology, associated with instability of the facial vasculature, facial flushing and the secondary development of inflamed papules and pustules, particularly affecting the cheeks, chin and central forehead. Coffee, spicy foods, alcohol and adverse weather are precipitants to avoid. It responds to oral antibiotics (e.g. tetracycline, erythromycin or metronidazole). Long-term cosmetic damage to the nose (enlargement with discoloration—rhinophyma) and facial telangiectasia can occur if not treated.

Hidradenitis suppurativa
Hidradenitis suppurativa is the apocrine equivalent of acne vulgaris. In mild forms, patients have recurrent boils in apocrine areas (axillae, groins, breasts, behind the ears). Staphylococcal carriage and diabetes mellitus should be excluded. Chronic nodulocystic involvement of the groins with suppuration and fistula formation can occur. Hidradenitis can respond indifferently to oral antibiotics, hormonal manipulation and isotretinoin. It may be necessary to resort to surgical excision.

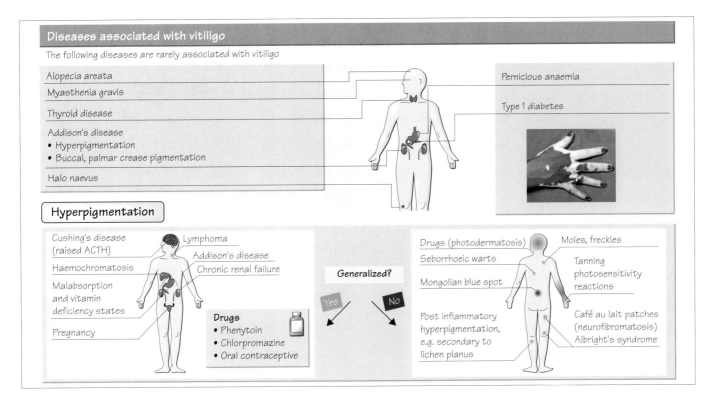

Excess or diminished pigmentation is usually due to excess/diminished melanocyte activity in the skin, although deposition of other pigments can be involved. Melanocyte activity is influenced by solar UV light. Both hypo- and hyperpigmentation are common complications of inflammatory dermatoses and are more pronounced in racially pigmented skin.

Hyperpigmentation

Congenital diseases associated with patches of hyperpigmented skin include melanocytic naevi, and Fanconi's and Albright's syndrome. Café-au-lait patches are also found in neurofibromatosis.

Acquired diseases can give rise to localized or generalized hyperpigmentation:
• Localized hyperpigmentation: many inflammatory skin diseases can leave patches of hyperpigmentation. Chloasma is patchy facial hyperpigmentation, due to endogenous or exogenous steroids, sunlight, drugs (e.g. antibiotics) and depilation.
• Generalized hyperpigmentation can result from acquired endocrine or systemic illness (see figure) or drugs, particularly photosensitive reactions to drugs, chemicals and plants.

Hypopigmentation

Hypopigmentation may be:
• Congenital and generalized, as in the genetic disease of albinism, where melanization cannot occur as a result of tyrosinase deficiency, or localized, such as the hypopigmented ash-leaf patches found in tuberous sclerosis.

• Acquired: post-inflammatory hypopigmentation (common, can occur after any cause of skin inflammation, e.g. contact dermatitis), with leprosy (depigmented anaesthetic areas). A common cause is vitiligo (below). A very rare cause is pituitary failure (generalized loss of skin pigment, often with loss of secondary sex characteristics).

Vitiligo

This is a common (1% of the population) autoimmune condition affecting all races, of unknown aetiology and associated with anti-melanocytic antibody production and organ-specific autoimmune disease.

Clinical features

Depigmented macules appear on sun-exposed areas, areas previously hyperpigmented (e.g. face, axillae, groins) and areas exposed to trauma or friction (an example of the Koebner phenomenon). Areas of vitiligo are readily demonstrated by ultraviolet (UV) radiation (Wood's light). Hairs within a lesion become amelanotic (white).

Management and prognosis

Treatment is unsatisfactory, but the priorities are:
• Protection from the sun to avoid skin cancer and to minimize the contrast between affected and unaffected skin.
• Cosmetic camouflage.

Of younger patients, 20% may repigment spontaneously, but it is usually unsatisfactory patchy and perifollicular. Some patients respond to phototherapy.

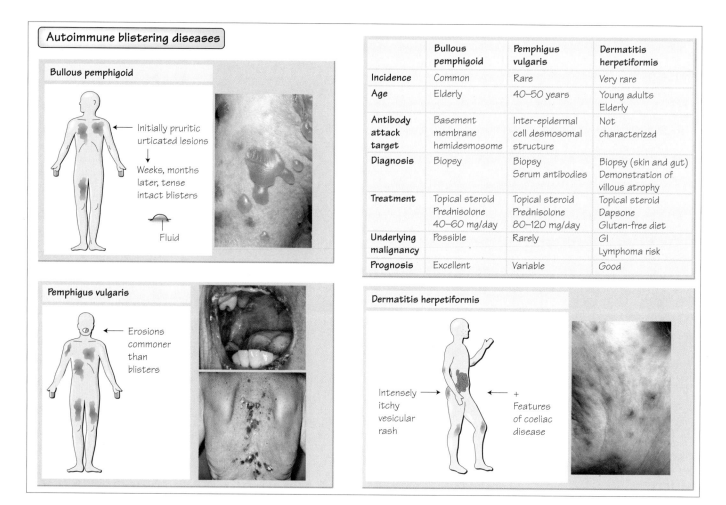

Autoimmune blistering diseases

Bullous pemphigoid

Initially pruritic urticated lesions

↓

Weeks, months later, tense intact blisters

Fluid

Pemphigus vulgaris

Erosions commoner than blisters

Dermatitis herpetiformis

Intensely itchy vesicular rash

+ Features of coeliac disease

	Bullous pemphigoid	Pemphigus vulgaris	Dermatitis herpetiformis
Incidence	Common	Rare	Very rare
Age	Elderly	40–50 years	Young adults Elderly
Antibody attack target	Basement membrane hemidesmosome	Inter-epidermal cell desmosomal structure	Not characterized
Diagnosis	Biopsy	Biopsy Serum antibodies	Biopsy (skin and gut) Demonstration of villous atrophy
Treatment	Topical steroid Prednisolone 40–60 mg/day	Topical steroid Prednisolone 80–120 mg/day	Topical steroid Dapsone Gluten-free diet
Underlying malignancy	Possible	Rarely	GI Lymphoma risk
Prognosis	Excellent	Variable	Good

Blisters are common, e.g. acute eczema, herpes, impetigo or insect bites. Some drug eruptions are bullous, e.g. toxic epidermal necrolysis (see below), as are some systemic diseases, e.g. porphyria cutanea tarda and amyloid. There are also primary bullous skin diseases (below).

Congenital blistering diseases

Several very rare non-infective diseases are associated with blisters from an early age (e.g. epidermolysis bullosa).

Toxic epidermal necrolysis—Lyell's syndrome

This serious, life-threatening idiosyncratic reaction can be the result of a drug reaction or an intercurrent illness. The 'full-blown' disease is rare, but milder 'forme fruste' cases, usually caused by drug reactions, are much more common. Clinically, there is widespread skin loss, compromising cutaneous homoeostasis. There is severe systemic upset. Cardiovascular collapse, infection and failure of thermoregulation contribute to a high mortality. Mucocutaneous involvement is common. Scarring may occur if the patient survives. Intravenous γ-globulins and ciclosporin can be used. The role of systemic steroids is controversial.

Bullous pemphigoid

Bullous pemphigoid is a common disease of elderly people, arising from an autoimmune attack on the hemidesmosome of the basement membrane. Circulating antibodies to the basement membrane zone (BMZ) are often found. There may be an association between seronegative disease, where mucosal lesions are more common, and malignancy. Clinically, the illness can start not as blisters but as erythematous, eczematous and urticated areas on the trunk and limbs. Tense blisters appear later in these sites. The diagnosis is confirmed by histology and tissue immunofluorescence. Most patients respond well to prednisolone 40–60 mg daily and azathioprine.

Pemphigus vulgaris

This is a rare disease, most common in the 45–50 age group, resulting from antibody-mediated attack on the interepidermal cell desmosomal structure. Clinically, the presenting lesion may be confined to the oral mucosa. The blisters are intraepithelial and rupture readily, leaving raw erosions. Skin lesions may not appear for some months. Circulating antibodies are found in the serum. Histology shows an intraepidermal blister with acantholysis (rupture of prickle cells). Direct immunofluorescence demonstrates intercellular IgG and C3. Before the use of systemic corticosteroids, pemphigus vulgaris was fatal. High doses (80–120 mg)

Diseases and Treatments at a Glance

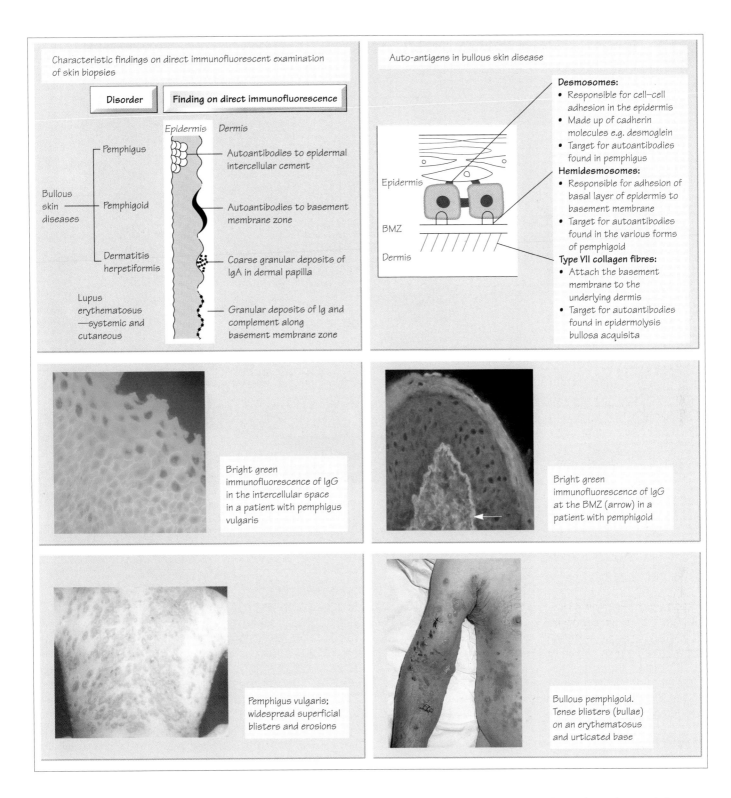

Characteristic findings on direct immunofluorescent examination of skin biopsies

Disorder	Finding on direct immunofluorescence

Bullous skin diseases:
- Pemphigus — Autoantibodies to epidermal intercellular cement
- Pemphigoid — Autoantibodies to basement membrane zone
- Dermatitis herpetiformis — Coarse granular deposits of IgA in dermal papilla
- Lupus erythematosus —systemic and cutaneous — Granular deposits of Ig and complement along basement membrane zone

Auto-antigens in bullous skin disease

Desmosomes:
- Responsible for cell–cell adhesion in the epidermis
- Made up of cadherin molecules e.g. desmoglein
- Target for autoantibodies found in pemphigus

Hemidesmosomes:
- Responsible for adhesion of basal layer of epidermis to basement membrane
- Target for autoantibodies found in the various forms of pemphigoid

Type VII collagen fibres:
- Attach the basement membrane to the underlying dermis
- Target for autoantibodies found in epidermolysis bullosa acquisita

Bright green immunofluorescence of IgG in the intercellular space in a patient with pemphigus vulgaris

Bright green immunofluorescence of IgG at the BMZ (arrow) in a patient with pemphigoid

Pemphigus vulgaris; widespread superficial blisters and erosions

Bullous pemphigoid. Tense blisters (bullae) on an erythematosus and urticated base

of prednisolone are life saving but often produce side effects, which contribute to the mortality. Potent topical steroids are used for the mucocutaneous lesions.

Dermatitis herpetiformis

This is a very rare illness of young adults, with a second peak in old age. Patients almost always have a gluten-sensitive enteropathy (coeliac disease). It is strongly associated with certain HLA haplotypes. Clinically, intensely itchy groups of small blisters on an urticarial base occur over the elbows, knees, buttocks or face—often only excoriations may be seen. Investigations for coeliac disease may be positive: endomysial antibody, intestinal biopsy or tests for malabsorption (full blood count [FBC], serum iron, and folate and red cell folate). Skin biopsy shows IgA deposition on the dermal papillae. The eruption responds to dapsone within a few days. A gluten-free diet allows most patients to discontinue dapsone. Follow-up requires awareness of the risk of agranulocytosis and haemolytic anaemia on dapsone and intestinal lymphoma complicating coeliac disease.

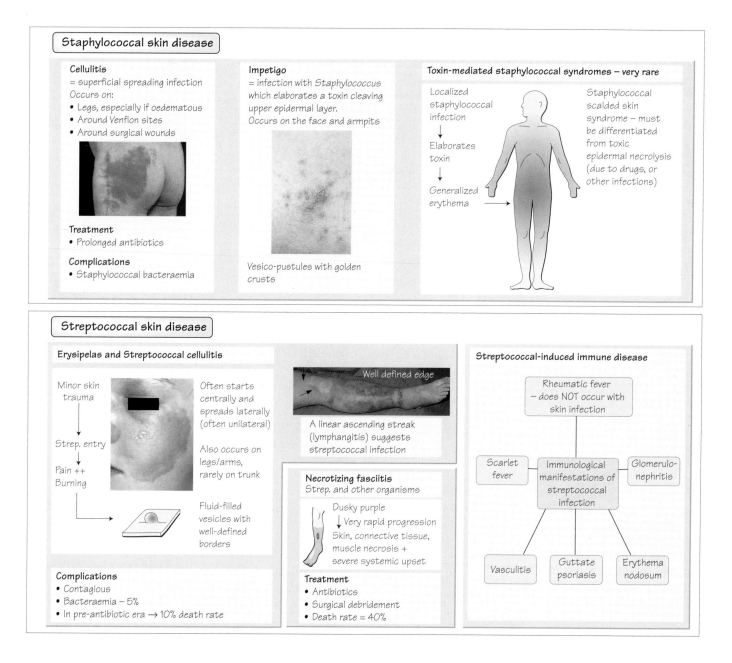

Staphylococcal skin disease

Cellulitis
= superficial spreading infection
Occurs on:
• Legs, especially if oedematous
• Around Venflon sites
• Around surgical wounds

Treatment
• Prolonged antibiotics

Complications
• Staphylococcal bacteraemia

Impetigo
= infection with *Staphylococcus* which elaborates a toxin cleaving upper epidermal layer.
Occurs on the face and armpits

Vesico-pustules with golden crusts

Toxin-mediated staphylococcal syndromes – very rare

Localized staphylococcal infection
↓
Elaborates toxin
↓
Generalized erythema

Staphylococcal scalded skin syndrome – must be differentiated from toxic epidermal necrolysis (due to drugs, or other infections)

Streptococcal skin disease

Erysipelas and Streptococcal cellulitis

Minor skin trauma
↓
Strep. entry
↓
Pain ++
Burning

Often starts centrally and spreads laterally (often unilateral)

Also occurs on legs/arms, rarely on trunk

Fluid-filled vesicles with well-defined borders

Well defined edge

A linear ascending streak (lymphangitis) suggests streptococcal infection

Necrotizing fasciitis
Strep. and other organisms

Dusky purple
↓ Very rapid progression
Skin, connective tissue, muscle necrosis + severe systemic upset

Treatment
• Antibiotics
• Surgical debridement
• Death rate = 40%

Complications
• Contagious
• Bacteraemia – 5%
• In pre-antibiotic era → 10% death rate

Streptococcal-induced immune disease

Rheumatic fever – does NOT occur with skin infection

Scarlet fever

Immunological manifestations of streptococcal infection

Glomerulo-nephritis

Vasculitis

Guttate psoriasis

Erythema nodosum

Staphylococci

Staphylococcal infection of the skin results in spreading superficial infections, deeper infection with abscesses or toxin-mediated damage:
• **Cellulitis**, often on the leg, is predisposed by trauma, tinea pedis or chronic oedema.
• **Impetigo** is caused by a toxin cleaving the upper layers of the epidermis; usually on the face and presents as pustules and golden crusts.
• **Abscesses** may be small and localized to hair follicles (folliculitis), or larger and deeper in the skin, causing boils (furunculosis), which may be extensive (carbuncles). Boils/carbuncles require incision and drainage. If they recur, nasal carriage of staphylococci and/or diabetes should be considered. All suspected skin infections should be swabbed for microbiology. Treatment is usually with systemic antibiotics.

• Staphylococcal scalded skin syndrome (SSSS) is a reaction to a toxin produced by staphylococci, characterized by generalized erythema and exfoliation in an unwell child or immunocompromised adult. It must be distinguished, usually by biopsy, from toxic epidermal necrolysis. The organism cannot be cultured from the skin. Systemic antistaphylococcal treatment and intravenous fluid replacement are given.

Streptococci

Streptococci commonly produce skin and throat infection, and more rarely muscle, joint or heart infection. Damage may result directly, or from toxin elaboration. Organisms may not always be cultured in streptococcal disease and diagnosis is clinical with retro-spective rises in the

Diseases and Treatments at a Glance

antistreptolysin O (ASO) and anti-DNAase titres. A portal of entry should be sought.

• **Erysipelas** is a superficial skin infection, of abrupt onset; it is painful and results in systemic upset. There is erythema, peeling and lymphangitis. Intravenous antibiotics are indicated.

• **Scarlet fever** is caused by upper respiratory tract infection with streptococci which elaborate an erythrogenic toxin, resulting in cutaneous vasodilatation.

• **Necrotizing fasciitis** is a serious, often mixed infection involving streptococci, staphylococci, enterobacteriaceae and obligate anaerobes, or *Streptococcus pyogenes* alone. Often there is no obvious portal of entry in a healthy individual, although the infection may begin in a wound in an unwell patient. The first sign is dusky induration with rapid progressive painful necrosis of skin, connective tissue and muscle. Prompt diagnosis is essential, intravenous antibiotics are rarely sufficient and surgical debridement is necessary. There is an appreciable mortality. The infection often occurs on a limb or the scrotum (Fournier's gangrene), or in a postoperative wound (Meleney's progressive synergistic gangrene).

• **Nephritis**, but not rheumatic fever, may follow streptococcal skin infections, so all streptococcal skin infections should be treated with systemic antibiotics. Hypersensitivity reactions to streptococci have been implicated in erythema nodosum, some types of vasculitis and guttate psoriasis.

Herpes skin infections
Herpes simplex
Any skin or mucosal site may be infected with, and show recurrence of, herpes simplex virus (HSV) infection. Herpetic lesions are painful vesicles and crusts on an erythematous base. They resolve over 2 weeks. Extra-genital disease is usually caused by HSV 1 and genital infections are usually caused by HSV 2. The diagnosis is clinical, supported by viral culture, electron microscopy and serology. Management: aciclovir orally/intravenously and antibiotics for secondary infection.

Herpes zoster (varicella) virus
This causes chickenpox or shingles. Shingles results from reactivation of herpes zoster virus (HZV). Physical trauma to the involved dermatome may be the most common trigger. If immune deficiency is present (e.g. lymphoproliferative disorders), zoster may be severe and recurrent. Paraesthesiae and pain precede the eruption. Very rarely, there is pain and no eruption (zoster sine herpete). The rash is variable, but usually asymmetrical. Erythematous oedematous papules and vesicles arise in one crop, become haemorrhagic and necrotic, and then scab and heal with superficial scarring. Outlying lesions are found in most patients. Recurrent zoster is rare and rarely at the same site.

Diagnosis is clinical, but shingles can be confused with HSV, so viral culture, electron microscopy and serology are useful. Mild analgesics control the pain of the prodrome and the illness. A topical antibiotic is often needed for secondary infection and topical steroids suppress the cutaneous inflammation. Post-herpetic neuralgia is a consequence of nerve involvement in zoster and is deservedly notorious for its intractability. A short course of oral prednisolone from the beginning of the disease may reduce the risk. Oral aciclovir reduces the time course of the cutaneous eruption, but does not prevent post-herpetic neuralgia. Zoster affecting the ophthalmic branch of the trigeminal nerve may cause conjunctivitis or rarely optic neuritis, and expert advice should be sought. Zoster of S2 and below may cause acute retention of urine and constipation, and be complicated by haemorrhagic cystitis. Systemic aciclovir is indicated in these and immunosuppressed patients.

Table 211.1 Human papillomavirus serotypes and associated diseases.

HPV serotype	Associated disease
HPV1	Deep verrucas, common warts
HPV2	Common warts, mosaic verrucas
HPV3	Plane warts
HPV4	Common warts and verrucas
HPV6, 11	Condylomata acuminata (genital warts)
HPV16, 18	Penile cancer, vulval cancer, cervical dysplasia and cancer, Bowen's disease, Bowenoid papulosis

Warts
Warts are due to human papillomavirus (HPV), of which there are many types (Table 211.1).

HPV has a fastidious requirement for human epidermal cells in a particular stage of differentiation. It causes a proliferation of keratinocytes, which partially keratinize and therefore sequester the virus from immunological elimination. Lesions may be sporadic, recurrent or persistent. Treatment is with keratolytics (such as salicylic acid or retinoic acid), or cryotherapy. Cautery and surgical excision may result in lower treatment success rates. Persistent warts can be treated by laser or intralesional bleomycin.

Mollusca are due to a poxvirus. The typical lesion is an umbilicated dome-shaped papule or nodule. Lesions are common on the trunk in children and usually resolve spontaneously. Cryotherapy is the treatment of choice in adults and is occasionally tolerated by a child.

Fungal infections
• **Candidosis** is usually an intertriginous infection (i.e. affecting the axillae, submammary folds, crurae and digital clefts). It is a common cause of vulvovaginitis in women. In the immunoincompetent, it may also affect the mucosa and genitalia. It is treated with topical nystatin or imidazole or clioquinol.

• **Pityriasis versicolor** is a superficial infection of the horny layer by the yeast *Pityrosporum orbiculare*. It is characterized by small, confluent, scaly depigmented patches, which are often apparent for the first time after tanning. Treatment is with a topical imidazole or with selenium sulphide. Occasionally an oral antifungal such as itraconazole is used.

• **Dermatophytosis** is the term for ringworm infection (tinea). Lesions are red, scaly and itchy. The groins, feet and axillae are common sites; the lesions are then not necessarily circular and scaly, but are macerated and moist with a scaly edge. The nails may be involved (onychomycosis). Scarring may occur on the scalp due to an infected inflammatory plaque called a kerion. *Microsporum* spp. form spores around hair (ectothrix) and fluoresce green under Wood's lamp, whereas *Trichophyton* spp. invade the hair shaft (endothrix) and do not fluoresce. Classical treatment is with a topical imidazole or griseofulvin orally. Systemic therapy is necessary for scalp or nail infections. Oral ketoconazole is not widely prescribed because of liver toxicity. Newer imidazoles are safer. The allyamine terbinafine is a newer fungicidal drug that has efficacy against dermatophytes.

Parasitosis
• **Scabies** must always enter the differential diagnosis of pruritus. Typically the rash is symmetrical, involving the fingers backs of hands, axillae, breasts and buttocks. Most lesions may be excoriated papules and nodules, but with care burrows are usually identified. Sites to ex-

amine carefully are digital clefts, around the nipples and the genitalia. By taking a skin scraping, burrow contents may be examined under a microscope. The presence of the female mite (*Sarcoptes scabiei*) or her eggs confirms the diagnosis. Only brief apposition of skin surfaces is needed to transmit the infestation; sexual contact is a common means of spread. Treatment: topical insecticides to cool dry skin all over the body. Secondary eczema and infection should also be treated. In adult scabies (without HIV) the head can be omitted. It is mandatory to treat partners and co-habitants at the same time after concomitant sexually diseases have been excluded.

• **Head lice** infestation is the result of *Pediculus humanus*, which sucks blood from the scalp and lays eggs cemented to the hair shaft (nits).

• **Vagabond's disease** (a widespread itchy excoriated dermatosis) is caused by *Pediculus humanus corporis*, which lives in the seams of clothing and lays its eggs there.

• **Crab louse** (*Pthirus pubis*) is named because of its appearance and tenacious adherence to skin whereas feeding causes pediculosis pubis.

Mycobacteria and the skin
• **Cutaneous tuberculosis** is common in the developing world but rare in the UK. It may be seen in elderly patients and in immigrants. A chest X-ray, tuberculin testing and skin biopsy are needed.
• **Atypical mycobacterial infection** is a common cause of skin lesion in people with AIDS or who are immunologically suppressed.
• Infection with *Mycobacterium marinum* can result in an indolent granulomatous ulcer. If contracted in a swimming bath it is called swimming pool granuloma; if seen in a pet fish keeper it is called fish-tank granuloma. *M. ulcerans* is an important cause of leg or arm ulceration in Africa (Buruli ulcer) or Australia (Searle's ulcer).
• Mycobacterium leprae – see figure.

| **Leprosy** | Tuberculoid TT | Borderline | | | Lepromatous LL | General features of leprosy |
		BT	BB	BL		
Immunological responsiveness	High (+ve lepromin test)	Intermediate			Low (−ve lepromin test)	Leprosy (Hansen's disease) results from infection (probably acquired through the respiratory tract) with *Mycobacterium leprae*. Infected patients shed the bacillus from infected nasal secretions; only 1% of contacts develop the disease. Incubation period 2–6 years. The clinical course depends on the host's immunity (see left); skin involvement is a prominent feature, as is peripheral nerve involvement, resulting in hypopigmented patches and anaesthesia. Diagnosis: clinical, finding bacilli in skin smears, culturing bacilli in mice food pad. Lepromin test: intra-dermal injection of dead bacilli – early reaction (Fernandez) < 48 hours = sensitivity to leprosy protein, late reaction (Mitsuda) 4–5 weeks resistance of host to infection. Treatment is with multiple drugs. Treatment reactions include: • Erythema nodosum leprosum – usually in LL leprosy, painful tender nodules on extensor surfaces • Allergic response to mycobacteria, causing further nerve damage • Iritis Treatment reactions can result in permanent injury – treat promptly with thalidomide
Organisms in lesions	Few – hard to find	Some			Many – easy to find	
Infectivity	Non-infectious	Slightly infectious			Infectious	
Extent of lesions	Localized	Scattered			Generalized	
Involvement	Skin & nerves only				Many tissues	
Skin lesions	1–2 only; commonly on face				Innumerable & widespread	

Tuberculoid leprosy: subtle depigmentation with a palpable erythematous rim at the upper edge

Borderline leprosy (BL). Borderline tuberculoid (BT) downgrading to BL. Showing typical well-defined hypopigmented macules of BT and many small lesions, some of which are papular

The 'leonine' facies of lepromatous leprosy

Nerve involvement	Thickened nerves in vicinity of skin lesions	Most peripheral nerves thickened
Anaesthesia distribution	Lesions hypoanaesthetic/no sweating	Lesions not hypoanaesthetic – but glove & stocking anaesthesia; trophic ulcers of periphery; muscle nerve paralysis
Clinical course	Disease localized; patients usually not very troubled by the disease – good prognosis, and spontaneous recovery may occur	Patients disabled by the disease with widespread organ involvement

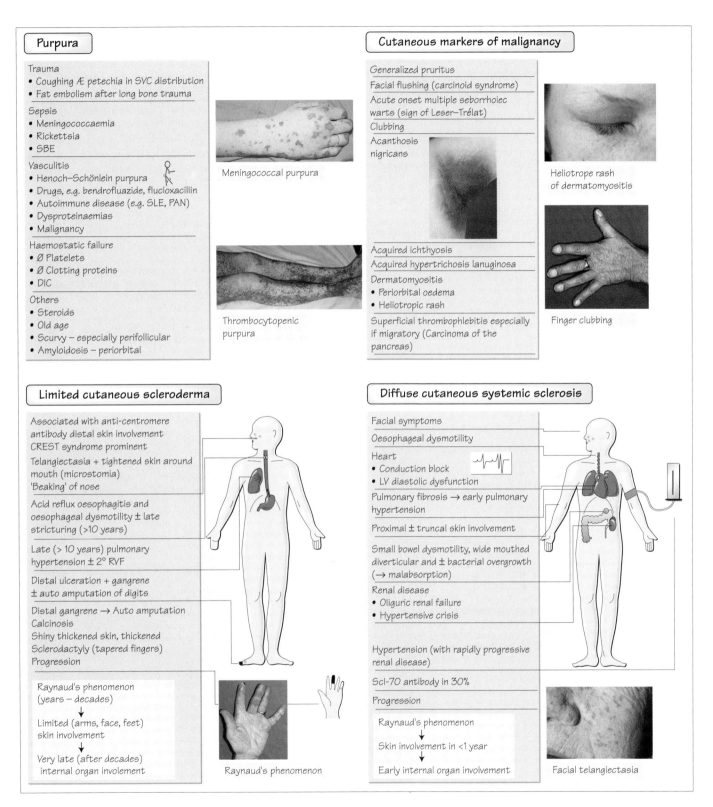

Purpura

Trauma
- Coughing Æ petechia in SVC distribution
- Fat embolism after long bone trauma

Sepsis
- Meningococcaemia
- Rickettsia
- SBE

Vasculitis
- Henoch–Schönlein purpura
- Drugs, e.g. bendrofluazide, flucloxacillin
- Autoimmune disease (e.g. SLE, PAN)
- Dysproteinaemias
- Malignancy

Haemostatic failure
- Ø Platelets
- Ø Clotting proteins
- DIC

Others
- Steroids
- Old age
- Scurvy – especially perifollicular
- Amyloidosis – periorbital

Meningococcal purpura

Thrombocytopenic purpura

Cutaneous markers of malignancy

Generalized pruritus

Facial flushing (carcinoid syndrome)

Acute onset multiple seborrhoiec warts (sign of Leser–Trélat)

Clubbing

Acanthosis nigricans

Acquired ichthyosis

Acquired hypertrichosis lanuginosa

Dermatomyositis
- Periorbital oedema
- Heliotropic rash

Superficial thrombophlebitis especially if migratory (Carcinoma of the pancreas)

Heliotrope rash of dermatomyositis

Finger clubbing

Limited cutaneous scleroderma

Associated with anti-centromere antibody distal skin involvement CREST syndrome prominent

Telangiectasia + tightened skin around mouth (microstomia)
'Beaking' of nose

Acid reflux oesophagitis and oesophageal dysmotility ± late stricturing (>10 years)

Late (> 10 years) pulmonary hypertension ± 2° RVF

Distal ulceration + gangrene ± auto amputation of digits

Distal gangrene → Auto amputation
Calcinosis
Shiny thickened skin, thickened
Sclerodactyly (tapered fingers)
Progression

Raynaud's phenomenon (years – decades)
↓
Limited (arms, face, feet) skin involvement
↓
Very late (after decades) internal organ involement

Raynaud's phenomenon

Diffuse cutaneous systemic sclerosis

Facial symptoms

Oesophageal dysmotility

Heart
- Conduction block
- LV diastolic dysfunction

Pulmonary fibrosis → early pulmonary hypertension

Proximal ± truncal skin involvement

Small bowel dysmotility, wide mouthed diverticular and ± bacterial overgrowth (→ malabsorption)

Renal disease
- Oliguric renal failure
- Hypertensive crisis

Hypertension (with rapidly progressive renal disease)

Scl-70 antibody in 30%

Progression

Raynaud's phenomenon
↓
Skin involvement in <1 year
↓
Early internal organ involvement

Facial telangiectasia

The skin can be involved in or react to many systemic disease processes.

Drug eruptions

Drug reactions are very commonly seen in acute internal medicine. Regard any drug as capable of causing any cutaneous reaction. Some reactions are predictable (striae with steroids), some likely (photosensitivity with amiodarone, β-blockers exacerbating psoriasis) and some unpredictable or idiosyncratic (erythema multiforme with antibiotics).

Vasculitis

Conditions producing a vasculitic reaction in the skin include:
• Infection: meningococcaemia, bacterial endocarditis.
• Systemic vasculitis (e.g. systemic lupus erythematosus [SLE], polyarteritis nodosa [PAN]) is suspected when internal organs such as the kidneys and/or lungs are involved. Immunology and skin biopsy may be diagnostic, as may renal/lung histology.
• Other causes, including drugs, connective tissue disease, paraneoplastic phenomena, clotting abnormalities and cryoglobulinaemia.
• Erythema nodosum (EN): painful palpable lesions on the lower legs, arising from a vasculitis of the deep dermis. Although no cause may be found, EN is associated with infection (streptococcal sore throat, mycobacteria, etc.), drugs, sarcoidosis and inflammatory bowel disease. Resolution typically occurs over 5–6 weeks.
• Skin infarcts, affecting particularly the extremities, e.g. nail-bed 'splinter haemorrhages' (caused by circulating immune complexes) occur in many acute and chronic infections, including bacterial endocarditis.
• Purpura has a wide differential diagnosis (see figure). Two common causes are:
  • Henoch–Schönlein purpura (HSP) (anaphylactoid purpura) occurs mainly in children as a result of an abnormal response to a viral infection. A purpuric rash occurs on the extensor aspects of the lower limbs. Nephritis may develop. HSP normally resolves without sequelae; very occasionally chronic renal damage occurs.
  • Leukocytoclastic or allergic vasculitis may be confined to the skin. The most common clinical pattern is acute self-limiting palpable purpura (other lesion may occur), which may be chronic or recurrent and usually affects the limbs with fever, malaise, arthralgia and gastrointestinal symptoms. The cause is often not discovered but infections, neoplasia and drugs should be excluded.

Skin markers of internal malignancy

There are a number of cutaneous stigmata of internal malignancy:
• Pruritus: lymphoma, polycythaemia rubra vera.
• Ichthyosis (dry skin).
• Acanthosis nigricans: velvety hyperkeratotic plaques found in flexures and intertriginous areas; also caused by endocrine disorders (acromegaly, Cushing's disease, Addison's disease, hypothyroidism, insulin-resistant diabetes mellitus, polycystic ovary disease), drugs (steroids) or obesity, or rarely it is familial.
• Dermatomyositis: skin involvement consists of erythematous plaques over the knuckles, finger joints, elbows and knees. Nail cuticles are ragged. Eyelids are swollen and are discoloured violet (see p. 413). Of patients aged > 50 years, 30% have an underlying cancer.
• Migratory superficial thrombosis often relates to pancreatic cancer.
• Secondary deposits in the skin, e.g. Sister Joseph's nodule (periumbilical deposit from an intra-abdominal malignancy) or Virchow's node (left supraclavicular fossa lymph node deposit from gastric cancer).

The scalp is a common site for cutaneous metastasis from internal solid cancers.

Raynaud's phenomenon

Raynaud's phenomenon is episodic, painful, digital ischaemia in response to cold or emotional stimuli, characterized by classic sequential colour changes of white to blue to red. The disorder may be primary and idiopathic or secondary to underlying disease (see Table 212.1):
• Idiopathic Raynaud's phenomenon is diagnosed in young women who have no features of an underlying disorder on clinical evaluation or investigation.
• Raynaud's phenomenon is more likely to be secondary, usually to systemic sclerosis, if it is especially severe (with digital skin changes)

Table 212.1 Causes of Raynaud's phenomenon.

Cervical rib
Vibrating tools
Vasculitis and connective tissue diseases
    Systemic sclerosis
    Sjögren's syndrome, systemic lupus erythematosus (SLE), dermatomyositis
    Rheumatoid arthritis
Cryoglobulinaemia
Cold agglutinins
Hyperviscosity syndromes
Drugs (β-blockers, ergot alkaloids, cytotoxics)

Table 212.2 Cutaneous manifestations of HIV infection and AIDS.

Inflammatory dermatoses
Seroconversion toxic erythema
Psoriasis
Seborrhoeic dermatitis
Severe drug reactions
Eosinophilic pustular folliculitis
Papular pruritic eruption

Infections
Tinea and onychomycosis
Candidosis
Hairy leucoplakia (EBV)
Atypical primary, secondary and late syphilis
Bacillary haemangiomatosis
Condyloma acuminata (viral warts)
Molluscum contagiosum
Cutaneous atypical mycobacterial infection
Kaposi's sarcoma (HHV 8)
Herpes simplex
Herpes zoster
Severe aphthous stomatitis

Other skin manifestations
Cutaneous and nail hyperpigmentation
Porphyria cutanea tarda
Acquired ichthyosis and keratoderma
Yellow nail syndrome

Neoplasia
Kaposi's sarcoma (HHV 8)
Cutaneous lymphoma
Melanoma and non-melanoma skin cancer

and persistent, or if it begins for the first time in early adulthood, in a male and is unilateral.

Investigations when indicated should include a chest X-ray (cervical rib), autoantibodies (antinuclear antibodies [ANA], double-stranded DNA (dsDNA), antineutrophil cytoplasmic antibody [ANCA]), cryoglobulins, cold agglutinins and erythrocyte sedimentation rate (ESR). Treatment: avoidance of cold, heated gloves and nifedipine. If severe, sympathectomy can be considered.

Systemic sclerosis

Systemic sclerosis ('hard skin') is an autoimmune disease damaging the skin and internal organs, which occurs in two forms: *limited cutaneous scleroderma* localized to the skin and *diffuse cutaneous systemic sclerosis* when internal viscera are involved. Scleroderma also occurs in a localized form (morphoea) and in malignancies (e.g. breast cancer), porphyria cutanea tarda, phenylketonuria and in the carcinoid syndrome.
• Limited cutaneous scleroderma (morphoea) skin lesions are circumscribed plaques. They can occur anywhere, or may involve the forehead (*en coup de sabre*). Systemic involvement is rare and occurs later.
• Diffuse cutaneous systemic sclerosis: female > male. Raynaud's phenomenon precedes cutaneous sclerosis, with puffy swelling of the hands and feet, leading to atrophic thinning of ulcerated digital tips and nailfold involvement. Muscle weakness occurs (disuse atrophy or muscle involvement). Perioral involvement produces very tight skin around the mouth, restricting opening, and may require lateral release (commissurotomy). Dry eyes and mouth (keratoconjunctivitis sicca and xerostomia—Sjögren's syndrome) occur. Oesophageal involve-

ment leads to difficulty swallowing, and small bowel disease produces abdominal pain and diarrhoea (caused by bacterial overgrowth). Pulmonary fibrosis produces shortness of breath (restrictive pattern on lung function testing). An erosive arthritis may cause joint pains. Renal failure occurs and is associated with a worse prognosis. Antinuclear antibodies are found in > 90% and anticentromere antibody in 70% with CREST (**c**alcinosis, **R**aynaud's, o**e**sophagitis, **s**clerodactyly **t**elangiectasia). No agent reliably arrests disease activity. Treatment is for symptom relief only. Digital vascular insufficiency is treated by cold avoidance, vasodilators (e.g. nifedipine, intravenous prostacyclin or intravenous calcitonin gene-related peptide). In severe cases, digital amputation may be necessary. Oesophageal reflux responds to proton pump inhibitors. The prognosis is generally good, even with some organ involvement, although renal or pulmonary disease can be fatal.

HIV

Skin disease is an important corollary of AIDS and HIV infection (see Table 212.2). The incidence of several cutaneous diseases is increased in people who are HIV positive or who have AIDS. The percentage of people with HIV who have skin manifestations, and the number of manifestations, increase as HIV infection progresses. The incidence and severity sometimes correlates with the absolute numbers of T-helper cells and the prognostic significance of some disorders is well recognized. HIV infection may affect the behaviour of other dermatological conditions such as psoriasis. Generally, HIV-related skin diseases improve with HAART (highly active antiretroviral therapy).

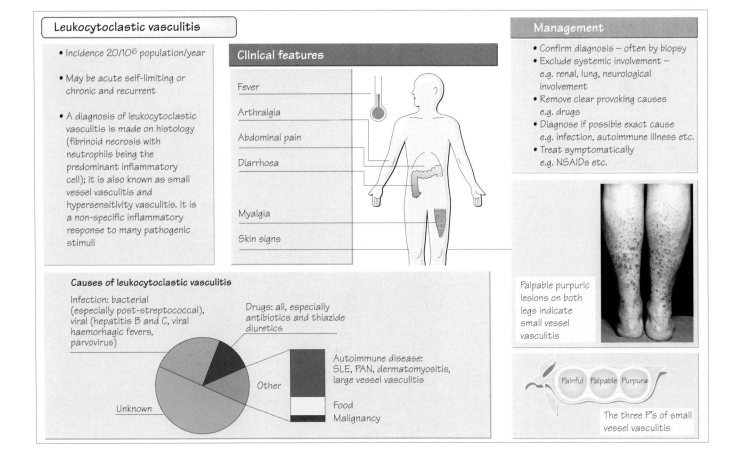

Leukocytoclastic vasculitis

• Incidence 20/10⁶ population/year

• May be acute self-limiting or chronic and recurrent

• A diagnosis of leukocytoclastic vasculitis is made on histology (fibrinoid necrosis with neutrophils being the predominant inflammatory cell); it is also known as small vessel vasculitis and hypersensitivity vasculitis. It is a non-specific inflammatory response to many pathogenic stimuli

Clinical features

Fever
Arthralgia
Abdominal pain
Diarrhoea
Myalgia
Skin signs

Management

• Confirm diagnosis – often by biopsy
• Exclude systemic involvement – e.g. renal, lung, neurological involvement
• Remove clear provoking causes e.g. drugs
• Diagnose if possible exact cause e.g. infection, autoimmune illness etc.
• Treat symptomatically e.g. NSAIDs etc.

Palpable purpuric lesions on both legs indicate small vessel vasculitis

Causes of leukocytoclastic vasculitis

Infection: bacterial (especially post-streptococcal), viral (hepatitis B and C, viral haemorrhagic fevers, parvovirus)

Drugs: all, especially antibiotics and thiazide diuretics

Other

Unknown

Autoimmune disease: SLE, PAN, dermatomyositis, large vessel vasculitis

Food
Malignancy

Painful Palpable Purpura

The three P's of small vessel vasculitis

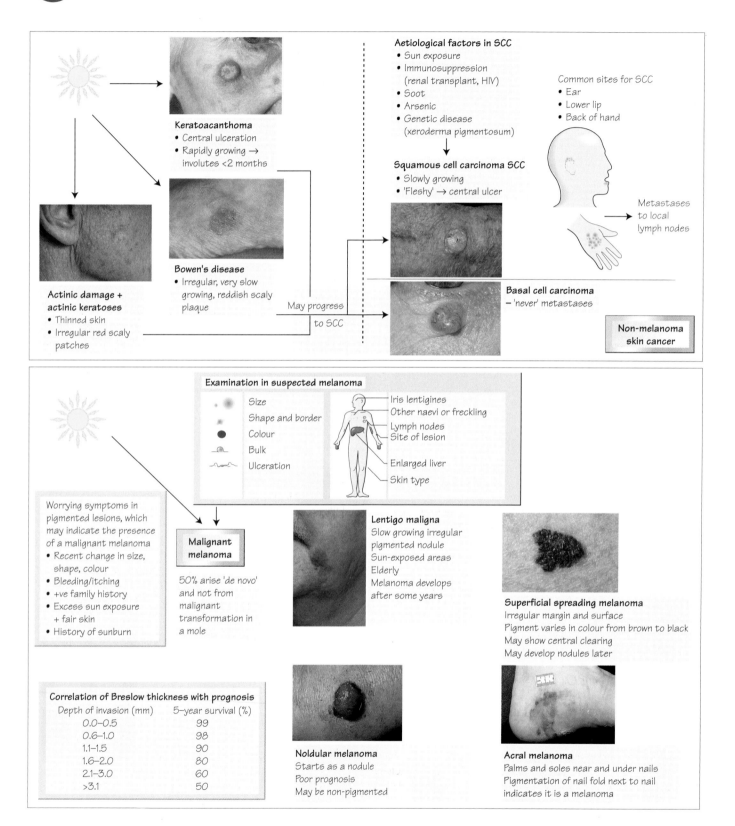

Keratoacanthoma
• Central ulceration
• Rapidly growing →
  involutes <2 months

Aetiological factors in SCC
• Sun exposure
• Immunosuppression
  (renal transplant, HIV)
• Soot
• Arsenic
• Genetic disease
  (xeroderma pigmentosum)

Common sites for SCC
• Ear
• Lower lip
• Back of hand

Squamous cell carcinoma SCC
• Slowly growing
• 'Fleshy' → central ulcer

Metastases
to local
lymph nodes

Bowen's disease
• Irregular, very slow
  growing, reddish scaly
  plaque

Basal cell carcinoma
– 'never' metastases

May progress
to SCC

**Actinic damage +
actinic keratoses**
• Thinned skin
• Irregular red scaly
  patches

**Non-melanoma
skin cancer**

Examination in suspected melanoma

Size
Shape and border
Colour
Bulk
Ulceration

Iris lentigines
Other naevi or freckling
Lymph nodes
Site of lesion
Enlarged liver
Skin type

Worrying symptoms in
pigmented lesions, which
may indicate the presence
of a malignant melanoma
• Recent change in size,
  shape, colour
• Bleeding/itching
• +ve family history
• Excess sun exposure
  + fair skin
• History of sunburn

**Malignant
melanoma**

50% arise 'de novo'
and not from
malignant
transformation in
a mole

Lentigo maligna
Slow growing irregular
pigmented nodule
Sun-exposed areas
Elderly
Melanoma develops
after some years

Superficial spreading melanoma
Irregular margin and surface
Pigment varies in colour from brown to black
May show central clearing
May develop nodules later

Correlation of Breslow thickness with prognosis

Depth of invasion (mm)	5–year survival (%)
0.0–0.5	99
0.6–1.0	98
1.1–1.5	90
1.6–2.0	80
2.1–3.0	60
>3.1	50

Noldular melanoma
Starts as a nodule
Poor prognosis
May be non-pigmented

Acral melanoma
Palms and soles near and under nails
Pigmentation of nail fold next to nail
indicates it is a melanoma

Diseases and Treatments at a Glance

Skin cancers are the most common cancers in the UK, with over 100 000 cases per annum. Sun exposure is a common aetiological factor.

Benign lesions

Solar or actinic keratoses are flat, scaly, often erythematous lesions, which show epidermal dysplasia on histology and have a low risk of developing into Bowen's disease or squamous carcinoma. They are usually associated with actinic (sun) damage. Treatment is with cryotherapy, curettage, topical 5-fluorouracil cream or diclofenac cream.

Keratoacanthoma is a rapidly growing nodular lesion on the light-exposed skin of the hand or face. It reaches its maximum size at < 1–2 months and appears as a smooth dome-shaped lesion with a central crater filled with keratinaceous material. It can spontaneously involute to leave scarring, but is best excised, as it is probably a form of squamous cell carcinoma (SCC).

Premalignant disease

Bowen's disease (intraepidermal carcinoma *in situ*) is a single, red, scaly patch that may be mistaken for eczema or psoriasis, but neither itches nor responds to topical steroids. Sometimes there are multiple lesions. Aetiological factors and treatment are as above, but include surgical curettage or excision. The condition may progress to invasive SCC.

Congenital melanocytic naevi are large pigmented lesions present from birth. They are common anywhere, but a bathing trunk distribution is recognized. There is a significant risk of malignant melanoma developing in lesions larger than 5 cm.

Dysplastic naevi may be associated with an increased risk of melanoma. The **dysplastic naevus syndrome** is the presence of many moles (dysplastic naevi), often abnormally distributed (scalp, buttocks, feet), usually larger than 0.5 cm, and iris lentigines in the context of a personal or first-degree family history of melanoma.

Malignant disease

Basal cell carcinoma/epithelioma (BCC/BCE) is an extremely common neoplasm, often on the face, head and neck of older people. BCEs 'never' metastasize, but indolent growth can lead to delayed presentation and deep invasion, leading to high rates of recurrence after conventional treatments. Sun damage is the greatest risk factor for BCE, but sometimes multiple BCEs are associated with previous X-ray treatment for ankylosing spondylitis (spine) and tinea capitis (scalp). Usual treatments are excision, curettage and cautery or radiotherapy, all with a 5–10% recurrence rate. Tumours around the eye and nasal furrows have a 20% recurrence rate, as a result of infiltration along embryological fusion lines. A 99.5% cure rate can be achieved using micrographic surgery (Mohs' procedure). Late presentation or failed treatment is complicated by fungation, involvement of other structures (such as the eye and lacrimal apparatus), and deep invasion with destruction of cartilage and bone, which may all represent incurable disease.

Squamous carcinoma occurs in sun-exposed areas in elderly people or as multiple tumours in very young people with xeroderma pigmentosum, a defect in the DNA-repair mechanism. Other risk factors include smoking (lip tumours) and chronic inflammation, e.g. associated with chronic venous ulceration (Marjolin's ulcer of the leg). The best-known occupational cancer was cancer of the scrotum in chimney sweeps, which in the nineteenth century was related to exposure to the hydrocarbons in soot. Squamous carcinoma most commonly presents as an irregular ulcer or as a slowly growing nodule. It may be very destructive locally, and can also metastasize to the lymph nodes. Treatment must therefore be ablative (i.e. excision or radiotherapy) and long-term follow-up is necessary.

Lentigo maligna (Hutchinson's melanotic freckle) is a slow-growing, pigmented macule on the face in older people. Histologically, it is an intraepidermal melanoma, but it can become invasive at any stage (lentigo maligna melanoma). Biopsy establishes the diagnosis. Treatment is by excision. Plastic repair may be necessary.

Malignant melanoma: in the UK there are 6000 new cases and 2000 deaths per year, with rates doubling every decade. Predisposing factors include (susceptibility to) ultraviolet light exposure: congenital naevi, family history of melanoma, large numbers of acquired naevi, any number of atypical naevi, freckles, previous episodes of sunburn, significant sun exposure before the age of 20 years.

Melanoma is rare in African-Caribbean and Asian individuals, and common in Scottish and Australian individuals. Three types of melanoma are recognized clinically: superficial spreading, nodular and acral lentiginous. Superficial spreading and nodular are the most common types and present in early adulthood. In men, the upper back is a common area, but in women it is the lower leg. Some melanomas do not arise from an existing mole. The earliest growth of superficial spreading melanoma is in the horizontal plane, so presentation is usually as a new or changing mole. Melanoma invades locally and metastasizes to lymph nodes early on. On examination, look for actinic damage, freckles, and numbers, types and distribution of moles (and iris lentigines—dark-brown macules), and check the local and distant lymph nodes and the liver. The crucial diagnostic investigation and treatment is excisional histopathology. Multidisciplinary management is appropriate.

The depth of the lesion on first presentation correlates with the prognosis (see figure). Melanoma is conventionally excised with wide margins. For extensive disease, surgical or laser debulking, amputation, isolated limb perfusion with chemotherapy, systemic chemotherapy, including with cytokines, and radiotherapy are used. Treatment of metastatic melanoma is not curative and the prognosis is grim.

Kaposi's sarcoma: AIDS-related neoplasm.

Lymphoma

Mycosis fungoides is a cutaneous T-cell lymphoma where there is slowly evolving infiltration of the skin with T-helper cells. The cause is not known but HTLV-1 was first isolated from a patient with Sézary syndrome (erythroderma, lymphadenopathy and abnormal Sézary cells with cerebriform nuclei in the blood). The differential diagnosis of erythroderma is given on p. 125.

The following stages are recognized:
- Fixed itchy scaly patches (like eczema or psoriasis)
- Fixed geographical plaques
- Nodules, tumours and ulcers
- Lymph node or systemic organ involvement.

It is possible that at an early stage malignant change has not occurred and the prognosis with gentle treatment (topical steroids, PUVA, topical nitrogen mustard, electron beam therapy) is good. With more advanced disease, therapy is more radical (radiotherapy, chemotherapy, extracorporeal photochemotherapy) and the outlook is bleak.

Adult T-cell lymphoma/leukaemia is a cutaneous prodrome of granulomatous papules and nodules (from which proviral DNA can be recovered) precedes and accompanies adult T-cell lymphoma/leukaemia (ATLL) due to HTLV-1.

Hodgkin's disease and non-Hodgkin's lymphoma may involve the skin and, it is argued, may originate in the skin.

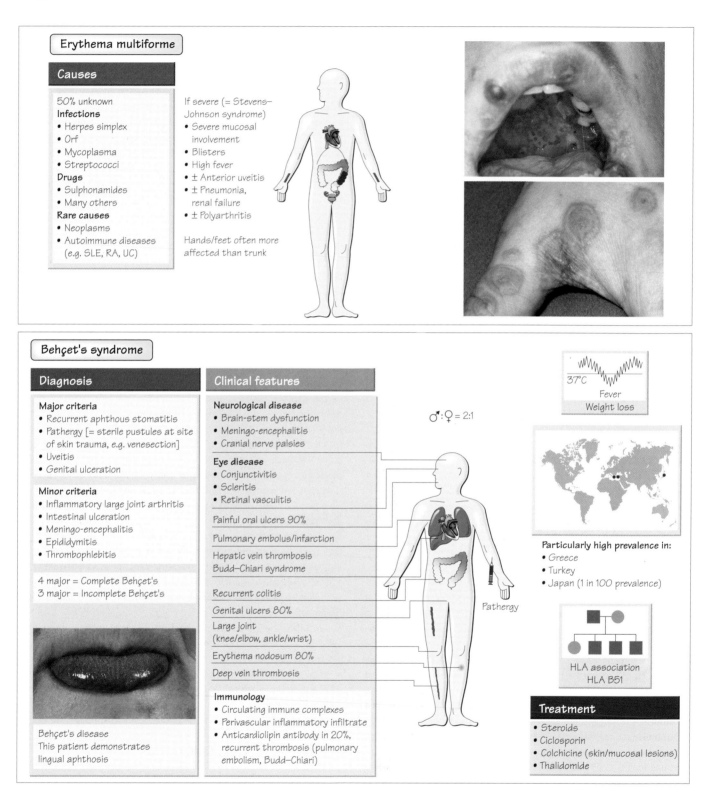

Erythema multiforme

Causes

50% unknown
Infections
- Herpes simplex
- Orf
- Mycoplasma
- Streptococci

Drugs
- Sulphonamides
- Many others

Rare causes
- Neoplasms
- Autoimmune diseases (e.g. SLE, RA, UC)

If severe (= Stevens–Johnson syndrome)
- Severe mucosal involvement
- Blisters
- High fever
- ± Anterior uveitis
- ± Pneumonia, renal failure
- ± Polyarthritis

Hands/feet often more affected than trunk

Behçet's syndrome

Diagnosis

Major criteria
- Recurrent aphthous stomatitis
- Pathergy [= sterile pustules at site of skin trauma, e.g. venesection]
- Uveitis
- Genital ulceration

Minor criteria
- Inflammatory large joint arthritis
- Intestinal ulceration
- Meningo-encephalitis
- Epididymitis
- Thrombophlebitis

4 major = Complete Behçet's
3 major = Incomplete Behçet's

Behçet's disease
This patient demonstrates
lingual aphthosis

Clinical features

Neurological disease
- Brain-stem dysfunction
- Meningo-encephalitis
- Cranial nerve palsies

Eye disease
- Conjunctivitis
- Scleritis
- Retinal vasculitis

Painful oral ulcers 90%

Pulmonary embolus/infarction

Hepatic vein thrombosis
Budd–Chiari syndrome

Recurrent colitis

Genital ulcers 80%

Large joint
(knee/elbow, ankle/wrist)

Erythema nodosum 80%

Deep vein thrombosis

Immunology
- Circulating immune complexes
- Perivascular inflammatory infiltrate
- Anticardiolipin antibody in 20%, recurrent thrombosis (pulmonary embolism, Budd–Chiari)

♂:♀ = 2:1

Pathergy

37°C
Fever
Weight loss

Particularly high prevalence in:
- Greece
- Turkey
- Japan (1 in 100 prevalence)

HLA association
HLA B51

Treatment

- Steroids
- Ciclosporin
- Colchicine (skin/mucosal lesions)
- Thalidomide

Diseases and Treatments at a Glance

Oral disorders

• **Oral ulceration**: the most common cause is idiopathic aphthous ulceration. Oral pemphigus is very rare but serious, and frequently diagnosed late (see p. 420). Examination of all patients with oral ulcers should include examination of other mucocutaneous sites and a search for lymphadenopathy. Investigations include microbiology and virology, and a biopsy with immunofluorescence. Treatment of aphthae concentrates on improving oral hygiene, antibiotic and antifungal mouthwashes, and topical steroids.

• *Candida* is an extremely common intraoral commensal, which acts as an opportunistic pathogen in those immunosuppressed from infection (e.g. HIV), disease (e.g. diabetes mellitus) or drugs (e.g. oral antibiotics or cytotoxics). White detachable deposits and plaques are the usual physical signs. Mouthwashes or nystatin lozenges and a systemic imidazole are effective treatments, but candidosis may recur depending on the context.

• **Leukoplakia** is a non-specific common disturbance of oral mucosal keratinization. Smoking and poor dental hygiene are associated factors. It may result from a syphilitic atrophic glossitis, but small white mucuus patches may occur anywhere in the oral cavity during secondary syphilis; 5% undergo malignant transformation.

• **Erythroplakia** describes red patches in the mouth. They are more likely to be malignant than leukoplakia and should therefore be biopsied.

• **Lichen planus** is characterized by lilac erythematous patches topped by lacy white striae (Wickham's striae). It is more common on the buccal mucosa than the tongue, although all intraoral sites may be involved. Of patients with the condition, 30% have extraoral lichen planus, and 10–50% of all patients with lichen planus have oral lesions. Erosive or atrophic lichen planus may progress to malignancy.

Vulval disorders

The vulva can be affected by dermatoses such as seborrhoeic dermatitis, psoriasis, lichen sclerosus and lichen planus, or sexually transmitted disease (STD). Patients may be severely symptomatic with itch irritation, dyspareunia and somatopsychic symptoms.

• Vulval warts are usually caused by human papilloma virus (HPV) types 6 and 11. All patients and their partners should be screened for STDs. Colposcopy and a cervical smear examination are indicated. Treatment is with liquid nitrogen therapy, topical podophyllin or topical imiquimod.

• Lichen simplex refers to a chronic eczematous process exaggerated and propagated by scratching in response to itch. Treatment is with topical steroids and night-time sedation, possibly with tricyclic antidepressants.

• Lichen sclerosus is an idiopathic chronic inflammatory dermatosis with subsequent atrophy, which causes intense itching. Lesions are shiny white and red-rimmed with central telangiectasia, purpura and erosions. There may be loss of architecture of the labia and burying of the clitoris. Potent topical steroids relieve the itch. Biopsy and continued monitoring are important because intraepithelial neoplasia and frank invasive carcinoma may develop.

• Vulval intraepithelial neoplasia (VIN) is suspected when hard white plaques or erosions are seen. The invasive potential of VIN is small. Cryotherapy and topical imiquimod can be used. Multidisciplinary management (gynaecologists, oncologists, etc.) is desirable.

• Additional causes of vulval itching include urinary incontinence and vaginal discharge, often as a result of candidosis. All women with pruritus vulvae should be screened for diabetes mellitus.

Penile disorders

The penis is a common site for seborrhoeic dermatitis, psoriasis, lichen sclerosus, lichen planus and viral warts. Balanitis due to *Candida* or other microbials may be a presenting feature of diabetes mellitus.

• Lichen sclerosus of the penis may result in phimosis and even retention of urine. The severest form of damage is balanitis xerotica obliterans. Circumcision should be considered in anyone presenting with phimosis.

• Zoon's balanitis is an irritant mucositis of the uncircumscribed male. It presents with moist raw patches and is treated by circumcision.

• Erythroplasia of Queyrat is the eponym for Bowen's disease (squamous cell carcinoma *in situ*) of the penis and is suspected if there are fixed red lesions of the penis. Biopsy is diagnostic. Treatment options include topical 5-fluorouracil, topical imiquimod, cryotherapy, radiotherapy or surgery. Follow-up (for malignancy detection) is essential.

Genital ulceration
Aetiology

Genital ulcers can be caused by dermatoses, sexually transmitted disease or other infections, Behçet's disease, pyoderma gangrenosum, artefact or, most importantly, squamous carcinoma.

Investigations

These include microbiology (including mycology) and skin biopsy.

Treatment

Genital hygiene, emollient, and topical antibiotic, antifungal and steroid applications.

Orogenital syndromes

Certain diseases result in simultaneous lesions in the mouth and genitalia. These include:

• Severe erythema multiforme: the cause of erythema multiforme is often unknown, but includes herpes simplex infection, other infections such as those caused by *Mycoplasma* spp. and drug reactions. In mild-to-moderate disease, involvement is limited to the skin. Lesions characteristically start as pleomorphic red eruptions on the arms and legs, which spread centrally to the trunk. Spontaneous remission is usual, although topical steroids may improve itch. In severe disease (the Stevens–Johnson syndrome) lesions occur in the mouth, conjunctiva and genitalia as well. Treatment is systemic steroids and antimicrobials for any infection.

• Behçet's syndrome (see figure) is characterized by painful oral (90–100%) and genital (60–90%) ulceration and variable involvement of other systems as follows:
  • Ocular manifestations (keratitis, uveitis, optic neuritis) (50–90%)
  • Pustules, pyoderma gangrenosum, erythema nodosum, arthritis (20–50%)
  • Central nervous system involvement (e.g. vasculitis, thrombophlebitis) (10–20%)
  • Pulmonary infarction (10–40%)
  • Renal involvement (10%)
  • Budd–Chiari syndrome (10%).

There are no diagnostic tests for Behçet's syndrome. Treatment is with systemic steroids; occasionally thalidomide is used. Many patients have mild disease and do well. However, cerebral/renal involvement is associated with severe treatment-resistant disease and a worse prognosis.

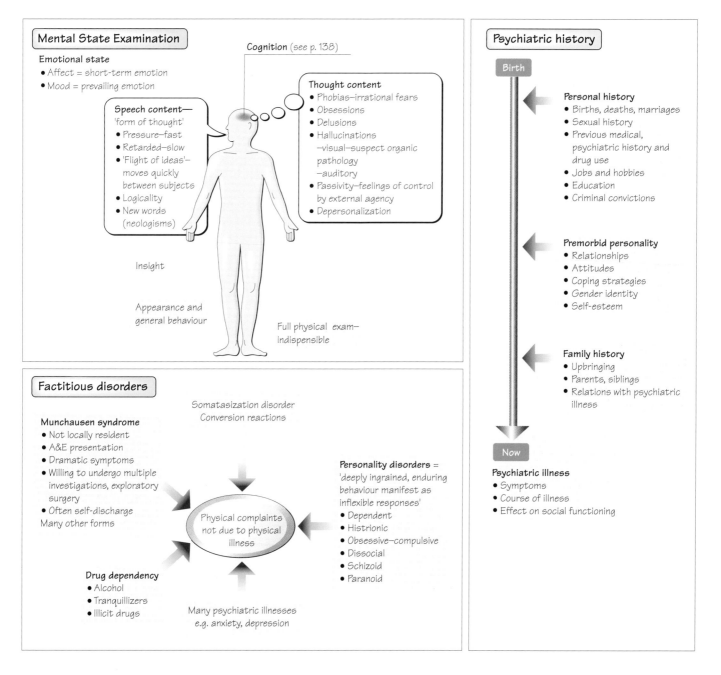

Psychological illnesses cause symptoms similar to those of organic disease, and may obscure an organic diagnosis or complicate its management. Of acute medical admissions 5–10% require formal psychiatric review.

Neurotic diseases are an exaggeration of normal emotional responses. Psychotic illnesses have symptoms outside the range of normal human experience.

Common psychological illnesses seen in medical practice

• Anxiety disorders cause psychological symptoms (apprehension, fear of impending doom/disaster, irritability, depersonalization) and phy-

sical ones (sweating, tremor, palpitations, 'dizziness', inability to sleep and poor concentration), which can be confused with certain diseases (e.g. thyrotoxicosis, alcohol intoxication/withdrawal, hypoglycaemia and, extremely rarely, phaeochromocytoma). Symptoms may be situation dependent, e.g. phobic disorders (particular objects or animals trigger attacks) or more commonly free floating, appearing without reason. Symptoms may appear in short overwhelming episodes ('panic attacks') —occasionally triggered by bad news, e.g. an untreatable diagnosis— or as longer, lower-intensity anxiety states. Treatment is psychological (explanation, reassurance, relaxation techniques). Short courses of benzodiazepines have a limited role.

• Abnormal illness behaviour: exaggerated anxiety, inappropriate adoption of the 'sick' role and prolonged illness denial are all common. Abnormal psychological reactions need to be identified and treated in order to treat any underlying organic disease effectively.

• Somatization disorders: psychic distress (often depression or anxiety) manifests as physical symptoms, and is common. Psychic symptoms are often denied or minimized and physical symptoms exaggerated. These disorders cause immense difficulty because the patient is convinced that a physical illness underlies the symptoms. Patients may attend the same department frequently (if the symptom complex remains unchanged) or multiple different departments (if the symptom complex varies) to establish an organic diagnosis. An important diagnostic clue is thick notes without any 'cast-iron' organic diagnosis. Treatment involves excluding physical illness, where possible identifying the underlying psychic symptoms and applying psychological treatments, including reassurance.

• Conversion reactions (hysterical disorders): psychic distress manifest as physical signs, e.g. paralysis, pseudo-seizures, blindness, etc. They are rare. Organic disease should be excluded using a minimum of investigation. The physician should refrain from further investigations, otherwise the patient incorrectly perceives that an organic disorder defying diagnosis is present. Treatment (from a psychiatrist specialized in conversion reactions) comprises reassurance that there is no underlying pathology and that symptoms will improve over time. Direct confrontation is unhelpful.

Schizophrenia

This is characterized by a set of beliefs, symptoms and behaviour outside normal experience. Highly suggestive first-rank symptoms are:

• Auditory hallucinations, often abusive, repeating the patient's words, or commenting on their behaviour or personality.

• Thought withdrawal, insertion and broadcasting: external agencies or people can remove, insert or listen in to their thoughts.

• Delusional beliefs, i.e. ideas outside the social norms of that society. For example, a belief in a deity is often not delusional, but the belief that a deity can actually perform miracles can be.

• External control of thoughts, emotions or actions.

Symptoms are positive, when delusional beliefs and floridly abnormal behaviour predominate, or negative, when inaction, apathy and social withdrawal predominate. Schizophrenic patients come to the attention of acute medical services through:

• Bizarre behaviour leading to accident and emergency attendance. Organic disease or drug intoxication may need to be excluded.

• Attempted (and successful) suicide is common in psychosis—all self-harm cases should have psychotic illness excluded.

If schizophrenia is suspected, immediate psychiatric review should be requested. The diagnosis is made from the mental state examination (see figure). Treatment is with antipsychotic drugs, which inhibit dopamine subtype D1- and D2-receptors and/or central nervous system (CNS) serotonin traffic. They improve positive symptoms, but have less impact on negative ones. Similar symptoms occasionally arise from organic mental disorders, caused by drugs (e.g. 'street' drugs, steroids, rarely other drugs) or physical illness (e.g. temporal lobe epilepsy, brain tumours). These may need to be actively excluded.

Affective (mood) disorders

• **Depression** results in a low mood and unhappiness. Conversation is slow, quiet and monotonous, with depressive ideation, low self-esteem, unworthiness and wretchedness. The intellect can be impaired. Physical symptoms can predominate. Somatic features of severe depression are: early morning waking, appetite and weight loss, constipation and loss of libido/sexual prowess. In psychotic depression, symptoms are profound and derogatory or abusive auditory hallucinations can occur. Depression complicates most physical illnesses (especially stroke) and amplifies physical symptoms, resulting in great distress and frequent physician consultations. Treatment is psychological (mild-moderate cases) and with antidepressant drugs, which prolong the action of noradrenaline (norepinephrine) and/or serotonin in neuronal synapses. Electroconvulsive therapy (ECT) acts quickly and is used for severe depression.

• **Mania** results in mental restlessness with mood elevation, fast and disinhibited speech, with 'flight of ideas' (never dwelling on one topic for long), over-confident self-belief, with delusions about intellectual, physical, financial or sexual prowess or omnipotence. Sufferers are physically restless and may not eat or sleep. Hypomania, a mild form of mania, comprises mild euphoria, overactivity and disinhibition. Mania can alternate with depression—a bipolar illness. Severe mania is treated with major tranquillizers, and subsequent attacks prevented by the mood-stabilizer lithium.

• **Personality disorders**, manifest as lifelong inflexible responses, cause management difficulties (see figure).

Substance misuse

This results in medical, social and economic problems.

• Cigarettes: highly addictive. Smokers die some 8 years before non-smokers (of ischaemic heart disease, cancer). Smoking ages skin (facial wrinkling). Counselling, nicotine replacement therapy and anti-depressants have a minor role in cessation.

• Alcohol: can cause problem drinking (social disruption) or physical dependence (cessation leads to the withdrawal syndrome—tremor, sweating, tachycardia, anxiety, confusion, hallucinations, seizures, which are treated with chlordiazepoxide and vitamins).

• Minor or major tranquillizers.

• Opiates: common, often injected (HIV, hepatitis infection from shared needles). Premature death from infection or accidental overdose. Addicts may express opiate-seeking behaviour and commit petty larceny on hospital wards. Withdrawal causes sweating, shivering, tachycardia, hypertension and diarrhoea.

• Ecstasy: occasionally causes acute confusion, cardiac arrhythmias, memory loss or 'malignant' hyponatraemia and lethal cerebral oedema.

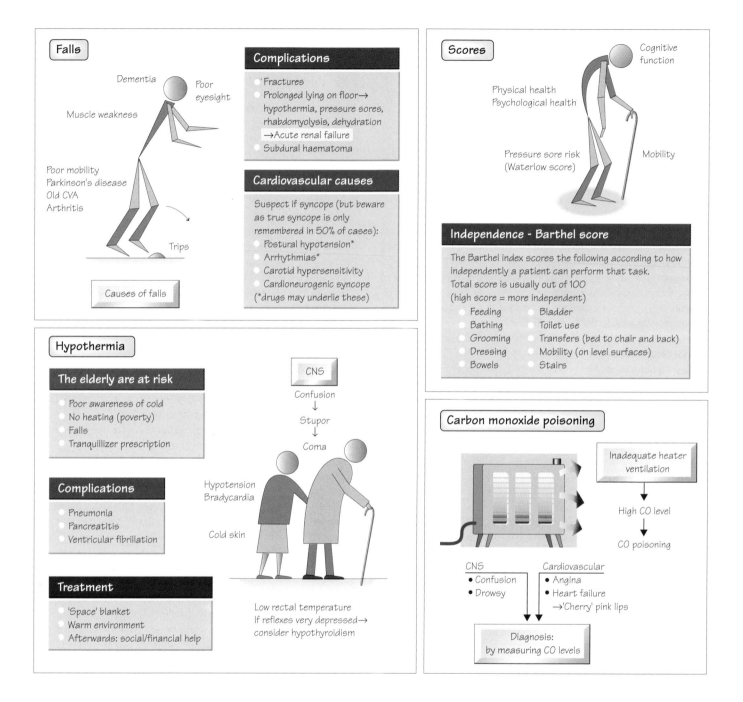

Falls

Dementia
Poor eyesight
Muscle weakness
Poor mobility
Parkinson's disease
Old CVA
Arthritis
Trips

Causes of falls

Complications

- Fractures
- Prolonged lying on floor→ hypothermia, pressure sores, rhabdomyolysis, dehydration →Acute renal failure
- Subdural haematoma

Cardiovascular causes

Suspect if syncope (but beware as true syncope is only remembered in 50% of cases):
- Postural hypotension*
- Arrhythmias*
- Carotid hypersensitivity
- Cardioneurogenic syncope
(*drugs may underlie these)

Scores

Cognitive function
Physical health
Psychological health
Pressure sore risk (Waterlow score)
Mobility

Independence – Barthel score

The Barthel index scores the following according to how independently a patient can perform that task.
Total score is usually out of 100
(high score = more independent)
- Feeding
- Bathing
- Grooming
- Dressing
- Bowels
- Bladder
- Toilet use
- Transfers (bed to chair and back)
- Mobility (on level surfaces)
- Stairs

Hypothermia

The elderly are at risk

- Poor awareness of cold
- No heating (poverty)
- Falls
- Tranquillizer prescription

Complications

- Pneumonia
- Pancreatitis
- Ventricular fibrillation

Treatment

- 'Space' blanket
- Warm environment
- Afterwards: social/financial help

CNS
Confusion
↓
Stupor
↓
Coma

Hypotension
Bradycardia

Cold skin

Low rectal temperature
If reflexes very depressed→ consider hypothyroidism

Carbon monoxide poisoning

Inadequate heater ventilation
↓
High CO level
↓
CO poisoning

CNS
- Confusion
- Drowsy

Cardiovascular
- Angina
- Heart failure →'Cherry' pink lips

Diagnosis: by measuring CO levels

Sick elderly people should in many respects be treated identically to young people, although there are important differences:
- Premorbid condition is often worse from multiple ongoing illnesses, multiple medications, varying degrees of dementia, poverty and social isolation. Thus, the rehabilitation potential following the acute illness may be more limited. Additional home support should be planned early on during hospital admission.
- Clinical presentation is often atypical and not classical.

- The differential diagnosis is usually broader.
- The risk to life from any illness is greater.
- Recovery is prolonged and may require substantial support.

Premorbid condition

It is vital to establish the premorbid condition, because this is the target to aim for in subsequent rehabilitation. How independent were they? Several scoring systems (e.g. of activities of daily living) can be used to ascertain functional status—the Barthel score is commonly used to measure independence and thus rehabilitation potential and progress (see figure).

Polypharmacy

Elderly people are often prescribed multiple drugs for multiple pathologies. This leads to compliance issues (disease progression) and side effects. Always ask whether the current illness can be explained by a side effect of medication.

Differential diagnosis

In young patients, 'Occam's razor'* applies: 'the least number of diagnoses needed to explain all the symptoms and signs establishes the correct diagnosis'. In elderly people, multiple pathologies often co-exist, e.g. heart failure, leg ulcers, diabetes and its complications, occult cancer, etc. A single unifying diagnosis is often not possible.

Clinical presentations and diseases

Presentations are often atypical, such as 'unwellness' without specific features, a decline in functional or cognitive capacity, rather than with organ-specific symptoms. The differential diagnosis is broader than in many younger patients. For example:
• Acute confusion is a common presentation of many diseases. As the febrile response is diminished, infections often present with minor fever and minor constitutional upset, and major confusion. Abscesses, e.g. subphrenic and pelvic, may present as 'unwellness', without localizing symptoms/signs.
• Many diseases present with decreased function/cognition or apathy and weight loss, rather than more classically. Diseases that may present in this manner include thyrotoxicosis, depression, temporal arteritis and cancer.
• Tuberculosis is not uncommon in elderly people, and may present quite atypically, e.g. with non-specific 'unwellness', loss of appetite, etc.
• Diseases may relate to poverty: there are many examples, including accidental carbon monoxide (CO) poisoning resulting from ill-maintained heaters, which is underdiagnosed. CO binds to haemoglobin, decreasing oxygen transport. Presentation is with central nervous system (CNS–headache, agitation, confusion, occasionally coma) and/or cardiac symptoms (heart failure, unstable angina)—common symptoms in elderly people that are often attributed to other pathology. Diagnosis is by measuring CO levels in blood. Treatment is high-dose hyperbaric (i.e. high-pressure) oxygen in severe cases (contact Royal Navy diving centres) and, crucially, heater maintenance.
• Hypothermia—see figure.

Specific issues

Falls are common. The cause should always be sought, as specific therapy may be effective:
• Musculoskeletal conditions, such as osteoarthritis or age-related decline in muscle strength, are a common causes of falls. Physical rehabilitation, a Zimmer frame or other walking aid, and adjustment of the home environment may prevent falls and consequent fractures.
• Cardiovascular diseases causing recurrent falls include postural hypotension, cardioneurogenic syncope, carotid hypersensitivity syndrome, intermittent arrhythmias (bradyarrhythmias such as complete heart block, occasionally ventricular tachycardia). Carotid sinus massage, tilt-table testing, and 24-h ECG taping may provide important clues to the presence of cardiovascular disease.
• Neurological disease, especially disability from a previous stroke, Parkinson's disease, peripheral neuropathy (e.g. diabetic), cervical myelopathy. Epilepsy rarely underlies recurrent falls.
• Dementia often underlies or contributes to falls and immobility.
  The consequence of falls also should be considered:
• Fractures, which may be lessened by treating osteoporosis, providing hip protectors and adjusting the home environment.
• Assistance may be needed to get up—various alarms are available. Regular visits by friends/neighbours play a vital role.

Diagnostic issues

As clinical symptoms and signs may be less reliable, investigations should be broad. All elderly patients admitted acutely should have:
• Full blood count, electrolytes (K^+, Na^+ and Ca^{2+}), renal and liver function, inflammatory markers (both erythrocyte sedimentation rate [ESR] and C-reactive protein).
• Chest X-ray and ECG.
• Urine dipstick and, if abnormal, culture.
• Blood cultures unless infection has been ruled by establishing an alternative diagnosis.

Special issues

• Special diagnostic clinics for falls, dementia, syncope, etc. allow for optimal care and treatment.
• The threshold for 'blind' abdomen/pelvis computed tomography is low even without localizing symptoms/signs, because cancer and intra-abdominal/pelvic abscesses are common.
• A therapeutic trial of steroids is diagnostic in temporal arteritis if symptoms resolve ≥ 48 h after starting steroids.

Consequence and treatment of illness

The risk to life from any illness (e.g. pneumonia, especially myocardial infarction, etc.) is greater with increasing age, justifying aggressive medical therapy. Age alone is *not a* bar to high-technology intervention, such as cardiac surgery (aortic valve replacement is feasible in many aged 85 years or more), abdominal surgery, intensive care, etc. Aggressive treatments, although often having more benefit, equally often have greater risk. This calls for careful clinical judgement in deciding the most appropriate therapy. Cardiac arrest is associated with a poorer outcome in very elderly people (≥ 85 years). Decisions on the appropriateness of cardiopulmonary resuscitation (CPR) should be made on admission in conjunction with the patient or, if they are incapacitated, their relatives.

Rehabilitation

It is vital that, in order to optimize outcome, specialists in old-age medicine, rather than general physicians, undertake rehabilitation, using multidisciplinary teams, including:
• Physiotherapists
• Occupational therapists
• Social workers.
  The aim should be to return the patient to a stable long-term environment of his or her choice.

---

* From William of Occam (1285–1347)—literally 'entities are not to be multiplied beyond necessity', i.e. the principle of parsimony; one should not make more assumptions than the minimum needed.

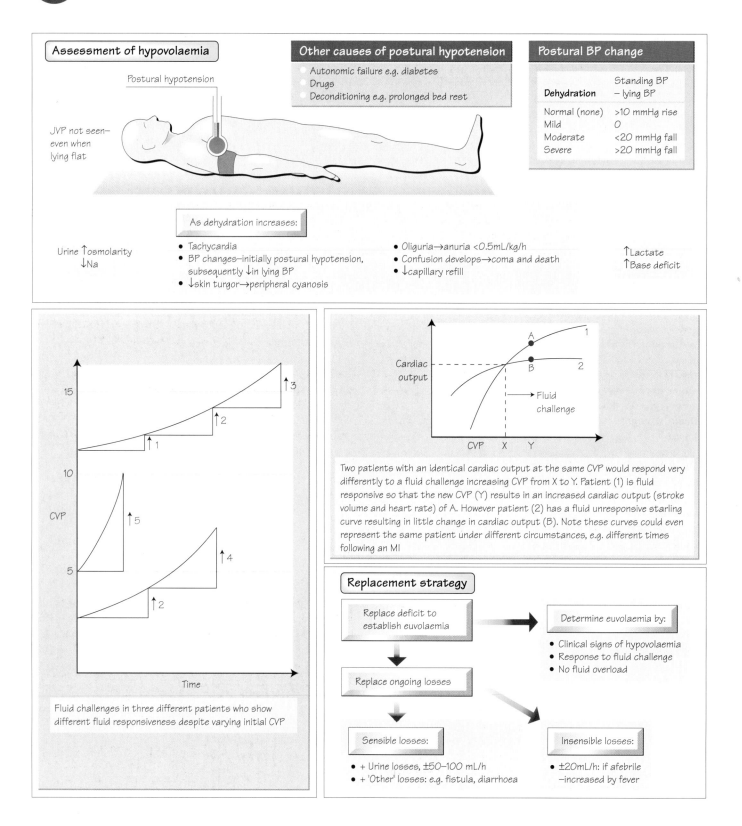

Assessment of hypovolaemia

Postural hypotension

JVP not seen—
even when
lying flat

Other causes of postural hypotension
- Autonomic failure e.g. diabetes
- Drugs
- Deconditioning e.g. prolonged bed rest

Postural BP change

Dehydration	Standing BP – lying BP
Normal (none)	>10 mmHg rise
Mild	0
Moderate	<20 mmHg fall
Severe	>20 mmHg fall

Urine ↑osmolarity
↓Na

As dehydration increases:
- Tachycardia
- BP changes–initially postural hypotension, subsequently ↓in lying BP
- ↓skin turgor→peripheral cyanosis

- Oliguria→anuria <0.5mL/kg/h
- Confusion develops→coma and death
- ↓capillary refill

↑Lactate
↑Base deficit

Fluid challenges in three different patients who show different fluid responsiveness despite varying initial CVP

Two patients with an identical cardiac output at the same CVP would respond very differently to a fluid challenge increasing CVP from X to Y. Patient (1) is fluid responsive so that the new CVP (Y) results in an increased cardiac output (stroke volume and heart rate) of A. However patient (2) has a fluid unresponsive starling curve resulting in little change in cardiac output (B). Note these curves could even represent the same patient under different circumstances, e.g. different times following an MI

Replacement strategy

Replace deficit to establish euvolaemia → **Determine euvolaemia by:**
- Clinical signs of hypovolaemia
- Response to fluid challenge
- No fluid overload

Replace ongoing losses

Sensible losses:
- + Urine losses, ±50–100 mL/h
- + 'Other' losses: e.g. fistula, diarrhoea

Insensible losses:
- ±20mL/h: if afebrile –increased by fever

Fluid may be required either for maintenance of euvolaemia or replacement of losses in hypovolaemic patients. The oral route for is optimal for maintenance. Patients unable to eat and drink normally can be fed by either a nasogastric or a percutaneous endoscopically placed gastric feeding tube. Occasionally, the enteral route is unavailable (recent gastrointestinal surgery, ileus); intravenous crystalloid may be administered for short periods to provide water and electrolytes, though parenteral nutrition needs to be considered if long-term maintenance is required.

Assessment of hypovolaemia

Profound hypovolaemia will eventually lead to tissue hypoperfusion and multiorgan failure. It may result from absolute losses (haemorrhage, diarrhoea, vomiting, burns, polyuria) or redistribution of fluid, sometimes known as 'third space' loss (sepsis, anaphylaxis, pancreatitis, trauma, spinal cord injury, ascites). The renin-angiotensin and sympathetic nervous systems are important in regulating the volume of the extracellular space. These compensatory mechanisms may make it difficult to detect mild hypovolaemia. The signs of hypovolaemia are:
• Reduced skin turgor, decreased capillary refill, tachycardia, low jugular venous pressure (JVP).
• Low urine output (< 0.5 mL/kg/hour), with high osmolality, low urine Na and urine urea:creatinine ratio > 40 and eventual abnormal urea and creatinine levels in blood. Plasma urea is disproportionably high in dehydration and GI haemorrhage. It may be low in patients with liver disease even in the presence of substantial hypovolaemia.
• Hypotension: reduction in blood pressure is a late feature. An apparently 'normal' blood pressure may be low if the patient suffers from untreated hypertension. Compensatory mechanisms mask significant hypovolaemia in the supine position, therefore hypotension may only become apparent on sitting or standing (postural hypotension). Such patients often complain of dizziness or syncope when erect. Hypovolaemia in the supine position may also be unmasked by raising the legs for 30 seconds (to increase venous return) and monitoring the effect on heart rate, blood pressure and JVP (or CVP).
• Reduced weight.
• Lactate and base deficit rise when there is significant tissue hypoperfusion.

As with many critically ill patients, the signs above may be non-specific and are not by themselves diagnostic, but taken together with the patient's history and diagnosis one may make an assessment of volume status. In some patients this is easy; for example a young man with 4 days diarrhoea who has not been drinking. If examination shows tachycardia, reduced capillary refill, hypotension, reduced JVP and oliguria there would be little doubt the patient is severely dehydrated. However, if the patient is elderly with pre-existing heart failure and is admitted with acute pancreatitis, the assessment is far more complex. **The fluid challenge is extremely useful in the diagnosis and treatment of hypovolaemia.**

Fluid challenge

The response to a fluid challenge may be assessed by changes in pulmonary artery occlusion pressure (reflecting left atrial pressure), stroke volume or CVP (reflecting right atrial pressure). The latter is most frequently used outside of the intensive care unit. Traditionally one is taught 'normal' values of right and left atrial pressures, however absolute values are of little use in guiding fluid therapy because they vary with ventricular compliance and venous tone. An absolute CVP value of 10 mmHg may represent hypovolaemia, euvolaemia or hypervolaemia in three different patients.

A fluid challenge involves giving a relatively small volume of crystalloid or colloid over a short period of time and monitoring the haemodynamic effects. Typically between 200 and 500 mL of fluid is given over a period of 10–20 minutes. The change in CVP depends on the volume status of the patient. In a hypovolaemic patient there is little increase in CVP following a fluid challenge (< 3 mmHg), which may then be repeated. A rise of 3 mmHg in the CVP following a challenge implies an adequate circulating volume, whilst a rise > 3 mmHg suggests hypervolaemia. The patient should also be monitored for improvements in other haemodynamic variables ($\downarrow$ heart rate, $\uparrow$ blood pressure, $\uparrow$ capillary refill) and tissue perfusion ($\uparrow$ urine output, $\uparrow$ GCS, reduction in acidosis/lactate), whilst avoiding signs of hypervolaemia.

Management of severely hypovolaemic patients

As with all critically ill patients there needs to be good vascular access (ideally central venous) and appropriate monitoring which should include ECG, pulse oximetry, hourly urine output, blood pressure (arterial catheter if severe hypotension or shock), respiratory rate and GCS. A pulmonary artery catheter, oesophageal Doppler or pulse contour analysis may be required in some patients.

Which fluid should be chosen?

Blood is required in acute haemorrhage, but colloid is given to maintain the circulation until this is available. Crystalloids equilibrate within the extracellular space (interstitial and intravascular) and so have less immediate effect on plasma expansion than colloids. Typically colloid expands plasma volume by three times as much as the same volume of crystalloid, but this effect is not maintained over time, particularly in critically ill patients with increased vascular permeability.

Crystalloids
Normal saline or lactated Ringer's solution (Hartmann's solution)
• Cheap compared to colloids. Less efficient plasma expansion than colloid.
• Hyperchloraemic acidosis with large volumes of saline (see below).

Colloids
Albumin 4.5% or 20% salt poor (mw 66.5 kDa). Most expensive. Some controversy in past, however recent multi-centre trial shows no difference in safety compared to saline.

Dextrans Examples include Dextran 40 or 70 (molecular weight in kDa). Less commonly used of all colloids in Europe. Decreases platelet aggregation.

Gelatins Gelatins (Gelofusine, Haemaccel) are derived from hydrolysed animal collagen (mw 30–35 kDa). Short duration of action. Highest risk of anaphylactoid reactions.

Hydroxyethyl starches Hydroxyethyl starches (HAES-Steril, eloHAES) are derived from maize. Various (high) molecular weights. May effect haemostasis. Long-term storage in tissues can cause pruritus.

Hyperchloraemic acidosis
Colloids contain osmotically active molecules in normal saline. Administration of large volumes of chloride-rich saline leads to a metabolic acidosis. This phenomenon is not observed with Hartmann's solution which is a physiologically balanced solution containing much less chloride. Patients with hyperchloraemic acidosis suffer with nausea, abdominal pain, and reduced urine output (hyperchloraemia reduces GFR). Future developments will undoubtedly see the wider introduction of colloids in physiological solutions.

218 Chronic tiredness and other medically unexplained symptoms

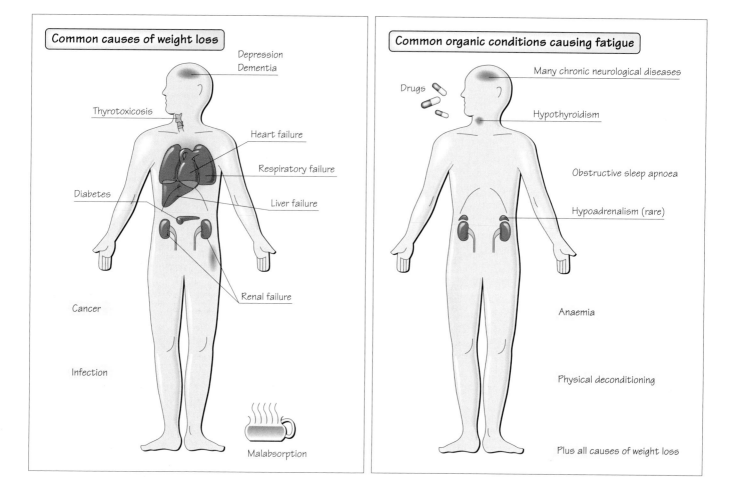

Common causes of weight loss

Depression
Dementia

Thyrotoxicosis

Heart failure

Respiratory failure

Diabetes

Liver failure

Cancer

Renal failure

Infection

Malabsorption

Common organic conditions causing fatigue

Drugs

Many chronic neurological diseases

Hypothyroidism

Obstructive sleep apnoea

Hypoadrenalism (rare)

Anaemia

Physical deconditioning

Plus all causes of weight loss

Chronic fatigue

Fatigue is a complex and common sensation accounting for 20% of GP consultations. Tiredness results from:
- Many (indeed most) organic diseases (see figure).
- Psychological distress.
- Social stresses.
- Psychiatric illness: of tired patients, 20–80% have a psychiatric disorder (depression, anxiety or somatization disorder).
- Tiredness may be a medically unexplained symptom (MUS): the diagnoses applied may vary between this, chronic fatigue syndrome (CFS—see below), post-viral fatigue (especially if there have been symptoms in the past 6 months suggesting a viral infection), and myalgic encephalomyelitis (ME). The variation in the diagnosis made for long-standing fatigue largely follows medical and social styles, rather than reflecting any real change in the epidemiology of the aetiology of this symptom.

From this list, it can be seen that almost any illness or psychic distress can cause tiredness. Accordingly the diagnosis of the cause of any fatigue rests on identifying associated symptoms, as well as on the demographics (patient's age and sex: male sex and increasing age are

associated with serious disease). Features suggestive of an underlying organic illness include:
- Weight loss—unintentional weight loss usually has a serious cause (see figure).
- Fevers, night sweats.
- Malaise.
- Persistent pains localized to one area.
- Persistent symptoms of new onset.
- Age ≥ 35 years.

It is important that serious organic or psychiatric pathology is diagnosed and treated; other causes of tiredness are usually diagnosed by exclusion (Table 218.1). Accurate diagnosis relies on the history and examination, although investigations are also important. A normal full blood count, renal and liver function and inflammatory markers (C-reactive protein, erythrocyte sedimentation rate) are reassuring, but *do not* exclude all serious inflammatory/malignant disease (disseminated cancer can present as fatigue with normal blood tests—the diagnostic clue is often weight loss and age ≥ 50 years). One-third of patients with fatigue have no identifiable organic or psychiatric disorder (including CFS).

Table 218.1 Physical disorders associated with fatigue.

- Vital organ failure (heart, lung, kidney, liver, bone marrow, skin)
- Chronic inflammation or infection
- Viral infections may cause *postviral fatigue* lasting < 6 months.
- Malignancy
- Endocrine disease (particularly thyroid disease, adrenal disease)
- Anaemia
- Sleep disorders (obstructive sleep apnoea)
- Neurological disease (multiple sclerosis, Parkinson's disease)
- Drugs, e.g. β-blockers.

Management and prognosis

These depend on the cause. If psychological stresses are significant, counselling may help. Of patients with non-specific fatigue, 25–50% still complain of fatigue a year later. Chronic fatigue for ≥ 6 months or associated with multiple associated somatic symptoms has a poorer long-term outlook. Most cases of fatigue are helped by physical reconditioning (a commonly advised exercise prescription is for 20-minute sessions of aerobic exercise, sufficiently intense to induce breathlessness, repeated three times a week); this is true whether or not organic illness is present, and so can be applied without prejudice as to the diagnosis.

Medically unexplained symptoms

These are an enormous workload on all doctors:

- Medically unexplained symptoms may account for up to 50% of new patient diagnoses in some specialties, such as gastroenterology, or neurology.
- Some symptoms are a marker for physical or sexual abuse—for example, pseudo-seizures is a fairly strong marker for childhood sexual abuse.
- Any associated psychological disease should be rapidly diagnosed and treated.
- When the diagnosis of MUS is suspected, it is important to exclude serious illness using the minimum of tests.
- Equally, it is crucial to explain to patients, before the results of the test are known, that it is highly likely that these investigations will be normal, indeed, that they are primarily being done to reassure the patient, and not because the doctor believes they will be abnormal. This will avoid the patient believing that normal results mean that the physician should look harder for a underlying organic illness.
- It is best to acknowledge to the patient that the symptoms are medically unexplained, that these symptoms are frequently seen (thus the individual physician and profession have considerable experience and knowledge of them), and that they have a benign prognosis.

- It is not wise to offer mechanistic explanations that are based on guess work, as these can often be disproved—leading to the patient losing confidence in their physician. Patients then seek help elsewhere; some patients seek large numbers of opinions (patients with MUS in neurology clinics have been seen in about six previous specialties), and not surprisingly receive multiple different explanations for their symptoms, leading them to lose faith in doctors generally.
- There is some evidence that labelling these symptoms as functional, rather than medically unexplained, offends fewer patients.
- Dealing with symptoms, rather than seeking an underlying unifying interpretation, may help, e.g. drugs to help constipation or diarrhoea, exercise to help tiredness, anxiolytics to help anxiety, cognitive therapy to help worries about the future, etc., when patients are amenable.

Somatization disorder

The definition of somatization disorder includes:

- ≥ 2 years of medically unexplained symptoms
- Persistent refusal to accept advice and reassurance for symptoms
- Impaired level of functioning.

Various specialties classify clusters of MUS symptoms together: non-cardiac chest pain, fibromyalgia, irritable bowel syndrome, chronic fatigue syndrome (see below), and repetitive strain injury. There is evidence that it is best not to give patients' symptoms such a name, as, while it helps to legitimize their symptoms as an illness (which patients find attractive), it may also help perpetuate their symptoms. Cognitive therapy may help, as can treating any of the commonly associated depression and/or anxiety states.

Chronic fatigue syndrome

Many, if not most, patients with *isolated* tiredness do not have serious organic pathology—some have the chronic fatigue syndrome, defined as 'new onset of persistent/relapsing, debilitating fatigue without previous fatigue, which does not resolve with bed rest and is severe enough to reduce daily activity to 50% of its premorbid level for ≥ 6 months'. It afflicts twice as many women as men and is very common—the overall incidence of tiredness in the general population is 1.5%. Such patients often have multiple other symptoms, each of which varies greatly from day to day. Patients with CFS are often keen on an 'organic' diagnosis —this is almost a hallmark of the condition, and it is important not to be drawn into endless cycles of negative investigations. This is best done by explaining that the diagnosis is CFS *before* investigations are ordered, so that negative results come as a reassurance, not as a surprise, or as a sign that the physician should look harder for any underlying pathology. Physical deconditioning often exacerbates symptoms, and regular exercise may have a role. Cognitive therapy and antidepressants likewise may help.

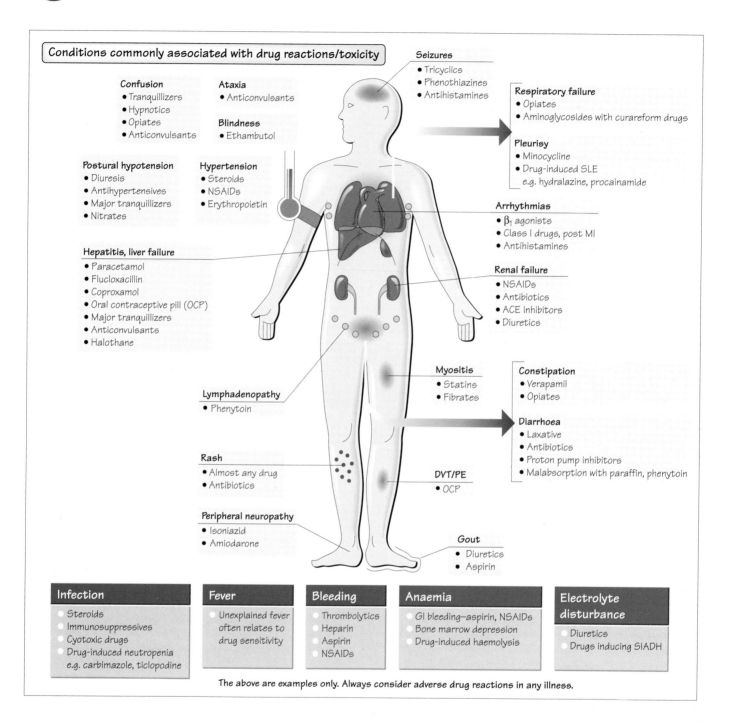

Conditions commonly associated with drug reactions/toxicity

Confusion
- Tranquillizers
- Hypnotics
- Opiates
- Anticonvulsants

Ataxia
- Anticonvulsants

Blindness
- Ethambutol

Postural hypotension
- Diuresis
- Antihypertensives
- Major tranquillizers
- Nitrates

Hypertension
- Steroids
- NSAIDs
- Erythropoietin

Hepatitis, liver failure
- Paracetamol
- Flucloxacillin
- Coproxamol
- Oral contraceptive pill (OCP)
- Major tranquillizers
- Anticonvulsants
- Halothane

Lymphadenopathy
- Phenytoin

Rash
- Almost any drug
- Antibiotics

Peripheral neuropathy
- Isoniazid
- Amiodarone

Seizures
- Tricyclics
- Phenothiazines
- Antihistamines

Respiratory failure
- Opiates
- Aminoglycosides with curareform drugs

Pleurisy
- Minocycline
- Drug-induced SLE e.g. hydralazine, procainamide

Arrhythmias
- β_1 agonists
- Class I drugs, post MI
- Antihistamines

Renal failure
- NSAIDs
- Antibiotics
- ACE inhibitors
- Diuretics

Myositis
- Statins
- Fibrates

Constipation
- Verapamil
- Opiates

Diarrhoea
- Laxative
- Antibiotics
- Proton pump inhibitors
- Malabsorption with paraffin, phenytoin

DVT/PE
- OCP

Gout
- Diuretics
- Aspirin

Infection
- Steroids
- Immunosuppressives
- Cyotoxic drugs
- Drug-induced neutropenia e.g. carbimazole, ticlopodine

Fever
- Unexplained fever often relates to drug sensitivity

Bleeding
- Thrombolytics
- Heparin
- Aspirin
- NSAIDs

Anaemia
- GI bleeding–aspirin, NSAIDs
- Bone marrow depression
- Drug-induced haemolysis

Electrolyte disturbance
- Diuretics
- Drugs inducing SIADH

The above are examples only. Always consider adverse drug reactions in any illness.

Adverse reactions to drugs are so common that it is crucial to determine whether any new symptom relates to a drug prescribed for another condition. Adverse reactions are classified as follows.

Predictable side effects

Predictable side effects at normal doses arise from those mechanisms responsible for therapeutic action. The paragraphs below are not comprehensive, but do give a number of different examples.

Interference with normal physiological function—drugs used in normal doses

- β-Receptor stimulation dilates peripheral blood vessel and β-blockade leads to vasoconstriction (cold peripheries).
- Bleeding with thrombolytic therapy.
- Immunosuppression from steroid therapy, presenting as severe/ unusual infection. Oral candida infection with inhaled steroids for asthma. Bone marrow suppression, with anaemia, infection and bleeding as a result of antineoplastic agents.

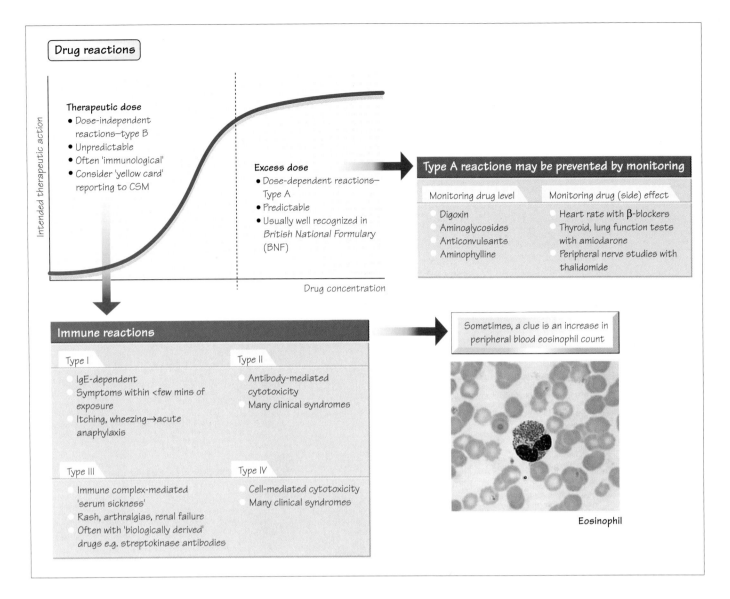

Drug reactions

Therapeutic dose
- Dose-independent reactions—type B
- Unpredictable
- Often 'immunological'
- Consider 'yellow card' reporting to CSM

Intended therapeutic action (vertical axis)

Drug concentration (horizontal axis)

Excess dose
- Dose-dependent reactions—Type A
- Predictable
- Usually well recognized in *British National Formulary* (BNF)

Type A reactions may be prevented by monitoring

Monitoring drug level	Monitoring drug (side) effect
Digoxin	Heart rate with β-blockers
Aminoglycosides	Thyroid, lung function tests with amiodarone
Anticonvulsants	Peripheral nerve studies with thalidomide
Aminophylline	

Immune reactions

Type I
- IgE-dependent
- Symptoms within <few mins of exposure
- Itching, wheezing→acute anaphylaxis

Type II
- Antibody-mediated cytotoxicity
- Many clinical syndromes

Type III
- Immune complex-mediated 'serum sickness'
- Rash, arthralgias, renal failure
- Often with 'biologically derived' drugs e.g. streptokinase antibodies

Type IV
- Cell-mediated cytotoxicity
- Many clinical syndromes

Sometimes, a clue is an increase in peripheral blood eosinophil count

Eosinophil

- Daytime sleepiness with nocturnal hypnotics.
- Movement disorders arising from long-term antiparkinsonian drugs.

Interference with normal physiological function—when drugs used in high concentrations (or when excretion impaired)

- Excess inhaled **β-receptor agonists** in asthma leads to palpitations: β-receptor stimulation increases the strength and rate of cardiac contraction.
- Diarrhoea with broad-spectrum antibiotics, from altered bowel flora.
- **Hypothyroidism** from antithyroid drugs or thyrotoxicosis from excess thyroxine.
- Hypoglycaemia from insulin.
- Hypercalcaemia with vitamin D.

Diseases enhancing drug side effects

There are a number of examples of this:
- β-blockade leading to bronchoconstriction in people with asthma; in phaeochromocytomas β-blockers lead to unopposed α-adrenergic stimulation, which produces intense vasoconstriction and increases peripheral resistance so raising blood pressure, which may result in heart failure or stroke.
- Pre-existing heart failure may be exacerbated in those given verapamil, a negatively inotropic calcium channel blocker; negative inotropism with calcium channel blockers partly correlates with negative chronotropism, i.e. the less they lower heart rate the less negative inotropism occurs.
- Class I antiarrhythmics drugs can cause (lethal) ventricular arrhythmias in those with structural heart disease, e.g. previous myocardial infarction.
- In bilateral renal artery stenosis, acute renal failure occurs if angiotensin-converting enzyme (ACE) inhibitors are given; constriction of the post-glomerular arteriole is mediated by angiotensin II. In renal artery stenosis this is critical in maintaining a high glomerular filtration pressure; if this vasoconstriction decreases, glomerular membrane filtration pressure is lost, and renal excretory function falls; if both kidneys have stenosed renal arteries, acute renal failure results.
- Paracetamol is more toxic in those with chronic liver disease, e.g. alcoholism.

Serotonin syndrome

Causes of serotonin syndrome	Clinical features
Any drug which increases serotonergic neuron activity, either administration or removal of serotonergic drugs; also if drugs which inhibit cytochromes CYP2D6/CYP3A4 are added to those already taking serotonergic drugs	Clinical triad of: • Mental state changes • Autonomic hyperactivity • Neuromuscular abnormalities
• Selective serotonin reuptake inhibitors: all • Antidepressant drugs: all • Monoamine oxidase inhibitors: all • Anticonvulsants: valproate • Antiemetics: ondansetron, metoclopramide • Analgesics: fentanyl, tramadol • Antitussives: dextromethorphan • Antibiotics: linezolide (MAO inhibitor), ritonavir • Some 'street' drugs: LSD, MDMA • Dietary supplements: St Johns Wort, ginseng, tryptophan. • Lithium	Incidence; 0.4 cases per 1000 patient-months for many serotonergic drugs Probably about 2–5000 cases/year in the UK, and 20–80 deaths Occurs in 15% of SSRI overdoses
Severe serotonin syndrome is especially likely when combinations of the above drugs are taken	Pathophysiology: relates to ↑serotonergic neuron activity, possibly 5-HT$_{2A}$, and 5HT$_{1A}$; also ↑CNS noradrenaline (norepinephrine) activity may be relevant

Features of the serotonin syndrome — a spectrum, with subtle symptoms/signs in mild cases, usually occurring ≤ few minutes after new medication or change in dose

		Mild	Moderate	Severe
Mental state		Normal	Mild agitation, hypervigilance, pressured speech	Delirious, great agitation
Autonomic changes	Heart rate	↑	↑↑	↑↑↑
	Sweating	+	++	+++
	Pupil dilatation	+	++	+++
	Blood pressure	Normal – ↑	↑	↑↑ → frank shock
	GI tract		↑bowel sounds Diarrhoea	↑↑ bowel sounds
Temperature		Normal	↑ to 40°C	High – up to 41°C
Neuromuscular changes	Muscle findings	Tremor	Inducible clonus	Rigid muscles (especially lower limbs)
	Reflexes	↑	↑↑	↑↑↑
Laboratory tests				Acidosis ↑Muscle enzymes
Therapy	REMOVE PROVOKING DRUG(S)	Supportive Benzodiazepines	Rehydrate, cool; 5-HT$_{2A}$ antagonists	If temp ≥ 41°C, neuromuscular paralysis and intubation/ventilation

Diagnosis; needs 1) knowledge that a serotonergic agent given ≤ 5 weeks ago 2) 1 or more of:
• Tremor with hyperreflexia
• Spontaneous clonus
• Muscle rigidity & T°C ≥38; and ocular or inducible clonus
• Ocular clonus & agitation or sweating
• Inducible clonus and agitation or sweating

Differential diagnosis: anticholinergic syndrome, neuroleptic malignant syndrome (page 67), malignant hyperthermia (page 67).

Electrolyte abnormalities increasing the likelihood of drug toxicity

• Hypokalaemia increases the action of digoxin (see below), and increases the likelihood of proarrhythmia occurring as a side effect of antiarrhythmic, antidepressant or antihistamine drugs.

• Chronic hyponatraemia predisposes to saline-induced brain-stem damage (central pontine myelinosis).

Age increasing drug side effects

• Cardiovascular compensatory reflexes are diminished in elderly

people, so postural hypotension is more common with antihypertensive therapy; this may present as fractured neck of femur or as recurrent falls.
• Renal tubular function declines in elderly people, so hyponatraemia from diuretics is more common; this may present as confusion.
• Increasing age diminishes brain reserve, so increasing the sensitivity to hypnotics and sedatives.

Sex increasing the possibility of side effects
Gynaecomastia in men treated with oestrogens.

Increased tissue action of the drug
Side effects arising from increased tissue action of the drug, from increased tissue sensitivity (see above) or from overdosage may result from:
• A narrow therapeutic range: small changes in drug metabolism/dosage can easily produce toxic levels. Monitoring drug concentration where possible helps prevent this, e.g. digoxin, anticonvulsants, and aminoglycosides.
• Renal or hepatic failure can slow metabolism of a drug or an active metabolite resulting in toxicity. In renal or/and hepatic failure, prescribe sparingly and always determine from the *British National Formulary* whether the dose should be adjusted.

Increased tissue action due to renal failure
• **Digoxin** is renally excreted and is commonly given with diuretics to elderly people with heart failure. Old age, renal failure and hypokalaemia all predispose to toxicity, manifest as (any) cardiac arrhythmia, visual disturbance (objects appear yellow), confusion, nausea and vomiting; the last produces dehydration and pre-renal renal failure, further increasing digoxin levels and exacerbating toxicity. Treatment: wait for renal elimination and normalize potassium. If symptoms are life threatening give dialysis or digoxin antibodies.
• **Lithium** is renally excreted. If toxic levels develop (excess dosage, dehydration, deliberate overdose), ataxia, confusion (which may progress to coma), convulsions and nephrogenic diabetes insipidus occur. Circulating fluid is lost, producing pre-renal renal failure, so lithium levels rise further, exacerbating toxicity. Treatment: intravenous fluids and withholding lithium. Dialysis is occasionally needed.
• **Aminoglycosides** are renally excreted and used in severe infections, which themselves may cause renal failure. Drug levels should be very carefully monitored to avoid toxicity, which is manifest as vestibulo-cochlear nerve damage (deafness, difficulty with balance) and renal failure. Furosemide (frusemide) if given as a rapid high-dose intravenous 'push' can result in a similar ototoxicity.
• **Opiate poisoning** occurs in renal failure (opiates are excreted renally), in cardiac failure (which impairs renal function), in elderly people (increased tissue sensitivity), in type II respiratory failure (CO_2 retention increases the sensitivity of the respiratory centre to respiratory depression induced by opiates and other central nervous system [CNS] depressants), and with excess opiates (inadvertent or deliberate overdose). Opiate overdose impairs conscious level, which may lead to coma, depress respiratory centre function, producing hypoventilation and leading to apnoea. Patients are often drowsy and hyperventilating with pinpoint pupils. Intravenous naloxone, a specific opiate receptor antagonist, rapidly improves conscious level and ventilatory function. Beware: as the half-life of naloxone in the circulation ($\pm$ 30 min) is less than that of opiates (up to several hours), naloxone administration may need to be repeated.

Toxicity arising from predictable drug–drug interactions
Often it is the way one drug interacts with another that results in toxicity:
• Altered drug concentration through inhibition/induction of cytochrome P450 (CYP): drugs inhibiting CYP isoforms increase the concentration of other drugs that depend on CYP for elimination. This may lead to toxicity, e.g. macrolide antibiotics inhibit CYP, slowing cisapride (a now withdrawn gut prokinetic agent) elimination, leading to toxic levels and ventricular arrhythmias. CYP induction by anticonvulsants decreases the effect of the oral contraceptive pill (OCP). Racial and familial differences in drug metabolism may be mediated by CYP isoform polymorphisms.
• Altered P-glycoprotein expression: P-glycoprotein decreases gastrointestinal drug absorption, increases CNS and kidney drug excretion, and extrudes drugs from cells, e.g. antineoplastic agents. Drugs that inhibit P-glycoprotein alter the concentration of other drugs, e.g. verapamil increases the concentration of ciclosporin.
• Altered protein binding: decreased protein binding increases levels of highly protein-bound drugs, e.g. antibiotics compete for the albumin binding of warfarin, increasing warfarin levels and anticoagulant effect. Antibiotics also kill gut bacteria, decreasing vitamin K production (the natural antagonist to warfarin), so increasing warfarin's effect.
• Administration of drugs with complementary function. Antiplatelet agents promote bleeding in those on warfarin. Drowsiness results from polypharmacy with antipsychotics, nocturnal hypnotics and sedating antihistamines. Excessive bradycardia or asystole results from the combination of verapamil and β-blockers.
• Other interactions, e.g. amiodarone doubles the plasma levels of digoxin, and so may cause toxicity.

Toxicity arising from other predictable mechanisms
• Genetic interactions: factor V Leiden dramatically increases the risk of OCP-induced venous thrombosis. Glucose-6-phosphate dehydrogenase deficiency produces haemolysis with many drugs. Many drugs may precipitate acute porphyric attacks.
• Inhibition of related enzyme systems: non-steroidal anti-inflammatory agents (NSAIDs) inhibit cyclo-oxygenase enzyme (COX) isoforms 1 and 2. COX-1 produces gastric mucosal protection factors, whereas COX-2 inhibition is responsible for the therapeutic efficacy of the drug. Early NSAIDs inhibited both isoforms, promoting gastrointestinal bleeding. Recent NSAIDs are more selective and may cause fewer gastrointestinal bleeds. NSAID-induced renal failure results from inhibition of prostaglandin production and is more likely in those with pre-existing renal failure. Chronic NSAID consumption can produce chronic renal failure (with prominent tubular damage and a salt-wasting nephropathy), papillary necrosis and uroepithelial cancer.
• Toxicity from other drug constituents: thyroid dysfunction with amiodarone relates to the high levels of contained iodine. Amiodarone commonly induces hypothyroidism in areas with normal environmental iodine levels, and less commonly hyperthyroidism.
• Long-term toxicity is often predictable. Use of chronic high-dose steroids leads to Cushing's syndrome, with osteoporosis, easy bruising, and excess cardiovascular morbidity and mortality from hypertension and an adverse lipid profile. Anticancer drugs produce a significant late, i.e. 10-year incidence of secondary tumours, often haematological, from the long-term effects of DNA damage.

Immune reactions

Immune reactions producing drug toxicity are subdivided according to the underlying mechanism:

• **Type I hypersensitivity reactions** usually occur after the third or fourth exposure to the drug. The sensitizing drug activates mast cell-bound IgE antibodies, causing degranulation, mild itching, urticaria and angioedema or anaphylaxis. Treatment: antihistamines, bronchodilators and steroids. Anaphylactoid reactions result when drugs cause direct mast cell degranulation, e.g. opiates, contrast medium or aspirin. Reactions are not mediated by immunoglobulin, so previous exposure is not required. Some less severe reactions are sporadic, occur long after the start of treatment, and are difficult clinically to associate with drug therapy, e.g. intermittent angioedema with angiotensin-converting enzyme inhibitors.

• **Type II hypersensitivity reactions** to drugs are rare. The most common example is penicillin-induced haemolytic anaemia, where red cell membrane-bound penicillin comes under IgG or IgM antibody-directed attack, so activating complement and producing cell lysis.

• **Type III hypersensitivity—serum sickness**: offending drugs bind with specific IgG producing antigen-antibody complexes, e.g. penicillin, streptokinase, horse sera and sulphonamides. Immune complex deposition and subsequent inflammation within tissues cause the clinical features of fever, arthralgias, vasculitic skin rashes and renal impairment. Serum complement C3 and C4 are low. Eosinophilia may occur. Skin biopsies show a 'leukocytoclastic' vasculitis. No specific IgE to the antigen can be demonstrated, although specific IgG may be detected.

• **Type IV hypersensitivity reactions** are unusual causes of drug allergy. Frequent exposure sensitizes CD4+ T lymphocytes to a drug, e.g. topically applied penicillin. Lymphocytes migrate to the site of exposure and recruit other cells including neutrophils and macrophages. Contact dermatitis occurs. This responds rapidly to steroids. Exposure to the offending agent via a patch test induces a diagnostic localized dermatitis after 48 h.

Unpredictable and other mechanisms giving rise to toxicity

Unfortunately much drug toxicity falls into this category. The common ones should be learnt, but the clinician must always be aware of the potential for new and unexpected reactions. Examples include:

• Pneumonitis with high-dose amiodarone is manifest as breathlessness, sometimes with a non-productive cough, and can be misinterpreted as worsening heart failure. Chest X-ray shows diffuse infiltrates. The carbon monoxide transfer factor is decreased. The diagnosis is confirmed by high-resolution computed tomography (HRCT) of the chest. Treatment: steroids (little evidence that they improve outcome), time because improvement is contemporaneous with amiodarone leaving the body, which, given its very long *in vivo* half-life of about 30 days, is often several months.

• Drug-induced skin rashes are often immunologically mediated (see above), although other mechanisms also operate, e.g. β-blockers exacerbating psoriasis.

• Anticonvulsant hypersensitivity syndrome from carbamazepine or phenytoin presents as fever, rash, lymphadenopathy, malaise and hepatitis. Re-challenge with either drug is often fatal if the first illness involved hepatitis.

• Malabsorption with phenytoin.

• Myositis on statin therapy.

Diagnosis

A full clinical history of the reaction and all drugs administered, including details about previous exposure and time from exposure to symptom onset. Eosinophils may be raised.

Management

• Discontinue the offending drug/agent. Avoid subsequently.

• Advise on any cross-reacting drugs.

• Medic-Alert bracelet for severe drug allergies.

• Inform the Committee on Safety of Medicines (CSM—BNF yellow card).

• In immune reactions drug desensitization (exposure to escalating doses of the drug on multiple occasions) for essential agents, e.g. insulin, but not if alternative treatments are available.

Index